Oxygen Uptake Kinetics in Sport, Exercise and Medicine

When we get up from a chair, run to catch a ball or bus, or participate in any athletic event, the energetic demands of our muscles change rapidly. In the transition from rest to movement, the pulmonary, cardiovascular and muscular systems increase the oxygen supply to muscle mitochondria, allowing aerobic respiration and energy production to increase in turn. If an individual can 'switch on' this aerobic energy system quickly, he or she will fatigue less rapidly and be better able to tolerate the demands of any exercise or physical activity. These oxygen uptake dynamics, or kinetics, can be improved by exercise training, but are impaired as a result of ageing and a variety of disease states.

Understanding the principal determinants of oxygen uptake kinetics is fundamental to improving both human performance in sport and quality of life in disease states. This book provides a comprehensive overview of the current state of knowledge within this emerging and buoyant field of study. Topics covered include: introduction to oxygen uptake kinetics and historical development of the discipline; measurement and analysis of oxygen uptake kinetics; control of and limitations to oxygen uptake kinetics; applications of oxygen uptake kinetics in human populations.

Oxygen Uptake Kinetics in Sport, Exercise and Medicine contains contributions from leading researchers in the field. The text is richly illustrated and structured to enable easy access to information. It represents an invaluable resource for students and researchers in sport and exercise physiology, as well as for respiratory physiologists and pulmonary clinicians.

Andrew M. Jones is Professor of Applied Physiology at Manchester Metropolitan University, UK.

David C. Poole is Professor of Kinesiology, Anatomy and Physiology at Kansas State University, USA.

Oxygen Uptake Kinetics in Sport, Exercise and Medicine

Edited by
Andrew M. Jones and
David C. Poole

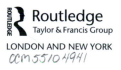

Routledge
Taylor & Francis Group

LONDON AND NEW YORK

First published 2005
by Routledge
2 Park Square, Milton Park, Abingdon, Oxon OX14 4RN

Simultaneously published in the USA and Canada
by Taylor & Francis Inc
270 Madison Ave, New York, NY 10016

Routledge is an imprint of the Taylor & Francis Group

Typeset in Goudy by
Newgen Imaging Systems (P) Ltd, Chennai, India
Printed and bound in Great Britain by
TJ International Ltd, Padstow, Cornwall

British Library Cataloguing in Publication Data
A catalogue record for this book is available from the British Library

Library of Congress Cataloging in Publication Data
A catalog record for this book has been requested

ISBN 0–415–30560–8 (hbk)
ISBN 0–415–30561–6 (pbk)

To my family: Mum, Dad and James,
I hope this makes you proud; Emma, Amy,
and baby Dylan, you make me proud.
This is for you.

A.M.J.

To my parents, Peter and Gwyneth; my wife, Katherine;
and children, Shayna, Connor and Kelton, now and always.

D.C.P.

'*Nullius in Verba*'
'Take nobody's word for it, see it for yourself'
Motto of The Royal Society

Contents

Illustrations

Figures

Tables

Contributors

Thomas J. Barstow, PhD Department of Kinesiology, Kansas State University, Manhattan, Kansas, 66506-0302, USA.

Brad J. Behnke, PhD Department of Health and Kinesiology, Texas A&M University, College Station, Texas 77843, USA.

Mark Burnley, PhD Department of Sport and Exercise Science, University of Wales Aberystwyth, SY23 3DA, UK.

Helen Carter, PhD Chelsea School Research Centre, University of Brighton, Eastbourne, BN20 7SP, UK.

Bruno Grassi, MD PhD Dipaerimento di Scienze e Tecnologie Biomediche, School of Medicine, University of Milan, I-20090 Segrate (MI), Italy.

Franklyn A. Howe, PhD Department of Biochemistry, St. George's Hospital Medical School, Tooting, London, SW17 0RE, UK.

Richard L. Hughson, PhD Department of Kinesiology, University of Waterloo, Waterloo ON, Canada.

Andrew M. Jones, PhD Department of Exercise and Sport Science, Manchester Metropolitan University, Alsager, ST7 2HL, UK.

Casey A. Kindig, PhD Division of Physiology, Department of Medicine, University of California San Diego, La Jolla, CA 92093-0623, USA (Deceased).

Shunsaku Koga, PhD Applied Physiology Laboratory, Kobe Design University, Kobe 651-2196, Japan.

Narihiko Kondo, PhD Laboratory for Applied Human Physiology, Kobe University, Kobe 657-8501, Japan.

Katrien Koppo, PhD Department of Movement and Sports Sciences, Ghent University, 9000 Ghent, Belgium.

David C. Poole, PhD DSc. Departments of Kinesiology, Anatomy and Physiology, Kansas State University, Manhattan, Kansas, 66506-0302, USA.

Jamie S.M. Pringle, PhD Chelsea School Research Centre, University of Brighton, Eastbourne, BN20 7SP, UK.

Harry B. Rossiter, PhD Division of Physiology, Department of Medicine, University of California San Diego, La Jolla, CA 92093-0623, USA.

Barry W. Scheuermann, PhD Department of Kinesiology, The University of Toledo, Toledo, OH 43606, USA.

Tomoyuki Shiojiri, MSc. Exercise Physiology Laboratory, Faculty of Science, Yokohama City University, Yokohama 236-0027, Japan.

Susan A. Ward, DPhil. School of Sport and Exercise Sciences, University of Leeds, Leeds, LS2 9JT, UK.

Brian J. Whipp, PhD DSc. Division of Respiratory and Critical Care Physiology and Medicine, Harbor-UCLA Medical Center, Torrance, CA 90509-2910, USA.

Preface

Without skeletal muscles and the energetic processes that power them, we humans would be immobile creatures very much at the mercy of our immediate environment. Skeletal muscles facilitate movement and the capacity to perform work and as such possess an extraordinarily large range of metabolic demands almost all of which must be met either immediately or at some later time by oxidative phosphorylation. Other than at rest or when performing a contrived activity such as constant work-rate exercise in the research laboratory, the sum total energetic (and therefore oxygen, O_2) demands of the body are rarely constant. Movement or exercise in humans involves rather sudden transitions from one metabolic rate to another. For example, a person walking for a bus may need to begin running before it pulls away and an athlete toeing the start line at the beginning of a race may need to increase his or her metabolic rate several times over within a few strides after the gun fires to meet the new energetic requirements. How well an individual copes with the exercise challenge will depend, in part, upon the rate at which oxygen uptake ($\dot{V}O_2$) rises in the transition from that at rest or near-rest to exercise. A rapid increase in $\dot{V}O_2$ requires a superb coordination among the respiratory, cardiovascular and muscular systems that regulate the flux of O_2 and substrates to the working muscle and remove heat, carbon dioxide and other products of the energetic processes. The faster these $\dot{V}O_2$ dynamics or kinetics, the less lactic acid will be produced in the exercising muscles, and fatigue may be delayed or avoided.

Differences in the speed of $\dot{V}O_2$ kinetics helps explain the range of athletic capabilities. Trained athletes have faster $\dot{V}O_2$ kinetics than untrained individuals who, in turn, have faster $\dot{V}O_2$ kinetics than patients with disease (e.g. heart failure, emphysema, diabetes). During continuous, moderate-intensity exercise in healthy individuals, the $\dot{V}O_2$ rises to reach a 'steady-state' or plateau within about three minutes. In contrast, during heavier exercise, the $\dot{V}O_2$ may either take longer to reach a 'steady-state' or alternatively, may continue to increase until the maximum $\dot{V}O_2$ is achieved or the exercise is terminated. This continued rise in $\dot{V}O_2$ over time during heavy or severe exercise has been termed the '$\dot{V}O_2$ slow component' and is closely related to the fatigue process. The mechanisms responsible for the development of the $\dot{V}O_2$ slow component are presently unknown and are the subject of lively debate.

This book is organized into four parts. The first of these, 'Introduction', provides a brief historical perspective of O_2 and some of the major steps taken in identifying the gas, its passage from mouth to muscle and the role of O_2 in energy metabolism. This part identifies key scientists whose efforts have developed the field of research into $\dot{V}O_2$ kinetics and highlights the importance of $\dot{V}O_2$ kinetics to exercise performance. The second part, 'Theory and practice of measuring $\dot{V}O_2$ kinetics', provides essential practical information on the approach to take in the measurement of $\dot{V}O_2$ kinetics either for the purpose of research or diagnosis. Both the theory of modelling the three phases of the $\dot{V}O_2$ kinetic response at the onset of exercise and the techniques that are currently available will be outlined. This part also contains chapters on differences in $\dot{V}O_2$ kinetics in humans performing various types of exercise and highlights species-specific characteristics of the response. The third part, 'Mechanistic bases of $\dot{V}O_2$ kinetics', reviews the control of, and the mechanistic limitations to, $\dot{V}O_2$ kinetics and identifies current controversies in the field. This part examines the validity of drawing inferences concerning muscle $\dot{V}O_2$ from measurements made at the mouth and reviews the evidence concerning the role of both central (i.e. O_2 delivery) and peripheral (i.e. intramuscular) factors in determining the $\dot{V}O_2$ kinetic response. The influence of muscle fibre type on $\dot{V}O_2$ kinetics is also covered. The fourth and final part, 'Practical applications to the study of $\dot{V}O_2$ kinetics', returns to the practical application of research in kinetics to the understanding of exercise tolerance and exercise performance. The effects of age, fitness and disease on the $\dot{V}O_2$ kinetics are discussed in light of the likely limitations to the responses introduced in the previous part. The effects of interventions such as exercise training on $\dot{V}O_2$ kinetics in these diverse populations are explored. Whereas the four parts of this book are self-contained, they are clearly linked to one another. Each of the parts, and each of the chapters, has been carefully planned to allow the reader to 'dip into' the book when searching for information on a particular aspect of $\dot{V}O_2$ kinetics. While each chapter covers a very specific topic, this book as a whole is designed to provide a comprehensive coverage of the field of $\dot{V}O_2$ kinetics.

Pioneering physiologists such as A.V. Hill, August Krogh and Erik Hohwu-Christensen in the early twentieth century appreciated the rapidity with which the cardiorespiratory processes could respond at the onset of exercise (Chapter 1: 'Introduction to oxygen uptake kinetics and historical development of the discipline'). In more recent years, there has been an enormous increase in the study of the features of the $\dot{V}O_2$ kinetic response to exercise, and of their determinants. This interest has been spurred on by the advent of rapidly responding gas analysers and breath-by-breath technology. Using this technology, scientists such as Karl Wasserman and Brian J. Whipp have provided insight into some of the central underlying control processes that facilitate the rapid and precise physiological alterations that occur in response to altered metabolic demands (Chapter 2: 'Measuring $\dot{V}O_2$ kinetics: the practicalities' and Chapter 3: 'The kinetics of oxygen uptake: physiological inferences from the parameters'). Such measurements have provided an invaluable window through which to view and understand metabolic function in health and dysfunction in disease. In addition, the study of $\dot{V}O_2$ kinetics and resolution of those kinetics across or within the exercising muscles (Chapter 6: 'Relationship between $\dot{V}O_2$ responses at the mouth and across the exercising muscles') has focused attention on the control of intracellular energetic processes (Chapter 7: 'Intramuscular phosphate and pulmonary $\dot{V}O_2$ kinetics during exercise: implications for control of skeletal muscle oxygen consumption) and generated scientifically valuable controversy (compare Chapter 8: 'Limitation of $\dot{V}O_2$ on-kinetics by O_2 delivery' with Chapter 9: 'Limitation of skeletal muscle $\dot{V}O_2$ on-kinetics by inertia of cellular respiration', and see Chapter 12: 'Towards an understanding of the mechanistic bases of $\dot{V}O_2$ kinetics'). Clearly, the metabolic response and resultant $\dot{V}O_2$ kinetics are dependent, in part, on the exercise modality (Chapter 4: 'Effect of exercise modality on $\dot{V}O_2$ kinetics'), the muscles recruited (Chapter 11: 'Influence of muscle fibre type and motor unit recruitment on $\dot{V}O_2$ kinetics) and factors such as proximity to previous exercise bouts (Chapter 10: ' "Priming exercise" and $\dot{V}O_2$ kinetics'). Whereas exercise training speeds the dynamic adjustments of O_2 uptake at the onset of exercise, we now acknowledge that age-ing (Chapter 13: '$\dot{V}O_2$ kinetics: effects of maturation and ageing') as well as many major chronic diseases (Chapter 14: '$\dot{V}O_2$ kinetics in different disease states') impair those kinetics. Indeed, measurement of $\dot{V}O_2$ kinetics in clinical medicine is becoming accepted as a powerful diagnostic tool that can provide important information about the severity and progression or regression of specific pathologies. In contrast to the deficits in O_2 transport and $\dot{V}O_2$ kinetics that arise from disease processes, exercise training up-regulates key facets of the cardiorespiratory and muscular systems that result in the speeding of kinetics (Chapter 15: 'Effect of training on $\dot{V}O_2$ kinetics and performance'). Interspecies comparisons from the crab and salamander to the Thoroughbred racing horse provide a far broader range of metabolic capacities than available in humans and help position our species appropriately within the vertebrate world as well as providing unique insights into metabolic control. Chapter 5, '$\dot{V}O_2$ dynamics in different species', adopts a comparative physiological approach that examines $\dot{V}O_2$ dynamics found across diverse mammalian, amphibian and invertebrate species.

Today, the study of $\dot{V}O_2$ kinetics is a particular growth area within the broad field of exercise physiology, with mainstream journals featuring papers on $\dot{V}O_2$ kinetics in almost every issue and major scientific conferences sponsoring symposia and special sessions on the subject. However, this text represents the first textbook to deal specifically with the subject. It is the purpose of this book to provide a practical and theoretical resource base for students of exercise physiology and researchers who are interested in this field of study. We hope that this book will be accessible to students of exercise physiology and sports science and also of value to respiratory physiologists, pulmonary clinicians, and expert researchers in $\dot{V}O_2$ kinetics. To achieve these goals, the opening chapters pro-vide a gentle introduction to the key issues and present information on the measurement of $\dot{V}O_2$ kinetics in practical settings. Subsequently, these issues are developed in several chapters that contain highly detailed, current, cutting-edge material written by world-leading scientists. While some of this content may be challenging to the casual reader, we believe that it is necessary to satisfy the needs of serious researchers in this field. Wherever possible, we have emphasized the use of straightforward, clear visual presentation of data and concepts in the form of graphs and diagrams.

From many perspectives, this book is a call to abandon the notion that analysis of $\dot{V}O_2$ kinetics is 'too difficult'. There are literally hundreds or possibly even thousands of scientists/students/clinicians with access to metabolic carts capable of collecting data suitable for kinetics analysis. Many of these individuals may have already collected such data but either have not analysed it correctly, or even at all. This is a criminal shame and we hope that this book can help facilitate moving such valuable data from the filing cabinet or computer disk to the scientific and public arenas.

Andrew M. Jones and David C. Poole
January 2004

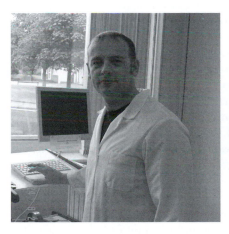 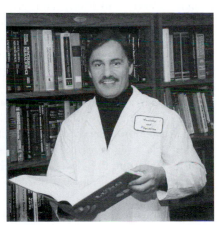

Acknowledgements

I would like to take this opportunity to thank my doctoral (Jo Doust) and post-doctoral (Tom Barstow, Richard Casaburi, Karl Wasserman) teachers and mentors for providing me both with excellent training and with the opportunity to pursue a topic I love: in many ways, this book is the culmination of your investment. I would also like to thank Brian Whipp for support and encouragement over several years; your exemplary scholarship remains an inspiration to me. I have had the good fortune to have been associated with a number of excellent students (Nik Berger, Mark Burnley, Helen Carter, Katrien Koppo, Jamie Pringle, Daryl Wilkerson) and great colleagues (Jacques Bouckaert, Iain Campbell, Keith Tolfrey) and I would like to publicly acknowledge their contributions to my work. Daryl: David and I are particularly grateful to you for your tireless efforts on our behalf with the graphics in this book; Mark and Katrien: you have both been tremendously supportive throughout this project. I am, of course, grateful to all the chapter authors for their good-natured and (generally) timely delivery of excellent chapters. Finally, I would like to thank my co-editor, David Poole, for his dedicated and conscientious work throughout all stages of the production of this book. This book would certainly not have been possible without his involvement. His professionalism, productivity and personal qualities make him the ideal role model for any aspiring scientist.

Andrew M. Jones

I am indebted to my wonderful colleague, Andy Jones who initially conceived the idea of this text and whose great drive and capabilities helped make it a reality. My gratitude goes also to an unbroken chain of brilliant mentors, colleagues, friends and students who have made my passage in science challenging, rewarding and most important of all, fun. In chronological order, these include Ronald J. Maughan, Thomas P. Reilly, Gerald W. Gardner, Glenn A. Gaesser, Susan A. Ward, Lindsey C. Henson, Peter D. Wagner, Odile Mathieu-Costello, John B. West, Michael C. Hogan, David F. Wilson, Timothy I. Musch, William L. Sexton, Laurie H. Manciet, Russell S. Richardson, Bruno Grassi, Walter Schaffartzik, Thomas J. Barstow, Michael B. Reid, Peter B. Raven, M. Roger Fedde, Howard H. Erickson, Andrew M. Jones, Shunsaku Koga, Casey A. Kindig, Paul McDonough, David W. Hill, Brad J. Behnke, Danielle K. Padilla and Yutaka

Kano. At the head of this pantheon is Professor Brian J. Whipp who represents the epitome of mental acuity and logical argument. He is a latter day 'William of Occam' whose influence will touch generations of scientists. A significant portion of the scientific research detailed in this text was supported by grants from the National Institute of Health, Heart, Lung and Blood Institute and the American Heart Association.

David C. Poole

Part I
Introduction

1 Introduction to oxygen uptake kinetics and historical development of the discipline

Andrew M. Jones and David C. Poole

A brief note on the history of oxygen and modern man

Today, we live in an atmosphere that contains 20.9% oxygen (O_2). In contrast, when the solar system was created approximately 4.6 billion years ago (Dickerson, 1978), the atmosphere of the Earth was completely devoid of both O_2 and ozone (O_3). In the absence of a protective high-altitude O_3 layer, the sun's ultraviolet radiation bombarded the surface of the earth. This radiation synthesized organic compounds (amino acids) from water, carbon dioxide (CO_2), methane, hydrogen and ammonia – the so-called 'primordial soup' that generated the first self-replicating chains of molecules. Fossils dating back over 3.5 billion years provide evidence of synthetic processes that enabled living organisms to capture solar energy and fabricate organic molecules such as glucose. Anaerobic fermentation (glycolysis) which powered these creatures may well have preceded all other biological energy-extracting pathways found on Earth. These ancient organisms released O_2 into the atmosphere and over the next two billion years an atmosphere was created where over one out of five molecules was O_2. In Shark Bay, Western Australia these algae-like micro-organisms known as cyanobacteria still cluster ~3 billion or so to the square metre in colonies on formations called stromalites. On close observation small streams of bubbles – molecular oxygen – can be seen rising from the stromalites. It is somewhat ironic that these cyanobacteria instigated life on Earth only to be eaten almost out of existence by their progeny.

Two of the most important effects of this O_2 atmosphere were as follows: (1) The formation of an O_3 layer in the upper atmosphere which effectively diminished the ultraviolet radiation reaching the Earth's surface. This halted non-biologic synthesis of organic matter. (2) O_2 may have reached toxic levels for many of the original O_2 producers and new metabolic pathways developed that utilized O_2 as a hydrogen acceptor. Solar energy in the visible wavelengths still reached the Earth and supported biologic photosynthesis.

The earliest and most simple form of aerobic life appeared about 1.5 billion years ago. This unicellular organism was eukaryotic (i.e. had a nucleus) and performed some of the fundamental functions that characterize cellular activity today, that is metabolism, excitability, locomotion and reproduction (Vidal, 1984). These organisms possessed DNA-containing mitochondria and from this point on, these mitochondria would be present in nearly all forms of life on Earth (Dickerson, 1980a,b; Astrand and Rodahl, 1986). Today, the storage and exchange of energy necessary to power these functions in most living organisms relies principally upon adenosine triphosphate (ATP). Energy is released when ATP is hydrolysed by water into adenosine diphosphate (ADP) and phosphate ion. Intracellular ATP stores are very limited, in part, because ATP is extremely heavy. For example, an active person could easily expend his/her own body weight in ATP each day. To sustain cellular function and integrity, it is crucial that ATP concentrations are maintained within very tight limits and hence, phosphocreatine (PCr) stores which are typically several fold higher than those of ATP, fall in response to increased energetic demands and in so doing, regenerate and stabilize ATP concentrations. The contraction-induced perturbation of the intracellular milieu ($\downarrow$PCr, $\uparrow$Cr, $\uparrow$ADP$_{free}$, $\uparrow$inorganic phosphate, $\uparrow$calcium) and accelerated glycolytic activity stimulate mitochondrial (aerobic) ATP resynthesis and enable the transition to greater metabolic rates that can be sustained for prolonged periods, providing that the commensurate supply of O_2 and substrates and the removal of heat and metabolic waste is achieved.

One major limit to increasing body size is the problem imposed by O_2 and substrate diffusion. This is effective over distances of microns but not millimetres or more. Beginning about 700 million years ago, larger animals began to develop (Valentine, 1978); but they could do so only after the O_2 diffusion problem had been surmounted. This was achieved by retaining a relatively small individual cellular mass, piling many of these cells together and developing cells dedicated to a particular function. Within the human body there are over 200 different cell types and specialized structures, the genes, provide a hierarchical control over cellular proliferation, structure and function.

As individual cells lost intimate contact with the external environment, transporting necessary supplies of energy substrates and structural components to each cell and removing metabolic wastes became a supreme challenge. Moreover, for many multicellular creatures, the external environment changed from water to air. The solution to both problems was solved by bathing each cell in interstitial fluid, which closely replicated the composition of the ancient seas, and developing a conduction system for substrate and metabolite transport over distances from several millimetres to many metres. Over the ensuing aeons, animals have evolved diverse strategies for enabling efficient gas exchange. Insects developed infoldings of their body walls forming networks of tubular airways (tracheae) which bring air into close proximity with the cells that require O_2 and CO_2 exchange. Fish have gills that project out into the water environment and which dry out rapidly if exposed to air. Mammals have a respiratory apparatus that is turned inwards, the lungs, and inspired air is warmed and humidified before arriving at the alveolar gas-exchange structures.

Muscle itself is an ancient tissue with the earliest animal fossil remains evidencing burrowing behaviour (which must have been powered by muscles) in the Precambrian seabed ~700 million years ago. Mammals first appeared in the Mesozoic era 250 million years ago whereas the first primates emerged

60–70 million years ago at a time when dinosaurs still ruled the earth. This latter period saw an evolutionary explosion that included the appearance of a multitude of birds, mammals and flowering plants. The hominids branched off the primate family tree 6–8 million years ago and eventually produced *Homo sapiens sapiens* which is the only surviving hominid.

Facilitated by bipedal adaptations that included pelvic alterations enabling an upright posture and bipedal gait with arms free, the hominids, after several abortive attempts, finally forsook life in the trees to forage and hunt on the ground. The brain size of one such hominid, Australopithecus approached 550 cubic centimetres (similar to a gorilla) and facilitated eventual tool and weapon design, and the development of cunning, intelligence and cooperation. These facilities heralded our (*Homo sapiens sapiens*) eventual success and dominance over all other species. In the ensuing 4 million years, brain size increased inexorably: *Homo habilis* (2.3–1.5 million years ago), 600–800 cubic centimetres; *Homo erectus* (first 'true' man, made fire, 1.6 million years ago), 1,050 cubic centimetres; *Homo sapiens* (wise man) neanderthalensis (250,000–35,000 years ago), possessed a larger brain than modern man, over 1,300 cubic centimetres. Despite possessing a very large brain, great manual dexterity, a common language among tribal groups and massive musculoskeletal structure, the Neanderthals died out 35,000 years ago. They were replaced by *Homo sapiens sapiens* who are basically designed for mobility with a locomotory apparatus and service organs that constitute the major bulk of the body mass.

Skeletal muscles today are powered, in part, by the same metabolic pathways that developed when the air was devoid of O_2, that is glycolysis. Pyruvic acid formed via glycolysis in our muscles is removed either by oxidation within the mitochondria or conversion to lactic acid which, in turn, may be oxidized or used as a glyco- or gluco-neogenic precursor in muscle or other tissues. Skeletal muscle has an astonishing capacity to increase its metabolic rate some 50–100 fold above resting which presents a major challenge for the O_2 delivery/utilization and metabolite removal systems. Furthermore, a tight control over the intramyocyte milieu is crucially important if heavy muscular exercise is to be sustained. The focus of this text is aimed at exploring the superb coordination among the pulmonary, cardiovascular and muscular systems at the onset of exercise. It is this coordination that facilitates effective matching of O_2 delivery to O_2 requirements and limits the reliance on glycolysis and other finite non-O_2 energy stores (comprising the O_2 deficit). Diseases such as heart failure disrupt effective O_2 delivery and muscle oxidative function such that the O_2 deficit is increased at exercise onset, eliciting a greater intracellular perturbation and reducing exercise tolerance (Chapter 14).

Historical development of the anatomy, physiology and chemistry of oxygen utilization

The following brief section presents a linear history of major scientific advances in our knowledge of O_2 and its movement through the body. In many ways this could be viewed as controversy between the vitalists (who believed that living things possessed a vital principal which was essential for life and which set animate beings apart from inanimate objects) and those who believed that respiration merely constituted ordinary chemical processes that obeyed simple laws. This remarkable argument, which in certain respects pitted unsubstantiated dogma against scientific observation began as early as the fifth century BC and was still continuing into the twentieth century AD.

No such history would be complete without a quick consideration of a few of the major bungles in the area. For example, 'respiration' itself is a misnomer stemming from the Greeks' belief that the energetic processes of the body, that is mitochondrial function, occurred in the lungs. The acknowledgement of such bungles is valuable in many respects because: (1) It is humbling in that it demonstrates how even the most brilliant of minds can be lead astray. Several major advances listed here were made by those individuals who also are guilty of severe 'bungles'. (2) It makes us appreciate the tremendous power of the experimental method and opens our minds to accepting new knowledge. (3) We are reminded that, no matter how reinforced dogma is, it remains exactly that. Bungles are *italicized*.

By necessity, historical perspectives of this nature must be derivative and the reader is referred to the following excellent works: Singer (1959); Goodfield (1960); Perkins (1964); West (1980, 1996).

Empedocles (c.490–430 BC) *considered that all matter was composed of four elements: earth, air, fire and water and that the purpose of respiration was solely to cool the heart and blood. In turn, the blood served to supply 'innate heat' from the heart to the different organs.*

Aristotle (384–322 BC; Figure 1.1) *tutor to Alexander the Great (356–323 BC) taught that the arteries normally contain air and that all illnesses resulted from an imbalance of the four humours (blood, phlegm, black bile, yellow bile).*

Erasistratus of Cos (c.330–250 BC) considered the possibility that pores linked the systemic arteries and the veins (disputed by Galen).

Galen (c.130–199 AD) established the fundamentals of pulmonary gas exchange, namely that blood was enriched with a vital element from the inspired air and distributed to the peripheral tissues by the arteries. Waste materials were eliminated from the blood by the lungs. *Galen originated the 'pneumatic' theory of respiration. He taught that blood was produced and imbued with 'natural spirit' in the liver from whence it flowed to the right ventricle from which a portion nourished the lungs via the pulmonary artery and the remainder passed through invisible pores in the interventricular septum and mixed with 'pneuma' from the inspired air. The product was 'vital spirit' which was distributed to the peripheral tissues via the arterial blood. Due to the unavailability of human corpses for dissection, Galen's anatomical descriptions were taken from animals and, despite gross errors, were the standard medical references for the next fourteen hundred years until corrected in* **Andreas Vesalius's (1514–1564)** *classic 'De Humani Corporis Fabrica'.*

Ibn An-Nafis (c.1210–1288) held that blood transited the lungs from the pulmonary artery to the vein (in direct contradiction to Galen's notion that blood passed through pores in the interventricular septum). This information remained hidden from the western world until the twentieth century.

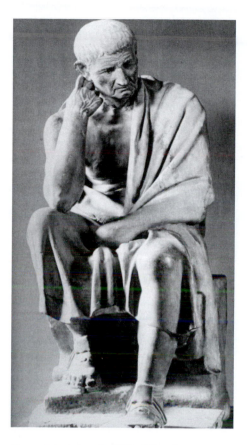

Figure 1.1 Aristotle (384–322 BC).

Michael Servetus (1511–1553) independently discovered the transit of blood through the lungs and noted that blood became 'reddish-yellow' as it passed through the lungs. Both Catholics and Calvinists considered his book (Christianismi Restitutio, 1553) to be heretical and he was burned at the stake in Geneva.

William Harvey (1578–1657) in 'De Motu Cordis et Sanguinis' (On the Motion of the Heart and Blood, 1628) described the key elements of the circulation and elucidated the functions of the heart and lungs.

Marcello Malpighi (1628–1694; Figure 1.2) was a superb microscopist who in 1661 established the anatomical basis for gas exchange in the lung by describing (in frogs) the movement of blood through the pulmonary capillaries and their relationship to the alveoli. *Unfortunately, although he observed individual red blood cells in the capillaries, he thought that they were fat globules.*

Anton van Leewenhoek (1632–1723) recognized the true nature of red blood cells.

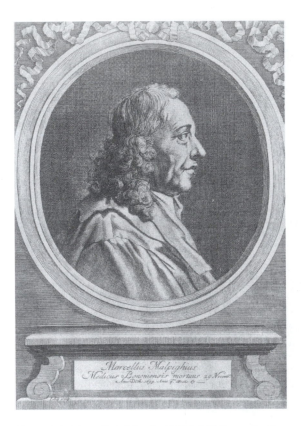

Figure 1.2 Marcello Malpighi (1628–1694) was the first person to see red blood cells
flowing through capillaries (~1666). Reproduced from West (1996) with
kind permission from the American Physiological Society.

Robert Boyle (1627–1691) and **Robert Hooke (1635–1703)** proposed that
the purpose of respiration was to supply a life-giving substance present in the
air to the body and that the respiratory movements themselves were of secondary importance. Unlike Empedocles and Galen, they verified this notion
experimentally, keeping a dog alive by blowing air through the lungs via holes
made in the pleural surface.

Richard Lower (1631–1691) proved that blood in the pulmonary vein turned
red before it reached the left heart unless the trachea was obstructed.

John Mayow (1643–1679) considered that air contained a 'nitro-aerial spirit'
that was essential for combustion and respiration. He showed that in an
enclosed jar an animal's death was accelerated in the presence of a burning
lamp. Mayow further argued that it was this 'nitro-aerial spirit' that entered
the blood via the lungs which facilitated muscular contraction.

Georg Ernst Stahl (1660–1734) *posited that all combustible substances consist of ash and 'phlogiston' (Greek for 'fire') and that phlogiston escaped on burning. The fact that the weight of metals increases during ashing lead to the assertion that phlogiston had negative weight!*

Joseph Black (1728–1799) rediscovered (initial discoverer, Jan Baptiste van Helmont [1577–1644]) carbon dioxide (CO_2) and determined its production by processes such as respiration, fermenting beer and also burning charcoal.

Joseph Priestly (1733–1804) and **Carl Wilhelm Scheele (1742–1786)** independently discovered oxygen (between 1772 and 1774). Each communicated his discovery to Antoine Lavoisier in Paris.

Antoine Laurent Lavoisier (1743–1794; Figure 1.3) in 1777, some three years after Priestley's visit, wrote 'Eminently respirable air that enters the lung,

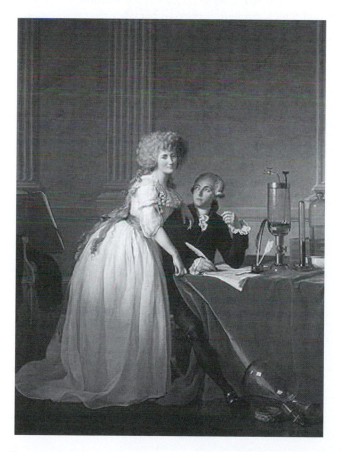

Figure 1.3 The great French chemist, Antoine Laurent Lavoisier (1743–1794) pictured with his wife in their laboratory. Tragically, Lavoisier was guillotined on 8 May 1794. This portrait was painted by David and hangs in the Metropolitan Museum of Art in New York. Reproduced from West (1996) with kind permission from the American Physiological Society.

leaves it in the form of chalky aeroform acids (CO_2)...in almost equal volume.' He recognized that respiration acts only on that 'portion of pure air that is eminently respirable' and that the 'mephitic portion' (nitrogen, N_2) was not utilized. Subsequently, he named the 'eminently respirable' air 'oxygine' for its acid-forming properties. This finally sounded the death knell of Stahl's phlogiston theory that had hamstrung respiratory physiological advancement for several decades. *However, like the ancients, Lavoisier concluded that respiratory combustion took place in the lungs and that the heat evolved was passed to the blood for transport around the body.*

Humphrey Davy (1778–1829) in 1799 was the first to prove that blood contained both O_2 and CO_2.

Heinrich Gustav Magnus (1802–1870; Figure 1.4) constructed a blood-gas analyser and showed that arterial blood contained more O_2 and less CO_2 than venous blood which strongly supported the idea that respiration occurred in the peripheral tissues. This conclusion was also advanced by **von Helmholtz (1821–1894)** after observing that a single twitch of an isolated muscle liberated heat.

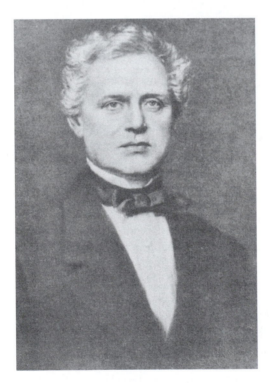

Figure 1.4 Heinrich Gustav Magnus (1802–1870) invented blood gas analysis and demonstrated that gas exchange occurred in the muscles (~1837). Reproduced from West (1996) with kind permission from the American Physiological Society.

Eduard Pfleuger (1829–1910) published definitive papers (1872 and 1875) demonstrating conclusively that metabolism occurs in peripheral tissues and that the blood merely transported the respiratory gases.

Max Rubner (1854–1932) (and also J. Geppert and N. Zuntz 1888, see later) performed direct calorimetry on intact animals and demonstrated the relationship between O_2 utilization and heat production.

Nathan Zuntz (1847–1920) with his colleague J. Geppert measured O_2 and CO_2 exchange in running dogs and also developed the eponymous 'Haldane transformation' some years before Haldane!

August Krogh (1874–1949) with his colleague J.L. Lindhard documented the very fast cardiovascular responses at the onset of exercise (1913).

J.S. Haldane (1860–1936) *and J.G. Priestly in line with the notion of the 'vitalism' espoused by Aristotle two millennia previously, as late as 1935 considered that the lungs actively secreted O_2 against its partial pressure gradient. Indeed, in 1919, Christian Bohr had argued vehemently that as much as 60% of the $\dot{V}O_2$ of an animal occurred in the tissues of the lung.*

Archibald Vivian Hill (1886–1977; Figure 1.5, left panel) demonstrated the clear exponential nature of the $\dot{V}O_2$ response at exercise onset.

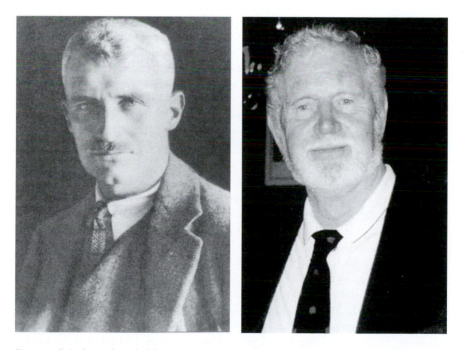

Figure 1.5 Left panel: Nobel laureate Archibald Vivian Hill pictured in 1927. *Right panel*: Brian J. Whipp pictured in 2002. These two individuals have done much to further our understanding of metabolic control.

Brian J. Whipp (Figure 1.5, right panel) and **Karl Wasserman** demonstrated the elegant and physiologically insightful three-phase $\dot{V}O_2$ response at exercise onset and provided its mechanistic physiological basis. They also described the relationship between $\dot{V}O_2$ kinetics and exercise intensity. In collaboration with W.L. Beaver, Lamarra and Wasserman (Beaver *et al.*, 1981) developed equations for measurement of breath-to-breath alveolar gas exchange that are used in many commercial gas analysis systems today.

Some of the founders of the field of '$\dot{V}O_2$ kinetics'

The study of $\dot{V}O_2$ kinetics is inextricably entwined within the broader field of exercise physiology. For example, the incomparable eighteenth-century French chemist Antoine Lavoisier and the great nineteenth-century German physiologists such as Nathan Zuntz and his colleague J. Geppert used muscular exercise to revolutionize our understanding of respiration and metabolism. The English Nobel laureate, Archibald Vivian Hill studied the dynamics of metabolic processes in muscles isolated from small animals and used these data to develop his ideas about energetics within human athletes. In the 1920s, Hill and his colleagues, C.N.H. Long and H. Lupton were to generate some of the first $\dot{V}O_2$ measurements at the onset of dynamic exercise in humans that demonstrated the rapidity and exponential nature of the $\dot{V}O_2$ response (see 'Historical Development' earlier and also Chapter 7, p. 154). As recounted by Brooks and colleagues (2000), it was A.V. Hill's lectures at Cornell University in 1926 that lead to the foundation of the Harvard Fatigue Laboratory at Harvard University. This laboratory was to bring Rodolfo Margaria (University of Milan), H.T. Edwards and David Bruce Dill together to study the metabolic responses during the non-steady-state conditions presiding during exercise.

In the late 1960s and early 1970s the physician scientist Karl Wasserman and brilliant Welshman, Brian J. Whipp (see Chapter 3) were to capitalize on advances in technology that facilitated breath-to-breath measurements of ventilation and pulmonary gas exchange. It was these individuals, with their team at Harbor-UCLA Medical Center and a string of eminent collaborators and visiting scientists, who would establish the field of $\dot{V}O_2$ dynamics to which this text is dedicated. At the same time as Wasserman and Whipp in California were beginning their studies into $\dot{V}O_2$ kinetics, Paolo Cerretelli and Pietro Di Prampero (Milan, Italy) and also Leon Farhi (Buffalo, USA) were to relate pulmonary $\dot{V}O_2$ to cardiac output dynamics at exercise onset. In many regards, the above-mentioned individuals may be considered among the pioneers of the study of $\dot{V}O_2$ kinetics. It was they who are largely responsible for laying the requisite groundwork for the next generation of physiologists for whom the study of $\dot{V}O_2$ kinetics would provide a fruitful window through which to gain a greater understanding of metabolic control and physiologic function. Indeed, as a parameter of physiological function, measurement of $\dot{V}O_2$ kinetics is poised to become a standard laboratory measurement.

Oxygen uptake kinetics

What is $\dot{V}O_2$ and what are $\dot{V}O_2$ kinetics?

As can be seen in the previous section, early descriptions and study of '$\dot{V}O_2$ kinetics' upon exertion began in the early part of the twentieth century. The term 'kinetics' can be defined as 'the science of the action of force in producing or changing motion' (*Chambers English Dictionary*). The study of $\dot{V}O_2$ kinetics, therefore, could be considered to involve the study of the physiological mechanisms responsible for the dynamic $\dot{V}O_2$ response to exercise and its subsequent recovery. The study of $\dot{V}O_2$ and its regulation is important because oxidative metabolism is the principal means by which the human organism generates energy to do work in all but the most short-lived of activities. Factors such as the highest attainable $\dot{V}O_2$ ($\dot{V}O_{2\,max}$), the $\dot{V}O_2$ required to perform sub-maximal exercise (i.e. the economy or efficiency of exercise), and the rate at which $\dot{V}O_2$ rises in the transition to an activity with a higher energetic requirement to reach the requisite steady-state level, will all influence an individual's tolerance to physical activity.

The consumption of oxygen by biological tissue can be described with the Fick equation:

$$\dot{V}O_2 = \dot{Q}_T \times (CaO_2 - CvO_2)$$

where $\dot{Q}_T$ represents tissue blood flow and CaO_2 and CvO_2 represent arterial and venous O_2 contents respectively. $\dot{Q}_T$ will depend upon cardiac output (the product of heart rate and stroke volume) and the degree of vasodilatation in the tissue vascular beds as well as the pressure differential acting across the tissue. CaO_2 is related to haemoglobin concentration and the degree of saturation of haemoglobin with O_2. The difference between CaO_2 and CvO_2 represents the amount of oxygen extracted from the arterial blood by the tissue in order to support oxidative phosphorylation in the cells' mitochondria. The $\dot{V}O_2$ of any tissue therefore depends both upon 'central' factors (i.e. the delivery of O_2 to the tissue) and 'peripheral' factors (i.e. the extraction and utilization of O_2 in the tissue). In exercise physiology, the tissue of greatest interest is often the exercising muscle. However, while direct measurements of muscle $\dot{V}O_2$ are certainly possible (see Chapter 6), they are invasive and technically challenging. Therefore, in studies of exercise metabolism, $\dot{V}O_2$ is commonly measured at the mouth either via the collection and subsequent analysis of expired air in Douglas bags or through the use of automated gas analysis systems (MacFarlane, 2001). The $\dot{V}O_2$ measured at the mouth represents the gross rate of oxygen uptake by the entire body and in the steady state may be equated with oxygen consumption. The $\dot{V}O_2$ at rest depends principally on body size but is around $0.25\,l \cdot min^{-1}$ in young adults, while the $\dot{V}O_2$ during exhaustive exercise (i.e. the $\dot{V}O_{2\,max}$) can be as high as $6\,l \cdot min^{-1}$ in male endurance athletes, particularly cross-country skiers. The human body therefore has an extraordinary capacity to increase its metabolic rate in response to energetic challenges. The $\dot{V}O_2$ measured at the mouth during exercise obviously reflects the elevated $\dot{V}O_2$ in the exercising muscles in addition to the elevated $\dot{V}O_2$ associated with 'support processes' (e.g. increased heart rate and pulmonary ventilation; lactate catabolism). However, while there is inevitably a degree of 'contamination' in measurements of respiratory gas exchange at the mouth, the measurement of pulmonary $\dot{V}O_2$ broadly reflects muscle $\dot{V}O_2$ during exercise (Chapter 6).

Parameters of aerobic energy metabolism

The $\dot{V}O_{2\ max}$ (normally obtained during an incremental exercise test performed to exhaustion; note that we make no distinction here between $\dot{V}O_{2'max'}$ and $\dot{V}O_{2\ 'peak'}$; see Day *et al.*, 2003) can provide important information on the integrated capacity of the pulmonary, cardiovascular and neuromuscular systems to perform exercise both in health and disease (Wasserman *et al.*, 1994). The $\dot{V}O_{2\ max}$ represents the maximal rate at which ATP can be synthesized aerobically, and therefore provides a ceiling for athletic performance in endurance athletes and for functional capacity in sedentary and patient populations. For exercise at sea level requiring more than about one-third of the total muscle mass, it is generally considered that the $\dot{V}O_{2\ max}$ is limited principally by the maximal cardiac output since the supply of additional O_2 to muscle can increase the $\dot{V}O_{2\ max}$ (Wagner, 2000). However, the $\dot{V}O_{2\ max}$ achieved will always depend upon both O_2 delivery and peripheral O_2 extraction (which in itself is determined by the O_2 diffusing capacity of the active muscle), and the limiting factor in the pathway of oxygen conductance from the mouth to the mitochondrion will depend also on the exercise mode (i.e. engagement of small vs large muscle mass; Chapter 4), the environment (i.e. altitude) and subject characteristics (i.e. age, training status and disease status; Chapters 13–15) (Bassett and Howley, 2000; Wagner, 2000).

The principal determinants of the exercising $\dot{V}O_2$ response are internal work, external work and efficiency. Internal work includes the resting metabolic rate and, for example during cycle ergometry, the internal work performed by moving the legs at a particular pedal rate with no external load. Pedal rates of 50–70 $\text{rev} \cdot \text{min}^{-1}$ elevate pulmonary $\dot{V}O_2$ to ~500 $\text{ml} \cdot \text{min}^{-1}$ whilst very high pedal rates (>90 $\text{rev} \cdot \text{min}^{-1}$) may require 1,000 $\text{ml} \cdot \text{min}^{-1}$. For walking or running on a level surface, internal work over and above the resting metabolism is performed as the body mass is raised. During cycle exercise, 'delta' exercise efficiency is 25–30% and is similar in principle to exercise economy which is the increase in $\dot{V}O_2$ above baseline per unit increase in work rate and usually corresponds to ~10 ml of O_2 consumed per minute of exercise per Watt of external power output (i.e. ~10 $\text{ml} \cdot \text{min}^{-1} \cdot \text{W}^{-1}$) during cycle exercise. Under conditions where no $\dot{V}O_2$ slow component is present (i.e. constant work rate (CWR) tests performed below the lactate threshold (LT) or during incremental cycle exercise), this value is relatively constant across 'sub-maximal' exercise intensities and in different subjects (although some inter-individual variability does exist which appears to be of physiological origin; Barstow *et al.*, 2000a,b; Mallory *et al.*, 2002). Exercise economy and $\dot{V}O_{2\,max}$ can be established using a series of discrete CWR exercise bouts, or by using an incremental exercise test in which the external work rate is progressively increased to the limit of tolerance. The steady-state increase in $\dot{V}O_2$ above baseline during sub-maximal exercise can be used to calculate exercise economy, whereas the attainment of the same $\dot{V}O_2$ despite continued increases in the work rate applied in the exercise bouts indicates the attainment of $\dot{V}O_{2\,max}$. In the case of the latter, that is incremental exercise which brings the subject to exhaustion in ~10 minutes, the slope of the regression line describing the $\dot{V}O_2$ – work-rate relationship gives the exercise economy while the $\dot{V}O_2$ attained in the last 30 s or so of the exercise test is the $\dot{V}O_{2\,max}$. Although a plateau in $\dot{V}O_2$ is not always evident during incremental exercise tests, the $\dot{V}O_{2\,max}$ attained is nevertheless consistent with that attained during a series of CWR bouts (Day *et al.*, 2003) such that an incremental test obviates the requirement for the performance of a series of discrete and time-consuming CWR tests for the assessment of $\dot{V}O_{2\,max}$. Longer incremental tests can give rise to a $\dot{V}O_2$ profile with upward curvilinearity later in the test (Hansen *et al.*, 1988; Zoladz *et al.*, 1995). The 'excess' $\dot{V}O_2$ (i.e. the $\dot{V}O_2$ exceeding that predicted from extrapolation of the $\dot{V}O_2$ – work-rate relationship established in the early part of the test) presumably has similar mechanistic origins to the $\dot{V}O_2$ 'slow component' that arises during high intensities of sub-maximal exercise (see Figure 1.6).

In addition to providing information on exercise economy and $\dot{V}O_{2\,max}$, the pulmonary gas exchange responses to incremental exercise can be used to estimate the $\dot{V}O_2$ at which the 'lactate threshold' occurs (Figure 1.6). The LT is the metabolic rate at which blood [lactate] begins to increase above baseline values. While this event does not necessarily signify an appreciable increase in anaerobic energy supply, it does indicate alterations in the cellular redox and phosphorylation potentials to drive mitochondrial respiration (Connett *et al.*, 1990). Bicarbonate buffering of the lactic acidosis results in the generation of non-metabolic CO_2 and an increase in $\dot{V}CO_2$ (and $\dot{V}_E$) measured at the mouth. The LT can therefore be estimated non-invasively by determination of the gas exchange threshold (GET) using for example the V-slope method (Beaver *et al.*, 1986). The GET typically occurs at 45–60% $\dot{V}O_{2\,max}$ but can be as low as ~35% $\dot{V}O_{2\,max}$ in patients and as high as ~80% $\dot{V}O_{2\,max}$ in athletes. These differences are important in 'normalizing' exercise intensity across individual subjects. For example, exercise at 60% $\dot{V}O_{2\,max}$ might be above the GET in one subject but below the GET in another, with the result that the metabolic and gas exchange responses to exercise are quite different. For this reason, in most of the studies that have investigated $\dot{V}O_2$ kinetics during CWR exercise, the '%Δ' concept has been used to normalize exercise intensity. This procedure takes into account both the $\dot{V}O_2$ at the GET and the $\dot{V}O_{2\,max}$ in the calculation of relative exercise intensity. For example, 40%Δ refers to the work rate requiring a $\dot{V}O_2$ that is 40% of the difference between the $\dot{V}O_2$ at the GET and $\dot{V}O_{2\,max}$ under conditions specified within a given testing regimen. The %Δ concept is useful in helping to

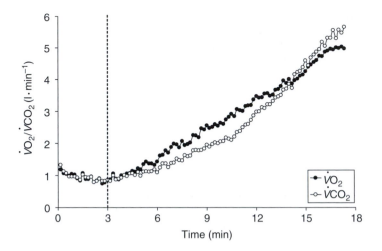

Figure 1.6 The response of $\dot{V}O_2$ and $\dot{V}CO_2$ to an incremental exercise test on a cycle ergometer in a well-trained subject. The test was preceded by a 3-min period of cycling at 20 W, after which work rate was increased by 30 $W \cdot min^{-1}$ resulting in termination of the test after ~17 min. Note the essentially linear increase in $\dot{V}O_2$ with work rate (this relationship has a slope of ~10 $ml \cdot min^{-1} \cdot W^{-1}$) until the maximum is reached. Note also that the previously linear relationship between $\dot{V}CO_2$ and work rate is lost at a particular sub-maximal $\dot{V}O_2$. This 'disproportionate' increase in CO_2 output (and $\dot{V}_E$), that is above the so-called 'gas exchange threshold' (GET), provides a non-invasive means for estimating the $\dot{V}O_2$ at the lactate threshold (LT).

ensure that subjects are exercising within the correct exercise intensity 'domain' (see later) in studies of $\dot{V}O_2$ kinetics.

Constant work-rate exercise

Other than when sleeping or being completely immobile, humans are rarely in a metabolic steady state; rather, we shift dynamically across a range of metabolic requirements (see Chapter 13, Figure 13.1). At the onset of movement or dynamic exercise such as cycling or running, the energetic requirements of the contracting muscles increase immediately with the first contraction in what has been termed a 'square-wave' fashion. However, as demonstrated in Figure 1.7, neither the increase in pulmonary nor muscle $\dot{V}O_2$ have 'square-wave' response profiles. Rather, the response demonstrates considerable inertia and, depending on the health or fitness of the individual and the exercise intensity, may take from 2 to 15 or more min to achieve the steady-state values (Figures 1.8 and 1.9). 'Square-wave' or 'step' exercise tests, in which the external work rate given by the ergometer is increased abruptly from a baseline of rest or unloaded exercise, permit the gathering of important information on the dynamic responses of

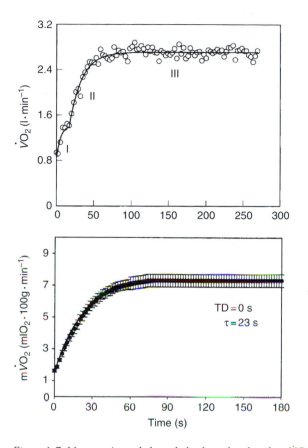

Figure 1.7 Upper: Actual breath-by-breath alveolar $\dot{V}O_2$ response across the transient from unloaded cycling (0 W) to a moderate work rate (no sustained lactic acidosis) for a representative subject (data from Grassi *et al.*, 1996). Notice the distinct phasic response (Phases I, II and III) that correspond to distinct physiological events (see text for details). *Lower:* Increase in muscle $\dot{V}O_2$ ($m\dot{V}O_2$) at the onset of muscle contractions (time 0) in rat spinotrapezius measured directly from capillary red blood cell flux and microvascular O_2 pressures (Behnke *et al.*, 2002). τ is the time constant (time required to reach 63% of the final response) of the mono-exponential. Note that $\dot{V}O_2$ increases immediately with the first contractions, however, it does not approach the steady state for about 80 s.

pulmonary gas exchange which reflects the integrated response of the ventilatory, cardiovascular, and neuromuscular systems to the exercise challenge. Measurement of $\dot{V}O_2$ kinetics has become an important tool in the evaluation of the extent of dysfunction and in some instances the mechanism behind that dysfunction in many major chronic disease conditions (see Table 1.1). The capability for $\dot{V}O_2$ kinetics determination to provide mechanistic insights into

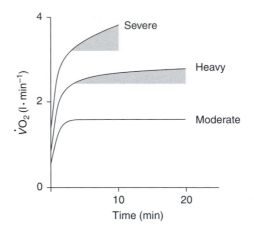

Figure 1.8 Schematic representation of the $\dot{V}O_2$ response to constant work-rate exercise in the moderate (below lactate threshold), heavy (above the lactate threshold) and severe (above the asymptote of the power–time relationship for high-intensity exercise, critical power, CP) exercise domains. For clarity, the $\dot{V}O_2$ response occurring at exercise onset (Phase I, see Figure 1.7) has been omitted. Note that for moderate intensity exercise, $\dot{V}O_2$ increases mono-exponentially (Phase II) to the steady state (plateau, Phase III), which in healthy subjects is achieved within 3 min. In contrast, for heavy and severe intensity exercise, the steady state is either delayed (heavy) or not achieved (severe) because of the slow component (shaded area) which occurs only above the lactate threshold. Traditionally, the magnitude of this slow component has been approximated as the increase in $\dot{V}O_2$ from minute 3 to end-exercise. The slow component elevates $\dot{V}O_2$ above that predicted for the work rate. Within the severe exercise domain, $\dot{V}O_2$ achieves its maximum value ($\dot{V}O_{2\,max}$) at or before fatigue.

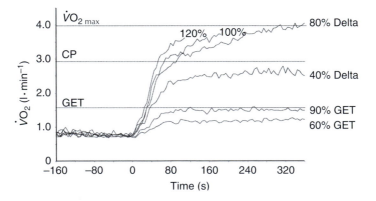

Figure 1.9 Actual $\dot{V}O_2$ response to moderate, heavy, severe and extreme intensity exercise in a representative subject. The lines represent an average of the $\dot{V}O_2$ response to several repetitions at each work rate. Note that for moderate work rates (<GET), a steady state is reached rapidly; for heavy work rates (>GET but <CP), a delayed but elevated steady state is attained; for severe work rates (>CP but <$\dot{V}O_{2\,max}$), a steady state is never attained and $\dot{V}O_2$ may attain its maximum given sufficient time; and for extreme work rates (>$\dot{V}O_{2\,max}$), exercise duration becomes so short that $\dot{V}O_{2\,max}$ cannot be attained.

Table 1.1 Chronic disease conditions evaluated using measurement of $\dot{V}O_2$ kinetics

Disease/condition	Publication(s)
Chronic obstructive pulmonary disease and emphysema	Palange *et al.*, 1995; Puente-Maestu *et al.*, 2000; Somfay *et al.*, 2002
Cystic fibrosis	Kusenbach *et al.*, 1999
Coronary artery disease	Adachi *et al.*, 2000
Mitral stenosis	Lim *et al.*, 1998
Congenital heart disease	McManus and Leung, 2000
Chronic heart failure	Hepple *et al.*, 1999
Atrial fibrillation	Lok and Lau, 1997
Dilated cardiomyopathy	deGroote *et al.*, 1996
Primary pulmonary hypertension	Riley *et al.*, 2000
Peripheral arterial disease	Bauer *et al.*, 1999
HIV	Stringer, 2000
Spinal cord injury	Barstow *et al.*, 2000; Fukuoka *et al.*, 2002
Chronic fatigue syndrome	Inbar *et al.*, 2001
Prolonged immobility	Convertino *et al.*, 1984

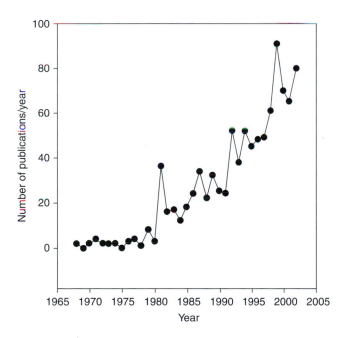

Figure 1.10 Number of $\dot{V}O_2$ kinetics publications per year from 1968 to present.

Source: PubMed database from the National Center for Biotechnology Information, National Library of Medicine, USA.

physiologic function and pathophysiologic dysfunction accounts in large part for the recent explosion in publications in this area (Figure 1.10). It should be noted here that in additional to incremental/ramp and CWR exercise tests, other types of forcing functions including impulse, sinusoidal and pseudo-random binary sequence may also be used for the analysis of $\dot{V}O_2$ kinetics (e.g. Hughson et al., 1988, 1990). However, relatively few studies now utilize these approaches and the interested reader is directed to the excellent review articles of Lamarra (1990) and Swanson (1990).

The pulmonary $\dot{V}O_2$ response following the onset of exercise has been well characterized (Whipp and Wasserman, 1972; Linnarsson, 1974; Whipp et al., 1982). At the onset of CWR exercise, there is an early rapid increase that is typically initiated within the first breath (Phase I, Figure 1.7). This initial increase in Phase I is followed by a rapid exponential increase in $\dot{V}O_2$ (Phase II) with a time constant or τ of some 20–45 s (healthy individuals) that drives $\dot{V}O_2$ to the actual, or towards the initially anticipated, steady-state value (Phase III) within 3 minutes. Phase I represents the O_2 exchange associated with the initial elevation of cardiac output and thus pulmonary blood flow. Phase II reflects the arrival at the lung of venous blood draining the exercising muscles (note that the Phase II $\dot{V}O_2$ response is variously described as the 'fast component', the 'primary component', or the 'fundamental component' in the $\dot{V}O_2$ kinetics literature). The pulmonary $\dot{V}O_2$ kinetics in Phase II therefore largely reflect the kinetics of O_2 consumption in the exercising muscles, although there is a temporal lag between events at the muscle and those recorded at the lung (Chapters 3 and 6). For moderate intensity exercise, the onset of Phase III corresponds to the point at which cardiac output plateaus and venous O_2 content reaches its nadir. At higher exercise intensities, the attainment of a steady state might be delayed or absent.

In the transition from rest or unloaded exercise to a work rate with a $\dot{V}O_2$ requirement below that at the LT, the vertical distance between the actual $\dot{V}O_2$ at a given moment and that required in the steady state represents the energy requirement that must be met from energy stores within the muscle. These stores consist principally of energy released through phosphocreatine hydrolysis and anaerobic glycolysis, with a small contribution from O_2 stores (myoglobin, venous blood). The total O_2 equivalent of the shaded area in Figure 1.11 is termed the O_2 deficit. As can be appreciated in that figure, the absolute size of this deficit is the product of the increase in $\dot{V}O_2$ ($\Delta\dot{V}O_2$) across the transient and the speed of the $\dot{V}O_2$ response denoted by the time constant (τ) of the $\dot{V}O_2$ response from the onset of exercise (τ represents the time taken to achieve 63% of $\Delta\dot{V}O_2$): O_2 deficit = $\Delta\dot{V}O_2 \times \tau$ where $\Delta\dot{V}O_2$ is given in $L \cdot min^{-1}$ and τ in fractions of a minute. [Note that in modelling pulmonary $\dot{V}O_2$ kinetics, it is the τ of the Phase II response (see Figure 1.7) that approximates the τ for muscle oxygen consumption; the sum of the duration of the Phase I response and the τ in Phase II (i.e. the mean response time, MRT) may be used to estimate the O_2 deficit]. Thus, for a given $\Delta\dot{V}O_2$ the faster the $\dot{V}O_2$ response (smaller τ), the smaller is the O_2 deficit that will be incurred. In contrast, extremely unfit or unhealthy individuals will have a very slow response (larger τ) and will incur a high O_2 deficit and thus a greater degree of intracellular perturbation (increased lactic acid, decreased PCr, Figure 1.11). Slow $\dot{V}O_2$ kinetics mandate a greater depletion of intramuscular [PCr] and a greater rate of glycogenolysis leading to greater accumulation of lactate and protons and a greater utilization of the finite

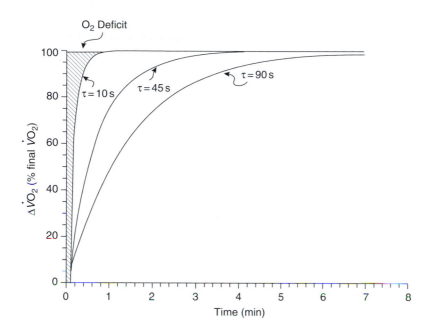

Figure 1.11 Schematic demonstration of the effect of altering the speed of $\dot{V}O_2$ kinetics (τ) on the O_2 deficit. The range of τ's given represent those measures in a race-horse (10 s), sedentary human (45 s), and a cardiac patient (90 s). The shaded area represents the size of the O_2 deficit for $\tau = 10$ s. Note that this area becomes systematically larger as $\dot{V}O_2$ kinetics become slower (increasing τ).

intramuscular glycogen reserves, all factors which predispose to a reduced exercise tolerance. Slow on-transient $\dot{V}O_2$ kinetics have the same deleterious effects at higher exercise intensities too, although it should be noted that greater complexity in the $\dot{V}O_2$ kinetics make the computation of the O_2 deficit at higher work rates more problematic (Whipp *et al.*, 2002; see Chapter 3).

Exercise intensity domains

As intimated earlier, the metabolic and gas exchange responses to CWR exercise can be defined in relation to a number of identifiable exercise intensity domains, namely: moderate, heavy, severe and extreme.

   Moderate exercise encompasses all work rates that are below the LT. For moderate intensity CWR cycle exercise, blood lactate is not elevated and steady state (Phase III) $\dot{V}O_2$ increases with a 'gain' of 9–11 ml $\cdot$ min$^{-1} \cdot$ W^{-1} above that found during unloaded pedalling. Within the moderate intensity domain, the speed of the Phase II $\dot{V}O_2$ kinetics has been generally shown to be invariant with work rate, but is accelerated by exercise training and slowed by ageing, prolonged inactivity and/or chronic diseases (see Chapters 13–15).

Heavy exercise comprises those work rates lying between the LT and the asymptote of the power–duration curve for high-intensity exercise, that is the critical power (CP; Monod and Scherrer 1965; Moritani *et al.* 1981). CWR exercise in the heavy intensity domain results in an elevated but stable blood [lactate] over time such that there is a balance between the rates of appearance of lactate in the blood and the rate of its removal from the blood. The upper boundary for the heavy domain is defined as the highest $\dot{V}O_2$ at which blood lactate (and $\dot{V}O_2$) can be stabilized, that is the maximal lactate steady state (MLSS). The MLSS broadly corresponds to the CP, both typically occurring at ~ 50%Δ (Smith and Jones, 2001; Pringle and Jones, 2002). There is some evidence that the Phase II $\dot{V}O_2$ kinetics may be slowed at the onset of heavy compared with moderate intensity exercise, although the bulk of the available literature has not demonstrated a significant difference from the response to moderate intensity exercise (Chapter 12). The gain of the primary component ($\Delta\dot{V}O_2/\Delta$WR) is similar to that observed during moderate intensity exercise. However, CWR exercise in the heavy domain does evidence a 'slow component' of the $\dot{V}O_2$ kinetics that becomes apparent after approximately two minutes following exercise onset and which is superimposed upon the primary $\dot{V}O_2$ response. Figures 1.8 and 1.12 illustrate that this slow component elevates the $\dot{V}O_2$ *above* rather than *towards* the $\dot{V}O_2$ that would be calculated for a particular work rate by extrapolation of the $\dot{V}O_2$ response to moderate exercise. Depending on the characteristics of the slow component, achievement of the steady-state $\dot{V}O_2$ may be delayed by 10–15 min or more in the extreme.

Severe exercise comprises those work rates lying between the MLSS/CP and the $\dot{V}O_{2\,max}$ as assessed during an incremental exercise test in which fatigue is reached in ~10 min. In the severe domain, the slow component causes $\dot{V}O_2$ to increase to its maximum and blood [lactate] rises inexorably until the exercise is terminated. In the extreme (for the lowest work-rates in this domain), the $\dot{V}O_2$ slow component may achieve values of $1-1.5\ L \cdot min^{-1}$ (Figures 1.8 and 1.12). There is some evidence that the gain of the $\dot{V}O_2$ primary component falls below the typical $10\ ml \cdot min^{-1} \cdot W^{-1}$ during severe intensity exercise (Jones *et al.*, 2002; Pringle *et al.*, 2003; Scheuermann and Barstow, 2003) and that, as for heavy exercise, the primary $\dot{V}O_2$ kinetics might be slowed relative to that observed during moderate exercise. For the very highest work rates in the severe domain, no slow component is evident and $\dot{V}O_2$ may rise with a close to monoexponential profile that is truncated at $\dot{V}O_{2\,max}$. However, for all work rates in the severe domain, when exercise is continued to the point of exhaustion, $\dot{V}O_{2\,max}$ is attained. Consequently, the severe-intensity domain presents a broad range of work rates in which it is possible to attain $\dot{V}O_{2\,max}$.

The slow component rise in $\dot{V}O_2$ during heavy and severe CWR exercise means that $\dot{V}O_2$ changes as a function of time as well as work rate in these domains. Consequently, without precise stipulation of the test conditions and timing of measurements, in the heavy and severe domains it is not appropriate to define a given work rate as a percentage of $\dot{V}O_{2\,max}$. Unfortunately, this important conceptual and practical consideration is often ignored in the design of exercise studies and in their interpretation.

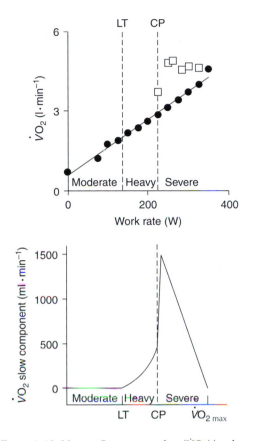

Figure 1.12 Upper: Oxygen uptake ($\dot{V}O_2$)/work rate relationship for incremental exercise, where work rate is increased by 25 W·min^{-1} to fatigue (solid symbols) and $\dot{V}O_2$ achieved during constant-load exercise (hollow symbols) for one healthy subject. The hollow symbol at left is at the upper limit of heavy exercise (24 min, non-fatiguing) whereas all other hollow symbols denote $\dot{V}O_2$ at fatigue during severe intensity exercise. LT identifies the lactate threshold and CP the asymptote of power of the power–time relationship for fatiguing high-intensity exercise and these parameters demarcate the moderate, heavy and severe domains. Notice that for all work rates >CP (5 upper hollow squares), $\dot{V}O_2$ achieves its maximum. *Lower:* Schematic illustration of the size of the $\dot{V}O_2$ slow component in proximity to LT, CP and $\dot{V}O_{2\,max}$. Notice the extraordinary magnitude of the $\dot{V}O_2$ slow component at the lower extremes of the severe exercise intensity domain.

Given the finite kinetics of $\dot{V}O_2$ it is inevitable that some work rates are so high that fatigue intervenes before $\dot{V}O_{2\,max}$ can be achieved. This domain has recently been termed '*extreme exercise*' (Hill *et al.*, 2002) and in an untrained population of college students corresponds to a work rate that is sufficiently high so as to limit the tolerable duration of exercise to <140 s (i.e. ~4 × a time constant of ~30 s). Obviously, fitter individuals will exhibit faster $\dot{V}O_2$ kinetics and it would therefore be expected that such individuals would require less time at these extreme work rates to reach their $\dot{V}O_{2\,max}$. Interestingly, due in part to the short duration of exercise before fatigue ensues, blood [lactate] at the end of exercise in this domain may not reach such high values as those recorded at the end of severe intensity exercise.

Note that this is not the only exercise-intensity categorization considered. For example, Figure 3.9 (p. 84) designates work rates that are $>CP$ but for which the primary or fundamental component projects below the subject's $\dot{V}O_{2\,max}$ as 'very heavy'. The higher 'severe' domain is reserved for work rates where the projected $\dot{V}O_2$ cost is $> \dot{V}O_{2\,max}$. In this schema, no discrimination is made for work rates so high that fatigue ensues before $\dot{V}O_2$ can reach $\dot{V}O_{2\,max}$.

The $\dot{V}O_2$ kinetics in the off-transient, that is during recovery from exercise, can provide additional information on gas exchange dynamics and can aid in interpretation of the physiological events underpinning the $\dot{V}O_2$ response in the on-transient. Surprisingly, relatively few studies have investigated the off-transient $\dot{V}O_2$ kinetics. It appears, however, that the linear first-order kinetics evidenced in moderate exercise (i.e. the $\dot{V}O_2$ response projects to essentially the same gain with essentially the same time constant irrespective of work rate) is also reflected in the recovery from exercise such that there is symmetry between the on- and off-kinetics (Paterson and Whipp, 1991; Ozyener et al., 2001). For higher exercise intensities, however, $\dot{V}O_2$ kinetics in the on- and off-transients become more complicated: for heavy exercise, a slow component term is observed in the $\dot{V}O_2$ on-response but not in the off-response; for severe exercise, a slow component is apparent both in the on- and off-transients; and for extreme exercise, a slow component exists in the off-transient but not the on-transient (Ozyener et al., 2001). These asymmetries may have important implications for interpreting the mechanisms responsible for the emergence of the $\dot{V}O_2$ slow component during heavy and severe exercise.

Model characterization of $\dot{V}O_2$ kinetics

It has been established that the $\dot{V}O_2$ response in Phase II is essentially exponential in character (Hill et al., 1924; Henry, 1951; Mahler, 1980). An exponential response of a system is consistent with the existence of an initial 'error signal' (i.e. a difference between the instantaneous and required value, in this case of $\dot{V}O_2$) and feedback control of the response until the error signal is eliminated (Figure 1.13). An exponential function has an amplitude and a time constant (τ, the equivalent of the reciprocal of the rate constant $(1/k)$; Whipp, 1971) which reflects the time required for the attainment of 63% of the total amplitude. The exponential nature of the $\dot{V}O_2$ response in Phase II can therefore be described with the following equation:

$$\dot{V}O_2\,(t) = \dot{V}O_2\,(b) + A\,(1 - e^{-(t - TD)/\tau})$$

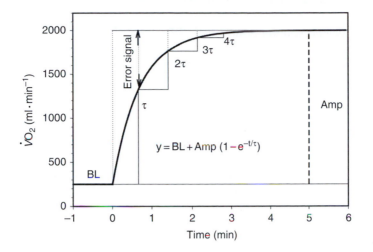

Figure 1.13 Schematic illustration of the exponential increase in muscle $\dot{V}O_2$ following the onset of exercise. The authors thank R.L. Hughson for this figure which was produced for Chapter 8. See text for further details.

where $\dot{V}O_2$ (*t*) is the $\dot{V}O_2$ at any point in time, $\dot{V}O_2$ (*b*) is the baseline $\dot{V}O_2$ before the commencement of the step transition to a higher work rate, A is the steady-state amplitude of the $\dot{V}O_2$ response, and $(1 - e^{-(t - TD)/\tau})$ is the exponential function describing the rate at which $\dot{V}O_2$ is rising towards the steady-state amplitude. In this exponential function, *t* is time, TD is the time delay before the start of the exponential term and τ is the time constant.

Therefore, for a τ of 30 s: 63% of the response amplitude is attained after 30 s; 86% of the response amplitude is attained after 60 s (i.e. 2 × τ; 1.0 − 0.63 = 0.37; (0.37 × 0.63) + 0.63 = 0.86); 95% of the response amplitude is attained after 90 s (3 × τ); 98% of response amplitude is attained after 120 s (4 × τ); and >99% of the response amplitude is attained after 150 s (5 × τ). It is generally considered that the response is essentially complete after four time constants have elapsed.

The exponential increase of pulmonary $\dot{V}O_2$ following the onset of muscular exercise is essentially a 'mirror image' of the exponential reduction of intramuscular [PCr], once the 'muscle to mouth' transport delay time has been accounted for (Rossiter *et al.*, 1999, 2002). This strongly suggests that muscle $\dot{V}O_2$ kinetics are principally under feedback control from one or more of the products of high-energy phosphate splitting (Whipp and Mahler, 1980). Models of respiratory control are addressed in detail in Chapter 7.

It is important to remember that, in the non-steady state, the relationship between muscle and pulmonary $\dot{V}O_2$ is distorted by at least three factors: the transit delay between the muscle and the lung; muscle and venous O_2 stores; and the kinetics of cardiac output (a given a-vO_2 difference at the muscle will be associated with a faster blood flow when it reaches the lung 5–20 s later). However, modelling studies predict (Barstow *et al.*, 1990) and direct experimental measurements confirm (Grassi *et al.*, 1996) that the Phase II pulmonary $\dot{V}O_2$ kinetics provide a close approximation of the kinetics (amplitude and time constant) of increased muscle O_2 consumption following the onset of exercise. If the goal of the analysis of pulmonary $\dot{V}O_2$ kinetics is to provide a non-invasive window on muscle energetics in different circumstances, then it is important that the Phase II component of the pulmonary signal is isolated since inclusion of part of the Phase I response can obscure the results obtained (Whipp *et al.*, 1982). The most appropriate approach for accounting for the Phase I response is debated and is split between those that fit an exponential term to Phase I in order to determine the Phase I–Phase II transition, and those that delete the first ~20 s of data following the onset of exercise to isolate the Phase II response (Chapter 3).

For heavy and severe intensity exercise, an additional exponential term is required for satisfactory fitting of the $\dot{V}O_2$ on-response following the completion of Phase I:

$$\dot{V}O_2\,(t) = \dot{V}O_2(b) + A_p\,(1-e^{-\,(t_p-TD_p)/\tau_p}) + A_s\,(1-e^{-\,(t_s-TD_s/\tau_s})$$

where A_p and A_s are the amplitudes of the $\dot{V}O_2$ primary and slow components, respectively, TD_p and TD_s are the independent time delays before the commencement of the primary and slow components, respectively, and τ_p and τ_s are the time constants for the primary and slow components, respectively. It has been demonstrated that the $\dot{V}O_2$ kinetics in heavy and severe exercise are better fit with two exponential terms than with a single exponential term following the completion of Phase I (Barstow and Mole, 1991). In the case of the latter, the 'residuals' (i.e. the differences between the actual data points and the model fit) show non-Gaussian trends. Interestingly, the data are also better fit when the slow component is assigned its own independent time delay (Barstow *et al.*, 1993). This suggests (but does not prove) that the slow component does not 'commence' at exercise onset and 'appear' later in exercise; rather, the slow component only 'begins' some time following the onset of exercise. The time at which the slow component begins to develop (or, at least, emerges discernibly) depends on the exercise intensity (it begins earlier at higher work rates within the heavy and severe domains) but is normally at ~ 2 min following the onset of exercise (e.g. Barstow *et al.*, 1996; Burnley *et al.*, 2000). It should be noted here that it is presently unclear whether the slow component develops in an exponential or a linear fashion in the heavy and severe domains. Carter *et al.* (1999) reported that the slow component was statistically better described with an exponential instead of a linear function in 26 out of 30 subjects performing treadmill running at 50%Δ. However, it may be equally appropriate to quantify the magnitude of the slow component as the difference in $\dot{V}O_2$ between the asymptotic (i.e. final) amplitude of the primary component and the $\dot{V}O_2$ at the end of exercise, especially as the τ of the slow component should not be used to make mechanistic inferences. The magnitude of the $\dot{V}O_2$ slow component under different conditions has also been quantified as the difference between the $\dot{V}O_2$ at 3 min (the time at which $\dot{V}O_2$ is assumed to have reached the required steady-state value for the work rate) and the $\dot{V}O_2$ at 6 min (i.e. $\Delta\dot{V}O_2$ [6–3]) or at the end of exercise. However, at least in studies with young and/or physically fit subjects, the primary component is essentially complete within ~ 2 min of the onset of exercise and the slow component also emerges at around the same time, such that using $\Delta\dot{V}O_2$ [6–3] will tend to underestimate the true magnitude of the slow component.

The $\dot{V}O_2$ kinetics in recovery from exercise can be analysed in a similar way to those during exercise, with one exception. In analysing recovery kinetics, following Phase I, any slow component term is assigned the same time delay as the primary exponential term. The rationale for this is that the mechanisms responsible for the emergence of the slow component during exercise (e.g. muscle fibre activation, muscle temperature, lactate increase, O_2 cost of ventilation; see later chapters) would be expected to still be present early in the recovery phase from such exercise.

Key controversies in $\dot{V}O_2$ kinetics research

Key controversies in this field of research are addressed in detail in later chapters of this book and are summarized in Chapter 12. However, the following provides a brief introduction to these topics.

Which factor or factors limit the rate at which $\dot{V}O_2$ rises at exercise onset?

In order to avoid a catastrophic fall in intra-cellular [ATP], it is vital that the rate of ATP supply to the contractile elements in the muscle cells is precisely matched to the rate at which ATP is utilized to meet the energy requirements of exercise. The relationship between ATP turnover (the 'input') and cellular oxygen consumption (the 'output'), and the various factors that might interact to regulate this relationship, can be described with the following equation:

$$3 \text{ ADP} + 3 \text{ P}_i + \text{NADH} + \text{H}^+ + \tfrac{1}{2} O_2 \rightarrow 3 \text{ ATP} + \text{NAD}^+ + H_2O$$

The relative importance of the availability of oxidizable substrate (i.e. NADH), the availability of sufficient O_2, and the concentration of reactants associated with ATP hydrolysis (e.g. ADP and P_i) in setting or limiting the $\dot{V}O_2$ kinetics is the source of considerable debate. Putative 'feed-forward' control mechanisms include Ca^{2+}-activated increases in cytosolic ATP hydrolysis, NADH delivery to the electron transport chain (which, it has been argued, might be limited at the level of the pyruvate dehydrogenase complex; Timmons *et al.*, 1996), and the intra-mitochondrial PO_2 (see Tschakovsky and Hughson, 1999, for review). It is also possible that the O_2 available for consumption is limited by competition between nitric oxide and O_2 for the binding site at cytochrome c oxidase, the terminal electron acceptor in the electron transport chain (Kindig *et al.*, 2001; Jones *et al.*, 2003). 'Feedback' mechanisms involved in the control of oxidative phosphorylation include alterations in the concentrations of ATP, ADP, P_i, PCr and Cr. It has been shown both in isolated muscle preparations (Chance *et al.*, 1981) and in exercising humans (Rossiter *et al.*, 1999) that there is a strong reciprocal relationship between changes in high-energy phosphate concentrations and the rise in $\dot{V}O_2$ following the onset of contractions/exercise. Evidence for and against each of these principal metabolic controllers and the potential interaction between feed-forward and feedback respiratory control mechanisms are addressed in detail in Chapters 7–10 and summarized in Chapter 12.

Does the factor or factors that limit the rate at which $\dot{V}O_2$ rises at exercise onset depend upon the exercise intensity domain?

It is feasible that differences in the metabolic and gas exchange responses to exercise within the various exercise intensity domains are the result of differences in the control of, or limitations to, muscle $\dot{V}O_2$. It is unclear whether Phase II pulmonary $\dot{V}O_2$ kinetics evidence linear, first-order behaviour throughout the continuum of 'sub-maximal' exercise. A linear, first-order system obeys the law of superposition; that is, the 'output' (the primary $\dot{V}O_2$ response) can be accurately predicted from the 'input' (the work rate). In terms of $\dot{V}O_2$ kinetics during exercise, this means that the time constant and gain of the primary response should be the same irrespective of whether the work-rate is in the moderate, heavy or severe domain. Linear first-order kinetics (as are observed within the moderate exercise intensity domain) indicate that there is a single rate-limiting step to the speed and amplitude of the $\dot{V}O_2$ adaptation in the transition to a higher metabolic rate; higher-order responses indicate that the control of the response has additional complexity. There is presently no consensus on whether or not the time constant for the Phase II $\dot{V}O_2$ response is unchanged or becomes longer (i.e. the kinetics become slower) for work rates in the heavy/severe domains compared to the moderate domain. Some studies have reported no significant difference while others have reported a significant slowing of the Phase II $\dot{V}O_2$ kinetics at higher work rates (Chapter 12). The majority of studies appear to show a trend for Phase II $\dot{V}O_2$ kinetics to be slower at higher work rates, although this difference has often been non-significant possibly because of small (and heterogeneous) sample sizes and large standard deviations around the mean values. It may also be that the Phase II $\dot{V}O_2$ kinetics are slower at higher exercise intensities in some, but not all, individuals. The law of superposition also predicts that the 'gain' of the primary response will be invariant between moderate and heavy/severe work rates. However, a number of recent studies indicate that this may not always be true (Jones *et al.*, 2002; Pringle *et al.*, 2003; Scheuermann and Barstow, 2003). The presence of slower Phase II $\dot{V}O_2$ kinetics at higher work rates has been interpreted to indicate that O_2 availability becomes (increasingly) limiting (Hughson *et al.*, 2001; Chapter 8 this volume). However, it has recently been considered that the potential for slower Phase II $\dot{V}O_2$ kinetics and for a progressive fall in the primary component gain at higher work rates may be related to the metabolic properties of the muscle fibres recruited to meet the increased force requirement at these higher work rates (Jones *et al.*, 2002; Pringle *et al.*, 2003). Again, these issues are considered in later chapters and summarized in Chapter 12.

What is the physiological mechanism responsible for the development of the
$\dot{V}O_2$ slow component during heavy and severe exercise?

The cause of the reduction in muscle efficiency (as evidenced by the continued rise in $\dot{V}O_2$ beyond ~2–3 min of exercise) during continuous exercise at work rates above the LT is unclear. It has been debated for some time whether the increasing O_2 cost of exercise with time is related to an increasing ATP turnover in the muscle (with a similar ratio of ATP re-synthesized to O_2 molecules consumed; i.e. similar P-to-O ratio), or to an increasing O_2 cost for the same ATP turnover (i.e. reduced P/O ratio). However, recent studies indicate that there is a continued fall in intramuscular [PCr] during the development of the $\dot{V}O_2$ slow component (Rossiter *et al.*, 2002), that high intensity CWR exercise is associated with an increasing energy turnover with time (Bangsbo *et al.*, 2001), and that mitochondrial P/O is not altered by high-intensity exercise (Tonkonogi *et al.*, 1999). These data suggest that at least some, if not all, of the 'excess' $\dot{V}O_2$ represented by the slow component is related to an increased energy demand in the muscles. It has been demonstrated that the source of the majority of the $\dot{V}O_2$ slow component (~ 86%) is the exercising muscles (Poole *et al.*, 1991). This indicates that the additional $\dot{V}O_2$ associated with increasing rates of ventilation and cardiac work with time at higher work rates does not contribute appreciably to the $\dot{V}O_2$ slow component. Although the development of the $\dot{V}O_2$ slow component is associated with a metabolic (lactic) acidosis, neither direct infusion of lactate into exercising dogs (Poole *et al.*, 1994b) nor infusion of adrenaline (which raised blood [lactate]) in humans (Gaesser *et al.*, 1994) alters exercise $\dot{V}O_2$. It is generally considered therefore that factors intrinsic to the muscles themselves, which might include muscle fibre type distribution and motor unit recruitment patterns, are an important mediator of the $\dot{V}O_2$ slow component (Poole, 1994a; Whipp, 1994). It is also interesting to note, however, that experiments designed to alter muscle blood flow and O_2 availability tend to result in changes in the amplitude of the $\dot{V}O_2$ slow component (e.g. Gerbino *et al.*, 1996; Koga *et al.*, 1999). To what extent muscle fibre type distribution (and recruitment patterns) and O_2 availability interact to mediate the slow component is presently unclear. This issue is specifically addressed in Chapter 11 and summarized in Chapter 12.

In summary, it is clear that the scientific discipline of '$\dot{V}O_2$ kinetics' has a long and rich history. However, it is equally clear that research into $\dot{V}O_2$ kinetics is growing rapidly, with new investigators recognizing the crucial role of such research in enhancing our understanding of metabolic control and the limitations to exercise tolerance. There are manifold unanswered questions and there is much work to do! The following chapters provide a comprehensive summary of what we presently know and, perhaps more importantly, what we don't know in this exciting field of study.

Glossary of terms

A	amplitude of a response, for example, of the increase in $\dot{V}O_2$ above baseline
ADP	adenosine diphosphate
ATP	adenosine triphosphate
a-vO$_2$ difference	difference between arterial and mixed venous blood oxygen content
Ca^{2+}	calcium
CaO_2	arterial blood oxygen content
CvO_2	venous blood oxygen content
CO_2	carbon dioxide
CP	critical power
Cr	creatine
CWR	constant work rate
DNA	deoxyribonucleic acid
Δ	'delta', that is difference or change in a value
$\%\Delta$	% difference (in $\dot{V}O_2$) between gas exchange threshold and $\dot{V}O_{2\,max}$
$\Delta\dot{V}O_2$ [6–3]	difference in $\dot{V}O_2$ between 3 min and 6 min of exercise
GET	gas exchange threshold
LT	lactate threshold
MLSS	maximal lactate steady state
NAD	nicotinamide adenine dinucleotide
NADH	nicotinamide adenine dinucleotide reduced
O_2	oxygen
O_2 deficit	difference between energy required for the work rate and energy supplied through oxidative metabolism
PCr	phosphocreatine
P_i	inorganic phosphate
PO_2	partial pressure of oxygen
P-to-O ratio	ratio of ADP rephosphorylated to oxygen consumed
Subscript p	signifies 'primary', for example the primary $\dot{V}O_2$ response
Subscript s	signifies 'slow', for example the $\dot{V}O_2$ slow component
$\dot{Q}$	cardiac output
$\dot{Q}_T$	tissue blood flow
τ	time constant (time taken to reach 63% of the final amplitude in an exponential function)
TD	time delay
t	time

$\dot{V}O_2$	oxygen uptake
$\dot{V}O_{2\ max/peak}$	the maximum $\dot{V}O_2$ attained during for example an incremental exercise test to exhaustion
$\dot{V}CO_2$	carbon dioxide output
[ ]	denotes concentration

References

Adachi, H., Koike, A., Niwa, A., Sato, A., Takamoto, T., Marumo, F. and Hiroe, M. (2000). Percutaneous transluminal coronary angioplasty improves oxygen uptake kinetics during the onset of exercise in patients with coronary artery disease. *Chest*, **118**, 329–35.

Astrand, P.-O. and Rodahl, K. (1986). *Textbook of Work Physiology*, 3rd Edition. McGraw-Hill, New York.

Bangsbo, J., Krustrup, P., Gonzalez-Alonso, J. and Saltin, B. (2001). ATP production and efficiency of human skeletal muscle during intense exercise: effect of previous exercise. *American Journal of Physiology*, **280**, E956–64.

Barstow, T.J. and Mole, P.A. (1991). Linear and nonlinear characteristics of oxygen uptake kinetics during heavy exercise. *Journal of Applied Physiology*, **71**, 2099–106.

Barstow, T.J., Lamarra, N. and Whipp, B.J. (1990). Modulation of muscle and pulmonary O_2 uptakes by circulatory dynamics during exercise. *Journal of Applied Physiology*, **68**, 979–89.

Barstow, T.J., Casaburi, R. and Wasserman, K. (1993). O_2 uptake kinetics and the O_2 deficit as related to exercise intensity and blood lactate. *Journal of Applied Physiology*, **75**, 755–62.

Barstow, T.J., Jones, A.M., Nguyen, P.H. and Casaburi, R. (1996). Influence of muscle fiber type and pedal frequency on oxygen uptake kinetics of heavy exercise. *Journal of Applied Physiology*, **81**, 1642–50.

Barstow, T.J., Jones, A.M., Nguyen, P.H. and Casaburi, R. (2000a). Influence of muscle fibre type and fitness on the oxygen uptake/power output slope during incremental exercise in humans. *Experimental Physiology*, **85**, 109–16.

Barstow, T.J., Scremin, A.M., Mutton, D.L., Kunkel, C.F., Cagle, T.G. and Whipp, B.J. (2000b). Peak and kinetic cardiorespiratory responses during arm and leg exercise in patients with spinal cord injury. *Spinal Cord*, **38**, 340–5.

Bassett, D.R. Jr and Howley, E.T. (2000). Limiting factors for maximum oxygen uptake and determinants of endurance performance. *Medicine and Science in Sports and Exercise*, **32**, 70–84.

Bauer, T.A., Regensteiner, J.G., Brass, E.P. and Hiatt, W.R. (1999). Oxygen uptake kinetics during exercise are slowed in patients with peripheral arterial disease. *Journal of Applied Physiology*, **87**, 809–16.

Beaver, W.L., Lamarra, N. and Wasserman, K. (1981). Related breath-by-breath measurement of true alveolar gas exchange. *Journal of Applied Physiology*, **51**, 1662–75.

Beaver, W.L., Wasserman, K. and Whipp, B.J. (1986). A new method for detecting anaerobic threshold by gas exchange. *Journal of Applied Physiology*, **60**, 2020–7.

Behnke, B.J., Barstow, T.J., McDonough, P., Musch Ti and Poole, D.C. (2002). Dynamics of oxygen uptake following exercise onset in rat skeletal muscle. *Respiration Physiology and Neurobiology*, **133**, 229–39.

Brooks, G.A., Fahey, T.D., White, T.P. and Baldwin, K.M. (2000). *Exercise Physiology: Human Bioenergetics and Its Applications*, 3rd Edition. Mayfield Publishing Co., Mountain View, CA, pp. 10–15.

Burnley, M., Jones, A.M., Carter, H. and Doust, J.H. (2000). Effects of prior heavy exercise on phase II pulmonary oxygen uptake kinetics during heavy exercise. *Journal of Applied Physiology*, **89**, 1387–96.

Carter, H., Jones, A.M. and Doust, J.H. (1999). Linear versus exponential characterisation of the oxygen uptake slow component. *Journal of Physiology*, **521**, P106.

Chance, B., Eleff, S., Leigh, J.S. Jr, Sokolow, D. and Sapega, A. (1981). Mitochondrial regulation of phosphocreatine/inorganic phosphate ratios in exercising human muscle: a gated ^{31}P NMR study. *Proceedings of the National Academy of Science, USA*, **78**, 6714–18.

Connett, R.J., Honig, C.R., Gayeski, T.E. and Brooks, G.A. (1990). Defining hypoxia: a systems view of $\dot{V}O_2$, glycolysis, energetics, and intracellular PO_2. *Journal of Applied Physiology*, **68**, 833–42.

Convertino, V.A., Goldwater, D.J. and Sandler, H. (1984). $\dot{V}O_2$ kinetics of constant-load exercise following bed-rest-induced deconditioning. *Journal of Applied Physiology*, **57**, 1545–50.

Day, J.R., Rossiter, H.B., Coats, E.M., Skasick, A. and Whipp, B.J. (2003). The maximally attainable $\dot{V}O_2$ during exercise in humans: the peak vs. maximum issue. *Journal of Applied Physiology*, **95**, 1901–7.

de Groote, P., Millaire, A., Decoulx, E., Nugue, O., Guimier, P., Ducloux, G. (1996). Kinetics of oxygen consumption during and after exercise in patients with dilated cardiomyopathy. New markers of exercise intolerance with clinical implications. *Journal of the American College of Cardiology*, **28**, 168–75.

Dickerson, R.E. (1978). Chemical evolution and the origin of life. *Scientific American*, **239**, 70–86.

Dickerson, R.E. (1980a). Cytochrome c and the evolution of energy metabolism. *Scientific American*, **242**, 137–53.

Dickerson, R.E. (1980b). *Man's Place in Evolution*. Cambridge University Press, Cambridge.

Geppert, J. and Zuntz, N. (1888). Ueber die Regulation der Athmung. *Pflugers Archives*, **42**, 189–245.

Fukuoka, Y., Endo, M., Kagawa, H., Itoh, M. and Nakanishi, R. (2002). Kinetics and steady-state of $\dot{V}O_2$ responses to arm exercise in trained spinal cord injury humans. *Spinal Cord*, **40**, 631–8.

Gaesser, G.A., Ward, S.A., Baum, V.C. and Whipp, B.J. (1994). Effects of infused epinephrine on slow phase of O_2 uptake kinetics during heavy exercise in humans. *Journal of Applied Physiology*, **77**, 2413–19.

Gerbino, A., Ward, S.A. and Whipp, B.J. (1996). Effects of prior exercise on pulmonary gas-exchange kinetics during high-intensity exercise in humans. *Journal of Applied Physiology*, **80**, 99–107.

Goodfield, G.J. (1960). *The Growth of Scientific Physiology*. Hutchinson, London.

Grassi, B., Poole, D.C., Richardson, R.S., Knight, D.R., Erickson, B.K. and Wagner, P.D. (1996). Muscle O_2 uptake kinetics in humans: implications for metabolic control. *Journal of Applied Physiology*, **80**, 988–98.

Hansen, J.E., Casaburi, R., Cooper, D.M. and Wasserman, K. (1988). Oxygen uptake as related to work rate increment during cycle ergometer exercise. *European Journal of Applied Physiology*, **57**, 140–5.

Henry, F.M. (1951). Aerobic oxygen consumption and alactic debt in muscular work. *Journal of Applied Physiology*, **3**, 427–38.

Hepple, R.T., Liu, P.P., Plyley, M.J. and Goodman, J.M. (1999). Oxygen uptake kinetics during exercise in chronic heart failure: influence of peripheral vascular reserve. *Clinical Science*, **97**, 569–77.

Hill, A.V., Long, C.N.H. and Lupton, H (1924). Muscular exercise, lactic acid, and supply and utilization of oxygen. *Proceedings of the Royal Society (London) Series B*, **97**, 96–137.

Hughson, R.L., Sherrill, D.L. and Swanson, G.D. (1988). Kinetics of $\dot{V}O_2$ with impulse and step exercise in humans. *Journal of Applied Physiology*, **64**, 451–9.

Hughson, R.L., Winter, D.A., Patla, A.E., Swanson, G.D. and Cuervo, L.A. (1990). Investigation of $\dot{V}O_2$ kinetics in humans with pseudorandom binary sequence work rate change. *Journal of Applied Physiology*, **68**, 796–801.

Hughson, R.L., Tschakovsky, M.E. and Houston, M.E. (2001). Regulation of oxygen consumption at the onset of exercise. *Exercise and Sport Science Reviews*, **29**, 129–33.

Inbar, O., Dlin, R., Rotstein, A. and Whipp, B.J. (2001). Physiological responses to incremental exercise in patients with chronic fatigue syndrome. *Medicine and Science in Sports and Exercise*, **33**, 1463–70.

Jones, A.M., Carter, H., Pringle, J.S.M. and Campbell, I.T. (2002). Effect of creatine supplementation on oxygen uptake kinetics during sub-maximal cycle exercise. *Journal of Applied Physiology*, **92**, 2571–7.

Jones, A.M., Wilkerson, D.P., Koppo, K., Wilmshurst, S. and Campbell, I.T. (2003). Inhibition of nitric oxide synthase by L-NAME speeds phase II pulmonary $\dot{V}O_2$ kinetics in the transition to moderate-intensity exercise in man. *Journal of Physiology*, **552**, 265–72.

Kindig, C.A., McDonough, P., Erickson, H.H. and Poole, D.C. (2001). Effect of L-NAME on oxygen uptake kinetics during heavy-intensity exercise in the horse. *Journal of Applied Physiology*, **91**, 891–6.

Koga, S., Shiojiri, T., Shibasaki, M., Kondo, N., Fukuba, Y. and Barstow, T.J. (1999). Kinetics of oxygen uptake during supine and upright heavy exercise. *Journal of Applied Physiology*, **87**, 253–60.

Kusenbach, G., Wieching, R., Barker, M., Hoffmann, U. and Essfeld, D. (1999). Effects of hyperoxia on oxygen uptake kinetics in cystic fibrosis patients as determined by pseudorandom binary sequence exercise. *European Journal of Applied Physiology*, **79**, 192–6.

Lamarra, N. (1990). Variables, constants, and parameters: clarifying the system structure. *Medicine and Science in Sports and Exercise*, **22**, 88–95.

Lim, H.Y., Lee, C.W., Park, S.W., Kim, J.J., Song, J.K., Hong, M.K., Jin, Y.S. and Park, S.J. (1998). Effects of percutaneous balloon mitral valvuloplasty and exercise training on the kinetics of recovery oxygen consumption after exercise in patients with mitral stenosis. *European Heart Journal*, **19**, 1865–71.

Linnarsson, D. (1974). Dynamics of pulmonary gas exchange and heart rate changes at start and end of exercise. *Acta Physiologica Scandinavica*, **415**, 1–68.

Lok, N.S. and Lau, C.P. (1997). Oxygen uptake kinetics and cardiopulmonary performance in lone atrial fibrillation and the effects of sotalol. *Chest*, **111**, 934–40.

MacFarlane, D.J. (2001). Automated metabolic gas analysis systems: a review. *Sports Medicine*, **31**, 841–61.

McManus, A. and Leung, M. (2000). Maximising the clinical use of exercise gaseous exchange testing in children with repaired cyanotic congenital heart defects: the development of an appropriate test strategy. *Sports Medicine*, **29**, 229–44.

Mahler, M. (1980). Kinetics and control of oxygen consumption in skeletal muscle. In P. Cerretelli and B.J. Whipp (Eds) *Exercise Bioenergetics and Gas Exchange*. Elsevier Biomedical Press, Amsterdam, pp. 53–66.

Mallory, L.A., Scheuermann, B.W., Hoelting, B.D., Weiss, M.L., McAllister, R.M. and Barstow, T.J. (2002). Influence of peak $\dot{V}O_2$ and muscle fiber type on the efficiency of moderate exercise. *Medicine and Science in Sports and Exercise*, **34**, 1279–87.

Monod, H. and Scherrer, J. (1965). The work capacity of a synergic muscle group. *Ergonomics*, **8**, 329–38.

Moritani, T., Nagata, A., de Vries, H.A. and Muro, M. (1981). Critical power as a measure of critical work capacity and anaerobic threshold. *Ergonomics*, **24**, 339–50.

Ozyener, F., Rossiter, H.B., Ward, S.A and Whipp, B.J. (2001). Influence of exercise intensity on the on- and off-transient kinetics of pulmonary oxygen uptake in humans. *Journal of Physiology*, **533**, 891–902.

Palange, P., Galassetti, P., Mannix, E.T., Farber, M.O., Manfredi, F., Serra, P. and Carlone, S. (1995). Oxygen effect on O_2 deficit and $\dot{V}O_2$ kinetics during exercise in obstructive pulmonary disease. *Journal of Applied Physiology*, **78**, 2228–34.

Paterson, D.H. and Whipp, B.J. (1991). Asymmetries of oxygen uptake transients at the on- and offset of heavy exercise in humans. *Journal of Physiology*, **443**, 575–86.

Perkins, J.F. (1964). Historical development of respiratory physiology. In H. Rahn and W.O. Fenn (Eds) *Handbook of Physiology. Sect. 3: Respiration*, Vol. 1, American Physiological Society, Washington, DC, pp. 1–62.

Poole, D.C. (1994). Role of exercising muscle in slow component of $\dot{V}O_2$. *Medicine and Science in Sports and Exercise*, **26**, 1335–40.

Poole, D.C., Schaffartzik, W., Knight, D.R., Derion, T., Kennedy, B., Guy, H.J., Prediletto, R. and Wagner, P.D. (1991). Contribution of exercising legs to the slow component of oxygen uptake kinetics in humans. *Journal of Applied Physiology*, **71**, 1245–60.

Poole, D.C., Barstow, T.J., Gaesser, G.A., Willis, W.T. and Whipp, B.J. (1994a). $\dot{V}O_2$ slow component: physiological and functional significance. *Medicine and Science in Sports and Exercise*, **26**, 1354–8.

Poole, D.C., Gladden, L.B., Kurdak, S. and Hogan, M.C. (1994b). L-(+)-lactate infusion into working dog gastrocnemius: no evidence lactate per se mediates $\dot{V}O_2$ slow component. *Journal of Applied Physiology*, **76**, 787–92.

Pringle, J.S.M. and Jones, A.M. (2002). Maximal lactate steady state, critical power and EMG during cycling. *European Journal of Applied Physiology*, **88**, 214–26.

Pringle, J.S.M., Doust, J.H., Carter, H., Tolfrey, K., Campbell, I.T. and Jones, A.M. (2003). Oxygen uptake kinetics during moderate, heavy and severe intensity submaximal exercise in humans: influence of muscle fibre type and capillarisation. *European Journal of Applied Physiology*, **89**, 289–300.

Puente-Maestu, L., Sanz, M.L., Sanz, P., Ruiz de Ona, J.M., Rodriguez-Hermosa, J.L. and Whipp, B.J. (2000). Effects of two types of training on pulmonary and cardiac responses to moderate exercise in patients with COPD. *European Respiratory Journal*, **15**, 1026–32.

Riley, M.S., Porszasz, J., Engelen, M.P., Shapiro, S.M., Brundage, B.H. and Wasserman, K. (2000). Responses to constant work rate bicycle ergometry exercise in primary pulmonary hypertension: the effect of inhaled nitric oxide. *Journal of the American College of Cardiology*, **36**, 547–56.

Rossiter, H.B., Ward, S.A., Doyle, V.L., Howe, F.A., Griffiths, J.R. and Whipp, B.J. (1999). Inferences from pulmonary O_2 uptake with respect to intramuscular [phosphocreatine] kinetics during moderate exercise in humans. *Journal of Physiology*, **518**, 921–32.

Rossiter, H.B., Ward, S.A., Kowalchuk, J.M., Howe, F.A., Griffiths, J.R. and Whipp, B.J. (2002). Dynamic asymmetry of phosphocreatine concentration and O_2 uptake between the on- and off-transients of moderate- and high-intensity exercise in humans. *Journal of Physiology*, **541**, 991–1002.

Scheuermann, B.W. and Barstow, T.J. (2003). O_2 uptake kinetics during exercise at peak O_2 uptake. *Journal of Applied Physiology*, **95**, 2014–22.

Singer, C. (1959). *A Short History of Scientific Ideas to 1900*. Oxford University Press, London.

Smith, C.G. and Jones, A.M. (2001). The relationship between critical velocity, maximal lactate steady-state velocity and lactate turnpoint velocity in runners. *European Journal of Applied Physiology*, **85**, 19–26.

Somfay, A., Porszasz, J., Lee, S.M. and Casaburi, R. (2002). Effect of hyperoxia on gas exchange and lactate kinetics following exercise onset in nonhypoxemic COPD patients. *Chest*, **121**, 393–400.

Stringer, W.W. (2000). Mechanisms of exercise limitation in HIV+ individuals. *Medicine and Science in Sports and Exercise*, **3**, S412–21.

Swanson, G.D. (1990). Assembling control models from pulmonary gas exchange dynamics. *Medicine and Science in Sports and Exercise*, **22**, 80–7.

Timmons, J.A., Poucher, S.M., Constantin-Teodosiu, D., Worrall, V., MacDonald, I.A. and Greenhaff, P.L. (1996). Increased acetyl group availability enhances contractile function of canine skeletal muscle during ischemia. *Journal of Clinical Investigations*, **97**, 879–83.

Tonkonogi, M., Walsh, B., Tiivel, T., Saks, V. and Sahlin, K. (1999). Mitochondrial function in human skeletal muscle is not impaired by high intensity exercise. *Pflugers Archives*, **437**, 562–8.

Tschakovsky, M.E. and Hughson, R.L. (1999). Interaction of factors determining oxygen uptake at the onset of exercise. *Journal of Applied Physiology*, **86**, 1101–13.

Valentine, J.W. (1978). The evolution of multicellular plants and animals. *Scientific American*, **239**, 140–6.

Vidal, G. (1984). The oldest eukaryotic cells. *Scientific American*, **250**, 48–57.

Wagner, P.D. (2000). New ideas on limitation to $\dot{V}O_{2\ max}$. *Exercise and Sport Science Reviews*, **28**, 10–14.

Wasserman, K., Hansen, J.E., Sue, D.Y., Whipp, B.J. and Casaburi, R. (1994). *Principles of Exercise Testing and Interpretation*. Lea & Febiger, Philadelphia.

West, J.B. (1980). Historical development.In *Pulmonary Gas Exchange*, Vol. I. Academic Press, New York, pp. 1–32.

West, J.B. (1996). *Respiratory Physiology: People and Ideas*. Oxford University Press, New York.

Whipp, B.J. (1971). Rate constant for the kinetics of oxygen uptake during light exercise. *Journal of Applied Physiology*, **30**, 261–3.

Whipp, B.J. (1994). The slow component of O_2 uptake kinetics during heavy exercise. *Medicine and Science in Sports and Exercise*, **26**, 1319–26.

Whipp, B.J. and Mahler, M. (1980). Dynamics of pulmonary gas exchange during exercise. In J.B. West (Ed.), *Pulmonary Gas Exchange* (Vol. II) *Organism and Environment*, Academic Press, London, pp. 33–96.

Whipp, B.J. and Wasserman, K. (1972). Oxygen uptake kinetics for various intensities of constant-load work. *Journal of Applied Physiology*, **33**, 351–6.

Whipp, B.J., Ward, S.A., Lamarra, N., Davis, J.A. and Wasserman, K. (1982). Parameters of ventilatory and gas exchange dynamics during exercise. *Journal of Applied Physiology*, **52**, 1506–13.

Whipp, B.J., Rossiter, H.B. and Ward, S.A. (2002). Exertional oxygen uptake kinetics: a stamen of stamina? *Biochemistry Society Transactions*, **30**, 237–47.

Zoladz, J.A., Rademaker, A.C. and Sargeant, A.J. (1995). Non-linear relationship between O_2 uptake and power output at high intensities of exercise in humans. *Journal of Physiology*, **488**, 211–17.

Part II

Theory and practice of measuring $\dot{V}O_2$ kinetics

2 Measuring $\dot{V}O_2$ kinetics

The practicalities

Shunsaku Koga, Tomoyuki Shiojiri and Narihiko Kondo

Introduction

The common perception of $\dot{V}O_2$ kinetics analysis is that it is too complex and difficult to grasp. Consequently, in laboratories around the world a great deal of data has been collected and either incompletely analysed or ignored. This is an almost criminal shame because the dynamic phases of the gas exchange responses at exercise onset are a rich source of information that can provide unique insights into metabolic function and dysfunction. This chapter walks the reader through various analysis techniques for kinetics data from simple identification of some parameters of the $\dot{V}O_2$ response such as t_{50} (time to 50% of the final response) and t_{63} (τ, time to 63% of the final response) to calculation of these parameters using semi-logarithmic analysis. Finally, some of the complex models that require computer-driven least squares iterative techniques are presented. Over the past half-century, data collection techniques have progressed considerably from periodic collection (every 15, 30 or 60 s) and analysis of expired gases in Douglas bags to measurement of breath-to-breath gas exchange. In part, this progress has been facilitated by the development of rapidly responding gas analysers and economical flow meters (pneumotachographs, anemometers, turbines and ultrasonic flow probes) and has forced the development and refinement of efficient gas exchange algorithms that can estimate alveolar gas exchange by accounting for changes in lung gas stores between consecutive breaths (e.g. Auchincloss *et al.*, 1966; Linnarsson, 1974; Wessel *et al.*, 1979; Beaver *et al.*, 1981; Giezendanner *et al.*, 1983; Swanson and Sherrill, 1983; di Prampero and Lafortuna, 1989). Whereas breath-to-breath resolution of the metabolic responses at exercise onset is extremely powerful, it generates unique problems related to the often high variability between breaths that leads sometimes to a low signal-to-noise ratio. In addition, there is the desire to resolve multiple kinetics parameters (i.e. up to three time delays and three time constants) some of which may have a high degree of interdependence. The majority of these issues are dealt with in this chapter which interdigitates closely with Chapter 3.

Measurement of breath-by-breath $\dot{V}O_2$

$\dot{V}O_2$ measured at the mouth

Several methods have been developed for on-line breath-by-breath calculation of $\dot{V}O_2$. From the middle of the 1960s to 1980s, computer algorithms for measuring $\dot{V}O_2$ at the mouth over single respiratory cycles were developed:

(A)   The expiratory flow method as used for calculation of $\dot{V}O_{2E}$, requires measurement of expiratory flow and expired gas fractions and assumes nitrogen (N_2) balance at the mouth (i.e. inspired N_2 volume = expired N_2 volume, open-circuit method) (Beaver *et al.*, 1973) (Figure 2.1). However, due to breath-by-breath changes in lung volumes, the assumption of nitrogen balance is invalid for single respiratory cycles, in particular during the transient state following exercise on- and off-set (Auchincloss *et al.*, 1966; Linnarsson, 1974; Wessel *et al.*, 1979; Beaver *et al.*, 1981; Giezendanner *et al.*, 1983; Swanson and Sherrill, 1983; di Prampero and Lafortuna, 1989).

(B)   Another algorithm for $\dot{V}O_2$ measurement at the mouth ($\dot{V}O_{2M}$) can be calculated as the difference between actually measured volumes of inspired

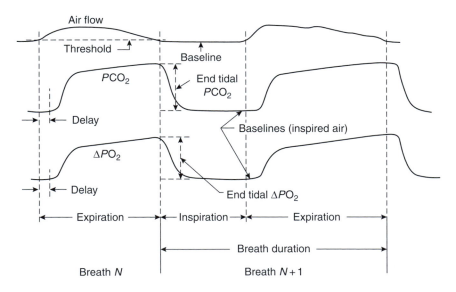

Figure 2.1 Profiles of expiratory flow and expired gas fractions across two consecutive breaths used for calculation of $\dot{V}O_{2E}$ (expiratory flow method). Beginning at the top, expired flow, CO_2 partial pressure (PCO_2), and difference in air and expired O_2 partial pressure (ΔPO_2). The gas concentration signals evidence a time delay with respect to the expired flow signal that arises from the time required to transport the sampled air from the mouthpiece to the sensors. This transit delay and the response time of the gas analysers must be accurately time-aligned with the appropriate instantaneous flow rate. From Beaver *et al.* (1973) with permission.

and expired O_2 ($V_IO_2 - V_EO_2$). However, for single respiratory cycles $V_I - V_E$ is primarily a function of N_2 exchange at the mouth and therefore, $\dot{V}O_{2M}$ is also affected by breath-by-breath changes in lung volumes (e.g. a deep expiration following a shallow inspiration results in negative $\dot{V}O_{2M}$. Interestingly, direct comparisons between $\dot{V}O_{2E}$ and $\dot{V}O_{2M}$ demonstrate that breath-by-breath fluctuation of $\dot{V}O_{2M}$ is larger than that of $\dot{V}O_{2E}$ (Beaver *et al.*, 1981; Giezendanner *et al.*, 1983; Barstow and Mole, 1987).

$\dot{V}O_2$ at the alveolar level

The volume of oxygen exchanged at the mouth during a breath (VO_{2E}, VO_{2M}) is equal to that taken up by pulmonary capillaries (VO_{2A}) only if lung oxygen stores are constant. Auchincloss *et al.* (1966) proposed an algorithm for $\dot{V}O_{2A}$ by correcting VO_{2M} for breath-by-breath changes in alveolar O_2 stores. This alveolar VO_2 method requires measurement of both inspired (I) and expired (E) breath volumes, gas fractions and estimation of changes in alveolar O_2 stores. The O_2 transfer at the alveolar level over a given breath (VO_{2Ai}) is the difference of VO_{2Mi} and the change of the alveolar O_2 store (S) over the same breath (ΔVO_{2Si}):

$$VO_{2Ai} = VO_{2Mi} - \Delta VO_{2Si}$$

$$VO_{2Mi} = V_IO_{2i} - \Delta V_EO_{2i}$$

$$\Delta VO_{2Si} = (F_AO_{2i} - F_AO_{2i-1})V_{Ai-1} + \Delta V_{Ai}F_AO_2$$

$$VO_{2Ai} = \dot{V}O_{2Mi} - (F_AO_{2i} - F_AO_{2i-1})V_{Ai-1} - \Delta V_{Ai}F_AO_{2i}$$

$$\Delta V_{Ai} = [VN_{2Mi} - (F_AN_{2i} - F_AN_{2i-1})V_{Ai-1}]/F_AN_{2i}$$

where V_{Ai-1} is the end-expiratory lung volume before the beginning of the breath i, F_AO_{2i} and F_AO_{2i-1} are the alveolar O_2 fractions in the current (i) and previous ($i - 1$) breath, respectively and ΔV_{Ai} (i.e. $V_{Ai} - V_{Ai-1}$) is the end-expiratory lung volume change over the current breath. Since ΔV_{Ai} can be calculated by assuming a net N_2 transfer across the alveolar–capillary membrane (VN_{2Ai}) equal to zero, the quantity not directly measurable breath-by-breath is V_{Ai-1}.

It has been reported that the estimates of $\dot{V}O_{2A}$ yield the same average value but greatly reduced breath-by-breath variability with respect to $\dot{V}O_2$ measured at the mouth (Auchincloss *et al.*, 1966; Wessel *et al.*, 1979; Beaver *et al.*, 1981; Giezendanner *et al.*, 1983; Swanson and Sherrill, 1983; Barstow and Mole, 1987; di Prampero and Lafortuna, 1989). During metabolic and respiratory transients, these differences often have significant influences on interpretation of the underlying physiology. For example, during Phase I following the onset of constant work-rate exercise, a pronounced difference between $\dot{V}O_{2A}$ and $\dot{V}O_{2E}$ is attributable to changes in alveolar O_2 stores (Beaver *et al.*, 1981) (Figure 2.2). Thus, a $\dot{V}O_{2A}$ algorithm should be adopted to quantify the immediate increase

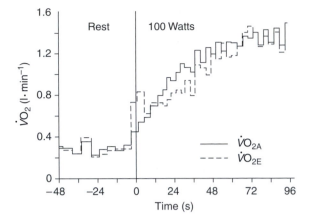

Figure 2.2 Time courses of $\dot{V}O_2$ calculated by the alveolar gas exchange ($\dot{V}O_{2A}$) and
expiratory flow ($\dot{V}O_{2E}$) methods. During Phase I following the onset
of exercise, a pronounced difference between $\dot{V}O_{2A}$ and $\dot{V}O_{2E}$ is attributable to changes in alveolar O_2 stores. From Beaver *et al.* (1981) with
permission.

in $\dot{V}O_2$ during Phase I, which provides an indirect estimate of pulmonary blood
flow (i.e. the cardiodynamic component) (Linnarsson, 1974; Whipp *et al.*, 1982;
Barstow and Mole, 1987; Whipp, 1994). Further, the $\dot{V}O_{2A}$ algorithm has
become a valuable tool for characterization of $\dot{V}O_2$ kinetics into discrete components, the initial- (Phase I), the primary- (Phase II), and the steady state or
slow component following the onset of exercise (Linnarsson, 1974; Hughson
et al., 1988, 2000; Casaburi *et al.*, 1989; Whipp and Ward, 1990; Paterson and
Whipp, 1991; Poole *et al.*, 1991; Barstow *et al.*, 1993, 1996; Engelen *et al.*, 1996;
Gerbino *et al.*, 1996; Grassi *et al.*, 1996; McCreary *et al.*, 1996; Koga *et al.*, 1997,
1999, 2001; MacDonald *et al.*, 1997, 1998, 2000; Scheuermann *et al.*, 1998;
Rossiter *et al.*, 1999, 2002; Özyener *et al.*, 2001) (see Chapters 1 and 6).

Ideal algorithms for breath-by-breath $\dot{V}O_{2A}$ are still being developed. One
pertinent question that must be addressed in this process is 'Why does breath-by-
breath $\dot{V}O_{2A}$ fluctuate even after correction for alveolar O_2 stores?' Possible reasons include key assumptions made for the algorithm. First of all, the
inappropriate assumption of end-expiratory lung volume (V_{Ai-1}) at the beginning of each breath produces fluctuations of breath-by-breath $\dot{V}O_{2A}$. Functional
residual capacity (FRC) at rest is often assumed as V_{Ai-1} (Auchincloss *et al.*,
1966; Beaver *et al.*, 1981; Giezendanner *et al.*, 1983). Several authors have
assigned to the V_{Ai-1} nominal values from zero (Wessel *et al.*, 1979) to the effective lung volume (Swanson and Sherrill, 1983) minimizing the variability in the
breath-by-breath $\dot{V}O_{2A}$. However, di Prampero and Lafortuna (1989)
showed that the $\dot{V}O_{2A}$ kinetics after exercise onset was influenced by the V_{Ai-1}

selected for the calculation and concluded that 'true' alveolar gas exchange remains elusive as long as the V_{Ai-1} cannot be measured for each single breath. In an attempt to circumvent these drawbacks, Grønlund (1984) proposed an alternative algorithm in which the respiratory cycle could be defined as the interval elapsing between two equal expiratory gas fractions in two successive breaths, without requiring any assumption about the V_{Ai-1}. Recently, Cautero *et al.* (2002, 2003) found that the Grønlund algorithm could assess $\dot{V}O_{2A}$ kinetics with a better precision than the widely used Auchincloss algorithm during exercise transients (Figure 2.3). Further, Aliverti *et al.* (2004) reported that opto-electronic plethysmography which measures breath-by-breath changes of absolute V_{Ai-1}, can be used to measure $\dot{V}O_{2A}$ accurately in conditions when V_{Ai-1} changes such as during on- and off-transients.

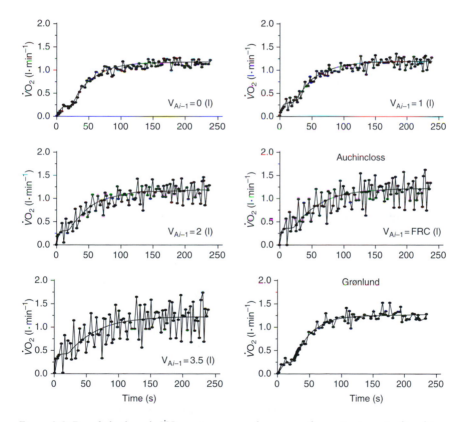

Figure 2.3 Breath-by-breath $\dot{V}O_{2A}$ response at the onset of exercise in a single subject. l is litres. The data were calculated by the algorithm of either Auchincloss *et al.* (1966) using different end-expiratory lung volumes (V_{Ai-1}) or Grønlund (1984). Note that when setting V_{Ai-1} = FRC (functional residual capacity) the Auchincloss algorithm produces larger fluctuations of breath-by-breath $\dot{V}O_{2A}$ compared with that of Grønlund. From Cautero *et al.* (2002) with permission.

Second, it has been argued whether breath-by-breath end-tidal gas fractions recorded at the mouth actually reflect ideal (mean) alveolar gas fractions, since distribution of ventilation/perfusion and/or dead space in the lung influence the true alveolar gas compositions (Swanson and Sherrill, 1983). In addition, the breath-by-breath respiratory pattern, the temporal and spatial variability in intrapleural pressures, and the degree of lung inflation may affect both pulmonary blood flow and blood volume and hence O_2 transfer at the pulmonary capillaries (di Prampero and Lafortuna, 1989). Further analysis and development of techniques for estimating true alveolar gas fractions is required.

Fortunately, except during the Phase I period, the transient responses have been reported to be similar between $\dot{V}O_{2A}$ and $\dot{V}O_{2E}$ (Linnarsson, 1974; Beaver et al., 1981). Therefore, the $\dot{V}O_{2E}$ algorithm is conventionally utilized for commercial gas exchange measurement systems to gain insight into individual components of $\dot{V}O_2$ kinetics beyond Phase I. However, due to the larger breath-by-breath variation in $\dot{V}O_{2E}$ than $\dot{V}O_{2A}$, the number of exercise transitions averaged when using the $\dot{V}O_{2E}$ estimate must be larger than for those using $\dot{V}O_{2A}$ estimates to obtain the required confidence in the kinetic parameters (i.e. time constants, time delays and amplitudes) (see section 'Analysis of breath-by-breath $\dot{V}O_2$ kinetics'). It should be noted here that an estimate of $\dot{V}O_{2A}$ can be obtained with the measurement of $\dot{V}O_{2E}$ and inspired flow (see equation A23 in appendix of Beaver et al., 1981).

A breath-by-breath system measures airflow or volume continuously and simultaneously determines instantaneous gas concentrations. To make accurate measurements, validation of these devices for ventilation (e.g. turbine flow meter and pneumotachograph) and gas concentrations (e.g. mass-spectrometer) is essential. When measuring gas flow rates and expired gas concentrations during exercise as seen in Figure 2.1, flow resistance, linearity, artifact noise, frequency response, and baseline drifts of the flow meter are important considerations. In addition, if a bi-directional flow meter (e.g. turbine, hot-wire anemometer or ultrasonic flow meter) is used to measure both inspiratory and expiratory gas flows, careful calibration and correction must be conducted for gas density and viscosity, temperature and water vapour pressure. For precise measurement of O_2 and CO_2 concentrations, care must be taken to maintain linearity and stability of the gas analysers and to avoid water vapour condensation and pressure change in the gas sampling tube. The gas transport delay time and the response time of the analysers are very important aspects of breath-by-breath gas exchange measurement systems. It is essential that the appropriate instantaneous flow rate and gas concentration are accurately time-aligned (see Figure 2.1). Further, in order to establish validity of the data acquisition software, errors in analog-to-digital sampling (amplitude- and time-quantization), the numerical integration of sample data and signal distortion must be minimized. For more specific details regarding these latter issues, the reader is referred to the following excellent works (e.g. Linnarsson, 1974; Pearce et al., 1977; Beaver et al., 1981; Hughson et al., 1991; Wasserman et al., 1994).

Analysis of breath-by-breath V̇O₂ kinetics

Data processing

Breath-to-breath resolution of the metabolic responses at exercise onset has become a valuable tool for characterization of V̇O₂ kinetics at the on- and off-set of exercise. However, it generates unique problems related to the often high variability between breaths that leads sometimes to a low signal-to-noise ratio (S/N). This has a significant influence on the confidence of the kinetic parameter estimates and their interpretation. This breath-by-breath 'noise' has previously been demonstrated to be an uncorrelated Gaussian stochastic process that is largely independent of metabolic rate (Lamarra et al., 1987; Lamarra, 1990). Lamarra et al. (1987) reported that the 95% confidence limit (Kn) for the estimation of the time constant for moderate exercise can be characterized by the equation,

$$Kn = L \cdot SD / (\Delta \dot{V}O_2 \cdot \sqrt{n})$$

where L is a constant that depends on the value of the underlying time constant and, hence, the amount of data relevant to the estimation, SD is the standard deviation of the breath-to-breath fluctuation in V̇O₂ and $\Delta \dot{V}O_2$ is the V̇O₂ amplitude above baseline level. The n is the number of exercise transitions. Thus, the Kn can be improved by (a) increasing the number of data points throughout the transient region utilized for the time constant estimation (i.e. effectively widening the fitting window of the model) and (b) increasing the S/N ratio, either by lowering SD/$\Delta \dot{V}O_2$ or by increasing n, or both (Lamarra et al., 1987; Lamarra, 1990) (Figure 2.4) (also see section of 'Confidence and

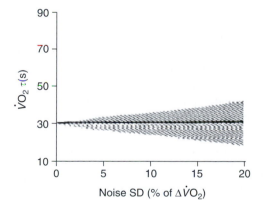

Figure 2.4 The 95% confidence intervals of the Phase II time constant (τ) as a function of the standard deviation (SD) of the breath-to-breath noise in V̇O₂. $\Delta \dot{V}O_2$ is the V̇O₂ amplitude above baseline level. The confidence intervals can be reduced by lowering SD/$\Delta \dot{V}O_2$. From Lamarra et al. (1987) with permission.

parameterization' in Chapter 3). For example, when four repetitions of the exercise test transition are performed, the Kn is reduced to one half of that of a single transition. For cycle exercise in healthy subjects, the number of repetitions normally averaged is four to eight for moderate-intensity (below lactate threshold (LT)) and two to four for heavy-intensity (above LT) exercise. In endurance trained subjects, the number of repetitions may be reduced due to greater values of $\dot{V}O_{2\,max}$ and LT (i.e. larger $\Delta\dot{V}O_2$ compared with sedentary subjects). However, in light of the smaller achievable $\Delta\dot{V}O_2$ response, a greater number of transitions are required to improve the S/N ratio in (a) children, subjects of low fitness, and patients with cardiovascular and pulmonary disease (Lamarra et al., 1987) and (b) small muscle mass exercise, such as plantar flexion or knee extension exercise (McCreary et al., 1996; Rossiter et al., 1999, 2002; Koga et al., 2001, 2004).

The Kn can be improved by the following (see also Table 2.1):

(a) Editing the collected data to eliminate occasional errant breaths arising from coughs, sighs or swallows, which are considered not to be reflective of the underlying kinetics; i.e. aberrant values greater than three or four SDs from the local mean are omitted (Lamarra et al., 1987; Bearden and Moffatt, 2001; Borrani et al., 2001; Özyener et al., 2001; Rossiter et al., 2002) (see section 'Fitting the data or characterizing the response?' in Chapter 3).

(b) Individual responses of breath-by-breath $\dot{V}O_2$ data are often time-interpolated using for example, $1 - $ s intervals (second-by-second values) or bin-averaged (e.g. 5, 15, or 30 s) (Figure 2.5).

(c) To further reduce the breath-by-breath fluctuation and enhance the fidelity of the underlying characteristics, interpolated data are time-aligned and averaged together using a number of repetitions of the same exercise protocol (Figure 2.6). In addition, some studies have utilized smoothing procedures that incorporate a moving average filter.

However, the investigator must be cautious when using the 'time-bin' averaging technique because the longer time-bins (e.g. 5 vs $1 - $ s) reduce the number of data points available for parameter estimation (see the equation for the 95% confidence limit [Kn] described on p. 45), which may compromise the fidelity of the true signals and the confidence of the estimates. Also, smoothing procedures sometimes result in distortion of the Phase I–II inflection points and detection of the slow component onset.

Table 2.1 Summary of techniques for improving confidence in model parameter estimates

- Increasing amount of data points through the transient region
- Lowering the $SD/\Delta\dot{V}O_2$
- Increasing the number of exercise transitions
- Editing of the measured $\dot{V}O_2$ data (elimination of aberrant values)
- Time-interpolation ($1 - $ s intervals or bin-averaged)
- Time aligning and averaging
- Smoothing procedure with moving average filter

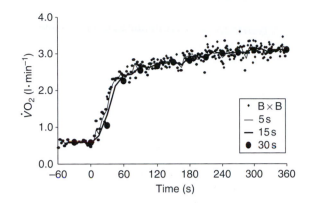

Figure 2.5 Individual responses of breath-by-breath V̇O₂ data (B×B) compared with bin-averaged data (5, 15 and 30 s) during a single heavy exercise transition. Note that the 'time-bin' averaging technique reduces the breath-by-breath fluctuation. However, the longer time-bins reduce the number of data points available for parameter estimation, which may compromise the fidelity of the true signals and the confidence in the derived parameter estimates.

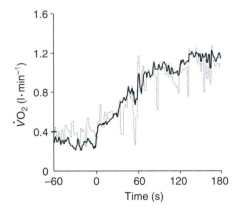

Figure 2.6 Time courses of breath-by-breath V̇O₂ data during a single exercise transition (dotted line) and the averaged 1 − s interpolated data (solid line, four exercise transitions). Note the reduction of the breath-by-breath variation using interpolation, time-aligning and averaging procedures.

The 95% confidence interval (C_{95}) of the parameter estimates can be calculated by commercially available software using the non-linear least-square regression method:

$$C_{95} = SE \cdot t_{dis}$$

where SE is the standard error of the parameter estimates, determined by fitting the response data of V̇O₂ to an exponential model function. The t_{dis} value is obtained from the *t*-distribution using the desired tail dimensions (i.e. 2.5% per tail for the 95% confidence interval). The degrees of freedom in the *t*-distribution table are set at 600, when 1 − s interpolated data are obtained from a 10 min exercise bout (e.g. 4 min of baseline followed by 6 min of constant-load exercise). A small confidence interval implies high confidence in the accuracy of the estimate.

Kinetics analysis techniques and modelling

Overall kinetics

Traditionally, the kinetics of $\dot{V}O_2$ have been determined by visual inspection in terms of the response time to achieve 50% of the change in $\dot{V}O_2$ from baseline to end-exercise (i.e. $t_{1/2}$, the half-time of the response) (Whipp and Wasserman, 1972; Cerretelli and di Prampero, 1987). Further, the mean response time (MRT) or effective time constant has been used, yielding a value that represents the time taken to attain 63% of the overall $\dot{V}O_2$ response (Linnarsson, 1974; Casaburi *et al.*, 1989; Whipp and Ward, 1990; Barstow *et al.*, 1993; Whipp, 1994; Gerbino *et al.*, 1996; Grassi *et al.*, 1996; Scheuermann *et al.*, 1998; Koga *et al.*, 1999, 2001; Rossiter *et al.*, 1999; Bearden and Moffatt, 2001; Burnley *et al.*, 2000; Fukuba *et al.*, 2002; Jones *et al.*, 2004) (Figure 2.7). Semi-logarithmic analysis also has been utilized to identify these kinetic parameters (Whipp and Wasserman, 1972; Whipp and Mahler, 1980; Hughson *et al.*, 2000;) (Figure 2.8). In recent years with the progressive development of computer technology, $\dot{V}O_2$ kinetics are modelled using iterative non-linear least-squares regression techniques in which minimizing the sum of squared error is the criterion for convergence. These computer fits are calculated by fitting the response data of $\dot{V}O_2$ to

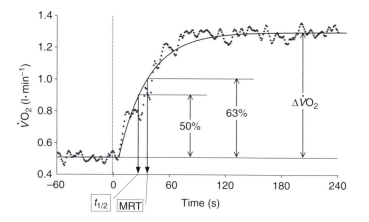

Figure 2.7 Overall kinetics of $\dot{V}O_2$ expressed as half-time ($t_{1/2}$, the response time to achieve 50% of change in $\dot{V}O_2$ between baseline and end-exercise) and the mean response time (MRT, the response time to attain 63% of the overall response from baseline to end-exercise).

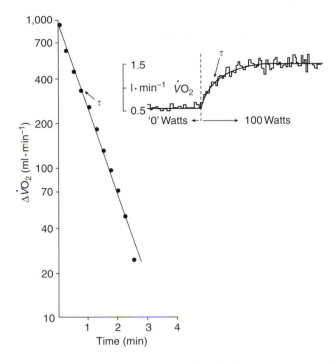

Figure 2.8 Use of semi-logarithmic analysis to identify the time constant (τ) of $\dot{V}O_2$ kinetics following the onset of moderate exercise. Redrawn from Whipp and Mahler (1980).

mono-exponential functions that includes a single amplitude and time constant with (MRT = time delay + time constant) or without a time delay, starting from the onset of the transition. Alternatively, the MRT may be calculated as the weighted sum of the time delay and time constant for each component partitioned by multiple term exponential function (Hughson *et al.*, 1996; MacDonald *et al.*, 1997, 1998, 2000; Perrey *et al.*, 2001).

Kinetics of individual components

Recently, the time course of the $\dot{V}O_2$ response after the onset of exercise has been described in terms of a mono- or multiple-component exponential function. For moderate intensity exercise, the time constant and amplitude of Phase II are obtained by fitting a mono-exponential function to Phase II. In order to infer muscle $\dot{V}O_2$ from pulmonary $\dot{V}O_2$ ($p\dot{V}O_2$), the Phase I (cardiodynamic) response is removed from the kinetics analysis. This serves to time-align the $m\dot{V}O_2$ and $p\dot{V}O_2$ responses as the initial, 'cardiodynamic' phase of the $p\dot{V}O_2$ response does not directly represent active muscle O_2 utilization (Linnarsson, 1974; Whipp *et al.*, 1982; Barstow and Mole, 1987; Barstow *et al.*, 1990; Grassi *et al.*, 1996) (see earlier text in this chapter and Chapter 6). In addition, deletion of Phase I $\dot{V}O_{2E}$ removes concerns related to the disparity between $\dot{V}O_{2A}$ and $\dot{V}O_{2E}$ and the effect of this disparity on the Phase II time constant (see Figure 2.2).

For heavy-intensity exercise, a two- or three-term exponential function that includes amplitudes, time constants and time delays has been adopted to partition $\dot{V}O_2$ kinetics into discrete components (a two-term exponential function is utilized after elimination of Phase I data; Figure 2.9). This is requisite in order to elucidate the mechanism by which the overall kinetics are slowed in heavy-intensity compared with moderate exercise (Barstow *et al.*, 1993, 1996; Engelen *et al.*, 1996; Scheuermann *et al.*, 1998, 2001; Koga *et al.*, 1999, 2001, 2004; Bearden and Moffatt, 2001; Burnley *et al.*, 2000; Carter *et al.*, 2000; MacDonald *et al.*, 2000; Bell *et al.*, 2001; Borrani *et al.*, 2001; Koppo and Bouckaert, 2001; Özyener *et al.*, 2001; Perrey *et al.*, 2001; Fukuba *et al.*, 2002; Rossiter *et al.*, 2002; Pringle *et al.*, 2003; Jones *et al.*, 2004). The three-term exponential function curve fitting procedure is described below.

The first exponential term is initiated at the onset of exercise and the second and third terms begin after independent time delays.

$$\dot{V}O_2(t) = \dot{V}O_2(b) + A_c \cdot (1 - e^{-t/\tau_c}) \quad \text{Phase I (cardiodynamic component)}$$
$$+ A_p \cdot [1 - e^{-(t - TDp)/\tau_p}] \quad \text{Phase II (primary component)}$$
$$+ A_s \cdot [1 - e^{-(t - TDs)/\tau_s}] \quad \text{slow component}$$

where $\dot{V}O_2(b)$ is the unloaded exercise baseline value; A_c, A_p, and A_s are the asymptotic amplitudes for the exponential terms; τ_c, τ_p, and τ_s are the time

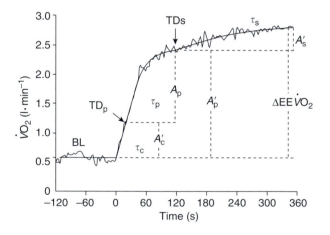

Figure 2.9 Schematic showing three-term exponential model that includes amplitudes, time constants, and time delays to partition $\dot{V}O_2$ kinetics into discrete components for heavy-intensity exercise. Redrawn from Koga *et al.* (1999). Please refer to text for definition of abbreviations. $\Delta EE\dot{V}O_2$, increase above baseline in $\dot{V}O_2$ at end exercise.

constants; and TD_p, and TD_s are the time delays. The Phase I $\dot{V}O_2$ at the start of Phase II (i.e. at TD_p) is assigned the value for that time (A'_c).

$$A'_c = A_c \cdot (1 - e^{-TD_p/\tau_c})$$

The physiologically relevant amplitude of the primary exponential component during Phase II (A'_p) is defined as the sum of $A'_c + A_p$. Because of concerns regarding the validity of using the extrapolated asymptotic value for the slow component (A_s) the value of the slow exponential function at the end of exercise, defined as A'_s is used. For both the responses during Phase I and for the slow component, the best fit to the data by the three-term exponential model sometimes results in unphysiologically large values of the amplitude and/or time constant. Engelen *et al.* (1996) suggested that when this occurred the region being described by the exponential term was best described by a linear function, the slope of which was the derivative of the exponential, A/τ (Casaburi *et al.*, 1989). For this reason, the relevant features of Phase I are the amplitude at the end of Phase I (A'_c) and the duration of Phase I (TD_p). Similarly, the relevant aspects of the slow component are the time of onset (TD_s) and the amplitude at the end of exercise (A'_s).

Since the $\dot{V}O_2$ response during moderate-intensity exercise reaches a new steady-state within 3 min after the onset of exercise in normal subjects, the slow exponential term invariably drops out during the iterative-fitting procedure. In addition, to facilitate comparison across subjects and different absolute work rates, the gain of the primary response ($G = A'_p$/work rate) and relative contribution of the slow component to the overall increase in $\dot{V}O_2$ at end-exercise $[A'_s/(A'_p + A'_s)]$ can be calculated. Further, the increment in $\dot{V}O_2$ between the third and sixth minute of the transition can be calculated as a simple rough estimate of the slow component of the $\dot{V}O_2$ kinetics.

The recovery $\dot{V}O_2$ kinetics (off-transient response) after moderate exercise are analysed by either a one- (omission of Phase I) or two-exponential component model as used for the on-transient response (Linnarsson, 1974; Hughson *et al.*, 1988; Paterson and Whipp, 1991; Engelen *et al.*, 1996; McCreary *et al.*, 1996; MacDonald *et al.*, 1997; Scheuermann *et al*, 1998, 2001; Koga *et al.*, 1999; Carter *et al.*, 2000; Cunningham *et al.*, 2000; Bearden and Moffatt, 2001; Özyener *et al.*, 2001). For the recovery kinetics after heavy exercise, several studies have utilized an exponential model where both the primary and slow exponential terms shared the same time delay (TD), equivalent to the Phase I duration in recovery (Linnarsson, 1974; Paterson and Whipp, 1991; Barstow *et al.*, 1996; Engelen *et al.*, 1996; MacDonald *et al.*, 1997; Koga *et al.*, 1999; Carter *et al.*, 2000; Cunningham *et al.*, 2000; Özyener *et al.*, 2001). However, a three-term exponential function has also been utilized, which contains separate time delays for the fast and slow exponential terms (Scheuermann *et al.*, 1998, 2001; Koga *et al.*, 1999). As described in Chapter 3, the higher-order fitting model, that is increasing the model order, can be justified only when the parameter confidences are superior compared with those of the lower-order fitting model.

The computation of best fit parameters is chosen by a commercially available software program (e.g. KaleidaGraph) so as to minimize the sum of the squared differences between the fitted function and the measured response (e.g. Koga et al., 2001; Özyener et al., 2001; Fukuba et al., 2002; Rossiter et al., 2002) (Figure 2.10). Thus, the curve-fitting procedure is iterated until any further modulation in the parameters does not reduce the mean squared error between the curve drawn from the model and the averaged data set. In addition to the C_{95} of the parameter estimates, two indices have been used to determine the goodness-of-fit: (1) the maintenance of a flat profile of the residual plot (i.e. signifying the lack of a systematic error in the model fit), as judged by visual inspection, and (2) the demonstration of a local 'threshold' in the chi-squared (χ^2) value (i.e. the sum of the squared errors) (Rossiter et al., 1999, 2002).

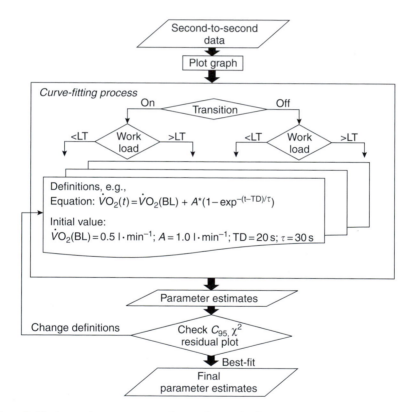

Figure 2.10 A step-by-step process for resolving the kinetic parameter estimates using non-linear least-squares regression curve-fitting techniques. The best-fit procedure is iterated until any further modulation in the parameters does not reduce the mean squared error between the curve drawn from the model and the measured data. The 95% confidence interval (C_{95}) of the parameter estimates, the maintenance of a flat profile of the residual plot, and the chi-squared (χ^2) value are used to determine the goodness-of-fit. Please refer to text for definition of abbreviations.

Measurement of muscle $\dot{V}O_2$ in humans

Muscle $\dot{V}O_2$ ($m\dot{V}O_2$) has been calculated from the Fick principle with measurement of muscle blood flow (MBF) and arteriovenous O_2 content difference (a-vO_2 diff.). To measure $m\dot{V}O_2$ on-kinetics at exercise onset, the time resolution should be adequate to follow non-steady state changes of MBF and a-vO_2 diff. Recently, simultaneous determination of muscle phosphocreatine (PCr) and $\dot{V}O_{2A}$ kinetics during whole body ^{31}P magnetic resonance spectroscopy has been utilized to investigate $m\dot{V}O_2$ kinetics following the onset of exercise (McCreary *et al.*, 1996; Rossiter *et al.*, 1999, 2002). This approach is based on the direct proportionality between the products of PCr splitting and $m\dot{V}O_2$ in animal muscles. Details of the measurement of PCr kinetics in humans are described in Chapter 7.

Muscle blood flow

The MBF kinetics are usually measured by the thermodilution method (Grassi *et al.*, 1996; Bangsbo *et al.*, 2000) or Doppler ultrasound (Shoemaker *et al.*, 1994; Hughson *et al.*, 1996; Rådegran, 1997; MacDonald *et al.*, 1998, 2000). This section describes the non-invasive Doppler ultrasound method for the femoral artery blood flow (LBF) kinetics at onset of knee extension exercise (KE). The LBF is considered to be proportional to the quadriceps MBF under normothermic conditions, assuming that the contribution of the skin blood flow to the LBF is very modest for short duration (e.g. 6 min) constant-load exercise. Further, it has been reported that the blood flow contribution from the lower leg muscles (gastrocnemius and tibialis anterior muscles) is relatively low during KE (Richardson *et al.*, 1993).

The LBF to the exercising muscles is obtained using pulsed and echo ultrasound Doppler to measure mean blood velocity (MBV) and femoral artery diameter from a site distal to the inguinal ligament and above the common femoral artery bifurcation into the superficial and profundus branches. The femoral artery MBV is obtained by using a pulsed-wave Doppler transducer probe with the lowest possible angle of insonation (direction of the transmitted sound-wave beam towards the site of measurement). Adjusting the sample volume width to cover the arterial diameter (Rådegran, 1997) and proper alignment of the ultrasound beam with the artery are required to minimize failure in Doppler insonation due to blood vessel movement during exercise. The audio-range signals for MBV and the ECG signal are sampled with analog-to-digital conversion. The spectrum of the audio-range signals is processed by Doppler signal processing software (Fast Fourier Transfer analysis (FFT)) to yield instantaneous MBV.

The longitudinal B-mode echo images of the femoral artery are recorded on videotape and subsequently analysed for artery diameter with on-screen calipers or visual imaging software. The diameter data are fit with a linear or exponential regression to obtain an average response so as to reduce random error (Hughson *et al.*, 1996; Rådegran, 1997; MacDonald *et al.*, 1998). Thus, mean LBF is calculated on a beat-by-beat basis by multiplying the MBV by the estimated diameter

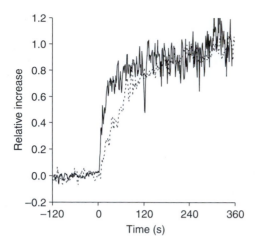

Figure 2.11 The relative increase in femoral artery blood flow (LBF, solid line) and
alveolar O_2 uptake ($\dot{V}O_{2A}$) (dotted line) responses for the transition
from unloaded knee extension exercise (KE) to heavy exercise in a
single subject. Redrawn from Koga *et al.* (2004). Note the far faster
kinetics for LBF compared with $\dot{V}O_{2A}$.

obtained from the regression equation for each time point. (A constant femoral
artery diameter at the onset of upright KE was observed by Shoemaker *et al.*
(1994), Rådegran (1997), MacDonald *et al.* (1998, 2000), and Koga *et al.*
(2004).) An example of LBF and $\dot{V}O_{2A}$ kinetics during the transition to heavy
KE exercise in the upright position is shown in Figure 2.11 (Koga *et al.*, 2004).

Validation of the Doppler ultrasound system for the LBF measurement is
conducted by (a) inputting a known Doppler-shift frequency with electric signals
that mimic the physiological response (validation of the FFT software), (b) *in vitro*
calibration of the ultrasound Doppler system utilizing either animal blood or
blood-mimicking test fluid and (c) simultaneous thermodilution blood flow
measurement (Rådegran, 1997).

a-vO₂ difference

Arterial and femoral venous blood samples during the KE exercise transition are
analysed for PO_2 and haemoglobin concentration and subsequently O_2 saturation and content are obtained using standard equations. (Non-invasive finger
oximetry is often utilized to estimate arterial O_2 saturation.) A constant arterial
O_2 content (CaO_2) has been reported from direct measurements of arterial blood
during KE exercise (Bangsbo *et al.*, 2000; MacDonald *et al.*, 2000), since KE
represents a relatively small cardiovascular challenge that does not compromise
arterial blood oxygenation in the lungs. Thus, a-vO₂ diff. is calculated from the
difference in CaO_2 and femoral venous O_2 content (CvO_2).

Muscle $\dot{V}O_2$

Leg $m\dot{V}O_2$ is calculated from the Fick principle as the product of LBF and a-vO_2 diff. The best fits to LBF responses are obtained by a non-linear least-squares curve-fitting to a one-, two-, or three-exponential function that includes amplitudes and time constants with time delays, starting from the onset of the transition. Values are then obtained from the best-fit regression for blood flow at those time points that correspond to the blood sampling for calculation of $m\dot{V}O_2$ (Hughson et al., 1996; MacDonald et al., 2000). Blood sampling from the femoral vein creates a transit time from capillaries to the venous sampling point. To achieve the most accurate match between LBF and O_2 extraction for the calculation of $m\dot{V}O_2$, correction for the capillary mean transit time is required. Bangsbo et al. (2000) recently found that after correcting for the transit time delay there was a delay of only a few seconds before $m\dot{V}O_2$ increased after the onset of intense KE. However, the presence of any delay in $m\dot{V}O_2$ at the onset of KE is not consistent with the immediate fall in PCr (e.g. Rossiter et al., 1999, 2002) (see Chapters 6 and 12 for a detailed discussion of this issue).

Recently, we characterized the time courses of pulmonary $\dot{V}O_2$ (p$\dot{V}O_2$) and $m\dot{V}O_2$ across the transition from unloaded to heavy KE exercise. The time course of the $m\dot{V}O_2$ was evaluated by the two-component exponential curve-fitting

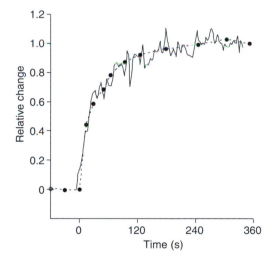

Figure 2.12 The relative changes in pulmonary $\dot{V}O_2$ (p$\dot{V}O_2$, solid line) and muscle $\dot{V}O_2$ (m$\dot{V}O_2$, dotted line) responses for the transition from unloaded knee extension exercise (KE) to heavy exercise in a representative subject. The p$\dot{V}O_2$ was time-aligned by omission of the Phase I p$\dot{V}O_2$ (i.e. Phase aligning of the Phase II p$\dot{V}O_2$ and m$\dot{V}O_2$). Note the close agreement of p$\dot{V}O_2$ and m$\dot{V}O_2$ kinetics for both the primary and the slow component during heavy KE. Redrawn from Koga et al. (2004).

procedure as detailed earlier. The first exponential term (primary component) started with the onset of exercise and the second term (slow component) began after an independent time delay. The time constant for the primary component of $m\dot{V}O_2$ during heavy KE was not significantly different from that of the Phase II $p\dot{V}O_2$. Moreover, the slow component of $p\dot{V}O_2$ evident for the heavy KE reflected the gradual increase in $m\dot{V}O_2$. This result addresses the mechanistic link between $p\dot{V}O_2$ and $m\dot{V}O_2$ kinetics for heavy KE (Figure 2.12; see also Chapter 6).

Conclusions

The dynamic phases of the pulmonary oxygen uptake responses at exercise on- and off-set are a rich source of information that can provide valuable insights into the fundamental mechanisms of metabolic function and dysfunction. This chapter has described algorithms for the determination of $\dot{V}O_2$ at the mouth- and alveolar-level, various analysis techniques for kinetics data, and measurement of muscle $\dot{V}O_2$ in humans. Since breath-by-breath variation of pulmonary $\dot{V}O_2$ often has a significant influence on interpretation of the underlying physiology during exercise transients, the number of exercise transition tests should be determined logically using the algorithms of $\dot{V}O_{2A}$ or the $\dot{V}O_{2E}$ (with omission of Phase I). Further, to obtain the required confidence in the kinetic parameters, adequate processing of the measured data, that is increasing the S/N ratio, editing, time-interpolation as well as time-aligning and averaging are requisite. In order to elucidate underlying mechanisms during exercise transients, precise characterization of $\dot{V}O_2$ kinetics into discrete components is necessary using efficient computerized curve-fitting techniques. Finally, measurement of muscle $\dot{V}O_2$ kinetics in humans provides useful information regarding the mechanistic link between pulmonary and muscle $\dot{V}O_2$ kinetics during exercise transients.

Glossary of terms

a-vO$_2$ diff.	arteriovenous O_2 content difference
C_{95}	95% confidence interval, a range of values for a parameter estimate which have 95% probability of containing the true value of the parameter
CaO_2, CvO_2	arterial and venous blood O_2 contents
E	expired
F	fractional concentration (e.g. F_AO_2 signifies fractional alveolar O_2 concentration)
FFT	fast Fourier transfer analysis
FRC	functional residual capacity
I	inspired
i	designates a given breath. $i - 1$ is the previous breath
KE	knee extension exercise

Kn	confidence limit (e.g. 95%)
L	a constant determined by the underlying kinetic parameter and therefore the quantity of data used to estimate the parameter
LBF	leg blood flow
LT	lactate threshold
MBF	muscle blood flow
MBV	mean blood velocity
MRT	mean response time, that is the time taken to achieve 63% of the difference between baseline and final value
n	number (e.g. of exercise transitions)
Parameter	a constant that characterizes the order of a system, for example, time constant
PCO_2	partial pressure of carbon dioxide
PCr	phosphocreatine
Phase I	initial increase in $\dot{V}O_2$ at exercise onset caused by elevated pulmonary blood flow (also called the cardiodynamic phase)
Phase II	the exponential increase in $\dot{V}O_2$ that is initiated when venous blood from the exercising muscles arrives at the lungs. Corresponds closely with muscle $\dot{V}O_2$ dynamics as demonstrated in this chapter.
Phase III	the steady-state phase of $\dot{V}O_2$ during moderate exercise
PO_2	partial pressure of O_2; ΔPO_2, change in PO_2
Residual	the difference between the measured and modelled response
SD	standard deviation
SE	standard error
S/N	signal-to-noise ratio
τ or tau	denotes time to 63% of final response
$t_{1/2}$	half-time of the response, that is time taken for the variable of interest, $\dot{V}O_2$, to achieve 50% of the difference between baseline and final value
t_{dis}	value obtained from the *t*-distribution for the derived tail dimensions and relevant degrees of freedom
V_{Ai}	end-expiratory lung (alveolar) volume before the beginning of breath, *i*
$\dot{V}O_2$	oxygen uptake
$p\dot{V}O_2$	pulmonary $\dot{V}O_2$ (may be expressed as $\dot{V}O_{2A}$ or $\dot{V}O_{2E}$ depending on individual study)
$m\dot{V}O_2$	muscle $\dot{V}O_2$
$\dot{V}O_{2A}$	calculated alveolar $\dot{V}O_2$ which approximates that occurring across the pulmonary capillaries
$\dot{V}O_{2E}$	$\dot{V}O_2$ measured from expired flow and gas analysis (assumes N_2 balance, that is inspired volume of N_2 = that expired)
$\dot{V}O_{2M}$	$\dot{V}O_2$ measured at the mouth from the difference between volumes of inspired and expired O_2 [$V_IO_2 - V_EO_2$]
$\Delta\dot{V}O_{2S}$	changes in alveolar O_2 store
$\Delta\dot{V}O_2$	$\dot{V}O_2$ amplitude above baseline

References

Aliverti, A., Kayser, B. and Macklem, P.T. (2004). Breath-by-breath assessment of alveolar gas stores and exchange. *Journal of Applied Physiology*, **96**(4), 1464–9.

Auchincloss, J.R., Gilbert, R. and Baule, G.H. (1966). Effect of ventilation on oxygen transfer during early exercise. *Journal of Applied Physiology*, **21**, 810–8.

Bangsbo, J., Krustrup, P., Gonzalez-Alonso, J., Boushel, R. and Saltin, B. (2000). Muscle oxygen kinetics at onset of intense dynamic exercise in humans. *American Journal of Physiology*, **279**, R899–906.

Barstow, T.J. and Mole, P.A. (1987). Simulation of pulmonary O_2 uptake during exercise transients in humans. *Journal of Applied Physiology*, **63**, 2253–61.

Barstow, T.J., Lamarra, N. and Whipp, B.J. (1990). Modulation of muscle and pulmonary O_2 uptakes by circulatory dynamics during exercise. *Journal of Applied Physiology*, **68**, 979–89.

Barstow, T.J., Casaburi, R. and Wasserman, K. (1993). O_2 uptake kinetics and the O_2 deficit as related to exercise intensity and blood lactate. *Journal of Applied Physiology*, **75**, 755–62.

Barstow, T.J., Jones, A.M., Nguyen P.H. and Casaburi, R. (1996). Influence of muscle fiber type and pedal frequency on oxygen uptake kinetics of heavy exercise. *Journal of Applied Physiology*, **81**, 1642–50.

Bearden, S.E. and Moffatt, R.J. (2001). $\dot{V}O_2$ and heart rate kinetics in cycling: transitions from an elevated baseline. *Journal of Applied Physiology*, **90**, 2081–7.

Beaver, W.L., Wasserman K. and Whipp, B.J. (1973). On-line computer analysis and breath-by-breath graphical display of exercise function tests. *Journal of Applied Physiology*, **34**, 128–32.

Beaver, W.L., Lamarra, N. and Wasserman, K. (1981). Breath-by-breath measurement of true alveolar gas exchange. *Journal of Applied Physiology*, **51**, 1662–75.

Bell, C., Paterson, D.H., Kowalchuk, J.M., Padilla, J. and Cunningham, D.A. (2001). A comparison of modelling techniques used to characterise oxygen uptake kinetics during the on-transient of exercise. *Experimental Physiology*, **36**, 667–76.

Borrani, F., Candau, R., Millet, G.Y., Perrey, S., Fuchslocher, J. and Rouillon, J.D. (2001). Is the $\dot{V}O_2$ slow component dependent on progressive recruitment of fast-twitch fibers in trained runners? *Journal of Applied Physiology*, **90**, 2212–20.

Burnley, M., Jones, A.M., Carter H. and Doust, J.H. (2000). Effects of prior heavy exercise on phase II pulmonary oxygen uptake kinetics during heavy exercise. *Journal of Applied Physiology*, **89**, 1387–96.

Carter, H., Jones, A.M., Barstow, T.J., Burnley, M., Williams, C.A. and Doust, J.H. (2000). Oxygen uptake kinetics in treadmill running and cycle ergometry: a comparison. *Journal of Applied Physiology*, **89**, 899–907.

Casaburi, R., Barstow, T.J., Robinson, T. and Wasserman, K. (1989). Influence of work rate on ventilatory and gas exchange kinetics. *Journal of Applied Physiology*, **67**, 547–55.

Cautero, M., Beltrami, P., di Prampero, P.E. and Capelli, C. (2002). Breath-by-breath alveolar oxygen transfer at the onset of step exercise in humans: methodological implications. *European Journal of Applied Physiology*, **88**, 203–13.

Cautero, M., di Prampero, P.E. and Capelli, C. (2003). New acquisitions in the assessment of breath-by-breath alveolar gas transfer in humans. *European Journal of Applied Physiology*, **90**, 231–41.

Cerretelli, P. and di Prampero, P.E. (1987). Gas exchange in exercise. In *Handbook of Physiology. The Respiratory System Gas Exchange*, Section 3, Vol. IV, American Physiological Society, Bethesda, MD, pp. 297–339.

Cunningham, D.A., Croix, C.M., Paterson, D.H., Özyener, F. and Whipp, B.J. (2000). The off-transient pulmonary oxygen uptake ($\dot{V}O_2$) kinetics following attainment of a particular $\dot{V}O_2$ during heavy-intensity exercise in humans. *Experimental Physiology*, **85**, 339–47.

di Prampero, P.E. and Lafortuna, C.L. (1989). Breath-by-breath estimate of alveolar gas transfer variability in man at rest and during exercise. *Journal of Physiology*, **415**, 459–75.

Engelen, M., Porszasz, J., Riley, M., Wasserman, K., Maehara K. and Barstow, T.J. (1996). Effects of hypoxic hypoxia on O_2 uptake and heart rate kinetics during heavy exercise. *Journal of Applied Physiology*, **81**, 2500–8.

Fukuba, Y., Hayashi, N., Koga, S. and Yoshida, T. (2002). $\dot{V}O_2$ kinetics in heavy exercise is not altered by prior exercise with a different muscle group. *Journal of Applied Physiology*, **92**, 2467–74.

Gerbino, A., Ward, S.A. and Whipp, B.J. (1996). Effects of prior exercise on pulmonary gas-exchange kinetics during high-intensity exercise in humans. *Journal of Applied Physiology*, **80**, 99–107.

Giezendanner, D., Cerretelli, P. and di Prampero, P.E. (1983). Breath-by-breath alveolar gas exchange. *Journal of Applied Physiology*, **55**, 583–90.

Grassi, B., Poole, D.C., Richardson, R.S., Knight, D.R., Erickson, B.K. and Wagner, P.D. (1996). Muscle O_2 uptake kinetics in humans: implications for metabolic control. *Journal of Applied Physiology*, **80**, 988–98.

Grønlund, J. (1984). A new method for breath-to-breath determination of oxygen flux across the alveolar membrane. *European Journal of Applied Physiology*, **52**, 167–72.

Hughson, R.L., Sherrill, D.L. and Swanson, G.D. (1988). Kinetics of $\dot{V}O_2$ with impulse and step exercise in humans. *Journal of Applied Physiology*, **64**, 451–9.

Hughson, R.L., Northey, D.R., Xing, H.C., Dietrich, B.H. and Cochrane, J.E. (1991). Alignment of ventilation and gas fraction for breath-by-breath respiratory gas exchange calculations in exercise. *Computational Biomedical Research*, **24**, 118–28.

Hughson, R.L., Shoemaker, J.K., Tschakovsky, M.E. and Kowalchuk, J.M. (1996). Dependence of muscle $\dot{V}O_2$ blood flow dynamics at onset of forearm exercise. *Journal of Applied Physiology*, **81**, 1619–26.

Hughson, R.L., O'Leary, D.D., Betik, A.C. and Hebestreit, H. (2000). Kinetics of oxygen uptake at the onset of exercise near or above peak oxygen uptake. *Journal of Applied Physiology*, **88**, 1812–19.

Jones, A.M., Wilkerson, D.P., Wilmshurst, S. and Campbell, I.T. (2004). Influence of L-NAME on pulmonary O_2 uptake kinetics during heavy-intensity cycle exercise. *Journal of Applied Physiology*, **96**, 1033–8.

Koga, S., Shiojiri, T., Kondo, N. and Barstow, T.J. (1997). Effect of increased muscle temperature on oxygen uptake kinetics during exercise. *Journal of Applied Physiology*, **83**, 1333–8.

Koga, S., Shiojiri, T., Shibasaki, M., Kondo, N., Fukuba, Y. and Barstow, T.J. (1999). Kinetics of oxygen uptake during supine and upright heavy exercise. *Journal of Applied Physiology*, **87**, 253–60.

Koga, S., Barstow, T.J., Shiojiri, T., Takaishi, T., Fukuba, Y., Kondo, N., Shibasaki, M. and Poole, D.C. (2001). Effect of muscle mass on $\dot{V}O_2$ kinetics at the onset of work. *Journal of Applied Physiology*, **90**, 461–8.

Koga, S., Poole, D.C., Shiojiri, T., Konda, N., Fukuba, Y., Miura, A. and Bartstow, T.J. (2004). A comparison of oxygen uptake kinetics during knee extension and cycle exercise. *American Journal of Physiology-Regulatory, Integrative and Comparative Physiology* (in press).

Koppo, K. and Bouckaert, J. (2001). The effect of prior high-intensity cycling exercise on the $\dot{V}O_2$ kinetics during high-intensity cycling exercise is situated at the additional slow component. *International Journal of Sports Medicine*, **22**, 21–6.

Lamarra, N. (1990). Variables, constants, and parameters: clarifying the system structure, *Medicine and Science in Sports and Exercise*, **22**, 88–95.

Lamarra, N., Whipp, B.J., Ward, S.A. and Wasserman, K. (1987). Effect of interbreath fluctuations on characterizing exercise gas exchange kinetics. *Journal of Applied Physiology*, **62**, 2003–12.

Linnarsson, D. (1974). Dynamics of pulmonary gas exchange and heart rate changes at start and end of exercise. *Acta Physiologica Scandinavica*, **415**, 1–68.

McCreary, C.R., Chilibeck, P.D., Marsh, G.D., Paterson, D.H., Cunningham, D.A. and Thompson, R.T. (1996). Kinetics of pulmonary oxygen uptake and muscle phosphates during moderate-intensity calf exercise. *Journal of Applied Physiology*, **81**, 1331–8.

MacDonald, M., Pedersen, P.K. and Hughson, R.L. (1997). Acceleration of $\dot{V}O_2$ kinetics in heavy submaximal exercise by hyperoxia and prior high-intensity exercise. *Journal of Applied Physiology*, **83**, 1318–25.

MacDonald, M.J., Shoemaker, J.K., Tschakovsky, M.E. and Hughson, R.L. (1998). Alveolar oxygen uptake and femoral artery blood flow dynamics in upright and supine leg exercise in humans. *Journal of Applied Physiology*, **85**, 1622–8.

MacDonald, M.J., Tarnopolsky, M.A. and Hughson, R.L. (2000). Effect of hyperoxia and hypoxia on leg blood flow and pulmonary and leg oxygen uptake at the onset of kicking exercise. *Canadian Journal of Physiology and Pharmacology*, **78**, 67–74.

Özyener, F., Rossiter, H.B., Ward, S.A. and Whipp, B.J. (2001). Influence of exercise intensity on the on- and off-transient kinetics of pulmonary oxygen uptake in humans. *Journal of Physiology*, **533**, 891–902.

Paterson, D.H. and Whipp, B.J. (1991). Asymmetries of oxygen uptake transients at the on- and offset of heavy exercise in humans. *Journal of Physiology*, **443**, 575–86.

Pearce, D.H., Milhorn, H.T., Holloman, G.H. and Reynolds, W.J. (1977). Computer-based system for analysis of respiratory responses to exercise. *Journal of Applied Physiology*, **42**, 968–75.

Perrey, S., Betik, A., Candau, R., Rouillon, J.D. and Hughson, R.L. (2001). Comparison of oxygen uptake kinetics during concentric and eccentric cycle exercise. *Journal of Applied Physiology*, **91**, 2135–42.

Poole, D.C., Schaffartzik, W., Knight, D.R., Derion, T., Kennedy, B., Guy, H.J., Prediletto, R. and Wagner, P.D. (1991). Contribution of exercising legs to the slow component of oxygen uptake kinetics in humans. *Journal of Applied Physiology*, **71**, 1245–53.

Pringle, J.S.M., Doust, J.H., Carter, H., Tolfrey, K. and Jones, A.M. (2003). Effect of pedal rate on primary and slow-component oxygen uptake responses during heavy-cycle exercise. *Journal of Applied Physiology*, **94**, 1501–7.

Rådegran, G. (1997). Ultrasound Doppler estimates of femoral artery blood flow during dynamic knee extensor exercise in humans. *Journal of Applied Physiology*, **83**, 1383–8.

Richardson, R.S., Poole, D.C., Knight, D.R., Kurdak, S.S., Hogan, M.C., Grassi, B., Johnson, E.C., Kendrick, K.F., Erickson, B.K. and Wagner, P.D. (1993). High muscle blood flow in man: is maximal O_2 extraction compromised? *Journal of Applied Physiology*, **75**, 1911–16.

Rossiter, H.B., Ward, S.A., Doyle, V.L., Howe, F.A., Griffiths, J.R. and Whipp, B.J. (1999). Inferences from pulmonary O_2 uptake with respect to intramuscular phosphocreatine kinetics during moderate exercise in humans. *Journal of Physiology*, **518**, 921–32.

Rossiter, H.B., Ward, S.A., Kowalchuk, J.M., Howe, F.A., Griffiths, J.R. and Whipp, B.J. (2002). Dynamic asymmetry of phosphocreatine concentration and O_2 uptake between the on- and off-transients of moderate- and high-intensity exercise in humans. *Journal of Physiology*, **541**, 991–1002.

Scheuermann, B.W., Kowalchuk, J.M., Paterson, D.H. and Cunningham, D.A. (1998). O_2 uptake kinetics after acetazolamide administration during moderate- and heavy-intensity exercise. *Journal of Applied Physiology*, **85**, 1384–93.

Scheuermann, B.W., Hoelting, B.D., Noble, M.L. and Barstow, T.J. (2001). The slow component of O_2 uptake is not accompanied by changes in muscle EMG during repeated bouts of heavy exercise in humans. *Journal of Physiology*, **531**, 245–56.

Shoemaker, J.K., Hodge, L. and Hughson, R.L. (1994). Cardiorespiratory kinetics and femoral artery blood velocity during dynamic knee extension exercise. *Journal of Applied Physiology*, **77**, 2625–32.

Swanson, G.D. and Sherrill, D.L. (1983). A model evaluation of estimates of breath-to-breath alveolar gas exchange. *Journal of Applied Physiology*, **55**, 1936–41.

Wasserman, K., Hansen, J.E., Sue, D.Y., Whipp, B.J. and Casaburi, R. (1994). 'Devices and systems for collecting and analyzing physiologic data' and 'Calculations, formulae, and examples', Appendix C and D. In *Principles of Exercise Testing and Interpretation*, 2nd edition, Williams & Wilkins, Media, PA, pp. 440–464.

Wessel, H.U., Stout, R.L., Bastanier, C.K. and Paul, M.H. (1979). Breath-by-breath variation of FRC: effect on $\dot{V}O_2$ and $\dot{V}CO_2$ measured at the mouth. *Journal of Applied Physiology*, **46**, 1122–6.

Whipp, B.J. (1994). The slow component of O_2 uptake kinetics during heavy exercise. *Medicine and Science in Sports and Exercise*, **26**, 1319–26.

Whipp, B.J. and Mahler, M. (1980). Dynamics of pulmonary gas exchange during exercise. In J.B. West (ed.) *Pulmonary Gas Exchange*, vol. II, *Organism and Environment*. Academic Press, New York, pp. 33–96.

Whipp, B.J. and Ward, S.A. (1990). Physiological determinants of pulmonary gas exchange kinetics during exercise. *Medicine and Science in Sports and Exercise*, **22**, 62–71.

Whipp, B.J. and Wasserman, K. (1972). Oxygen uptake kinetics for various intensities of constant-load work. *Journal of Applied Physiology*, **33**, 351–6.

Whipp, B.J., Ward, S.A., Lamarra, N., Davis, J.A. and Wasserman, K. (1982). Parameters of ventilatory and gas exchange dynamics during exercise. *Journal of Applied Physiology*, **52**, 1506–13.

3 The kinetics of oxygen uptake
Physiological inferences from the parameters

Brian J. Whipp and Harry B. Rossiter

Introduction

One of the major features of an effectively functioning physiological system is its ability to respond to a particular stressor with rapid response characteristics. For example, during muscular exercise the greater the aerobic contribution to the energy transformations that fuel the muscular contraction the less is the reliance on anaerobic mechanisms – which are major contributors to the fatigue process (e.g. Hepple, 2002; Westerblad *et al.*, 2002 for review). A rapid dynamic response profile of O_2 uptake is, consequently, a characteristic feature of subjects manifesting high exercise tolerance (e.g. Hagberg *et al.*, 1980; Powers *et al.*, 1985; Whipp *et al.*, 2001). In order to understand the mechanisms controlling O_2 uptake at the lung ($\dot{V}O_2$), the O_2 consumption in the skeletal muscle ($m\dot{V}O_2$), and the factors that can dissociate them, it is naturally important to establish a precise characterization of the time course in order to draw justifiable control inferences. $m\dot{V}O_2$, for example, is known to be controlled by enzymatic processes linked to high-energy phosphate turnover in the muscle: hence the 'expected' response profile is exponential (e.g. Chance *et al.*, 1955; Owen and Wilson, 1974; Holian *et al.*, 1977; Bessman and Geiger, 1981; Mahler, 1985; Saks *et al.*, 2001; and see Wilson, 1994 for review). And so the attention given to exponential analysis is not that it is simply a convenient fitting strategy – there are other models that would give a more or less adequate fit to the data – it is that the exponential provides the potential for establishing justifiable physiological equivalents of the response parameters. An understanding of the basic features of the exponential is therefore essential to making physiological inferences from exercise transients.

Basic features of the exponential

An exponential may be considered to be any process whose instantaneous rate of change is proportional to 'how far' it currently is from its target. This is true whether the target value, at that time, is constant as for a step change of demand or one that is changing as a ramp or sinusoid, for example. A mechanical example for a step change of demand is, perhaps, easiest to conceptualize. Consider that having inhaled (through inspiratory muscle action) to some lung volume

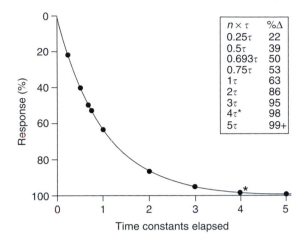

$n \times \tau$	%Δ
0.25τ	22
0.5τ	39
0.693τ	50
0.75τ	53
1τ	63
2τ	86
3τ	95
$4\tau^*$	98
5τ	99+

Figure 3.1 Schematic representation of the time course of an exponential process that is a function whose instantaneous rate of change is proportional to 'how far' it currently is from its 'target'. The time course can be characterized by the time constant (τ). After 1τ has elapsed the response will have attained 63% of its final value. The inset shows the percentage of the final value attained after $n\tau$ has elapsed.

above functional residual capacity (FRC – the lung volume that is attained when the respiratory muscles are not active) you then allow all the respiratory muscles to relax. The thorax will recoil back to the FRC at a rate that is initially high and which then progressively decreases (as a function of time) as the volume approaches FRC. Consequently, the lung (or thoracic) volume will decrease exponentially throughout the exhalation as shown in Figure 3.1.

Therefore, as for any physiological variable (y) which decreases as a function of time (t) with these characteristics, its rate of change is described by

$$-\frac{dy}{dt} = k \cdot y_{(t)} \tag{3.1}$$

where k is the proportionality constant or, more commonly, simply the rate constant, that is

$$\frac{dy}{dt} = -k \cdot y_{(t)} \tag{3.2}$$

But the exponential change can also be characterized by its time constant (τ), this is simply the inverse of the rate constant, that is as $\tau = 1/k$, then

$$\tau \cdot \frac{dy}{dt} = -y_{(t)} \tag{3.3}$$

One might ask, for example, how far will the exponential process have proceeded in one τ? To establish this it is necessary to make use of the more general mathematical formulation (derived in the Appendix) of the time course of such an exponential process:

$$y_{(t)} = y_{ss} \cdot e^{-t/\tau} \tag{3.4}$$

where e is the base for the natural logarithm and y_{ss} is the 'steady-state' or asymptotic amplitude of the response.

Note that after one time constant has elapsed, that is when $t = \tau$ then

$$\frac{y_{(t)}}{y_{ss}} = e^{-1} \tag{3.5}$$

which has a value of 0.37.

Therefore, in $1 \cdot \tau$ the exponential will have progressed to within 37% of its steady-state requirement – alternatively the process will have changed by 63% of the steady-state value. After the next τ it will have changed by another 63% of the remaining 37% and so on for each successively elapsed τ. The inset in Figure 3.1 shows the proportion of the steady-state change that is attained at various time constants of response.

Note that at the half-time ($t_{1/2}$) of the response, at which time $y_{(t)}/y_{ss} = 0.5$, then $0.693 \cdot \tau$ will have elapsed. This means that a very simple relationship exists between τ and the $t_{1/2}$

$$\tau = 1.44 \cdot t_{1/2} \tag{3.6}$$

or, for 'broad brush' purposes (although not where accurate quantification is needed) the time constant is roughly 1.5 times the half time.

Similarly if, instead of progressively decreasing as in the example of the spontaneous recoil of the lung, the function increases towards some higher steady-state value (y_{ss}) with these characteristics (such as $m\dot{V}O_2$ in response to step increase in work rate, for example Grassi et al., 1996 and 1998; Bangsbo et al., 2000) as shown in Figure 3.2A then,

$$\frac{dy}{dt} = k \cdot (y_{ss} - y_{(t)}) \tag{3.7}$$

And so,

$$\tau \cdot \frac{dy}{dt} = y_{ss} - y_{(t)} \tag{3.8}$$

for the increasing phase of the response. However, note that (as shown in Figure 3.2A) at the beginning of the response (i.e. $y_{(t)} = 0$) that

$$\tau \cdot \frac{dy}{dt} = y_{ss} \tag{3.9}$$

This means that the tangent to the exponential response at $t = 0$ meets the required steady-state value at a time corresponding precisely to one time constant.

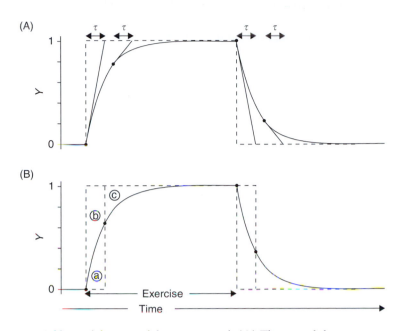

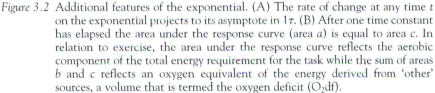

Figure 3.2 Additional features of the exponential. (A) The rate of change at any time *t* on the exponential projects to its asymptote in 1τ. (B) After one time constant has elapsed the area under the response curve (area *a*) is equal to area *c*. In relation to exercise, the area under the response curve reflects the aerobic component of the total energy requirement for the task while the sum of areas *b* and *c* reflects an oxygen equivalent of the energy derived from 'other' sources, a volume that is termed the oxygen deficit (O_2df).

However, as this exponential has the same characteristics throughout its time course, one could arbitrarily consider any point on the exponential to serve as $t = 0$ for the purpose of consideration. That is, the tangent (or the instantaneous rate of change at any such point) reaches the steady state in one time constant. Naturally, these same features apply at the off-transient (Figure 3.2A).

For the example of $m\dot{V}O_2$, the area under the response curve in Figure 3.2A reflects the aerobic component of the total energy requirement for the task. The area bounded by this curve and the dashed lines (i.e. the back-extrapolation of the steady-state $\dot{V}O_2$ to $t = 0$) reflects the oxygen equivalent of the energy derived from 'other' sources – although *presumably reflects* would be more accurate as it depends on the validity of the assumption inherent in the back-extrapolation. This volume is termed the oxygen deficit (O_2df; Krogh and Lindhard, 1913). In skeletal muscle, the 'other' sources are anaerobic, that is the energy generated from high-energy phosphate depletion (specifically, creatine phosphate; PCr) and that from lactate (L^-) and hydrogen ion (H^+) production. At the lung, an additional component is reflected by the O_2 utilized from the body O_2 stores during the transient. This is functionally represented by the reduction in mixed venous O_2 content (Whipp and Ward, 1982; see later).

It is of interest, therefore, to consider the relationship between the τ of $\dot{V}O_2$ and the size of the O_2df. If the total energy equivalent of the task is assumed to be $A \cdot t$ (where A is the amplitude of the response, i.e. the difference between the baseline and steady-state values of the response) then the total aerobic component of this energy equivalent can be shown to be

$$VO_2 = A \cdot \int_0^t (1 - e^{-t/\tau})dt \qquad (3.10)$$

Therefore,

$$O_2df = (A \cdot t) - A \cdot \int_0^t (1 - e^{-t/\tau})dt \qquad (3.11)$$

When t becomes substantially greater than τ, this simplifies to the useful expression:

$$O_2df = A \cdot \tau \qquad (3.12)$$

As a result, the O_2 deficit increases as a linear function of work rate for a given τ, a relationship that is valid over the range where the $\dot{V}O_2$–work-rate relationship is linear and τ is invariant.

The O_2 deficit can therefore be readily determined if A and τ are both known precisely; τ being normally determined from a high-density computation of $\dot{V}O_2$ throughout the transient (e.g. Whipp and Wasserman, 1972; Linnarsson, 1974; Hughson and Morrissey, 1982; Cerretelli and di Prampero, 1987; Barstow and Molé, 1991; Özyener *et al.*, 2001 and see later text). By extension therefore, the amount of O_2 used up to a particular time (t), or $\dot{V}O_2$, for this response profile can be computed as

$$\dot{V}O_2 = A \cdot t - \dot{V}O_2 \cdot \tau \qquad (3.13)$$

Apparently small 'errors' in the O_2df, however, can lead to surprisingly large changes in the estimated τ. For example, end-expiratory lung volume decreases during dynamic muscular exercise in normal subjects by some 0.51– in patients with chronic obstructive lung disease it can increase by at least that. It is crucial that this component be corrected for by an appropriately discriminating algorithm: all of those in current use are, however, rife with assumptions (including assumptions in addition to this volume issue), which pertain to what actually constitutes an 'alveolar' O_2 concentration and when 'it' occurs during the breath (e.g. see Beaver *et al.*, 1981; Cautero *et al.*, 2002 for discussion). But for this example, as the fractional concentration of alveolar O_2 is approximately 0.15, and assuming that mean alveolar PO_2 does not change in the steady state of moderate exercise, then the lung O_2 stores will change by approximately 75 ml from this end-expiratory lung volume effect – not much it might seem. But reference to Eqn (3.12) reveals that as A for a work rate of 75 W is approximately 750 ml $\cdot$ min^{-1} the τ will be different as a consequence by 75/750 min or an appreciable 6 s. Naturally, this will be less at higher work rates. This underscores the challenge of drawing appropriate physiological inferences from the parameters.

It is also useful to consider another feature of the exponential as schematized in Figure 3.2B. This shows that at an exercise time (t) equal to τ, the amount of O_2 utilized during the exercise is exactly equal to the remaining component of the O_2 deficit, that is

$$O_2df = A \cdot \tau = \text{area}(b) + \text{area}(c) \tag{3.14}$$

but,

$$A \cdot \tau = \text{area}(a) + \text{area}(b) \tag{3.15}$$

therefore,

$$\text{area}(a) = \text{area}(c) \tag{3.16}$$

This relationship is important, for example, in minimizing the error resulting from the instrumental response 'delay' during breath-by-breath analysis of pulmonary gas exchange (Beaver *et al.*, 1981; Lamarra and Whipp, 1995). The τ provides the best time to be added to the pure transport delay, in order to phase align the gas concentration signal to the functionally instantaneous airflow signal – assuming, of course, that the analyser responds exponentially. However, if the response profile of the analyser were sigmoid, for example, then the $t_{1/2}$ would give the best result.

Further consideration of Figure 3.2B also reveals that in area(b), the accumulated O_2 deficit (AOD) will, at any point on the exponential, be equal to the total O_2 deficit (assuming the work could be continued into the steady-state) minus the remaining component of the deficit, that is

$$\text{area}(b) = \text{area}(b + c) - \text{area}(c) \tag{3.17}$$

or, AOD up to any point in time, t:

$$AOD_t = A \cdot \tau - (A - \dot{V}O_{2(t)}) \cdot \tau \tag{3.18}$$

or,

$$AOD_t = \dot{V}O_{2(t)} \cdot \tau \tag{3.19}$$

that is, the AOD at any time during the response may be calculated from the product of the $\dot{V}O_2$ value at that time (t) and the time constant (τ) (Özyener *et al.*, 2003).

We could, however, consider that $\dot{V}O_{2(t)}$ represents the subject's actual $\dot{V}O_{2\,max}$. In this case, the accumulated O_2 deficit at $\dot{V}O_{2\,max}$ becomes equal to the $\dot{V}O_{2\,max} \cdot \tau$, that is

$$AOD_{max} = \dot{V}O_{2\,max} \cdot \tau \tag{3.20}$$

Note that the O_2 deficit for such a function up to the point of limitation by $\dot{V}O_{2\,max}$ (or, of course, cessation at that time for 'non-limiting' reasons) is independent of work rate or of the actual steady-state $\dot{V}O_2$ projected for that work rate. This presumably forms the basis for the concept of the maximum accumulated oxygen deficit (e.g. Medbø et al., 1988).

It is also instructive to consider both the magnitude and components of the physiological contributions to the O_2 deficit. Over the moderate work-rate range the O_2 deficit is determined predominantly by changes in the available high-energy phosphate stores and the accessible O_2 stores with a small transient lactate elevation (e.g. di Prampero and Margaria, 1968; Piiper et al., 1968; Cerretelli et al., 1979; di Prampero et al., 1983). At higher intensities the lactate-related contribution is proportionally greater.

Consider, for example, a subject with a 10 kg active muscle mass and an intramuscular PCr store which has decreased from a resting value of 20 or 25 mmol·kg^{-1} (wet wt) to as low as 2 mmol·kg^{-1}, at high-intensity exercise. The PCr pool depletion of some 20 mmol·kg^{-1} results in approximately 200 mmol of high-energy phosphate being contributory to the deficit – ATP concentration, does not decrease appreciably until extremely high work rates. Consequently, as $\sim P:O_2 \approx 6$, this results in approximately 33 mmol of O_2 equivalent and, as each mmol of O_2 is equivalent to 22.4 ml, then the O_2 equivalent of the total depletable high-energy phosphate pool is approximately 750 ml (i.e. $33 \cdot 22.4 \approx 750$). The O_2 taken from the O_2 stores provides the other alactic source of the O_2 deficit. In an adult with a 3 l venous blood volume, and a reduction in mixed venous O_2 content from 150 ml·l^{-1} at rest to 50 ml·l^{-1} during high-intensity exercise, the deficit equivalent of the O_2 stores utilized will be 300 ml (i.e. $3 l \cdot 100$ ml·l^{-1}). The myoglobin in the red muscle fibres, with its P_{50} of ~3.0 mmHg at physiological temperature (e.g. Schenkman et al., 1997; Richardson et al., 2002) is unlikely to contribute to this value until high levels of exercise. And even then, assuming that half of the total available myoglobin, at 25 mg·g^{-1} dry wt, in 10 kg of skeletal muscle (being liberal and assuming all the mass to be 'red') is depleted of its O_2, this would only contribute approximately 80 ml of O_2 to the deficit. The low O_2 solubility in plasma and muscle water (approximately 0.6 ml·l^{-1} muscle water · 20 mmHg reduction in muscle tissue PO_2) would provide only a trace additional quantity for this purpose. Consequently, the total O_2 deficit available for such exercise from these sources in the adult is only of the order of 1 l. The importance of the $\dot{V}O_2$ time constant becomes apparent from this example. For a subject with a τ of 30 s, the alactic sources of O_2 deficit will be depleted at a work rate of approximately 200 W: with a τ of 1 min, naturally, this would occur at approximately 100 W, making anaerobiosis obligatory. The effective oxidation of the consequent lactate production is vital for the continuation of the exercise.

Phases of the response

$\dot{V}O_2$ during constant-load exercise, however, does not change with the simple exponential characteristics described earlier (Figure 3.2). Rather, there is an early phase of $\dot{V}O_2$ (Phase I) which is determined by the increase in pulmonary blood flow prior to blood with greater O_2 extraction (as a result of the muscle contraction) reaching the lungs (Krogh and Lindhard, 1913; Whipp *et al.*, 1982). The subsequent and dominant (at all but very low work rates) component of the non-steady-state response (Phase II) results from the further effect on the mixed venous blood of the increased O_2 extraction in the blood perfusing the contracting muscles – as schematized in Figure 3.3 (e.g. Casaburi *et al.*, 1989; Grassi *et al.*, 1996). The pulmonary response therefore conflates the influence of the cardiac output (or more properly that of the pulmonary blood flow) and the changes in the mixed venous O_2 concentration (Figure 3.3) and characterized by the Fick equation:

$$\dot{V}O_2 = \dot{Q} \cdot (CaO_2 - C\bar{v}O_2) \tag{3.21}$$

When both time courses are complete a steady state is attained: this is termed Phase III.

Consequently, the two-phased feature of the non-steady-state $\dot{V}O_2$ response introduces, a delay-like component (TD) which influences the overall response characterization:

$$\dot{V}O_{2t} = \Delta\dot{V}O_{2ss} \cdot (1 - e^{-(t - TD)/\tau}) \tag{3.22}$$

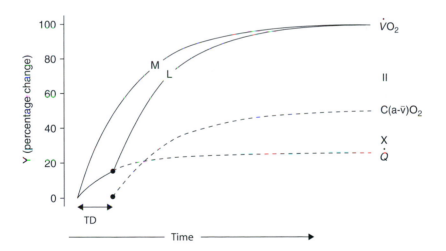

Figure 3.3 A schematic representation of the Fick equation (Eqn (3.21)), showing the idealized difference between muscle (M) and lung (L) gas exchange following the transition to constant-load exercise. Pulmonary O_2 uptake ($\dot{V}O_2$) is the product of blood flow ($\dot{Q}$) and arterial–mixed venous O_2 content difference ($C(a-\bar{v})O_2$). Therefore, the $\dot{V}O_2$ response conflates the influence of early increases in pulmonary perfusion (Phase I) with the subsequent reduced O_2 content in the venous blood as a result of the muscle contraction (Phase II). The arrival of O_2 extracted blood at the lung determines the delay (TD). The difference between muscle and lung blood flow at any fixed point in time (or at any fixed $C(a-\bar{v})O_2$) modulates $\dot{V}O_2$ at the lung from that seen at the muscle.

The difference between the oxygen consumption profile in the muscle and the oxygen uptake profile at the lung, as schematized in Figure 3.3, reflects the O_2 utilization from the O_2 stores. The TD in Figure 3.3 represents the time taken for the altered O_2 concentration in the venous effluent from the exercising muscle(s) to influence the O_2 concentration in the mixed venous blood entering the pulmonary capillary bed. Note here that this only represents the muscle-to-lung transit time if the O_2 concentration of the muscle venous blood changes in concert with the onset of exercise that is,

$$C\bar{v}O_2 = CaO_2 - \dot{V}O_2/\dot{Q} \tag{3.23}$$

This delay is signalled at the lung both by the gas exchange ratio (R) beginning to decrease as a consequence of the predominantly intra-muscular storage of CO_2 and the end-tidal PCO_2 beginning to increase and end-tidal PO_2 beginning to decrease as a result of the altered mixed venous gas partial pressures. This delay therefore has a physiological equivalent – but not the delay derived when Eqn (3.22) is applied to the pulmonary $\dot{V}O_2$ response using pre-exercise $\dot{V}O_2$ as the baseline (see later). This is because the TD in Eqn (3.22) describes the time at which the exponential (Phase II) component is required to begin, were it to start from the pre-exercise $\dot{V}O_2$ value. In reality the Phase I and Phase II components are intertwined, complicating the interpretation of the TD value from Eqn (3.22).

That there is an oxygen-stores component of the O_2 deficit at the lung has suggested to some that there must be an obligatory slowing of the time constant for pulmonary $\dot{V}O_2$ compared with $m\dot{V}O_2$ (e.g. see Cerretelli and di Prampero, 1987; Barstow et al., 1990). This is not necessarily the case. As schematized in Figure 3.4 there are two conditions in which pulmonary $\dot{V}O_2$ would have exactly the same time constant as that of the muscle (i.e. Figure 3.4A and B): One condition would be where $\dot{Q}$ increased in precise proportion to $\dot{V}O_2$ (Figure 3.4A). In this case, as evident in Eqn (3.21), there would be no Phase II as the entire response would be a cardiodynamic Phase I. An alternative would be if $\dot{Q}$ did not change (assuming the O_2 stores would be sufficient to allow the required O_2 uptake; Figure 3.4B). In this case there would be no increase in pulmonary $\dot{V}O_2$ during Phase I. In reality, however, the $\dot{V}O_2$ response is intermediate with a cardiodynamic phase preceding the Phase II response (Figure 3.4C and shown for a real response in Figure 3.5A). But what would the τ of this Phase II response be, relative to that of the muscle (e.g. the model fit shown in Figure 3.5B)? Not very different it turns out – to within 10% or so for this effect. This has been demonstrated by modelling the influences of plausible differences in on-transient $\dot{Q}$ profiles and venous capacitance volumes (Barstow et al., 1990). It has also been shown by direct analysis of the time course of pulmonary $\dot{V}O_2$ in concert with that of the exercising muscle O_2 consumption (Grassi et al., 1996). This required high-density determinations of the variables in the Fick equation (Eqn (3.21)) – a procedure presenting formidable technical challenges. Consequently, Phase II $\tau \dot{V}O_2$ (Figure 3.5B) is often used as a surrogate of the muscle τ – but with an 'uncertainty' level of up to 10%.

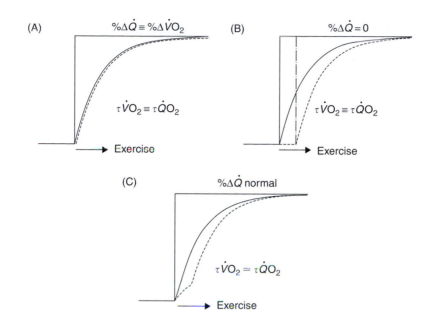

Figure 3.4 Idealized and actual differences between the kinetics of muscle and lung gas exchange. Panels A and B represent idealized schemes demonstrating the potential for the muscle and lung $\dot{V}O_2$ time-constants (τ) to be identical. (A) Muscle and lung blood flow ($\dot{Q}$) increase with the precise kinetics of muscle O_2 consumption. Here there is no change in $C(a\text{-}\bar{v})O_2$ and the entire dynamic is comprised of increased $\dot{Q}$, that is the pulmonary $\dot{V}O_2$ response is entirely Phase I. The muscle and lung τ values would therefore be identical with no delay separating them. (B) An instance where there is no increase in muscle or lung $\dot{Q}$. Here the $\dot{V}O_2$ response is entirely comprised of change in $C(a\text{-}\bar{v})O_2$, and again the muscle and lung τ values are identical, but this time separated by a pure delay where there is no change in $\dot{V}O_2$, that is the response is entirely Phase II. (C) A model of the actual pattern of $\dot{Q}$ and $C(a\text{-}\bar{v})O_2$ changes following the onset of constant-load exercise. Here the muscle and lung τ values are not identical, but typically differ by up to ~10%.

We stress 'up to' here as the values could in fact be the same in some circumstances – but one cannot at present 'know' with certainty.

While Eqn (3.22) provides a 'somewhat better' characterization of the $\dot{V}O_2$ response dynamics, it still does not yield an accurate reflection of the actual time course of $\dot{V}O_2$. This is because the fitting procedure minimizes the error between the model fit and the actual data over the entire time course of response. As shown in Figure 3.5, this gives a τ value that is smaller (Figure 3.5F) than when the model is fixed to begin at time zero (Figure 3.5D) but larger than that of the actual Phase II response (Figure 3.5B). Also the delay term (TD) resulting from Eqn (3.22) is shorter, in all cases, than that of the actual Phase I–Phase II

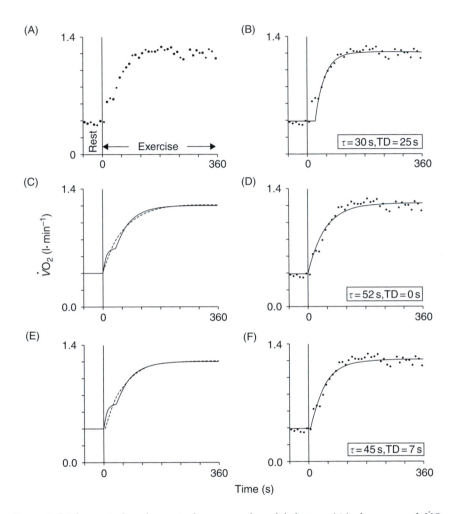

Figure 3.5 Theoretical and practical aspects of model fitting. (A) shows a real $\dot{V}O_2$ response obtained from a subject during moderate-intensity exercise. (B) demonstrates an exponential fit solely to the Phase II portion of this response, resulting in a time-constant estimation reflective (to within ~10%) of muscle O_2 consumption. (C) and (D) show the theoretical and actual response and models fit to the entire $\dot{V}O_2$ response (using Eqn (3.22)) where the exponential model is restricted to begin at exercise onset (i.e. TD = 0). This results in a longer τ than when the strategy in panel E is used to describe the response (panel F). However, the τ + TD from panel F is equal to τ in panel D: both of which have been termed the mean response time (MRT) or the effective time constant (τ'). The strategies used in panel C–F allow estimation of the appropriate τ for calculation of the O_2df (Eqn (3.24)).

transition time (Figure 3.5B, D and F). Interestingly however this least-squares fit does allow an accurate quantification of the O_2df, that is,

$$O_2df = \Delta\dot{V}O_{2ss} \cdot (\tau + TD) \tag{3.24}$$

as derived from Eqn (3.12) (e.g. Rossiter *et al.*, 1999, cf. Cerretelli and di Prampero, 1987). The sum of τ and TD in Eqn (3.22) has been termed the mean response time (MRT Linnarsson, 1974) or the 'effective' time constant (τ'; Whipp and Ward, 1990). As discussed later, the distinction between the actual τ and the τ' (or MRT) for the entire response has major implications for the inferences which can be drawn from the dynamics. Therefore, the O_2df may be computed from the product of the steady-state increment in $\dot{V}O_2$ required for the task and the effective time constant determined either from the model exponential-fit from time zero (Figure 3.5D), or modelled as described by Eqn (3.22) (because $\tau + TD = \tau'$; Figure 3.5F). But, it is important to reiterate that the time constant of this latter relationship is not an accurate depiction of the 'real' non-steady-state response and that, from a physiological standpoint, this TD is entirely factitious. This is one of the few cases where two erroneous values with respect to a mechanism sum to provide an appropriate value for a physiological construct.

Those interested in the control of the non-steady-state $\dot{V}O_2$ dynamics, however, need a more precise characterization of the response. Two approaches have been made to this problem, with little of practical import to choose between them. Some investigators attempt to characterize the entire non-steady response for moderate exercise with a model requiring six parameters (i.e. two delay terms, two time constants and two proportional gains). Others choose to delete the cardiodynamic phase (Phase I) of the response by constraining the fitting window for the parameter estimation to start not at exercise onset (i.e. $t = 0$) but rather some sufficient time after the exercise onset to ensure that the Phase II component is being manifest. Ideally, as mentioned earlier, this should be triggered by the start of the fall in the pulmonary gas exchange ratio ($R = \dot{V}CO_2/\dot{V}O_2$), which reflects the influence of the intra-muscular CO_2 storage. However, the beginning of this decrease is often not sufficiently clear for this purpose and so a value of at least 20 s is commonly used. This is to allay the concern, that starting the fit before Phase II has begun will allow a Phase I contribution to distort the goodness-of-fit. A physiological justification for the strategy of simply deleting the cardiodynamic Phase I $\dot{V}O_2$ component from the exponential fit, is based upon the reasoning that (a) there is no sufficiently sound evidence to support the exponentiality of the Phase I component and (b) that the asymptote of the physiological determinant of Phase I (see Figure 3.3 for example) is larger than the value attained at the time of the Phase I–Phase II transition. Both of these approaches, however, are designed to ensure that inferences for the control of $\dot{V}O_2$ during the non-steady-state of muscular exercise are based upon fitting procedures that appropriately characterize the time constant of the Phase II $\dot{V}O_2$ response.

There are separate, but related, concerns at the cessation of exercise. Here, Phase I for the off-transient is more complex than at the onset because it is made up of the product of a decreasing cardiac output and pulmonary blood flow (that decreases at a much slower rate than the corresponding increase at exercise onset) at a time when the mixed-venous O_2 concentration is still rising (owing to the influence of the limb-to-lung transit time). The uncertainty generated by these effects is generally dealt with by a similar omission of the first 20 s of the response from the fitted data at cessation. There is further concern when attempting to ascertain the influence of the slow component of $\dot{V}O_2$ at exercise cessation (see later).

Fitting the data or characterizing the response?

Modelling, as Steiner (1992) reminds us, often 'provides a kind of depth that is isolated from the contaminations of real context'. This is particularly appropriate regarding considerations of the $\dot{V}O_2$ transient. The problem being that the 'real' transient $\dot{V}O_2$ profile is rarely 'clean'. In addition to the 'normal' breath-to-breath fluctuations in $\dot{V}O_2$, which co-relate with the fluctuations in tidal volume and consequent changes in pulmonary blood flow resulting from the changes in pleural pressure, there are typically markedly large or small breaths resulting from 'sighs', 'swallows', 'coughs' etc. (e.g. Lamarra et al., 1987; Rossiter et al., 2000). These are unrelated to the metabolically-linked pattern of response and degrade the quality of the signal to be processed (for an example see section 'Confidence and parameterization'). The investigator must choose what to do about these errant breaths: to leave them in or edit them out.

Editing of the breath-by-breath file, though necessary to estimate the underlying pattern of response, strays perilously close to the brink of scientific ethics. The procedure should be approached with caution and criteria. The criteria for determining the presence of data points which could not reasonably be considered to be reflective of the system response dynamics should be established a priori. In this regard it is reasonable to assume that data points resulting from coughs, swallows, sighs or error in the breath-start criterion, for example, are not fundamental components of the response. The difference between not-editing and editing these 'errant' breaths is the difference between 'fitting the data' and 'fitting the physiological response of interest'. While 'pure', in a sense, the former can result in physiologically misleading values for the parameters that might suggest that two physiological functions may not be mechanistically related, or coupled, when in fact they are – or *vice versa*, of course. For example, mistriggered breaths can result in extremely high or low values, which, if included in the parameter estimation process, can lead to values that were extremely fast or extremely slow, respectively and, as such, distort the physiological interpretation. The value estimated from data fit by these criteria would reflect the kinetic properties of the data but not of the underlying physiological mechanism of interest. This would be akin to interpreting an ECG, during exercise, with a loose electrode. The concern naturally is for the criterion (or criteria) for establishing what is, or is not, a valid component of the response under consideration. While there is no absolute value for this decision we prefer to err on the side of stringency, for example, using the criterion that a datum that lies more than four standard deviations away from the local mean (i.e. with a probability less than 0.005; e.g. Rossiter *et al.*, 2000) has a disappearingly-small likelihood of being part of the physiological response of interest. Its inclusion however, can exert a major influence on the parameter estimation. We demonstrate this in Figure 3.6 for a 'pure' exponential response with a time constant of 30 s (panel A). When the response includes a single 'errant' value (of 300 ml·min^{-1} in this case) the best-fit time constant is influenced by a variable amount; depending on when the 'errant' value occurs. Such breaths early in the transient exert the greatest influence. In this case, reducing the time constant by approximately 3–4 s (panels B and C); there is little influence once the transient is functionally complete (i.e. panel D). As shown in panel E the influence of the errant point is also dependent on the underlying time constant itself (see Lamarra *et al.*, 1987): the response with the greatest τ (in this case 45 s) expresses the smallest percentage error. However, the duration of the influence is prolonged as the response takes more time to attain a functional steady state. Likewise the fastest response (here 20 s, consistent with that of $\dot{V}O_2$ in a healthy fit subject, for example) has the greatest 'error' as there is little data in the transient region and therefore the errant breath exerts a greater influence. A symmetrical high–low pairing of such breaths close in time will naturally tend to have offsetting effects on the fit.

When considering actual $\dot{V}O_2$ data, these potential errors are, in reality, magnified due to the influence of the 'normal' breath-to-breath fluctuations. The non-linear least-squares fitting procedure attempts to minimize the sum of the errors, such that the difference between the model fit throughout the time period considered is evenly distributed (i.e. the model is 'in error' by an equal degree both over and under the actual response for the time period in question). Therefore, the theoretical percentage error resulting from the inclusion of a breath that does not reflect the underlying physiological response in question (Figure 3.6E) when the actual response is a pure (noise-free) exponential is magnified when actual breath-to-breath fluctuations are included in the data. Figure 3.6F illustrates an actual $\dot{V}O_2$ response in a healthy subject to moderate-intensity constant load cycle ergometry exercise. Here the underlying exponential is partially obscured by the effects of the breath-to-breath fluctuation, and therefore, the best non-linear least-squares fit of this response results in a τ of ~27s which has a positive χ^2 value (unlike Figure 3.6A which has a χ^2 of 0). When an errant breath is included in the fit (i.e. a breath of similar magnitude to the above mentioned theoretic consideration) the effect of its inclusion is distributed throughout the entire response and the model results in a τ of ~19s. This dramatic alteration of ~30% clearly demonstrates the legitimacy of the decision to edit, but does not justify the criteria for it.

Confidence and parameterization

Without the benefit of a 'pure' exponential response unadulterated by 'noise', the parameter values established from model fitting of the $\dot{V}O_2$ response kinetics are

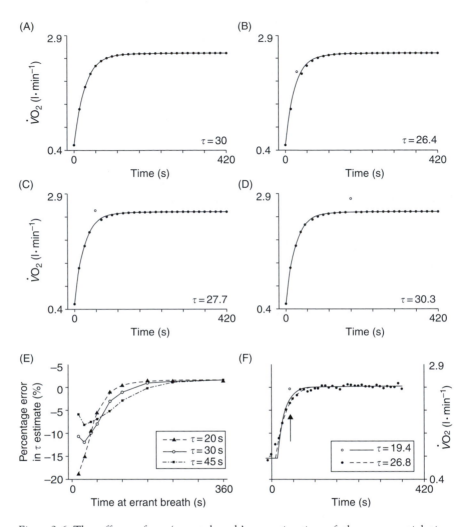

Figure 3.6 The effects of an 'errant breath' on estimation of the exponential time constant (τ). (A) A pure exponential response, with a fitted model. (B), (C) and (D) show the effects of a single 'errant breath' of $300\,ml \cdot min^{-1}$ magnitude appearing at different times during the transient (B: at $\sim\tau$; C: at $\sim2\tau$; D: at $> 5\tau$). When an 'errant breath' occurs early in the transition, its effects on τ estimation are more severe than when it occurs at a later stage. (E) Over a range of pure exponentials, this influence will be more extreme when associated with an exponential with a small τ (e.g. $\dot{V}O_2$) than those with longer τ values (e.g. $\dot{V}CO_2$ or ventilation). (F) The effects of 'errant breath' inclusion on fitting an actual data response. In fitting an actual data set, the 'error' of the errant breath is distributed among the 'errors' resulting from the normal breath-to-breath fluctuations. The result is a more extreme influence of the errant value (i.e. $\sim30\%$), on the estimated τ of real data, compared to the theoretical prediction in panel E. (Solid line includes 'errant breath'.)

necessarily estimates. While these estimates may be robust, in that the model provides an adequate characterization of the response, robust estimates need not be compelling. That is to say, the confidence in a particular parameter estimate of a model is not simply dependent on the goodness-of-fit. For a parameter to lend itself to convincing physiological implication it must also possess high confidence. Confidence in parameter values can, for example, be characterized by a 95% confidence interval (e.g. Rossiter *et al.*, 1999, 2002), which is akin to describing the range over which the value may vary with 95% probability. When attempting to extract a τ value from a typical $\dot{V}O_2$ response, factors that influence the confidence of the τ estimation are numerous, but of particular importance are signal-to-noise ratio and the number of parameters in the model. The 'noise' distribution around the underlying $\dot{V}O_2$ signal has been typically shown to be Gaussian with a standard deviation of $\sim\pm200$ ml·min^{-1} (Lamarra *et al.*, 1987; Rossiter *et al.*, 2000). The distribution seems not to be influenced by the metabolic rate and, as such, becomes a diminishing proportion of the entire response as the $\dot{V}O_2$ amplitude increases. Thus, the signal-to-noise (S/N) of the pulmonary $\dot{V}O_2$ data can be increased either by increasing S or by decreasing N, or both. High work rates require large increases in $\dot{V}O_2$. However, the degree to which the work rate can be incremented and $\dot{V}O_2$ still express the same characteristics for the particular subject is set by the domain thresholds (Whipp, 1996; see section 'Intensity domains'). It is also a common practice to increase S/N by decreasing the noise. This can be achieved by averaging together the responses of a number of repetitions of the same exercise protocol (Lamarra *et al.*, 1987). This is only justified when the noise is demonstrably Gaussian and stochastic (i.e. has low auto-correlation; as recently raised by Cautero *et al.* (2002), who showed that some algorithms commonly used to calculate $\dot{V}O_2$ have a high propensity to produce data with noise that has a highly auto-correlated component). When the breath-to-breath fluctuations are normally distributed around the mean and occur at random, the effect of averaging repeated-protocol responses is to average-out the variation. An example of this procedure is shown in Figure 3.7A and B. The model fit to the single transition (Figure 3.7A) appears to be a good characterization of the response with residuals that are evenly distributed and unsystematic: they are broad however. When the same protocol is repeated on three occasions and the responses averaged (i.e. the average of four transitions) the fit and residual is very similar to that seen with a single experiment (Figure 3.7B), but the confidence in the parameter estimation is improved by $\sim$3-fold. That τ $\dot{V}O_2$ did not change as a result of some experimental intervention, or was not different from that of some proposed mediator, means little if the confidence limits are so large that appreciable real differences could not possibly be discriminated. The outcome of the model fit in Figure 3.7B allows physiological inferences to be drawn with a greater, and possibly acceptable, degree of confidence.

The number of parameters in the model fit to the data will also affect the confidence in two key ways. First, it directly affects the confidence calculation by reducing the degrees of freedom, that is a large number of parameters reduces

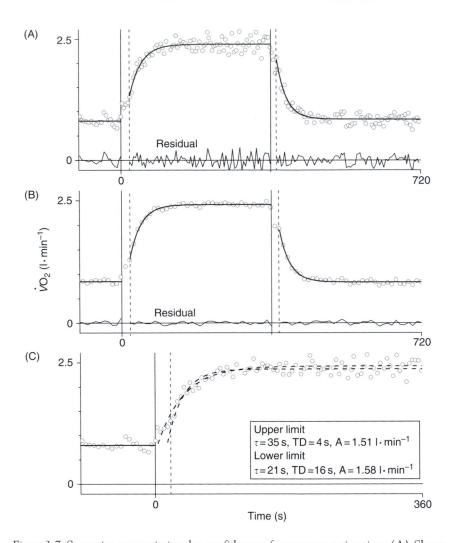

Figure 3.7 Strategies to maximize the confidence of parameter estimation. (A) Shows a $\dot{V}O_2$ response during moderate-intensity constant-load exercise. A model has been fitted to the data, excluding the Phase I response, in order to get an estimate of the τ for muscle O_2 consumption. While the fitted model shows good characterization the large breath-to-breath fluctuations in the response, lead to flat, but broad residuals to the fit. (B) The averaged response of four trials (with only two floating variables: τ and TD) allows far greater confidence in the parameter estimates. Here the residuals to the fitted model are similarly flat but narrow, and the confidence of the fit is improved ~3-fold. (C) Reducing the number of parameters in the model allows both confidence and dependency to be improved. The models fitted in panel C (the same data set as in panel A) show the extremes of 95% confidence interval of the panel A fit (where three variables/parameters are unfixed; i.e. τ, TD and A). While both models (i.e. represented by the two dashed lines through the data) appear to be reasonable representations of the response, the τ values vary markedly; by 65%! Compare this to the confidence of the fit in panel B where the upper and lower limits of confidence vary by only 8% (26 s vs 28 s).

the degrees of freedom and widens the confidence interval (lowering the confidence of the parameter estimates). Second, the number of parameters in the model affects the dependency of each of the parameters and variables within the model. This quantity describes the mutual dependency of one parameter with others in the model. This can be easily conceptualized by referring to Figure 3.5. If the experimenter wishes to select model C or E (Figure 3.5; i.e. a single exponential, with a delay term fit to the entire response – not limiting the fit to the Phase II response), they may wish to fix the delay term at $t = 0$ or allow it to be a freely floating parameter with a value to be decided by the fitting procedure. When TD is fixed it has no dependency (i.e. a value of 0) and τ has a higher confidence (e.g. see Figure 3.5; and Lamarra *et al.*, 1987). When τ and TD are both freely floating they share a high dependency that results in a quantifiable relationship between these values (in the example in Figure 3.5 the dependency of τ and TD is ~0.37; where dependency ranges from 0 to 1). In this example, were the 'true' delay (TD) to be 1 s less (i.e. 6 rather than 7 s) then τ would be 1 s greater (i.e. 46 rather than 45 s). In this simple illustration, τ and TD are the only two 'unknowns', however, when a model contains a large number of freely floating 'unknowns' (e.g. when using multi-exponential models to describe the $\dot{V}O_2$ response in high-intensity exercise) the mutual dependency may be shared over a large number of parameters and variables typically with dependency values closer to 1. The dependency, therefore, can be used to assess whether an equation is over-parameterized, in which case many of its operators will have a strong dependency.

Considering these influences on parameter confidence, models should be selected to maximize the confidence in the parameter(s) of interest. This is more straightforward when considering $\dot{V}O_2$ responses to moderate- rather than high-intensity exercise. During moderate-intensity constant work-rate exercise bouts the $\dot{V}O_2$ response typically attains a new steady-state within ~3 to 4 min (e.g. Whipp *et al.*, 1982 and Figure 3.7B). As the parameter of interest is typically τ, it is appropriate to maximize its confidence. For this moderate-intensity protocol the values from which, and to which, the $\dot{V}O_2$ projects can be very confidently established from fits of the steady-state regions over a relatively long duration. For instance, the 4 min preceding exercise and the last n minutes of exercise (where n is the exercise duration minus at least 4τ; see Figure 3.1) may reasonably be assumed to reflect steady-state $\dot{V}O_2$ and may be set as such. Having established these values, τ and TD of only the Phase II region may be estimated to the greatest confidence allowed by the data (this can be achieved by eliminating the cardiodynamic data from the fitted region, see section 'Phases of the response'). Adding parameters, either by allowing the $\dot{V}O_2$ asymptote to be freely floating, or by including a cardiodynamic term in the equation will both reduce the confidence of τ estimation. Figure 3.7C illustrates the effect of allowing three parameters/variables to vary (i.e. τ, TD and A (amplitude)) on the confidence of the fitted model, using the same data and fitting window as shown in Figure 3.7A. With this approach the model fit shown in Figure 3.7A possesses a wide 95% confidence interval, the limits of which are shown in Figure 3.7C. While these limits appear to be reasonable with respect to the data, note that the τ values of the upper and lower bounds vary by 65% (21 s vs 35 s); compare this to the confidence of the fit in Figure 3.7B (i.e. averaged and with only two floating variables, τ and TD) where the upper and lower limits of confidence only vary by 8% (26 s vs 28 s).

These considerations of confidence and parameterization become paramount during higher exercise intensities where the exponential $\dot{V}O_2$ response is supplemented by a second, slowly developing, phase of the response (Barstow and Molé, 1991; Paterson and Whipp, 1991). During work rates where $\dot{V}O_2$ continually increases (see section 'Intensity domains'), confident estimation of the Phase II asymptote is problematic as the projected steady-state is either obscured by the slow component or may be above $\dot{V}O_{2\,max}$. Here, estimation of Phase II τ necessitates three floating parameters and is therefore less confidently estimated (although the greater response amplitude improves the S/N properties of the response, compared to moderate intensity). If additional parameters are included in the model (i.e. a second linear or exponential term to describe the slow component) then the confidence is reduced further. At high intensities where a slow component is apparent, the situation is even complicated to a greater degree by the difficulty in discerning the interface (i.e. delay) between the fundamental and slow components. Here the fundamental response and the slow component delay are associated with doubt-bounds such that the discrimination of the interface between the two components becomes highly uncertain. The mutual dependency of these estimates conspires to significantly reduce the validity of the physiological interpretation of either parameter. In other words, during exercise in this domain there is considerable potential for the Phase II τ estimate to be influenced by an unassociated portion of the response.

The importance of this is perhaps exemplified by the disparate interpretations of the apparent speeding of the dynamic response to heavy-intensity exercise when it has been recently preceded by a prior heavy-intensity bout (Gerbino et al., 1996; Macdonald et al., 1997; Burnley et al., 2000). While there is no dispute that the slow component is reduced there are different views on the influence on the fundamental component. Equation (3.8) helps focus the concern to the model assumptions. The rate-of-change of $\dot{V}O_2$ ($d\dot{V}O_2/dt$) at a given $\dot{V}O_2$ during the transient is increased (e.g. Rossiter et al., 2001). But this increase could be associated with either a reduced τ, an increased asymptotic $\dot{V}O_2$ ($\dot{V}O_{2ss}$) or both. It was initially thought that (a) as the $\dot{V}O_2$ gain of the fundamental component was not discernibly different with or without the presence of a developing metabolic acidosis on a single bout; and (b) a prior high-intensity bout did not affect the response to subsequent moderate-intensity exercise, then a reduced τ was most likely – possibly resulting from the residual metabolic acidosis during the second bout improving muscle blood flow (Gerbino et al., 1996; Bohnert et al., 1998). Further studies (e.g. Burnley et al., 2000; Endo et al., 2003) with increased resolution of the fundamental dynamics, however, provided evidence for the $\dot{V}O_{2ss}$ being increased rather than τ being decreased – suggesting a different model entirely.

Additional concerns in this intensity domain are manifest when considering the time of onset of the slow phase of the kinetics. As discussed earlier, adding components to the model reduces the confidence of the estimation of the other parameters/variables in the model. This is particularly relevant when considering the delay term for the slow phase onset. This is a particularly difficult variable to characterize precisely because, unlike Phase I, its value cannot be verified from the response of a related variable such as that of the R profile. Furthermore, it is the onset time of a component that is small in amplitude (therefore manifesting large doubt-bounds), which is expressed at a time when the Phase II fundamental kinetics may not have attained their steady state. Teasing apart these compounding factors is difficult. While current modelling strategies result in a delay for the slow component, this delay may only reflect the time at which the slow component becomes discernible, and not the actual time at which it began. This poor confidence can dramatically affect the values and confidence of the other parameters in the model via dependency; and may reduce the confidence of Phase II τ beyond the bounds of acceptability. Interestingly, the extent to which the delay influences the model fit is not of such concern at the off-transient. That is, any fast or slow phases induced by the exercise are present from the beginning of the recovery and have the same delay that is TD = 0 for both.

In modelling $\dot{V}O_2$ responses, therefore, it is prudent to err on the side of simplicity in order that the estimation of the physiological parameter of interest (e.g. inferences for m $\dot{V}O_2$ dynamics from the Phase II τ) be of the highest confidence.

Physiological inferences from the parameters

The inference that the kinetics of the $\dot{V}O_2$ response to moderate-intensity exercise reflects (or not) the behaviour of a compartment with relatively uniform metabolic characteristics, is based largely upon the goodness-of-fit of the $\dot{V}O_2$ response to a mono-exponential. Two exponential compartments, with markedly different τ values, for example do not provide a good fit to a mono-exponential when summed to provide the overall response.

However, a structure with numerous compartments having a wide range of τ values can indeed sum to provide a well-fit mono-exponential response. For example, the summed response of a ten-compartment model with individual τ values varying from 20–65 s differs in only subtle ways from a 'pure' mono-exponential, as shown in Figure 3.8A (Whipp et al., 2002); the difference is so subtle in fact that the response would not be discernible with even a small component of breath-to-breath noise. Also, the 'actual' O_2 deficit, taken as the sum of the individual regional compartment deficits, is slightly greater than that determined from the single best-fit τ and the steady-state amplitude. This is also true if the gain of each compartment differs (Figure 3.8B; Brittain et al., 2001). And so, it is important to consider not simply what the well-fit τ reveals, but also what it might conceal. For example, two subjects with ostensibly the same overall τ could have either a small distribution or a large distribution of regional τ values. The potential for metabolic stress in the long time-constant units of the

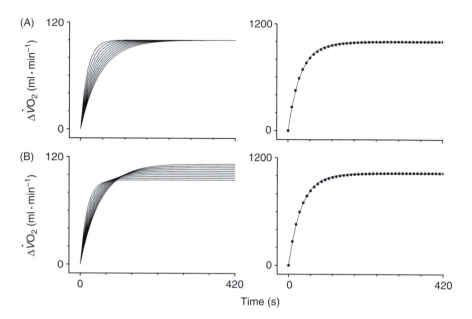

Figure 3.8 A ten-compartment model of muscle function during exercise (A) incorporating a wide range of time constants (20–65 s). The response is functionally indistinguishable from a 'pure' exponential. This is also true if the gain of each compartment also differs. (B) Two subjects with ostensibly the same overall τ $\dot{V}O_2$ could therefore have either a small or large distribution of regional intra-muscular τ values, and therefore different potentials for metabolic stress.

more widely distributed model would naturally be appreciably greater. This would consequently lead to an earlier and increased demand for supplemental regional energy transfer from L^--yielding mechanisms, presumably resulting in different regional lactate threshold (LT) values despite the same average τ $\dot{V}O_2$ for the kinetics (Whipp *et al.*, 2001).

Whether such regional variations in metabolic function are actually manifest in human muscle during exercise is not directly amenable to modelling: rather it requires experimental verification. In isolated muscle there appears to be substantial heterogeneity in the distribution of metabolic activity relative to perfusion. There is also a developing body of evidence in humans that metabolism is highly variable during muscular exercise (e.g. Meyer and Foley, 1996; Prior *et al.*, 1999; Piiper, 2000). Clearly, further work is needed on this important issue of distributed metabolic function under conditions for which uniformity might be assumed from the apparent goodness-of-fit to a particular control model. The mean response of a group of muscles or even a particular muscle (as determined by ^{31}P-NMR spectroscopy, for example, or from a femoral-venous blood sample) is likely to mask important regional variations; a spot (muscle biopsy) sample from an individual muscle may be just as misleading.

Intensity domains

While there is currently no generally agreed-upon definition of work intensity the $\%\dot{V}O_{2\,max}$ is, we contend, not a justifiable index; unfortunately, it continues to be used as if it were. The reason why this may be so assertively stated is that the profile of ventilatory, of muscle and pulmonary gas exchange, and of muscle and blood acid–base status are markedly different at a given $\%\dot{V}O_{2\,max}$ depending on whether $[L^-]$ and $[H^+]$ are unchanged from the control condition, whether they are elevated but not continuing to increase or are rising inexorably (Poole *et al.*, 1988; Whipp, 1996). Work-rate clusters of common intensity should be expected to have common profiles of stress response. In contrast, these responses show a consistent profile among subjects of variable 'fitness' levels when considered within what may be termed 'intensity domains' (Whipp, 1996; Özyener *et al.*, 2001).

The parameters that partition these intensity domains (the LT, the critical power and the $\dot{V}O_{2\,max}$) have highly variable relationships to each other in different subjects. Consequently, assigning intensity domains on the basis of a single parameter, such as $\%\dot{V}O_{2\,max}$ or $\%LT$, can lead to markedly different physiological stress characteristics in different subjects at what is apparently the same work intensity. In other words the 'intensity scale' is not linear with respect to $\%\dot{V}O_{2\,max}$. The profiles of metabolic and gas exchange response, however, do provide a means of assigning exercise intensity (Figure 3.9) which, to a large extent, overcomes these concerns. Naturally, while, an improvement, we believe, over the $\%\dot{V}O_{2\,max}$ or 'Met' increments even this will only provide a coarse characterization of intensity. Further refinements would likely have to include within-domain stratification; features (e.g. ventilatory) of the subjects' responses; and also perceptual or symptomatic considerations.

Work rates for which there is no sustained metabolic acidosis (i.e. <LT) can usually be sustained for long periods with a modest sense of effort. These are accompanied by steady-state increments in $\dot{V}O_2$ ($\Delta\dot{V}O_{2ss}$) that increase as a linear function of work rate with a slope or gain ($\Delta\dot{V}O_{2ss}/\Delta W$) of $\approx 10 \; ml \cdot min^{-1} \cdot W^{-1}$, on average, for cycle ergometry (Wasserman and Whipp, 1975; Hansen *et al.*, 1984). A steady state is usually attained within about 3 min in young healthy adults, but sooner in those of high aerobic fitness indices and considerably longer in older subjects and those with cardio-pulmonary dysfunction. These work rates may therefore be considered to be of 'moderate' intensity (Figure 3.9; also see Chapter 14). A higher range of work rates (i.e. >LT) can be identified in which there is a sustained metabolic acidosis, with increased arterial $[L^-]$ and $[H^+]$, but at which the variables either stabilize or decline back towards the baseline value. This 'heavy' intensity (i.e. between LT and what has been termed critical power; CP in Figure 3.9) is characterized by a $\dot{V}O_2$ steady-state that is attained after a considerable delay; as much as 10–15 min. While the eventual $\dot{V}O_2$ steady-state allows the work rate to be sustained it does so at a cost of appreciably greater glycogen utilization, and of muscular and ventilatory system stress. Furthermore, when $\dot{V}O_2$ does eventually stabilize, $\Delta\dot{V}O_{2ss}/\Delta W$ is

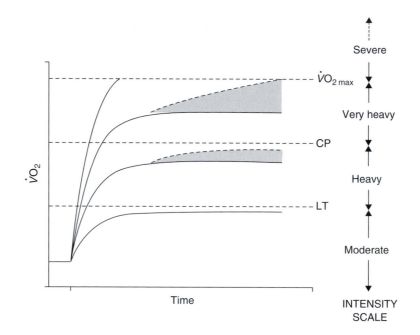

Figure 3.9 A scheme to represent the intensity domains of muscular exercise, delineated on the basis of $\dot{V}O_2$ profiles. Moderate-intensity exercise is below the lactate threshold (LT) and results in a mono-exponential response to the steady state. Above LT the kinetics become more complex, with the expression of the 'excess' of $\dot{V}O_2$ (grey shading), causing $\dot{V}O_2$ to increase above that predicted by the sub-LT $\dot{V}O_2$ to work-rate relationship. During heavy-intensity exercise (i.e. between LT and what has been termed critical power; CP) $\dot{V}O_2$ reaches a delayed steady-state only after the excess $\dot{V}O_2$ component has attained its asymptotic value. Very heavy-intensity exercise (between CP and $\dot{V}O_{2\,max}$) is characterized by a $\dot{V}O_2$ response that continues to increase throughout the test to, or towards, $\dot{V}O_{2\,max}$. Severe-intensity can be identified for work rates that are supra-maximal with respect to the expected $\dot{V}O_2$ requirement. [*Editors' note: the intensity schemes used here and in Chapter 1, for example, differ as there is currently no generally agreed-upon definition of work intensity.*]

markedly increased, and values of $13\,ml \cdot min^{-1} \cdot W^{-1}$ are not uncommon during tests of 10–15 min duration (e.g. Özyener *et al.*, 2001).

At even higher work rates, however, [L^-] and [H^+] are not only increased but continue to increase inexorably as the exercise continues: a profile signalling ensuing fatigue. We term this 'very heavy' exercise. In this domain $\dot{V}O_2$ also continues to increase throughout the test to, or towards, $\dot{V}O_{2\,max}$ (between CP and $\dot{V}O_{2\,max}$ in Figure 3.9). The consequence is extremely important as, in this domain, it is not possible for a subject to perform a constant work-rate that provides a particular percentage of $\dot{V}O_{2\,max}$. This %$\dot{V}O_{2\,max}$ can only be attained fleetingly, as $\dot{V}O_2$ continues to increase past the ostensible %$\dot{V}O_{2\,max}$ value. This also means that $\dot{V}O_{2max}$ is not associated with a unique 'maximal' work rate; rather, it is established over a range of work rates – many of which would be predicted to be sub-maximal (Özyener *et al.*, 2003). While all work rates above critical power are often considered to be of the same intensity (classified as 'very heavy' in some instances and 'severe' in others) we consider there to be justification for separating the work rates for which the projected fundamental component is less than the subjects $\dot{V}O_{2max}$ and those for which it is greater, that is these work rates are supra-maximal with respect to the 'expected' $\dot{V}O_2$ requirement (Figure 3.9). These we term 'very heavy' and 'severe', respectively, with the important distinction that it is the slow phase of the response that brings the subject to the $\dot{V}O_{2\,max}$ in the former case and either not, or not necessarily, so in the latter. Work rates of 'severe' intensity are usually only sustainable for a few minutes or so.

The highest work rate at which a sustainable $\%\dot{V}O_{2\,max}$ can be attained (i.e. with a steady state of $\dot{V}O_2$) coincides with the highest work-rate at which blood $[L^-]$ and $[H^+]$ do not continue to rise throughout the test. Furthermore, this work rate seems to correlate closely with the asymptote of the subject's power–duration curve (Poole *et al.*, 1988; Neder *et al.*, 2000). Above this 'critical power' or 'fatigue threshold', the more rapidly the slow component projects towards $\dot{V}O_{2\,max}$, the shorter will be the tolerable duration of the work rate. The mechanisms of the slow component remain to be convincingly elucidated: others consider the physiological issues elsewhere in this volume (Chapter 12). We shall address means of characterizing the response and the extent to which justifiable physiological inferences may be drawn from them.

The difference between the actual $\dot{V}O_2$ achieved in the quasi-steady state of 'heavy' or 'very heavy' exercise and the 'expected' steady-state value (i.e. projected from the sub-LT $\dot{V}O_2$ to work-rate relationship) is positive (Whipp and Mahler, 1980; Özyener *et al.*, 2003). This is true for the range of work rates above LT at which the steady state is projected to be less than the subject's $\dot{V}O_{2\,max}$. This additional increment in $\dot{V}O_2$ may, for convenience, be termed 'excess' $\dot{V}O_2$. This excess component has been shown to be a result of a slow component of the $\dot{V}O_2$ kinetics, which is superimposed upon the early 'fundamental' component of the $\dot{V}O_2$ response (see Poole *et al.*, 1994 for review). Furthermore, this superimposed component appears to be of delayed onset, beginning some minutes into the test. But while the slow phase manifests slow kinetics even by inspection, that it is of delayed onset is by no means as certain from the available data. That is, what we can tell, with some statistical justification, is that it emerges discernibly from the confidence interval of the usually continuing background component of the fundamental profile only after some delay. That it is of delayed onset implies that the conventional means of computing the O_2 deficit will be invalidated: the final asymptotic value will not provide an appropriate frame of reference for the early response dynamics.

The early component of the kinetics, however, not only remains exponential but projects to a steady-state value that gives approximately the same gain (i.e. $\Delta\dot{V}O_2/\Delta W$) and with a time constant that is little, if at all, different from that of sub-threshold exercise. The 'excess' $\dot{V}O_2$ is, therefore, considered to supplement what has been termed the 'fundamental' component of the response (Rossiter *et al.*, 1999, 2002). A consequence of the excess $\dot{V}O_2$ component being both slow and of delayed onset, is that its influence is virtually undetectable in the 'severe'-intensity domain (Özyener *et al.*, 2001).

The confidence of fitting the exponential at this severe intensity is necessarily reduced: the asymptote for the response may not be fixed from its attained steady-state value as for moderate exercise. Extrapolating the asymptote from the progression of steady-states attained by the fundamentals of lower work rates involves an assumption that, by its nature, cannot be verified even were it to be justified. And so, the fitting procedure must estimate both A and τ – and from a relatively sparse amount of data. Taking the maximally attained value as the asymptote, however, is not appropriate even if there is evidence of a plateau: because the earlier $\dot{V}O_2$ trajectory at this intensity is, by definition, to a higher value.

In the very heavy domain, the challenge is magnified, partly, as discussed earlier, because of the influence on the individual parameter confidence (see section 'Confidence and parameterization') resulting from the number of free parameters that are commonly estimated (e.g. Figure 3.10; with kind permission from the authors) to characterize the entire response, that is

$$\dot{V}O_{2t}=A_c \cdot (1 - e^{-(t - TDc)/\tau c}) + A_p \cdot (1 - e^{-(t - TDp)/\tau p}) + A_s \cdot (1 - e^{-(t - TDs)/\tau s})$$

$$(3.25)$$

where the subscripts c, p and s in the three exponential terms refer to the cardiodynamic (c), fundamental (p) and slow components (s) of the high-intensity response. TD is the time delay. But perhaps even more significant is the assumption of exponentiality of the slow phase. We are aware of no justification for this. That it is acceptably well-fit by such an equation is tautological, unless other acceptably well-fit profiles are ruled out on statistical, or better physiological, grounds. In some instances the slow phase τ is so great that even a linear profile is equally justified statistically – a model not compatible with an asymptote of constant amplitude. Parameter estimation, and model discrimination, therefore, should be kindred features of kinetic analysis. If, for example, the exponential characterization of the slow phase is interpreted in the same sense as for moderate exercise then it implies that the O_2 deficit for that component can be established from A'_s (Figure 3.10). Using this logic the O_2 deficit could be thought of as comprising two separate compartments; one bounded by exercise onset and A'_p, the other beginning at TD_s and bounded by A'_s (as depicted in Figure 3.11B; e.g. Scheuermann *et al.*, 2001). And while this may seem to be an improvement over the 'traditional' approach to quantifying the O_2 deficit (Figure 3.11A; Krogh and Lindhard, 1913; Hill, 1926) it bears a heavy burden of assumption – that being, that at any time during the slow phase $\dot{V}O_2$ has a trajectory towards the final exponential asymptote (A'_s in Figure 3.10). It is 'as though' a new compartment with relatively uniform metabolic characteristics is abruptly recruited (e.g. at time TD_s, in Figure 3.10). It should be recognized, however, that a well-fit mono-exponential response can be achieved by a wholly different model structure: this being one with progressively increasing gain and a single time constant,

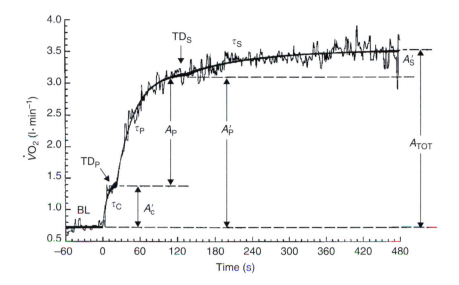

Figure 3.10 The fitting of a three-component model to the $\dot{V}O_2$ response during heavy or very heavy-intensity exercise. The three-exponential terms, each with a τ, TD, and A, correspond to the Phase I (subscript 'c'), Phase II (subscript 'p') and slow component (subscript 's') portions of the response. The end-exercise $\dot{V}O_2$ is taken at the value of the model at exercise cessation. A_{TOT} describes the end-exercise amplitude over the baseline (BL) value. A'_p corresponds to the amplitude (above BL) that Phase II $\dot{V}O_2$ attains at the onset of the slow component and A'_s is the difference between this value and the value at end-exercise. Reproduced, with permission from Scheuermann *et al.*, 2001.

for example, as shown in Figure 3.11C (Whipp *et al.*, 2002). The interesting feature of this model is that the actual underlying τ of the metabolic units generating this phase can be appreciably faster than that of the τ estimated from a fit to the data. In the case of Figure 3.11C, the fundamental τ was set to be 30 s and the 'real' slow phase τ (i.e. projecting to the varying asymptote) arbitrarily at 45 s. The changing gain and the relatively fast kinetics conflate to yield a well-fit mono-exponential component but with an apparent τ of 250 s. The consequent deficit for this phase will be appreciably smaller than for the procedure used in Figure 3.11B. While this underscores the fact that highly confident parameter estimation is a necessary but not sufficient feature of an appropriate model – especially when physiological inferences are being drawn – the actual time constant(s?) and gain profile of the slow phase naturally remain to be determined.

The multi-parameter approach depicted in Figure 3.10 is, however, utile in several respects. It provides a method of isolating the fundamental component of the response for optimum dynamic characterization. It also provides a convenient broad-brush description of the overall dynamic features. Whether each of the variables and parameters of the equation are system descriptors, with justifiable physiological equivalents, is currently by no means as clear.

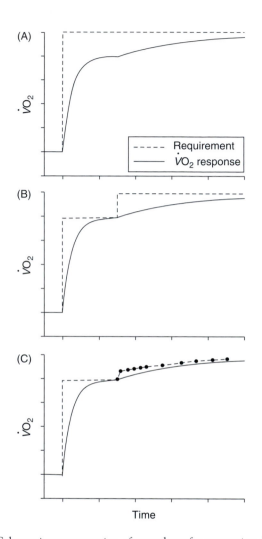

Figure 3.11 Schematic representation of procedures for computing the O_2 deficit during high-intensity exercise. (A) The 'traditional' model where the end-exercise or asymptotic $\dot{V}O_2$ is assumed to represent the O_2 equivalent of the energy requirement throughout the entire exercise bout. (B) A method which partitions the deficit into that from the fundamental and that from the slow component – the assumption being that the slow component can be treated in the same manner as that of the fundamental component as if a new compartment with relatively uniform metabolic characteristics is abruptly recruited (e.g. at time TD_s, in Figure 3.10). (C) A well-fit mono-exponential response can be achieved by progressively increasing the gain of the response expressed with a single time constant. Here the actual underlying τ of the metabolic units generating this phase (45 s) is faster than that of the τ estimated from a fit to the data (250 s). The changing gain and the relatively fast kinetics results in a response that appears mono-exponential, but with a consequent O_2 deficit for this phase that is appreciably smaller than for procedures A or B.

Appendix

Time course of a variable changing with an exponential profile

A process that decreases from a particular value y_{ss} to zero as a simple mono-exponential function of time (e.g. Figure 3.1) may be characterized as

$$-\frac{dy}{dt} \; \alpha \; y_{(t)}, \text{ or} \tag{i}$$

$$-\frac{dy}{dt} = k \cdot y_{(t)} \tag{ii}$$

where k is the proportionality constant termed the rate constant. Re-arranging this gives:

$$\frac{dy}{y_{(t)}} = -k \cdot dt \tag{iii}$$

Taking the integrals of both sides with respect to time results in

$$\ln [y_{(t)}] + C_1 = -kt + C_2 \tag{iv}$$

where C1 and C2 are constants of integration. The natural antilog gives

$$y_{(t)} \cdot C3 = e^{-kt} \cdot C4 \tag{v}$$

(note the 'add to multiply' shift between the log and antilog representations, but with new values for the constants). The constants may be collected as a new constant C5 (i.e. C4/C3), thus

$$y_{(t)} = C5 \cdot e^{-kt} \tag{vi}$$

But at $t = 0$, $e = 1$, therefore C5 is the original value of $y_{(t)}$, that is y_{ss}, therefore

$$y_{(t)} = y_{ss} \cdot e^{-kt} \quad \text{or,} \quad y_{(t)} = y_{ss} \cdot e^{-t/\tau} \tag{vii}$$

(where τ, the time constant, is the inverse of the rate constant). And for a function which increases asymptotically to a new steady state (y_{ss}) from 0 (e.g. Figure 3.2) the relationship becomes

$$y_{(t)} = y_{ss} - y_{ss} \cdot e^{-t/\tau} \tag{viii}$$

or,

$$y_{(t)} = y_{ss} \cdot (1 - e^{-t/\tau}) \tag{ix}$$

Note that if the function $y_{(t)}$ does not begin or end at 0 then the y_{ss} value will be the difference in the starting and ending values, that is,

$$y_{(t)} = \Delta y_{ss} \cdot (1 - e^{-t/\tau}) \tag{x}$$

Glossary of terms

A	the response amplitude [i.e. (steady-state) − (baseline)]
AOD	the accumulated (over time) oxygen deficit
BL	baseline
χ^2	the sum of the squares of the deviations of a theoretical fitted curve from the experimental data
CP	critical power
$C(a\text{-}\bar{v}O_2)$	difference between arterial and mixed venous blood oxygen content
e	the base for the natural logarithm
ECG	electrocardiogram
FRC	functional residual capacity (of lung volume)
k	the rate (or proportionality) constant
L^-	lactate
LT	lactate threshold
MRT	mean response time (equal to τ+TD from Eqn 3.22)
$m\dot{V}O_2$	skeletal muscle oxygen consumption
O_2df	the oxygen deficit
~P	high-energy phosphate
PCr	creatine phosphate (or phosphocreatine)
$\dot{Q}$	cardiac output
R	gas exchange ratio
S/N	signal to noise ratio
t	time
$t_{1/2}, t_{63}$	time to reach 50% or 63% of the response ($t_{63} = \tau$)
τ	the time constant of the exponential (equal to $1/k$)
TD	time delay
$\dot{V}CO_2$	pulmonary carbon dioxide output
$\dot{V}O_2$	pulmonary oxygen uptake
$\dot{V}O_{2\,max}$	maximum oxygen uptake
W	watts
$\Delta[x]$	change in [x]
$P[x]$	partial pressure
$[x]$	brackets denote concentration
$[x]_{ss}$	subscript denotes 'steady-state'

References

Bangsbo, J., Krustrup, P., Gonzalez-Alonso, J., Boushel, R. and Saltin, B. (2000). Muscle oxygen kinetics at onset of intense dynamic exercise in humans. *American Journal of Physiology*, **279**, R899–906.

Barstow, T.J. and Molé, P.A. (1991). Linear and non-linear characteristics of oxygen uptake kinetics during heavy exercise. *Journal of Applied Physiology*, **71**, 2099–106.

Barstow, T.J., Lamarra, N. and Whipp, B.J. (1990). Modulation of muscle and pulmonary O_2 uptakes by circulatory dynamics during exercise. *Journal of Applied Physiology*, **68**, 979–89.

Beaver, W.L., Lamarra, N. and Wasserman, K. (1981). Breath-by-breath measurement of true alveolar gas exchange. *Journal of Applied Physiology*, **51**, 1662–75.

Bessman, S.P. and Geiger, P.J. (1981). Transport of energy in muscle: the phosphorylcreatine shuttle. *Science*, **211**, 448–52.

Bohnert, B., Ward, S.A. and Whipp, B.J. (1998). Effects of prior arm exercise on pulmonary gas exchange kinetics during high-intensity leg exercise in humans. *Experimental Physiology*, **83**, 557–70.

Brittain, C.J., Rossiter, H.B., Kowalchuk, J.M. and Whipp, B.J. (2001). Pulmonary gas exchange kinetics within different regions of the moderate intensity exercise domain in humans. *European Journal of Applied Physiology*, **86**, 125–34.

Burnley, M., Jones, A.M., Carter, H. and Doust, J.H. (2000). Effects of prior heavy exercise on phase II pulmonary oxygen uptake kinetics during heavy exercise. *Journal of Applied Physiology*, **89**, 1387–96.

Casaburi, R., Daly, J., Hansen, J.E. and Effros, R.M. (1989). Abrupt changes in mixed-venous blood gas composition following the onset of exercise. *Journal of Applied Physiology*, **67**, 1106–12.

Cautero, M., Beltrami, A.P., di Prampero, P.E. and Capelli, C. (2002). Breath-by-breath alveolar oxygen transfer at the onset of step exercise in humans: methodological implications. *European Journal of Applied Physiology*, **88**, 203–13.

Cerretelli, P. and di Prampero, P.E. (1987). Gas exchange in exercise. In *Handbook of physiology. The respiratory system. Gas exchange.* American Physiological Society, Bethesda, MD, Sect. 3, Vol. IV, ch. 16, pp. 297–340.

Cerretelli, P., Pendergast, D.R., Paganelli, W.C. and Rennie, D.W. (1979). Effects of specific muscle training on $\dot{V}O_2$ on-response and early blood lactate. *Journal of Applied Physiology*, **47**, 761–9.

Chance, B. and Williams, C.M. (1955). Respiratory enzymes in oxidative phosphorylation. I. Kinetics of oxygen utilisation. *Journal of Biological Chemistry*, **217**, 383–93.

di Prampero, P.E. and Margaria, R. (1968). Relationship between O_2 consumption, high energy phosphates and the kinetics of the O_2 debt in exercise. *Pflugers Archives*, **304**, 11–19.

di Prampero, P.E., Boutellier, U. and Pietsch, P. (1983). Oxygen deficit and stores at onset of muscular exercise in humans. *Journal of Applied Physiology*, **55**, 146–53.

Endo, M., Tauchi, S., Hayashi, N., Koga, S., Rossiter, H.B. and Fukuba, Y. (2003). Facial cooling-induced bradycardia does not slow pulmonary $\dot{V}O_2$ kinetics at the onset of high-intensity exercise. *Journal of Applied Physiology*, **95**, 1623–31.

Gerbino, A., Ward, S.A. and Whipp, B.J. (1996). Effects of prior exercise on pulmonary gas-exchange kinetics during high-intensity exercise in humans. *Journal of Applied Physiology*, **80**, 99–107.

Grassi, B., Poole, D.C., Richardson, R.S., Knight, D.R., Erickson, B.K. and Wagner, P.D. (1996). Muscle O_2 uptake kinetics in humans: implications for metabolic control. *Journal of Applied Physiology*, **80**, 988–98.

Grassi, B., Gladden, L.B., Samaja, M., Stary, C.M. and Hogan, M.C. (1998). Faster adjustment of O_2 delivery does not affect $\dot{V}O_2$ on-kinetics in isolated in situ canine muscle. *Journal of Applied Physiology*, **85**, 1394–403.

Hagberg, J.M., Hickson, R.C., Ehsani, A.A. and Holloszy, J.O. (1980). Faster adjustment to and from recovery from submaximal exercise in the trained state. *Journal of Applied Physiology*, **48**, 218–24.

Hansen, J.E., Sue, D.Y. and Wasserman, K. (1984). Predicted values for clinical exercise testing. *American Review of Respiratory Disease*, **129**, S49–55.

Hepple, R.T. (2002). The role of O_2 supply in muscle fatigue. *Canadian Journal of Applied Physiology*, **27**, 56–69.

Hill, A.V. (1926). *Muscular Activity: The Herter Lectures for 1924*. Williams & Wilkins Co., Baltimore, USA. Ch. III–IV, pp. 87–111.

Holian, A., Owen, C.S. and Wilson, D.F. (1977). Control of respiration in isolated mitochondria: quantitative evaluation of the dependence of respiratory rates on [ATP], [ADP] and [Pi]. *Archives of Biochemistry and Biophysics*, **181**, 164–71.

Hughson, R.L. and Morrissey, M. (1982). Delayed kinetics of respiratory gas exchange in the transition from prior exercise. *Journal of Applied Physiology*, **52**, 921–9.

Krogh, A. and Lindhard, J. (1913). The regulation of respiration and circulation during the initial stages of muscular work. *Journal of Physiology*, **47**, 112–36.

Lamarra, N. and Whipp, B.J. (1995). Measurement of pulmonary gas exchange. In P.J. Maud, C. Foster (Eds) *Physiological Assessment of Human Fitness*. Human Kinetics, Champaign, IL, pp. 19–35.

Lamarra, N., Whipp, B.J., Ward, S.A. and Wasserman, K. (1987). Effect of interbreath fluctuations on characterising exercise gas exchange kinetics. *Journal of Applied Physiology*, **62**, 2003–12.

Linnarsson, D. (1974). Dynamics of pulmonary gas exchange and heart rate changes at the start and end of exercise. *Acta Physiologica Scandinavica*, **415**, 1–68.

Macdonald, M., Pedersen, P.K. and Hughson, R.L. (1997). Acceleration of $\dot{V}O_2$ kinetics in heavy submaximal exercise by hyperoxia and prior high-intensity exercise. *Journal of Applied Physiology*, **83**, 1318–25.

Mahler, M. (1985). First order kinetics of muscle oxygen consumption, and equivalent proportionality between $\dot{Q}\ O_2$ and phosphorylcreatine level. Implications for the control of respiration. *Journal of Applied Physiology*, **86**, 135–65.

Medbø, J.I., Mohn, A., Tabata, I., Bahr, R., Vaage, O. and Sejersted, O.M. (1988). Anaerobic capacity determined by maximal accumulated O_2 deficit. *Journal of Applied Physiology*, **64**, 50–60.

Meyer, R.A. and Foley, J.M. (1996). Cellular processes integrating the metabolic response to exercise. In L.B. Rowell and J.T. Shepherd (Eds) *Handbook of Physiology*, Sect. 12, Exercise: regulation and integration of multiple systems. American Physiological Society, Bethesda, MD, pp. 841–69.

Neder, J.A., Jones, P.W., Nery, L.E. and Whipp, B.J. (2000). Determinants of the exercise endurance capacity in patients with chronic obstructive pulmonary disease. The power–duration relationship. *American Journal of Respiratory and Critical Care Medicine*, **162**, 497–504.

Owen, C.S. and Wilson, D.F. (1974). Control of respiration by the mitochondrial phosphorylation state. *Archives of Biochemistry and Biophysics*, **161**, 581–91.

Özyener, F., Rossiter, H.B., Ward, S.A. and Whipp, B.J. (2001). Influence of exercise intensity on symmetry of the on- and off-transient kinetics of pulmonary oxygen uptake. *Journal of Physiology*, **533**, 891–902.

Özyener, F., Rossiter, H.B., Ward, S.A. and Whipp, B.J. (2003). Negative accumulated oxygen deficit during heavy and very-heavy intensity cycling erogmetry in humans. *European Journal of Applied Physiology*, **90**, 185–90.

Paterson, D.H. and Whipp, B.J. (1991). Asymmetries of oxygen uptake transients at the on- and offset of heavy exercise in humans. *Journal of Physiology*, **443**, 575–86.

Piiper, J. (2000). Perfusion, diffusion and their heterogeneities limiting blood-tissue O_2 transfer in muscle. *Acta Physiologica Scandinavica*, **168**, 603–7.

Piiper, J., di Prampero, P.E. and Cerretelli, P. (1968). Oxygen debt and high-energy phosphates in gastrocnemius muscle of the dog. *American Journal of Physiology*, **215**, 523–31.

Prior, B.M., Foley, J.M., Jayaraman, R.C. and Meyer, R.A. (1999). Pixel T2 distribution in functional magnetic resonance images of muscle. *Journal of Applied Physiology*, **87**, 2107–14.

Poole, D.C., Ward, S.A., Gardner, G.W. and Whipp, B.J. (1988). Metabolic and respiratory profile of the upper limit for prolonged exercise in man. *Ergonomics*, **31**, 1265–79.

Poole, D.C., Barstow, T.J., Gaesser, G.A., Willis, W.T. and Whipp, B.J. (1994). $\dot{V}O_2$ slow component: physiological and functional significance. *Medicine and Science in Sports and Exercise*, **26**, 1354–8.

Powers, S.K., Dodd, S. and Beadle, R.E. (1985). Oxygen uptake kinetics in trained athletes differing in $\dot{V}O_{2\,max}$. *European Journal of Applied Physiology*, **54**, 306–8.

Richardson, R.S., Noyszewski, E.A., Haseler, L.J., Bluml, S. and Frank, L.R. (2002). Evolving techniques for the investigation of muscle bioenergetics and oxygenation. *Biochemical Society Transactions*, **30**, 232–7.

Rossiter, H.B., Ward, S.A., Doyle, V.L., Howe, F.A., Griffiths, J.R. and Whipp, B.J. (1999). Inferences from pulmonary O_2 uptake with respect to intramuscular [PCr] kinetics during moderate exercise in humans. *Journal of Physiology*, **518**, 921–32.

Rossiter, H.B., Howe, F.A., Ward, S.A., Kowalchuk, J.M., Doyle, V.L., Griffiths, J.R. and Whipp, B.J. (2000). Inter-sample fluctuations of intramuscular [phosphocreatine] determination by ^{31}P-MRS on parameter estimation of metabolic responses to exercise in humans. *Journal of Physiology*, **528**, 359–69.

Rossiter, H.B., Ward, S.A., Kowalchuk, J.M., Howe, F.A., Griffiths, J.R. and Whipp, B.J. (2001). Effects of prior exercise on oxygen uptake and phosphocreatine kinetics during high-intensity knee-extension exercise in humans. *Journal of Physiology*, **537**, 291–303.

Rossiter, H.B., Ward, S.A., Kowalchuk, J.M., Howe, F.A., Griffiths, J.R. and Whipp, B.J. (2002). Dynamic asymmetry of phosphocreatine concentration and O_2 uptake between the on- and off-transients of moderate- and high-intensity exercise in humans. *Journal of Physiology*, **541**, 991–1002.

Saks, V.A., Kaambre, T., Sikk, P., Eimre, M., Orlova, E., Paju, K., Piirsoo, A., Appaix, F., Kay, L., Regitz-Zagrosek, V., Fleck, E. and Seppet, E. (2001). Intracellular energetic units in red muscle cells. *Biochemistry Journal*, **356**, 643–57.

Scheuermann, B.W., Hoelting, B.D., Noble, M.L. and Barstow, T.J. (2001). The slow component of O_2 uptake is not accompanied by changes in muscle EMG during repeated bouts of heavy exercise in humans. *Journal of Physiology*, **531**, 245–56.

Schenkman, K.A., Marble, D.R., Burns, D.H. and Feigl, E.O. (1997). Myoglobin oxygen dissociation by multiwavelength spectroscopy. *Journal of Applied Physiology*, **68**, 2369–72.

Steiner, G. (1992). *After Babel*. Oxford University Press, Oxford, p. 213.

Wasserman, K. and Whipp, B.J. (1975). Exercise physiology in health and disease. *American Review of Respiratory Disease*, **112**, 219–49.

Westerblad, H., Allen, D.G. and Lannergren, J. (2002). Muscle fatigue: lactic acid or inorganic phosphate the major cause? *News in Physiological Sciences*, **17**, 17–21.

Wilson, D.F. (1994). Factors affecting the rate and energetics of mitochondrial oxidative phosphorylation. *Medicine and Science in Sports and Exercise*, **26**, 37–43.

Whipp, B.J. (1996). Domains of aerobic function and their limiting parameters. In J.M. Steinacker and S.A. Ward (Eds) *The Physiology and Pathophysiology of Exercise Tolerance*. Plenum Press, New York, pp. 83–9.

Whipp, B.J. and Wasserman, K. (1972). Oxygen uptake kinetics for various intensities of constant load work. *Journal of Applied Physiology*, **33**, 351–6.

Whipp, B.J. and Mahler, M. (1980). Dynamics of gas exchange during exercise. In J.B. West (Ed.) *Pulmonary Gas Exchange*, Vol. II. New York: Academic Press, pp. 33–96.

Whipp, B.J. and Ward, S.A. (1982). Cardiopulmonary coupling during exercise. *Journal of Experimental Biology*, **100**, 175–93.

Whipp, B.J. and Ward, S.A. (1990). Physiological determinants of pulmonary gas exchange kinetics during exercise. *Medicine and Science in Sport and Exercise*, **22**, 62–71.

Whipp, B.J., Ward, S.A., Lamarra, N., Davis, J.A. and Wasserman, K. (1982). Parameters of ventilatory and gas exchange dynamics during exercise. *Journal of Applied Physiology*, **52**, 1506–13.

Whipp, B.J., Rossiter, H.B., Skasick, M. and Ward, S.A. (2001). The kinetics of $\dot{V}O_2$ as a determinant of maximum aerobic performance during exercise in humans. *Proceedings of The International Union of Physiological Sciences, Christchurch NZ*, 1664 pp.

Whipp, B.J., Rossiter, H.B. and Ward, S.A. (2002). Exertional oxygen-uptake kinetics: a stamen of stamina? *Biochemical Society Transactions*, **30**, 237–47.

4 Effect of exercise modality on $\dot{V}O_2$ kinetics

Andrew M. Jones and Mark Burnley

Introduction

The tools necessary for the accurate characterization of the transient oxygen uptake ($\dot{V}O_2$) response, namely a range of ergometers, gas analysers, flow meters and the mathematical techniques for data analysis, have been well developed throughout the last century. In recent years, experimental focus has shifted increasingly towards using these tools to characterize the $\dot{V}O_2$ time course at exercise onset and to address problems related to metabolic control. Of recent interest is that the $\dot{V}O_2$ response to exercise can be altered considerably when different ergometers are used to impose the desired work rate (Koga *et al.*, 1996; Billat *et al.*, 1998a; Jones and McConnell, 1999; Carter *et al.*, 2000b; Koga *et al.*, 2001; Koppo *et al.*, 2002; Pringle *et al.*, 2002). These findings imply that the $\dot{V}O_2$ response kinetics may be strongly influenced not only by metabolic factors and perhaps O_2 delivery to the working muscle (Tschakovsky and Hughson, 1999), but also by the muscle contraction regimen and the ensuing muscle fibre recruitment profile itself. This chapter will consider that latter factor in detail, where possible providing the likely physiological mechanisms that may explain the observed differences between exercise modalities. The focus is principally upon the $\dot{V}O_2$ response to exercise (i.e. the 'on'-kinetics) rather than to recovery (i.e. the 'off'-kinetics), largely because few studies have specifically addressed the relationship between the on- and off-transient kinetics across exercise modalities. However, it is evident that that there may be differences in the nature of the $\dot{V}O_2$ off-response across different exercise modalities relative to the on-response and across exercise intensity domains (Carter *et al.*, 2000b; Perrey *et al.*, 2002; Rossiter *et al.*, 2002), at least when compared to the characteristics of the on- and off-transient responses described for cycle exercise (Paterson and Whipp, 1991; Özyener *et al.*, 2001).

Hill and Lupton (1923) investigated the $\dot{V}O_2$ responses to various constant running speeds and for the first time established the O_2 deficit and debt concept in human subjects. Of retrospective interest is the inclusion of data demonstrating a 320 ml · min^{-1} increase in $\dot{V}O_2$ from 3 min to the end of exercise during 26 min of treadmill running at 14.4 km · h^{-1}. Though Hill and Lupton (1923) attributed this to 'a painful blister causing inefficient movement' (p. 155 of that publication), the fact that this running speed represented ~86% $\dot{V}O_{2\,max}$ suggests that these data may represent the first observation of the $\dot{V}O_2$ slow component phenomenon in the exercising human. The majority of the subsequent work in this field has been conducted using cycle ergometry (e.g. Henry, 1951; Whipp and Wasserman, 1972; Linnarsson, 1974), since this mode of exercise has distinct advantages over treadmill running for data acquisition and in particular work rate imposition (Fujihara *et al.*, 1973; Lamarra, 1990; see Margaria *et al.* (1965) for an example of kinetic analysis of treadmill exercise). Specifically, it is very much easier to collect gas and blood samples from a 'stationary' cycling subject than from a subject performing treadmill running. Further, the direct measurement of power output cannot be made during treadmill running, and hence the precise relation of work input to work output, a principal goal of kinetic characterizations of the $\dot{V}O_2$ response, is confounded.

Although the vast majority of studies in the field have been performed using cycle ergometry, it appears that the $\dot{V}O_2$ response to moderate, heavy and severe exercise is qualitatively similar among different modes of exercise. Data suitable for analysis of $\dot{V}O_2$ kinetics has been acquired during running (Billat *et al.*, 1998a; Jones and McConnell, 1999; Carter and Jones, 1999; Carter *et al.*, 2000a; 2002), knee extension exercise (Shoemaker *et al.*, 1994; MacDonald *et al.*, 1998), prone kicking exercise (Rossiter *et al.*, 2001, 2002), swimming (Demarie *et al.* 2001) handgrip exercise (Hughson *et al.*, 1996), arm cranking (Casaburi *et al.*, 1992; Koga *et al.*, 1996; Koppo *et al.*, 2002), supine cycling (Hughson *et al.*, 1993; Koga *et al.*, 1999), recumbent cycling (Williamson *et al.*, 1996), and single-legged cycling (Koga *et al.*, 2001). Each of these studies has confirmed the general character of the $\dot{V}O_2$ response seen during upright cycle exercise (Whipp and Wasserman, 1972; Whipp, 1994). In short, the initial cardiodynamic and primary exponential components are evident during moderate exercise, in which a steady state is rapidly attained and significant changes in blood [lactate] are absent. During heavy and severe exercise intensities, in which blood [lactate] is elevated (but stabilizes at that elevated level given sufficient time or rises inexorably to fatigue, respectively), the $\dot{V}O_2$ slow component emerges after a delay of ~100–120 s and results in a delayed and elevated steady state $\dot{V}O_2$ (heavy exercise) or continues to increase until exhaustion occurs (severe exercise; Gaesser and Poole, 1996). That these characteristic responses occur in a variety of exercise modes suggests that $\dot{V}O_2$ kinetics are essentially modulated by the same fundamental physiological mechanisms. This tenet is strengthened by the fact that the characteristic $\dot{V}O_2$ responses noted above are also evident in the exercising horse (Langsetmo *et al.*, 1997) and in electrically stimulated dog muscle (Grassi *et al.*, 1998), (see Chapter 5 for discussion). However, although the general characteristics of the response are similar between a number of exercise modalities, recent studies have uncovered subtle differences between them which might provide mechanistic insight.

While a number of studies have compared the physiological response to exercise across exercise modalities (e.g. Astrand and Saltin, 1961; Pendergast, 1989), relatively few have addressed the parameters of the transient $\dot{V}O_2$ response. The first study to compare the $\dot{V}O_2$ kinetics in two different modes of exercise was that of Cerretelli *et al.* (1977). These investigators demonstrated that the half time for the on-transient $\dot{V}O_2$ kinetics was significantly longer at the same absolute metabolic requirement for arm cranking compared to cycling, but was similar at the same relative exercise intensity. Cerretelli *et al.* (1979) further demonstrated that the $\dot{V}O_2$ kinetics were dependent upon the training status of the exercising muscle both between subjects (a sedentary subject had slower $\dot{V}O_2$ kinetics during arm cranking than a trained kayaker) and within the same subject (swimmers had faster $\dot{V}O_2$ kinetics during arm compared with leg exercise, whereas runners demonstrated the opposite trend). Further progress in the field was made almost exclusively using cycle ergometry (Figure 4.1), the exercise mode in which the modelling procedures currently used to characterize the $\dot{V}O_2$ response were developed (Whipp *et al.*, 1982) and continue to be studied (Bell *et al.*, 2001b). Treadmill running has been less frequently used for the evaluation of $\dot{V}O_2$ kinetics due, in part, to the potential introduction of movement and electronic artefacts to the data with this mode of exercise. Furthermore, ambulatory

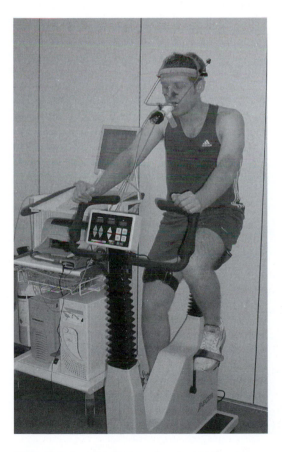

Figure 4.1 A volunteer performing cycle ergometry in the exercise physiology laboratory.

difficulties in some populations add to the complexities of data interpretation for this form of ergometry.

Comparison of $\dot{V}O_2$ kinetics in running and cycling

Whilst the study of $\dot{V}O_2$ kinetics in cycling has been pivotal to our understanding of the $\dot{V}O_2$ response dynamics, a clear understanding of the $\dot{V}O_2$ response to running exercise is important simply because the human has evolved bipedal locomotion, and hence the muscular, cardiovascular, ventilatory and neural mechanisms that operate during continuous exercise are perhaps most naturally expressed during running. Indeed, it could be argued that running exercise should be considered the control condition from the point of view of the $\dot{V}O_2$ kinetics. A number of recent studies have therefore set out to characterize the $\dot{V}O_2$ kinetics during treadmill running (Bernard *et al.*, 1998; Billat *et al.*, 1998a,b; Jones and McConnell, 1999; Carter *et al.*, 2000a,b, 2002; Williams *et al.*, 2001; Hill *et al.*, 2003, see Figure 4.2). It has been demonstrated that the primary component time constant (τ_p) is similar or tends to lengthen slightly, and that the primary component gain (G_p) is similar or tends to fall, as running speed is increased from moderate to heavy/severe running speeds (Carter and Jones, 1999; Carter *et al.*, 2000a,b; Williams *et al.*, 2001; Carter *et al.*, 2002). In addition, a $\dot{V}O_2$ slow component becomes evident as running speed exceeds the lactate threshold (LT). Therefore, the $\dot{V}O_2$ response to running has similar characteristics to those observed during cycling, and these responses can be appropriately described with the same modelling techniques (Carter and Jones, 1999).

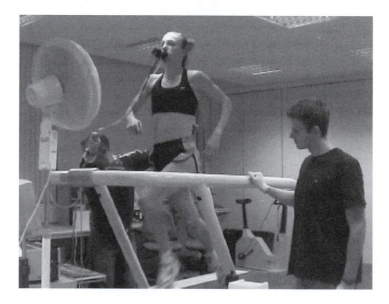

Figure 4.2 An athlete undergoing physiological assessment on the motorized treadmill in the exercise physiology laboratory.

However, subtle differences in the $\dot{V}O_2$ response to different modes of exercise, and to the physiological mechanisms responsible for these, are best revealed when direct comparisons are made in the same subjects. Billat *et al.* (1998b) compared the $\dot{V}O_2$ response to running and cycling exercise at 90% of the peak work rate in ten triathletes. They found that the $\dot{V}O_2$ slow component (measured from 3 min to the limit of tolerance) was ~270 ml $\cdot$ min^{-1} in cycling but only ~20 ml $\cdot$ min^{-1} in running, a figure smaller than the measurement error associated with modern gas analysis systems (Howley *et al.*, 1995). However, at least part of the reason for this difference lies in the fact that several subjects significantly exceeded their peak incremental $\dot{V}O_2$ values during constant work-rate cycling, and one subject showed a negative change in $\dot{V}O_2$ between 3 min and the end of exercise in running (Billat *et al.*, 1998b).

Further experimental work by Jones and McConnell (1999) demonstrated that the $\dot{V}O_2$ slow component measured from 3 to 6 min during running at 50% of the difference between the mode-specific lactate threshold and $\dot{V}O_2$ was ten times larger than the amplitude observed by Billat *et al.* (1998a,b). However, a difference in the $\dot{V}O_2$ slow component between the two modes of exercise (~290 ml $\cdot$ min^{-1} for cycling vs ~200 ml $\cdot$ min^{-1} during running) was still apparent. Whether the difference between the studies of Jones and McConnell (1999) and Billat *et al.* (1998b) reflected sampling differences or differences in the treadmill protocols (Jones and McConnell (1999) chose a 5% treadmill grade, which may have increased the amplitude of the $\dot{V}O_2$ slow component, see later) is not clear. Furthermore, in the work of both Billat *et al.* (1998b) and Jones and McConnell (1999) no further partitioning of the $\dot{V}O_2$ response into its kinetic components was attempted. It was unclear from these studies whether the τ_p was sensitive to the exercise mode, or precisely what fraction of the overall $\dot{V}O_2$ response was accounted for by the $\dot{V}O_2$ slow component in each exercise mode (since the primary $\dot{V}O_2$ amplitude was not determined).

The first study to compare running and cycling utilizing mathematical modelling methods that characterized the individual components of the $\dot{V}O_2$ response was conducted by Carter *et al.* (2000b). These investigators monitored the $\dot{V}O_2$ response during cycling and running at 80% LT and 25%, 50% and 75% of the difference between LT and $\dot{V}O_{2\,max}$. Using the modelling procedures of Barstow *et al.* (1996), Carter *et al.* (2000b) demonstrated that the $\dot{V}O_2$ slow component was indeed smaller in amplitude during running exercise compared to cycling. Furthermore, they demonstrated that the $\dot{V}O_2$ slow component accounted for a significantly smaller fraction (i.e. 3–10% vs 7–17%) of the overall $\dot{V}O_2$ response during running exercise, despite the fact that the absolute metabolic rate at an equivalent relative exercise intensity was consistently higher during running than cycling in their subjects. The τ_p was, however, similar between running and cycling at all the relative exercise intensities studied. In contrast to this, Hill *et al.* (2003) reported that τ_p was significantly faster in running compared to cycling (~14 vs ~25 s) during exercise that resulted in exhaustion in ~5 min such that $\dot{V}O_{2\,peak}$ was reached significantly earlier during running. Overall, the τ_p does appear to be somewhat faster in running (15–25 s; Carter *et al.*, 2000a,b,

2002; Hill *et al.*, 2003) compared to cycling (20–30 s; Barstow *et al.*, 1996; Carter *et al.*, 2000a,b; Hill *et al.*, 2003) in young healthy subjects. The reason for this difference is not entirely clear. However, in addition to differences in muscle contraction regimen (see later), it should be borne in mind that in most subjects, the muscles used in day-to-day activities (such as walking) are likely to be relatively better trained than those used in other exercise modes. Indeed, Chilibeck *et al.* (1996) used this rationale as an explanation for the significantly slower $\dot{V}O_2$ kinetics they observed in cycling compared to both treadmill walking and plantar flexion exercise in old (but not young) subjects (see Chapter 13).

The responses to running and cycling as described by Carter *et al.* (2000b) are shown in Figure 4.3 which reveals several features of interest. First, as mentioned earlier, the amplitude of the primary $\dot{V}O_2$ response is considerably higher during running than during cycling in both absolute and relative terms (Figure 4.3A). The subjects in the study of Carter *et al.* (2000b) were, like those in Jones and McConnell (1999), active but not highly trained. A higher $\dot{V}O_{2\,max}$ and LT in running compared to cycling would be expected in such a sample. Nevertheless, the use of the 'delta' concept to normalize the relative exercise intensities (see Chapter 1) was successful in equalizing the apparent metabolic stress of exercise (reflected by the end-exercise blood [lactate]). Interestingly, despite the similar exercise intensity, the $\dot{V}O_2$ slow component emerges at a lower relative $\dot{V}O_2$ for cycling than for running exercise, but accounts for a larger fraction of the end-exercise $\dot{V}O_2$.

Although running and cycling are both used for general fitness training, the difference in muscle contraction regime between them is obvious to anyone who has attempted to run or cycle any appreciable distance. Running involves relatively high impact forces during the stance phase, which results in eccentric work and a stretch-shortening cycle that very efficiently returns elastic energy during subsequent concentric work. Muscle activity during the stance phase seems to predominantly provide extensor support to allow the return of this elastic energy (Williams, 2000). The most vivid demonstration of this is the classic work of Dawson and Taylor (1973), which showed that $\dot{V}O_2$ in hopping kangaroos declined as treadmill speed was increased. One likely explanation for this is the storage and return of elastic energy in the exceptionally long hind limb tendons of these marsupials. In humans, manipulating the stiffness of the legs leads to marked and predictable changes in the mechanics and energetics of running. For example, McMahon *et al.* (1987) showed that increasing knee flexion during running ('Groucho' running) reduced the vertical ground reaction forces but increased the O_2 cost of running at any given speed (by ~20–30%).

In contrast to running, cycling involves little or no eccentric work or impact forces. Power output in cycling is determined by the product of torque applied to the crank and its angular velocity. Unlike the running action, where the stiffness of the legs (McMahon *et al.*, 1987; Ferris *et al.*, 1999) and range of motion of the lower limbs (Williams, 2000) can and do vary in order to minimize the

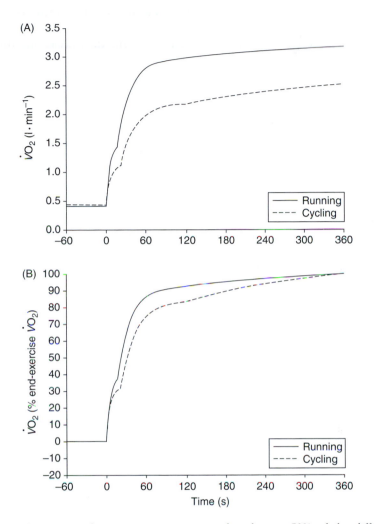

Figure 4.3 Superimposed responses to running and cycling at 50% of the difference between LT and $\dot{V}O_{2\,max}$. Curves are drawn from the mean data of Carter *et al.* (2000b). Panel A, absolute $\dot{V}O_2$ responses; panel B responses normalized to the end-exercise $\dot{V}O_2$. Notice the emergence of the $\dot{V}O_2$ slow component at a lower absolute $\dot{V}O_2$ in cycling (A) and the greater contribution it makes to the overall $\dot{V}O_2$ response (B).

O_2 cost of the work while the external power requirements increase, the cyclist cannot alter any biomechanical variables significantly to this end if a constant pedal rate is maintained. Instead, the only means by which power output can be increased is by increasing torque during the downstroke (Coyle *et al.*, 1991). This has important implications for the metabolic stress imposed during cycling because a greater torque will be accompanied by a greater intra-muscular pressure which could rhythmically impede blood flow (Rådegran and Saltin, 1998). At a constant pedal rate, therefore, a higher power output will be associated with a greater rate of ATP utilization, yet the duty cycle, and thus the duration of vascular occlusion (or partial occlusion), remains unaltered. The rate of fatigue may therefore be higher for cycling at any given relative exercise intensity, demanding additional motor unit recruitment as exercise proceeds. This may explain why the $\dot{V}O_2$ slow component develops at both a lower absolute $\dot{V}O_2$ and to a greater degree than during running in the same subjects (Carter *et al.*, 2000b; Hill *et al.*, 2003).

It has also been suggested that a larger $\dot{V}O_2$ slow component may occur in cycling due to the increased use of auxiliary muscles as the subject fatigues, when forceful gripping of the handlebars and rocking of the torso is sometimes observed (Jones and McConnell, 1999; Carter *et al.*, 2000). Although the vast majority of the slow component originates in the exercising limbs (Poole *et al.*, 1991), a significant portion of the $\dot{V}O_2$ response measured at the mouth during heavy and severe exercise may be attributable to forceful movements of the arms and torso during cycling as the subject fatigues. Indeed, Billat *et al.* (2000) reported that the addition of light arm crank exercise during severe cycle exercise actually reduced the magnitude of the $\dot{V}O_2$ slow component compared to when subjects gripped the handlebars. Furthermore, the preliminary work of Özyener *et al.* (1999) demonstrated significant desaturation of the forearm muscle during cycling at 80% of the difference between LT and $\dot{V}O_{2\,max}$, which was correlated with the amplitude of the $\dot{V}O_2$ slow component. Data such as these should be interpreted with caution, however, since it is not clear whether the desaturation observed reflected an increased O_2 extraction consequent to an increased arm muscle $\dot{V}O_2$, or a sympathetically mediated pressor reflex reducing arm blood flow and thus oxygenation (Hansen *et al.*, 1996) at a constant arm muscle $\dot{V}O_2$. Consistent with the latter interpretation, Musch *et al.* (1987) found a reduction in blood flow to the non-locomotive temporalis muscle during severe exercise in dogs. Indeed, it is common to observe a large $\dot{V}O_2$ slow component during cycling without any perceptible gripping of the handlebars or rocking of the torso, suggesting that the oxygenation data presented by Özyener *et al.* (1999) may indeed reflect a pressor reflex.

There are other differences between running and cycling exercise that could partially explain the differences in the $\dot{V}O_2$ kinetics between these exercise modes. For example, it is likely that O_2 consumption in the upper body makes a greater relative contribution to the whole body $\dot{V}O_2$ during running such that, for the same relative exercise intensity, the force and metabolic requirements are higher in the exercising muscles of the legs during cycle exercise. Again, this would be predicted to result in a greater recruitment of type II muscle fibres. Another difference is that both the LT (~75% vs ~55% $\dot{V}O_{2\,peak}$) and the critical power/velocity (CP/v; ~90% vs ~80% $\dot{V}O_{2\,peak}$) occur at a higher % $\dot{V}O_{2\,peak}$ in running compared to cycling, at least in individuals who are not specifically trained for either activity (Poole *et al.*, 1988; Jones and McConnell, 1999;

Smith and Jones, 2001). Therefore, if heavy or severe exercise is continued until $\dot{V}O_{2\,peak}$ is approached or attained, there will be more 'room' for the $\dot{V}O_2$ slow component to develop in cycling compared to running. This might also explain why highly trained runners are apparently able to attain a steady-state $\dot{V}O_2$ at running speeds requiring $\geq 90\%$ $\dot{V}O_{2\,peak}$ (Bernard *et al.*, 1998; Billat *et al.*, 1998a); unless the selected running speed clearly exceeds the CV, then no increase in $\dot{V}O_2$ with time should be expected after the initial 'steady-state' is achieved. The cause of the higher $\%$ $\dot{V}O_{2\,peak}$ at LT and CP/v in running compared to cycling is unclear, but might conceivably be related to the factors discussed previously, that is greater eccentric muscle action in running affording greater fatigue resistance, lower muscle forces, less impedance to blood flow and later or reduced recruitment of type II fibres.

Concentric vs eccentric exercise

As discussed earlier, the qualitatively similar but quantitatively dissimilar $\dot{V}O_2$ responses during running and cycling in the same subjects are, in part, reflective of fundamental differences in muscle contraction regimes between these two modes. Recent work by Perrey *et al.* (2001) supports this concept. In this study, subjects performed bouts of moderate and heavy exercise on an electrically braked cycle ergometer, which resulted in $\dot{V}O_2$ responses characteristic of these exercise intensity domains. However, when the same heavy intensity work rate (~ 317 W) was performed using a Monark ergometer attached to a motor which drove the pedals backwards, the $\dot{V}O_2$ was markedly lower than that noted during concentric exercise. In fact, the amplitude of the $\dot{V}O_2$ response to the heavy eccentric work rate was not different from concentric exercise performed at ~ 60 W. No $\dot{V}O_2$ slow component was noted in the eccentric exercise condition, suggesting that metabolic demand rather than external work rate, *per se*, is a crucial determinant of the presence or otherwise of the $\dot{V}O_2$ slow component (Henson *et al.*, 1989). Interestingly, the normalized integrated electromyogram only increased during the heavy concentric exercise bout in which a $\dot{V}O_2$ slow component was observed. These data suggest that the $\dot{V}O_2$ slow component is linked to increased motor unit recruitment with fatigue; the lower metabolic demand during eccentric exercise (Aura and Komi, 1986; Ryschon *et al.*, 1997) apparently limits the development of fatigue and the requirement for additional motor unit recruitment as exercise proceeds.

Pringle *et al.* (2002) reported results that were consistent with those of Perrey *et al.* (2001). In this study, subjects ran at the same relative exercise intensity with the treadmill set at 0% grade and with the treadmill set at 10% grade, in order to increase the proportion of concentric to eccentric muscle action (from $\sim 1{:}1$ to $\sim 9{:}1$; Minetti *et al.*, 1994). In keeping with the hypothesis, running at 10% grade was associated with a 40% greater amplitude of the $\dot{V}O_2$ slow component despite there being no difference in the amplitude of the primary $\dot{V}O_2$ response. From these studies, it is clear that differences in the muscle contraction regimen can impact significantly upon $\dot{V}O_2$ kinetics.

Posture and perfusion

It may be unreasonable to consider upright and prone or supine cycling as discrete exercise modalities. However, it is known that altering body position during the same exercise task can influence $\dot{V}O_2$ kinetics; indeed, studies that have altered muscle perfusion pressure by manipulating body position during exercise in this way have contributed to our understanding of the control and limitations to muscle $\dot{V}O_2$. The performance of exercise in the supine position (Convertino *et al.*, 1984; Hughson *et al.*, 1993; MacDonald *et al.*, 1998; Koga *et al.*, 1999) reduces muscle perfusion pressure by negating the 'gravitational assist' that exists during upright exercise. The reduction in the potential for muscle blood flow (and O_2 availability) in both supine (Convertino *et al.*, 1984; Hughson *et al.*, 1993; MacDonald *et al.*, 1998) and prone (Rossiter *et al.*, 2001, 2002) exercise generally results in a longer τ_p (i.e. slower kinetics) compared to upright exercise at the same work rate. The application of lower body negative pressure during supine exercise to facilitate muscle blood flow results in a speeding of the primary $\dot{V}O_2$ kinetics to a value that is similar to that observed during upright exercise (Hughson *et al.*, 1993). However, these observations should not, *per se*, be used as evidence for an O_2 delivery limitation to $\dot{V}O_2$ kinetics in the control (i.e. upright) position (see Chapter 12). For example, Williamson *et al.* (1996) demonstrated that the application of lower body positive pressure during recumbent cycle exercise did not alter the $\dot{V}O_2$ kinetics indicating that muscle blood flow is not limiting when the working muscle is below the level of the heart. It is also of interest that although slower $\dot{V}O_2$ kinetics during supine exercise are associated with slower estimated muscle blood flow kinetics compared to the upright condition, muscle blood flow kinetics are appreciably faster than $\dot{V}O_2$ kinetics in both conditions (MacDonald *et al.*, 1998, see Figure 4.4). Interestingly, Koga *et al.* (1999) recently reported that supine exercise resulted in a significantly longer mean response time for $\dot{V}O_2$ compared to the upright control condition during moderate and heavy exercise, but no difference in the τ_p between conditions. For heavy exercise, supine exercise caused a significant reduction of the primary component amplitude and a significant increase in the slow component amplitude, responses that are the exact opposite of the typical $\dot{V}O_2$ response observed when muscle blood flow is increased by the performance of prior heavy exercise (Burnley *et al.*, 2001, Chapter 10). These data may indicate that the amplitudes of the primary and slow components are themselves sensitive to alterations in muscle blood flow and that this may, in turn, influence motor unit recruitment patterns (see Chapter 12).

In an intriguing recent study, Koga *et al.* (2001) compared the $\dot{V}O_2$ response to one-legged and two-legged upright cycle exercise. A novel ergometer was constructed such that the activation of the leg muscles (as assessed by electromyography) was similar in the two conditions. The authors hypothesized that if O_2 availability were limiting in the two-legged cycling condition, then exercising a smaller muscle mass in the same exercise mode should result in faster primary component $\dot{V}O_2$ kinetics. The results demonstrated that the τ_p was not significantly

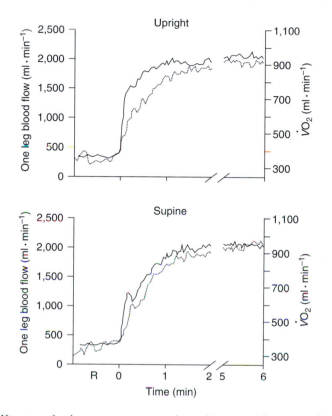

Figure 4.4 Kinetics of pulmonary oxygen uptake and leg blood flow during upright and supine cycle exercise. Figure reproduced with permission from MacDonald *et al.* (1998). Both $\dot{V}O_2$ kinetics (dotted lines) and leg blood flow kinetics (solid lines) were slower for supine compared to upright exercise. However, leg blood flow kinetics were faster than $\dot{V}O_2$ kinetics for both upright and supine exercise.

different between the two conditions for either moderate or heavy exercise (Figure 4.5). This finding is consistent with other studies that also demonstrated no difference in the τ_p when exercise requiring different lower limb muscle volumes were compared (Barstow *et al.*, 1994; Chilibeck *et al.*, 1996). However, the G_p was twice as large during one-legged as compared to two-legged cycling for both exercise intensities (i.e. ~20 vs ~10 ml·min^{-1}·W^{-1}). Although the primary component gain has been shown to exceed 10 ml·min^{-1}·W^{-1} for other types of exercise where a small muscle mass is engaged (Richardson *et al.*, 1993; Bell *et al.*, 2001a; Koppo *et al.*, 2002), it is possible that the elevated $\dot{V}O_2$ resulted, at least in part, from an additional O_2 cost of stabilising the trunk and upper body in the Koga *et al.* study.

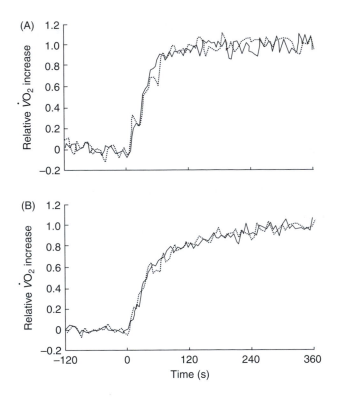

Figure 4.5 Pulmonary oxygen uptake response to one-legged (solid lines) and two-legged (dotted lines) cycle exercise of moderate (panel A) and heavy (panel B) intensity. Figure reproduced with permission from Koga *et al.* (2001). Data are scaled to the end-exercise $\dot{V}O_2$. Note that the $\dot{V}O_2$ kinetics are indistinguishable despite the potential for greater muscle perfusion in the one-legged cycle condition. These data suggest that muscle perfusion does not limit the $\dot{V}O_2$ on-kinetics during moderate or heavy intensity cycle exercise.

Arm exercise

A number of early studies established that, for the same absolute work rate, arm crank exercise (Figure 4.6) engenders a higher $\dot{V}O_2$ (Davies and Sargeant, 1974; Vokac *et al.*, 1975) and a slower kinetic response to the onset of work (Ceretelli *et al.*, 1977; Pendergast *et al.*, 1980) compared to leg exercise. However, because the $\dot{V}O_{2\,peak}$ and LT are also lower during arm compared to leg exercise, there tends to be a greater lactate accumulation for the same absolute work rate during arm exercise. Casaburi *et al.* (1992) compared responses to arm cranking and leg cycle exercise in the same subjects and reported that the apparently lower efficiency for arm cranking was correlated with the accumulation of lactate at lower work rates in this mode of exercise. However, even at work rates that did not elicit an elevated blood [lactate], the $\dot{V}O_2$ kinetics for arm exercise tended to be slower than for leg exercise.

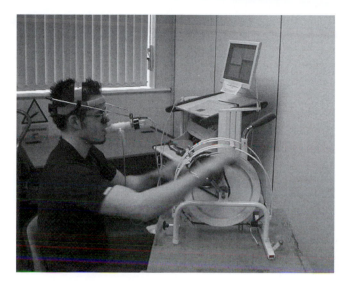

Figure 4.6 A volunteer performing arm crank exercise in the exercise physiology laboratory.

Recent studies have more clearly partitioned the $\dot{V}O_2$ response at the onset of arm exercise into its discrete components and compared these to the response at the onset of leg exercise of the same relative intensity (Koga *et al.*, 1996; Koppo *et al.*, 2002; Schneider *et al.*, 2002). Koppo *et al.* (1996) compared the $\dot{V}O_2$ kinetics during arm cranking (with the arms below the level of the heart) and leg cycle exercise at 90% $\dot{V}O_{2\,peak}$ (eliciting a blood [lactate] of ~8.5 mM in both exercise modes). The τ_p was significantly longer (~48 vs ~21 s), and the G_p was significantly greater (~12.1 vs ~9.2 ml·min^{-1}·W^{-1}) for arm exercise compared to leg exercise, although the contribution of the $\dot{V}O_2$ slow component to the end-exercise $\dot{V}O_2$ was similar (~20%) for the two exercise modes (Figure 4.7). Schneider *et al.* (2002) also reported significantly slower primary $\dot{V}O_2$ kinetics (arm: ~66 s vs leg: ~42 s) but found that the magnitude of the $\dot{V}O_2$ slow component was relatively higher (arm: ~24% vs leg: ~14%) during arm exercise compared to leg exercise at a relative exercise intensity of 50% Δ. During high-intensity front crawl swimming (an exercise mode that will primarily, though not exclusively, tax the upper body musculature) in a swim flume, the $\dot{V}O_2$ slow component has been reported to attain ~240 ml·min^{-1} (Demarie *et al.*, 2001). However, it is possible that a larger than normal fraction of this amplitude can be apportioned to the increased work of breathing against external resistance during swimming.

The cause of the slower $\dot{V}O_2$ kinetics in arm compared to leg exercise is unclear. On the one hand, there is some evidence from impedance cardiography that stroke volume is limited and that cardiac output kinetics might be slower for arm exercise (Koga *et al.*, 1996) such that the rate at which $\dot{V}O_2$ rises following

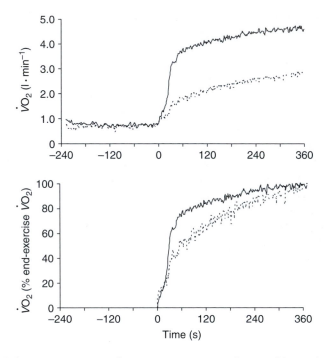

Figure 4.7 Pulmonary oxygen uptake response to arm cranking and leg cycle exercise in absolute terms (upper panel) and when scaled to the end-exercise $\dot{V}O_2$ (lower panel). Figure reproduced with permission from Koppo *et al.* (2002). Note the dramatically slower overall kinetics for arm exercise (dashed lines) compared to leg exercise (solid lines) despite the possibility that muscle perfusion was enhanced for arm crank exercise.

the onset of exercise is limited by muscle perfusion. In keeping with this suggestion, Hughson and Inman (1986) reported that $\dot{V}O_2$ kinetics following the onset of supine arm exercise were significantly faster when blood flow to non-working leg muscles was occluded in order to enhance O_2 availability to the arms. On the other hand, different studies suggest that muscle blood flow is higher per unit muscle mass for the same metabolic rate in arm compared to leg exercise (Clausen, 1976) and that there is no appreciable difference in muscle blood flow kinetics (Pendergast *et al.*, 1980), or oxygenation (Bhambhani *et al.*, 1998) between arm and leg exercise. Schneider *et al.* (2002) reported that although both heart rate kinetics and $\dot{V}O_2$ kinetics were slower during arm exercise than during cycling, there was no correlation between the time constant for the heart rate and the $\dot{V}O_2$ on-responses. Theoretically, if the arms are working below the level of the heart, one might expect enhanced perfusion in this small muscle group. In this case, the slower $\dot{V}O_2$ kinetics in arm exercise must be explained by factors other than inadequate O_2 delivery. One possible explanation is inherently slower kinetics as the result of the relatively high % type II fibres that exist in the muscles of the arms (Gollnick *et al.*, 1972; Johnson *et al.*, 1973), (see Chapters 11 and 12 for further discussion on the influence of muscle fibre type on $\dot{V}O_2$ kinetics), and/or earlier or greater recruitment of type II fibres as the result of higher intra-muscular tension development during arm exercise (Sawka *et al.*, 1983). Differences in the energetic properties of the muscle fibres contributing to force production could explain both the slower on-kinetics and the overall higher O_2 requirement during arm exercise compared to leg exercise. With this in mind, it is interesting to compare Figure 4.5 (from the one vs two-legged cycle study of Koga *et al.*, 2001) with Figure 4.7 (from the arm crank vs leg cycle study of Koppo *et al.*, 2002). In both situations, muscle perfusion should have been facilitated in the small muscle mass condition (i.e. one-legged cycling and arm cranking, respectively); however, only in the latter situation (i.e. arm vs leg exercise) would there have been a difference in muscle fibre type distribution. It is intriguing, therefore, that the $\dot{V}O_2$ kinetics were not altered with one-legged vs two-legged cycling but were substantially altered during arm exercise compared to leg exercise. This suggests that the fibre type characteristics of the muscle mass engaged in exercise may be an important determinant of the response profile (see Chapter 11 for discussion on the influence of muscle fibre type and recruitment patterns on $\dot{V}O_2$ kinetics).

In summary, it is clear that study of $\dot{V}O_2$ kinetics during different types of exercise has provided valuable insights into the physiological mechanisms which interact to determine the time course of the $\dot{V}O_2$ response in the transition to a higher metabolic rate. It is now apparent that the proportional contribution of concentric and eccentric muscle action during exercise has a significant influence on muscle efficiency and fatigue that, in turn, impact upon the parameters of the $\dot{V}O_2$ kinetics (Perrey *et al.*, 2001; Pringle *et al.*, 2002). In particular, the stretch-shortening cycle in running, perhaps along with the greater potential for making modifications to mechanics and differences in muscle tension and blood flow, appears to result in a reduction in the amplitude of the $\dot{V}O_2$ slow component (Jones and McConnell, 1999; Carter *et al.*, 2000b). Isometric muscle activity might make a small but important contribution to the development of the $\dot{V}O_2$ slow component during cycling (Billat *et al.*, 2000). Reducing muscle perfusion pressure by altering body position, for example during supine as compared to upright cycle exercise, results in an overall slowing of the $\dot{V}O_2$ response following the onset of exercise (Hughson *et al.*, 1993) along with an increased amplitude of the $\dot{V}O_2$ slow component (Koga *et al.*, 1999). However, attempts to improve muscle perfusion by reducing the volume of muscle mass engaged in the same type of exercise did not result in faster $\dot{V}O_2$ on-kinetics or a reduction in the slow component amplitude (Koga *et al.*, 2001). During arm crank exercise, the $\dot{V}O_2$ on-kinetics are slower and the O_2 cost of exercise is higher in comparison to leg cycle exercise (Casaburi *et al.*, 1992; Koppo *et al.*, 2002). Although possible differences in muscle training status, muscle pump effectiveness, and parasympathetic and sympathetic responses confound simple interpretation of these differences in $\dot{V}O_2$ kinetics between arm and leg exercise, the fact that $\dot{V}O_2$ kinetics are slower when muscle perfusion is likely to be higher during arm exercise, indicates that factors intrinsic to the muscle are of great importance in determining the time course of the $\dot{V}O_2$ response following the onset of exercise.

Glossary of terms

ATP	adenosine triphosphate
CP	critical power
CV	critical velocity
G_p	gain of the primary component (i.e. increase in $\dot{V}O_2$ per unit increase in external work rate)
LT	lactate threshold
O_2	oxygen
τ_p	time constant for the primary component (i.e. time to attain 63% of the final Phase II amplitude)
$\dot{V}O_2$	oxygen uptake

References

Åstrand, P.O. and Saltin, B. (1961). Maximal oxygen uptake and heart rate in various types of muscular activity. *Journal of Applied Physiology*, **16**, 977–81.

Aura, P.O. and Komi, P.V. (1986). Mechanical efficiency of pure positive and pure negative work with special reference to work intensity. *International Journal of Sports Medicine*, **7**, 44–9.

Barstow, T.J., Casaburi, R. and Wasserman, K. (1993). O_2 uptake kinetics and the O_2 deficit as related to exercise intensity and blood lactate. *Journal of Applied Physiology*, **75**, 755–62.

Barstow, T.J., Buchthal, S. Zanconato, S. and Cooper, D.M. (1994). Muscle energetics and pulmonary oxygen uptake kinetics during moderate exercise. *Journal of Applied Physiology*, **77**, 1742–9.

Barstow, T.J., Jones, A.M., Nguyen, P.H. and Casaburi, R. (1996). Influence of muscle fibre type and pedal frequency on oxygen uptake kinetics of heavy exercise. *Journal of Applied Physiology*, **81**, 1642–50.

Bell, C., Paterson, D.H., Kowalchuk, J.M., Moy, A.P., Thorp, D.B., Noble, E.G., Taylor, A.W., and Cunningham, D.A. (2001a). Determinants of oxygen uptake kinetics in older humans following single-limb endurance exercise training. *Experimental Physiology*, **86**, 659–65.

Bell, C., Paterson, D.H., Kowalchuk, J.M., Padilla, J. and Cunningham, D.A. (2001b). A comparison of modelling techniques used to characterise oxygen uptake kinetics during the on-transient of exercise. *Experimental Physiology*, **86**, 667–76.

Bernard, O., Maddio, F., Ouattara, S., Jimenez, C., Charpenet, A., Melin, B. and Bittel, J. (1998). Influence of the oxygen uptake slow component on the aerobic energy cost of high-intensity submaximal treadmill running in humans. *European Journal of Applied Physiology*, **78**, 578–85.

Bhambhani, Y., Maikala, R. and Buckley, S. (1998). Muscle oxygenation during incremental arm and leg exercise in men and women. *European Journal of Applied Physiology*, **78**, 422–31.

Billat, V., Binesse, V.M., Petit, B. and Koralsztein, J.P. (1998a). High level runners are able to maintain a $\dot{V}O_2$ steady-state below $\dot{V}O_{2\,max}$ in an all-out run over their critical velocity. *Archives of Physiology and Biochemistry*, **106**, 38–45.

Billat, V.L., Richard, R., Binesse, V.M., Koralsztein, J.P. and Haouzi, P. (1998b) The $\dot{V}O_2$ slow component for severe exercise depends on type of exercise and is not correlated with time to fatigue. *Journal of Applied Physiology*, **85**, 2118–24.

Billat, V.L., Hamard, L., Bocquet, V., Demarie, S., Beroni, M., Petit, B. and Koralsztein, J.P. (2000). Influence of light additional arm cranking exercise on the kinetics of $\dot{V}O_2$ in severe cycling exercise. *International Journal of Sports Medicine*, **21**, 344–50.

Burnley, M., Doust, J.H., Carter, H. and Jones, A.M. (2001). Effect of prior exercise and recovery duration on oxygen uptake kinetics during heavy exercise in humans. *Experimental Physiology*, **86**, 417–25.

Carter, H. and Jones, A.M. (1999). Mathematical modelling of oxygen uptake kinetics during treadmill running. *Journal of Physiology*, 518P, 98P.

Carter, H., Jones, A.M., Barstow, T.J., Burnley, M., Williams, C.A. and Doust, J.H. (2000a). Effect of endurance training on oxygen uptake kinetics during treadmill running. *Journal of Applied Physiology*, **89**, 1744–52.

Carter, H., Jones, A.M., Barstow, T.J., Burnley, M., Williams, C.A. and Doust, J.H. (2000b). Oxygen uptake kinetics in treadmill running and cycle ergometry: a comparison. *Journal of Applied Physiology*, **89**, 899–907.

Carter, H., Pringle, J.S.M., Jones, A.M. and Doust, J.H. (2002). Oxygen uptake kinetics during treadmill running across exercise intensity domains. *European Journal of Applied Physiology*, **86**, 347–54.

Casaburi, R., Barstow, T.J., Robinson, T. and Wasserman, K. (1992). Dynamic and steady state ventilatory and gas exchange responses to arm exercise. *Medicine and Science in Sports and Exercise*, **24**, 1365–74.

Cerretelli, P., Shindell, D., Pendergast, D. and Rennie, D.W. (1977). Oxygen uptake transients at the onset and offset of arm and leg work. *Respiration Physiology*, **30**, 81–97.

Cerretelli, P., Pendergast, D., Paganelli, W.C. and Rennie, D.W. (1979). Effects of specific muscle training on $\dot{V}O_2$ on-response and early blood lactate. *Journal of Applied Physiology*, **47**, 761–69.

Chilibeck, P.D., Paterson, D.H., Smith, W.D. and Cunningham, D.A. (1996). Cardiorespiratory kinetics during exercise of different muscle groups and mass in old and young. *Journal of Applied Physiology*, **81**, 1388–94.

Clausen, J.P. (1976). Circulatory adjustments to dynamic exercise and effect of physical training in normal subjects and in patients with coronary artery disease. *Progress in Cardiovascular Disease*, **18**, 459–95.

Convertino, V.A., Goldwater, D.J. and Sandler, H. (1984). Oxygen uptake kinetics of constant-load work: upright vs supine exercise. *Aviation Space Environmental Medicine*, **55**, 501–6.

Coyle, E.F., Feltner, M.E., Kautz, S.A., Hamilton, M.T., Montain, S.J., Baylor, A.M., Abraham, L.D. and Petrek, G.W. (1991). Physiological and biomechanical factors associated with elite endurance cycling performance. *Medicine and Science in Sports and Exercise*, **23**, 93–107.

Davies, C.T.M. and Sargeant, A.J. (1974). Physiological responses to standardised arm work. *Ergonomics*, **17**, 41–9.

Dawson, T.J. and Taylor, C.R. (1973). Energetic cost of locomotion in kangaroos. *Nature*, **246**, 313–4.

Demarie, S., Sardella, F., Billat, V., Magini, W. and Faina, M. (2001). The $\dot{V}O_2$ slow component in swimming. *European Journal of Applied Physiology*, **84**, 95–9.

Ferris, D.P., Liang, K. and Farley, C.T. (1999). Runners adjust leg stiffness for their first step on a new running surface. *Journal of Biomechanics*, **32**, 787–94.

Fujihara, Y., Hilderbrandt, J.R. and Hilderbrandt, J. (1973). Cardiorespiratory transients in exercising man I. Tests of superposition. *Journal of Applied Physiology*, **35**, 58–67.

Gaesser, G.A. and Poole, D.C. (1996). The slow component of oxygen uptake kinetics in humans. *Exercise and Sport Sciences Reviews*, **24**, 35–70.

Gollnick, P.D., Armstrong, R.B., Saubert, C.W., Piehl, K. and Saltin, B. (1972). Enzyme activity and fiber composition of skeletal muscle of untrained and trained men. *Journal of Applied Physiology*, **33**, 312–19.

Grassi, B., Gladden, L.B., Samaja, M., Stary, C.M. and Hogan, M.C. (1998). Faster adjustment of O_2 delivery does not affect O_2 on-kinetics in isolated in situ canine muscle. *Journal of Applied Physiology*, **85**, 1394–403.

Hansen, J., Thomas, G.D., Harris, S.A., Parsons, W.J. and Victor, R.G. (1996). Differential sympathetic neural control of oxygenation in resting and exercising human skeletal muscle. *Journal of Clinical Investigations*, **98**, 584–96.

Henry, F.M. (1951). Aerobic oxygen consumption and alactic debt in muscular work. *Journal of Applied Physiology*, **3**, 427–38.

Henson, L.C., Poole, D.C. and Whipp, B.J. (1989). Fitness as a determinant of oxygen uptake response to constant-load exercise. *European Journal of Applied Physiology*, **59**, 21–8.

Hill, A.V. and Lupton, H. (1923). Muscular exercise, lactic acid, and the supply and utilisation of oxygen. *Quarterly Journal of Medicine*, **16**, 135–71.

Hill, D.W., Halcomb, J.N. and Stevens, E.C. (2003). Oxygen uptake kinetics during severe intensity running and cycling. *European Journal of Applied Physiology*, **89**(6), 612–8.

Howley, E.T., Bassett, D.R. and Welch, H.G. (1995). Criteria for maximal oxygen uptake: review and commentary. *Medicine and Science in Sports and Exercise*, **27**, 1292–301.

Hughson, R.L. and Inman, M.D. (1986). Faster kinetics of $\dot{V}O_2$ during arm exercise with circulatory occlusion of the legs. *International Journal of Sports Medicine*, **7**, 22–5.

Hughson, R.L., Cochrane, J.E. and Butler, G.C. (1993). Faster O_2 uptake kinetics at onset of supine exercise with than without lower body negative pressure. *Journal of Applied Physiology*, **75**, 1962–7.

Hughson, R.L., Shoemaker, J.K., Tschakovsky, M.E. and Kowalchuk, J.M. (1996). Dependence of muscle $\dot{V}O_2$ on blood flow dynamics at onset of forearm exercise. *Journal of Applied Physiology*, **81**, 1619–26.

Johnson, M.A., Polgar, J., Weightman, D. and Appleton, D. (1973). Data on the distribution of fiber types in thirty-six human muscles: an autopsy study. *Journal of Neurological Science*, **18**, 111–29.

Jones, A.M. and McConnell, A.M. (1999). Effect of exercise modality on oxygen uptake kinetics during heavy exercise. *European Journal of Applied Physiology*, **80**, 213–19.

Koga, S., Shiojiri, T., Shibasaki, M., Fukuba, Y., Fukuoka, Y. and Kondo, N. (1996). Kinetics of oxygen uptake and cardiac output at onset of arm exercise. *Respiration Physiology*, **103**, 195–202.

Koga, S., Shiojiri, T., Shibasaki, M., Kondo, N., Fukuba, Y. and Barstow, T.J. (1999). Kinetics of oxygen uptake during supine and upright exercise. *Journal of Applied Physiology*, **87**, 253–60.

Koga, S., Barstow, T.J., Shiojiri, T., Takaishi, T., Fukuba, Y., Shibasaki, M. and Poole, D.C. (2001). Effect of muscle mass on $\dot{V}O_2$ kinetics at the onset of work. *Journal of Applied Physiology*, **90**, 461–8.

Koppo, K., Bouckaert, J. and Jones, A.M. (2002). Oxygen uptake kinetics during high-intensity arm and leg exercise. *Respiration Physiology and Neurobiology*, **133**, 241–50.

Langsetmo, I., Weigle, G.E., Fedde, M.R., Erickson, H.H., Barstow, T.J. and Poole, D.C. (1997). V̇O$_2$ kinetics in the horse during moderate and heavy exercise. *Journal of Applied Physiology*, **83**, 1235–41.

Lamarra, N. (1990). Variables, constants, and parameters: clarifying the system structure. *Medicine and Science in Sports and Exercise*, **22**, 88–95.

Linnarsson, D. (1974). Dynamics of pulmonary gas exchange and heart rate changes at start and end of exercise. *Acta Physiologica Scandinavica*, **415**, 1–68.

MacDonald, M.J., Shoemaker, J.K., Tschakovsky, M.E. and Hughson, R.L. (1998). Alveolar oxygen uptake and femoral artery blood flow dynamics in upright and supine leg exercise in humans. *Journal of Applied Physiology*, **85**, 1622–8.

McMahon, T.A., Valiant, G. and Frederick, E.C. (1987). Groucho running. *Journal of Applied Physiology*, **62**, 2326–37.

Margaria, R., Mangili, F., Cuttica, F. and Cerretelli, P. (1965). The kinetics of oxygen consumption at the onset of muscular exercise in man. *Ergonomics*, **8**, 49–54.

Minetti, A.E., Ardigo, L.P. and Saibene, F. (1994). Mechanical determinants of the minimum energy cost of gradient running in humans. *Journal of Experimental Biology*, **195**, 211–25.

Musch, T.I., Friedman, D.B., Pitekki, K.H., Haidet, G.C., Stray-Gunderson, J., Mitchell, J.H. and Ordway, G.A. (1987). Regional distribution of blood flow of dogs during graded dynamic exercise. *Journal of Applied Physiology*, **63**(6), 2269–77.

Özyener, F., Ward, S.A. and Whipp, B.J. (1999). Contribution of arm muscle oxygenation to the slow component of pulmonary oxygen uptake during leg-cycle ergometry. *Journal of Physiology*, **515**, 72P.

Özyener, F., Rossiter, H.B, Ward, S.A. and Whipp, B.J. (2001). Influence of exercise intensity on the on- and off-transient kinetics of pulmonary oxygen uptake in humans. *Journal of Physiology*, **533**(Pt 3), 891–902.

Paterson, D.H. and Whipp, B.J. (1991). Asymmetries of oxygen uptake transients at the on- and offset of heavy exercise in humans. *Journal of Physiology*, **443**, 575–86.

Pendergast, D.R. (1989). Cardiovascular, respiratory, and metabolic responses to upper body exercise. *Medicine and Science in Sports and Exercise*, **21**(5 suppl), S121–5.

Pendergast, D.R., Shindell, D., Cerretelli, P. and Rennie, D.W. (1980). Role of central and peripheral circulatory adjustments in oxygen transport at the onset of exercise. *International Journal of Sports Medicine*, **1**, 160–70.

Perrey, S., Betik, A., Candau, R., Rouillon, J.D. and Hughson, R.L. (2001). Comparison of oxygen uptake kinetics during concentric and eccentric cycle exercise. *Journal of Applied Physiology*, **91**, 2135–42.

Perrey, S., Candau, R., Borrani, F., Millet, G.Y. and Rouillon, J.D. (2002). Recovery kinetics of oxygen uptake following severe-intensity exercise in runners. *Journal of Sports Medicine and Physical Fitness*, **42**, 381–8.

Poole, D.C., Ward, S.A., Gardner, G.W. and Whipp, B.J. (1988). Metabolic and respiratory profile of the upper limit for prolonged exercise in man. *Ergonomics*, **31**, 1265–79.

Poole, D.C., Schaffartzik, W., Knight, D.R., Derion, T., Kennedy, B., Guy, H., Prediletto, R. and Wagner, P.D. (1991). Contribution of the exercising legs to the slow component of oxygen uptake kinetics in humans. *Journal of Applied Physiology*, **71**, 1245–53.

Pringle, J.S.M., Carter, H., Doust, J.H. and Jones, A.M. (2002). Oxygen uptake kinetics during horizontal and uphill treadmill running. *European Journal of Applied Physiology*, **88**, 163–9.

Rådegran, G. and Saltin, B. (1998). Muscle blood flow at onset of dynamic exercise in humans. *American Journal of Physiology*, **274**, H314–22.

Richardson, R.S., Poole, D.C., Knight, D.R., Kurdak, S.S., Hogan, M.C., Grassi, B. Johnson, E.C., Kendrick, K.F., Erickson, B.K. and Wagner, P.D. (1993). High muscle blood flow in man: is maximal O_2 extraction compromised? *Journal of Applied Physiology*, **75**, 1911–16.

Rossiter, H.B., Ward, S.A., Kowalchuk, J.M., Howe, F.A., Griffiths, J.R. and Whipp, B.J. (2001). Effects of prior exercise on oxygen uptake and phosphocreatine kinetics during high-intensity knee-extension exercise in humans. *Journal of Physiology*, **537**, 291–303.

Rossiter, H.B., Ward, S.A., Kowalchuk, J.M., Howe, F.A., Griffiths, J.R. and Whipp, B.J. (2002). Dynamic asymmetry of phosphocreatine concentration and O_2 uptake between the on- and off-transients of moderate- and high-intensity exercise in humans. *Journal of Physiology*, **541**, 991–1002.

Ryschon, T.W., Fowler, M.D., Wysong, R.E., Anthony, A. and Balaban, R.S. (1997). Efficiency of human skeletal muscle in vivo: comparison of isometric, concentric, and eccentric muscle action. *Journal of Applied Physiology*, **83**, 867–74.

Sawka, M.N., Foley, M.E., Pimental, N.A., Toner, M.M. and Pandolf, K.B. (1983). Determination of maximal aerobic power during upper-body exercise. *Journal of Applied Physiology*, **54**, 113–17.

Schneider, D.A., Wing, A.N. and Morris, N.R. (2002). Oxygen uptake and heart rate kinetics during heavy exercise: a comparison between arm cranking and leg cycling. *European Journal of Applied Physiology*, **88**, 100–6.

Shoemaker, J.K., Hodge, L. and Hughson, R.L. (1994). Cardiorespiratory kinetics and femoral artery blood velocity during dynamic knee extension exercise. *Journal of Applied Physiology*, **77**, 2625–32.

Smith, C.G.M. and Jones, A.M. (2001). The relationship between critical velocity, maximal lactate steady state velocity, and lactate turnpoint velocity in runners. *European Journal of Applied Physiology*, **85**, 19–26.

Tschakovsky, M.E. and Hughson, R.L. (1999). Interaction of factors determining oxygen uptake at the onset of exercise. *Journal of Applied Physiology*, **86**, 1101–13.

Vokac, H., Bell, E., Bautz-Holter, E. and Rodahl, K. (1975). Oxygen uptake/heart rate relationship in leg and arm exercise, sitting and standing. *Journal of Applied Physiology*, **39**, 54–9.

Whipp, B.J. (1994). The slow component of O_2 uptake kinetics during heavy exercise. *Medicine and Science in Sports and Exercise*, **26**, 1319–26.

Whipp, B.J. and Wasserman, K. (1972). Oxygen uptake kinetics for various intensities of constant load work. *Journal of Applied Physiology*, **33**, 351–6.

Whipp, B.J., Ward, S.A., Lamarra, N., Davis, J.A. and Wasserman, K. (1982). Parameters of ventilatory and gas exchange dynamics during exercise. *Journal of Applied Physiology*, **52**, 1506–13.

Williams, C.A., Carter, H., Jones, A.M. and Doust, J.H. (2001). Oxygen uptake kinetics during treadmill running in boys and men. *Journal of Applied Physiology*, **90**, 1700–6.

Williams, K.R. (2000). The dynamics of running. In V.R. Zatsiorski (Ed.) *Biomechanics in Sport*. Blackwell Science, London, pp. 161–83.

Williamson, J.W., Raven, P.B. and Whipp, B.J. (1996). Unaltered oxygen uptake kinetics at exercise onset with lower-body positive pressure in humans. *Experimental Physiology*, **81**, 695–705.

5 $\dot{V}O_2$ dynamics in different species

Casey A. Kindig, Brad J. Behnke and David C. Poole

Introduction

This book is focused principally on understanding $\dot{V}O_2$ kinetics in man. Where experiments on animals or animal muscles are presented within the various chapters, it is usually because the experimental modality is either not feasible, or cannot be conducted ethically, in humans. In contrast, this chapter adopts a comparative physiological approach that explores $\dot{V}O_2$ kinetics across extremely diverse species. As detailed in Chapter 15, $\dot{V}O_2$ kinetics are generally faster in fitter humans when compared with their sedentary or less-fit counterparts as judged by $\dot{V}O_{2\,max.}$ Moreover, after exercise training the speeding of $\dot{V}O_2$ kinetics in humans is associated with an increased $\dot{V}O_{2\,max.}$ These latter observations have been made over a relatively modest range (two- and three-fold, i.e. $20\text{--}70\,ml\cdot min^{-1}\cdot kg^{-1}$) of $\dot{V}O_{2\,max}$ values. By comparison, judicious selection of the poorly aerobic lungless salamander ($\dot{V}O_{2\,max}$ $<10\,ml\cdot min^{-1}\cdot kg^{-1}$) and the Thoroughbred horse (Figure 5.1) or deer mouse ($\dot{V}O_{2\,max}$ $160\text{--}220\,ml\cdot min^{-1}\cdot kg^{-1}$) permits analysis of this relationship over a much broader range of absolute and mass-specific $\dot{V}O_{2\,max}$ values (Figure 5.2). These species and several of intermediate $\dot{V}O_{2\,max}$ are examined in this chapter.

Application of rapidly responding gas analysers and development of high capacity ($\sim 10{,}000\,l\cdot min^{-1}$) flow-by or bias flow systems has facilitated resolution of $\dot{V}O_2$ kinetics in the running horse with a fidelity approaching that possible in humans. The results of these experiments are detailed later and suggest that whilst the magnitude and speed of the $\dot{V}O_2$ response is very different from that found in humans, there are substantial commonalities between these two species. These include the presence of (1) a discernible Phase I and Phase II response, and (2) a $\dot{V}O_2$ slow component that arises within 1–2 min after increasing running speed within the heavy or severe exercise intensity domains.

A further surprising feature of the on-transient $\dot{V}O_2$ response to moderate intensity exercise in the horse is preservation of the mono-exponential kinetics. This response occurs despite the presence of a massive ($\sim 14\,kg$) spleen, contraction of which at exercise onset can almost double arterial haemoglobin concentration and therefore arterial O_2 carrying capacity within 20–60 s.

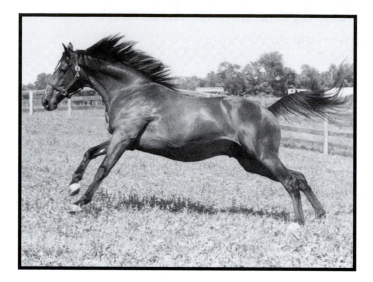

Figure 5.1 The Thoroughbred horse (*Equus caballus*), which through thousands of years of selective breeding, is one of the top athletes in the world. This animal has achieved maximal $\dot{V}O_2$ values exceeding 200 ml · min^{-1} · kg^{-1} (Young *et al.*, 2002).

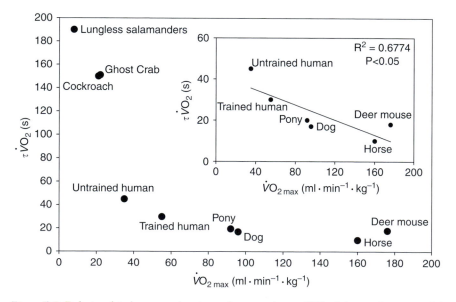

Figure 5.2 Relationship between the time taken to achieve 63% of the total increase (τ) of O_2 uptake and the mass-specific $\dot{V}O_{2\,max}$ in the different species featured in this chapter. These animals evidence a range of $\dot{V}O_{2\,max}$ values from <10 to ~180 ml · min^{-1} · kg^{-1}. Inset demonstrates the correlation between $\tau \dot{V}O_2$ and $\dot{V}O_{2\,max}$ in the mammalian species.

It is beyond the scope of this chapter to detail the specific anatomy and physiology of O_2 transport among all species presented herein. However, where pertinent to the central issue of understanding the possible control mechanisms for $\dot{V}O_2$ kinetics, discrete anatomical features will be explored briefly.

Horse

The equine (*Equus caballus*, Figure 5.1) athlete is distinctive in that it has been bred for its running performance for over 6,000 years. This has ultimately resulted in an animal (horse and pony) with a remarkably high oxidative metabolic capacity. From several perspectives, the horse may well be the most impressive aerobic athlete on the planet. In concert with the relationship between mass-specific $\dot{V}O_{2\,max}$ and the speed of the $\dot{V}O_2$ kinetics at exercise onset demonstrated in humans (Chapter 15), the Thoroughbred horse is capable of achieving maximal $\dot{V}O_2$ values near 200 ml $\cdot$ min^{-1} $\cdot$ kg^{-1} and the speed of the $\dot{V}O_2$ kinetic response is correspondingly rapid (Figure 5.2). $\dot{V}O_2$ kinetics were first measured in the pony in 1984 (Forster *et al.*, 1984) and subsequent investigations have studied $\dot{V}O_2$ kinetics in Standardbred, Thoroughbred and Quarter horses. However, it was not until recently, that a rigorous investigation was undertaken to formally characterize equine $\dot{V}O_2$ kinetics (Langsetmo *et al.*, 1997).

$\dot{V}O_2$ kinetics in the horse

While previous investigations had studied $\dot{V}O_2$ kinetics in equids (e.g. Rose *et al.*, 1989; Hodgson *et al.*, 1990), prior to the work of Langsetmo and colleagues (1997), $\dot{V}O_2$ was not measured rapidly enough to accurately assess $\dot{V}O_2$ kinetics. By obtaining gas exchange data on a second-by-second basis and studying $\dot{V}O_2$ kinetics strictly within the moderate and heavy work domains while horses were running on a high-speed treadmill, several principal findings were elucidated (Figures 5.3–5.5). First, in the moderate domain, $\dot{V}O_2$ kinetics were well fit by a two-phase exponential model (cardiodynamic + primary phases), the primary phase of which was very rapid (the τ was ~10 s). Second, for heavy exercise, the primary phase τ was still quite rapid (i.e. ~21 s) but markedly slowed compared with that during moderate running. Additionally, heavy exercise was attended (with one exception in that investigation) by a $\dot{V}O_2$ slow component which was detectable from ~135 s post-exercise onset.

The incredibly fast $\dot{V}O_2$ kinetics reported by Langsetmo *et al.* (1997) have subsequently been replicated by Geor and colleagues (2000) (Figure 5.6). In that investigation, in which Standardbred horses were transitioned almost instantaneously from a walk to supramaximal treadmill speeds (i.e. speeds 15% greater than that attained during $\dot{V}O_{2\,max}$ elicited via ramp protocol), the $\dot{V}O_2$ primary τ (Phase II) was ~23 s. This τ was shortened significantly to ~16 s when the exercise trial was preceded by a warm-up. For the horses in that investigation, the absolute $\dot{V}O_2$ approached 60 l $\cdot$ min^{-1} (150 ml $\cdot$ min^{-1} $\cdot$ kg^{-1})!

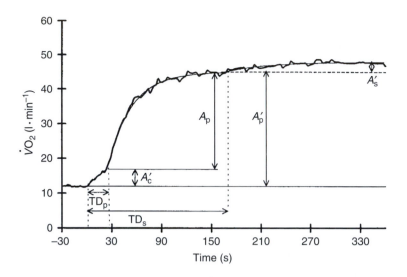

Figure 5.3 The dynamic profile of O_2 uptake ($\dot{V}O_2$) in the Thoroughbred horse at the onset of heavy-intensity exercise. Note the profile is very similar, albeit more rapid, than that of the human. Specifically, at exercise onset there is an initial cardio-dynamic phase (Phase I), followed by the primary fast exponential increase (Phase II). A'_c, A'_p, and A'_s denote the amplitudes of Phase I, Phase II and the slow component, respectively. TD_p and TD_s denote the time delays prior to the start of Phase II and the slow component. Adapted from Langsetmo *et al.* (1997).

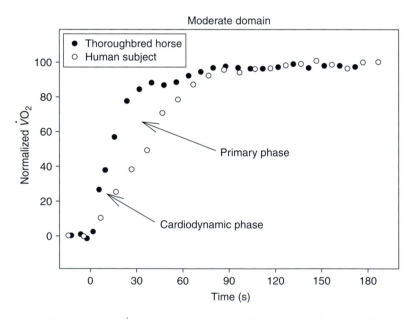

Figure 5.4 Comparison of $\dot{V}O_2$ kinetics (normalized) between the horse and human for moderate-intensity exercise. Note that the horse demonstrated much more rapid dynamics than the human, however, the horse still demonstrates three distinct phases (i.e. Phase I – cardiodynamic phase, Phase II – primary phase, and Phase III – steady state).

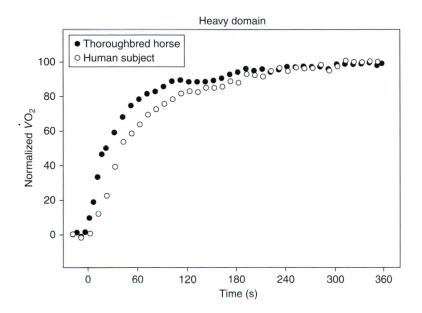

Figure 5.5 Comparison of $\dot{V}O_2$ kinetics (normalized) between the horse and human for heavy-intensity exercise. Note that the horse demonstrated much more rapid dynamics than the human and both horse and human demonstrate a slow-component at roughly the same point of exercise (~160–180 s after exercise onset).

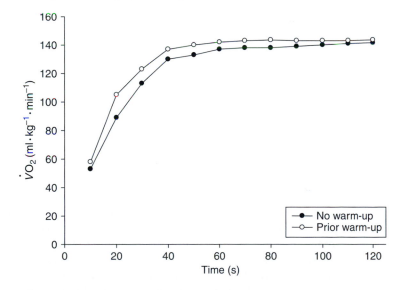

Figure 5.6 Effect of a warm-up exercise on $\dot{V}O_2$ kinetics in the moderate-intensity domain. By 'warming-up' or 'priming' the muscles with prior exercise, in the subsequent bout of exercise (of the same intensity) the speed of the $\dot{V}O_2$ kinetics is increased (hollow circles). Adapted from Geor et al. (2000).

$\dot{V}O_2$ kinetics in the pony

Equus caballus represents a unique diversity of within-species variability. Specifically, whereas the Thoroughbred and Standardbred horse have been bred over generations to attain peak running performance and correspondingly impressive aerobic capacities, other breeds such as the Shetland pony have not. Nevertheless, while the pony is considered less aerobically capable than its equine counterparts, the $\dot{V}O_{2\,max}$ of the pony can exceed $100\;ml \cdot min^{-1} \cdot kg^{-1}$ with training (Katz *et al.*, 2000). As mentioned earlier, the first study demonstrating the $\dot{V}O_2$ kinetic response for *Equus caballus* was actually performed on Welsh–Shetland mixed-breed ponies (Forster *et al.*, 1984). The ponies were run at varying speeds and inclines reaching 6 mph on a 3% grade. While the data were not modelled using least-squares iterative processes, in all instances, 95% of the final exercising $\dot{V}O_2$ response was reached within 60 s. Taking into account the initial time delay (cardiodynamic phase) and onset of the slow component (which was clearly evident), the τ can be approximated at ~20 s. Similarly, Powers and colleagues (1987) demonstrated in Welsh–Shetland ponies that the time to 50% of the rise in $\dot{V}O_2$ from rest to 2.6 mph ($70\;m \cdot min^{-1}$, 7% grade ~20% $\dot{V}O_{2\,max}$ for ponies of this size, Katz *et al.* 2000) was ~13.5 s. As the ponies in both of investigations reached a $\dot{V}O_2$ of only ~3 $l \cdot min^{-1}$ at the highest work intensity, this work rate was obviously well within their moderate domain.

Comparison of the horse and human

Despite the capacity to reach maximal relative $\dot{V}O_2$ values two- to three-fold greater than humans, the rapidity with which the horse responds energetically at the transition to higher running speeds is generally far superior to its human counterpart (Figures 5.3 and 5.4). Nonetheless, key underlying features of the equine $\dot{V}O_2$ kinetic response to an elevation in metabolic demand are remarkably similar to that in humans.

Figure 5.4 demonstrates $\dot{V}O_2$ kinetics normalized to end-exercise values in a running horse and a human performing cycle ergometer exercise across the transition to moderate-intensity exercise. While both the horse and human have proportionately sized cardiodynamic and primary phase amplitudes, the most striking feature is how much more rapid the rise in $\dot{V}O_2$ is in the horse compared to the human. Again, in the heavy domain (Figure 5.5), key features of the $\dot{V}O_2$ on-kinetic response (i.e. three distinct phases) are similar between the horse and human. As depicted in Figure 5.5, $\dot{V}O_2$ onset kinetics in the Thoroughbred horse are significantly faster than that reported in the human. However, Langsetmo *et al.* (1997) demonstrated a clear slowing of the equine $\dot{V}O_2$ on-kinetic response when running at speeds in the heavy vs moderate domain. Whether this slowing of the $\dot{V}O_2$ kinetics from moderate to heavy exercise occurs in humans is controversial (see Chapter 12). Specifically, a number of studies demonstrate that the speed of the primary $\dot{V}O_2$ amplitude rise is unchanged as work intensity increases from moderate to heavy in humans (e.g. Casaburi *et al.*, 1979; Barstow and Mole, 1991; Barstow *et al.*, 1993; Ozyener *et al.*, 2001; Rossiter *et al.*, 2002). In contrast, several investigations also studying human subjects have reported slowed $\dot{V}O_2$ on-transient kinetics in response to heavy compared with moderate exercise (e.g. Hughson and Morissey, 1982; Paterson and Whipp, 1991; Engelen *et al.*, 1996; Gerbino *et al.*, 1996; MacDonald *et al.*, 1997; Koga *et al.*, 1999; Carter *et al.*, 2002). It is certainly possible that oxidative capacity and/or fitness level of the subjects may play an important role in these disparate findings. However, with respect to the horse, its reliance on a contractile spleen to increase O_2 delivery via an augmented RBC influx during periods of increased metabolic demand may place a constraint on the speed of $\dot{V}O_2$ kinetics in the heavy domain that is unique to this species. There may also be fibre type recruitment profiles that may slow the $\dot{V}O_2$ response to heavy exercise that cannot be discounted at the present time. As shown in Figures 5.3 and 5.5, a clear slow component is evidenced in the equine profile, the magnitude of which is proportionately similar to that seen in humans. Interestingly, Langsetmo *et al.* (1997) reported that one of the horses did not display a slow component during heavy domain running. It is also true that some humans do not evidence a slow component during heavy exercise.

Why are $\dot{V}O_2$ kinetics so fast in the horse?

As mentioned previously, the Thoroughbred racehorse is a superlative model of mammalian oxidative function. The immense capacity to deliver and utilize O_2 culminates, ultimately, in prodigious maximal $\dot{V}O_2$ values. This demands a superb integration of pulmonary, cardiovascular and muscle function. Specifically, the horse has a large heart-to-body ratio which is capable of generating extraordinary cardiac outputs in excess of $300 \, l \cdot min^{-1}$ or $600 \, ml \cdot min^{-1} \cdot kg^{-1}$ (Kindig *et al.*, 2000). To place this in perspective, one would be hard-pressed to get half this flow of water (let alone blood with a haematocrit of ~70%) out of a high-pressure hose with the diameter of an equine atrioventricular valve! Next, the pulmonary system must be capable of achieving alveolar ventilation rates that will facilitate oxygenation of the prodigious cardiac output in order to maintain arterial O_2 saturation. To this end, during strenuous exercise the horse is capable of total ventilations in excess of $1700 \, l \cdot min^{-1}$ (estimated alveolar ventilation $>1400 \, l \cdot min^{-1}$, Butler *et al.*, 1993). However, despite these ventilatory rates, severe arterial hypoxemia nearing 60 Torr is incurred during intense running (Butler *et al.*, 1993; Kindig *et al.*, 2000). In addition to the short RBC transit times in the pulmonary capillaries, one contributing factor to this hypoxemia is the fact that the blood–gas barrier has to be thicker (~1 μm) than that of other mammals (~0.3 μm in man). This additional thickness helps protect against the very high pulmonary arterial pressures which may reach values in excess of 120 Torr during maximal exercise. Despite the thicker blood–gas barrier that must impede gas exchange, racehorses do experience exercise-induced pulmonary haemorrhage at the gallop to an extent that exceeds that found in any other species. Thus, the blood–gas barrier is effectively thickened by plasma exudates and RBCs in the alveolar space. In addition and as mentioned earlier, the horse (as well as some canine breeds) has a contractile spleen which is capable of increasing the number of circulating RBCs which dramatically augments O_2 carrying capacity (Persson *et al.*, 1973). Finally, in the Thoroughbred racehorse muscle comprises ~50% of the body mass and that muscle contains a dense capillary network and a correspondingly high mitochondrial volume density (e.g. Hoppeler *et al.*, 1987; Armstrong *et al.*, 1992).

Applications

It is apparent that the racehorse has evolved into a muscle, heart and lung machine capable of performing athletically at the highest level. As the horse adapts well to treadmill running and can tolerate headgear necessary to gather gas exchange data as well as arterial and venous lines even while running at speeds well in excess of 30 mph, the horse represents an excellent model to study control of $\dot{V}O_2$ kinetics and provides insights germane to the understanding of metabolic control and performance in humans and other species.

For example, the horse was used recently to elucidate issues key to understanding the mechanistic bases of the metabolic inertia manifested at exercise onset. Horses performed heavy-intensity exercise on a treadmill under control and systemic nitric oxide synthase (NOS) inhibition conditions. Whilst NO is necessary to attain peak cardiac outputs and systemic O_2 delivery in the horse (Kindig *et al.*, 2000), it also inhibits mitochondrial oxygen consumption by binding to cytochrome c oxidase. Kindig and colleagues (2001) demonstrated, in the face of a reduced cardiac output and presumably muscle blood flow, that $\dot{V}O_2$ kinetics were speeded significantly with NOS inhibition. Additionally, NOS inhibition resulted in an earlier onset of the slow component. These findings suggest that NO-inhibition of the mitochondrial O_2 consumption may contribute importantly to the mitochondrial inertia seen at the transition to increased metabolic demands. Interestingly, at the onset of heavy exercise, NOS inhibition sped $\dot{V}O_2$ kinetics near that seen during moderate-intensity running. Subsequent research shown in Figure 5.7, demonstrated that NOS inhibition sped $\dot{V}O_2$ kinetics ~30% at the onset of moderate running (NOS inhibition $\tau = 12$ s vs control = 18 s) (Kindig *et al.*, 2002). This represents some of the first data demonstrating that the rapidity of $\dot{V}O_2$ kinetics can be enhanced during moderate-intensity exercise.

Dog

The domestic dog (*Canidae*), like the horse, represents another extreme athlete, with $\dot{V}O_{2\,max}$ values almost double that of humans (i.e. ~100 ml $O_2 \cdot min^{-1} \cdot kg^{-1}$; Musch *et al.*, 1986). In addition, the dog as an experimental modality has played a pivotal role in filling the void between isolated single-fibre (usually amphibian) and whole organism (e.g. human) preparations. Specifically, canine $\dot{V}O_2$ kinetics have been studied within both the whole body and surgically isolated but otherwise intact isolated muscle groups. Whereas pulmonary and muscle $\dot{V}O_2$ can be measured simultaneously in the human (Andersen and Saltin, 1985;

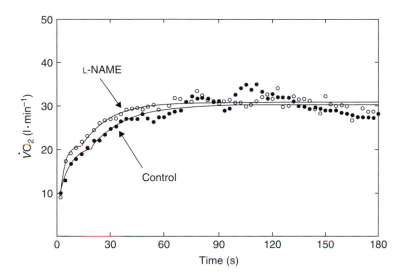

Figure 5.7 Effect of L-NAME (an inhibitor of nitric oxide synthase) administration on $\dot{V}O_2$ kinetics. L-NAME alleviated the NO-inhibition of mitochondrial O_2 consumption, thereby reducing the metabolic inertia at exercise onset and speeding $\dot{V}O_2$ kinetics. Adapted from Kindig *et al.* (2002).

Richardson *et al.*, 1995; Grassi *et al.*, 1996), the experimental conditions (e.g. blood O_2 content, blood flow dynamics) can be controlled to a greater extent in dog preparations. Accordingly, a substantial portion of our understanding of the regulation of $\dot{V}O_2$ kinetics has stemmed from research using the dog.

Whole body vs isolated muscle preparations

$\dot{V}O_2$ kinetics have been studied extensively in dog locomotory muscle groups (Piiper *et al.*, 1968; Casaburi *et al.*, 1979; Grassi *et al.* 1998a,b). However, few studies have focused on quantifying pulmonary $\dot{V}O_2$ kinetics in conscious, exercising dogs. One such study was performed by Marconi and colleagues (1982), which was the first to quantify the $\dot{V}O_2$ response at the onset of 'square-wave' exercise bouts in conscious dogs. With an experimental set-up similar to that used in humans (i.e. respiratory mask connected to a mass spectrometer), these researchers subjected dogs to different work intensities (constant load treadmill exercise) and measured the ensuing whole body $\dot{V}O_2$ on-kinetics. These investigators demonstrated that the dog has extremely rapid $\dot{V}O_2$ on-kinetics with a τ of ~20 s (Figure 5.8), apparently independent of workload at least up to 12 km · h^{-1} on a 10% incline. Notice the absence of a discernible slow component for any of the runs in that figure. At similar relative workloads, humans demonstrate a pronounced slow component as described in Chapter 1. One important finding in the Marconi *et al.* (1982) investigation was the similarity between whole

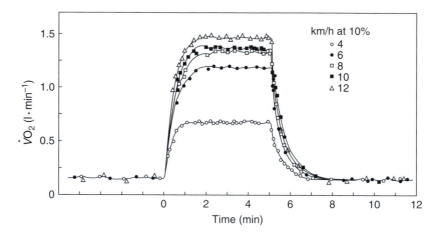

Figure 5.8 Pulmonary $\dot{V}O_2$ kinetics in the mongrel dog. Time zero represents the onset of exercise. Note the rapid $\dot{V}O_2$ dynamics ($\tau \sim 20$ s) for all running speeds (Marconi *et al.*, 1982).

body pulmonary $\dot{V}O_2$ on-kinetics, and those found in the dog isolated-gastrocnemius complex (τ pulmonary $\dot{V}O_2$ ~20 s, Marconi *et al.*, 1982; isolated gastrocnemius τ $\dot{V}O_2$ 15–17 s, Piiper *et al.*, 1968), thereby substantiating pulmonary $\dot{V}O_2$ kinetics as an accurate representation of that occurring within the active musculature. This finding corroborated the work of Casaburi *et al.* (1979) who, by measuring concomitantly pulmonary and muscle $\dot{V}O_2$ in anaesthetized dogs, demonstrated no difference in $\dot{V}O_2$ on-kinetics between pulmonary and muscle (both ~17 s) during electrical stimulation. The relationship between pulmonary and muscle $\dot{V}O_2$ kinetics is discussed further in Chapter 6.

Dog isolated muscle $\dot{V}O_2$ kinetics

Individual surgically isolated canine muscles or muscle groups (e.g. gastrocnemius–plantaris complex) in the dog have been used to study muscle energetics since the early twentieth century (Kramer and Quensel, 1938). One particularly attractive feature of this experimental model is that it allows a rapid and precise control of the blood flow into the muscle and alteration of the physiochemical properties (e.g. gas contents) of that blood. Specifically, the investigator can manipulate O_2 delivery independently of O_2 uptake (Grassi *et al.*, 1998a,b; or *vice versa*, see Grassi *et al.*, 2002) to elucidate the mechanisms governing the rate of $\dot{V}O_2$ increase. For example, using the dog isolated gastrocnemius complex (comprised of gastrocnemius–plantaris muscles) first described by Stainsby and Welch (1966), Grassi and colleagues have demonstrated that muscle $\dot{V}O_2$ on-kinetics for moderate-intensity contractions (yielding <60% $\dot{V}O_{2\,max}$) are not affected by (1) An increase in peripheral O_2 diffusion evoked via hyperoxia or hyperoxia concomitantly with a rightward shift of the haemoglobin–O_2 dissociation curve (via the drug RSR-13). Both of these paradigms act to increase the driving force for O_2 from the capillary to the myocyte thus facilitating enhanced transcapillary O_2 flux. The $\tau\dot{V}O_2$ was not altered by these manipulations being 24–26 s under all conditions (Grassi et al., 1998b, and (2) A faster adjustment of O_2 delivery at exercise onset by setting the pre-contracting blood flow to the same values attained during steady-state contractions. $\tau\dot{V}O_2$ was unchanged at 17–19 s for both a spontaneous and pre-adjusted increase in blood flow to the muscle (Grassi et al., 1998a). As can be seen from these two latter series of experiments, dog muscle demonstrates rapid $\dot{V}O_2$ on-kinetics which are not limited by O_2 delivery at least in the moderate-intensity domain. For a detailed explanation of mechanisms governing the speed of $\dot{V}O_2$ kinetics see Chapters 8, 9 and 12.

Mechanisms responsible for rapid $\dot{V}O_2$ on-kinetics in the dog

There are many adaptations in the dog that contribute to rapid $\dot{V}O_2$ kinetics. However, it is evident that the dog enjoys an extremely high mitochondrial volume density in most locomotory muscles (Parsons et al., 1985). Moreover, the kinetics of blood (and therefore O_2) delivery to these muscles is astonishingly fast and as in most models considered actually precedes the increase in $\dot{V}O_2$ (see Chapters 9 and 12).

Rodents

Compared to the horse and dog, there is very little known about pulmonary $\dot{V}O_2$ kinetics in rodents (e.g. mice and rats). Although $\dot{V}O_2$ steady states can be measured with high fidelity in both rats (Gleeson and Baldwin, 1981; Musch et al., 1988) and mice (Schefer and Talon, 1996), it is much more difficult to measure the rate of change or the dynamics of $\dot{V}O_2$ in these animals. Specifically, $\dot{V}O_2$ is usually measured in small animals by placing them in a relatively large chamber, and subsequently sampling the gases (CO_2 and O_2) during steady states. Therefore, due to a gross mismatching of tidal volume (extremely low in small rodents) to chamber volume size (thereby increasing the time required for proper mixing of the gases), the fidelity of $\dot{V}O_2$ measurements during non-steady states is greatly reduced. Nonetheless, Chappell (1984) has managed, through design of an open-circuit flow system, to collect $\dot{V}O_2$ kinetic data in the mouse. Thus, across the rest-to-running transition, the deer mouse (*Peromyscus maniculatus*) can increase its exercising $\dot{V}O_2$ with a τ ~20–25 s (Figure 5.9; Chappell, 1984). In addition to these rapid kinetics, an impressive $\dot{V}O_{2\,max}$ (~175 ml $O_2 \cdot min^{-1} \cdot kg^{-1}$) was measured. Apparently in these creatures, the same very high $\dot{V}O_{2\,max}$ can be achieved by either exercise or cold exposure. This observation raises the intriguing possibility that the rapid $\dot{V}O_2$ kinetics in the deer mouse may have resulted from environmental temperature challenges rather than exercise *per se*.

As for the mouse, very few studies have measured $\dot{V}O_2$ kinetics in the laboratory rat. It has been assumed, based on demonstrated high $\dot{V}O_{2\,max}$ values (70–80 ml $\cdot min^{-1} \cdot kg^{-1}$; Gleeson and Baldwin, 1981; Musch et al., 1988), that

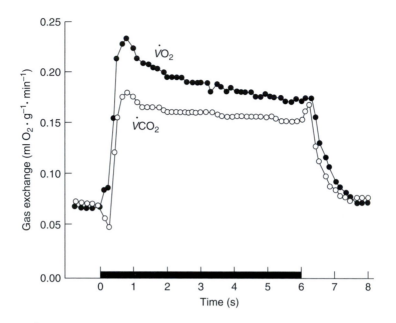

Figure 5.9 $\dot{V}O_2$ on-kinetics for the deer mouse (*Peromyscus maniculatus*). Time zero is the onset of exercise. Note the rapid increase in $\dot{V}O_2$ which overshoots the steady state (Chappell, 1984).

the rat would display rapid $\dot{V}O_2$ kinetics (as discussed in 'Introduction', in most cases $\tau \dot{V}O_2$ is proportional to $\dot{V}O_{2\,max}$). However, it was only recently that $\dot{V}O_2$ kinetics in the rat, or more specifically rat muscle have been described. Behnke *et al.* (2002) demonstrated that, across the rest to electrically-induced contractions, rat skeletal muscle (i.e. spinotrapezius) $\dot{V}O_2$ follows a mono-exponential time course to the steady state with a τ of ~20 s (Figure 5.10; Behnke *et al.*, 2002). This was the first study to demonstrate that $\dot{V}O_2$ increases almost immediately (i.e. no apparent time delay) at the onset of contractions, which is consistent with current concepts of metabolic control (see Chapter 12). In addition, the muscle studied in that investigation (i.e. spinotrapezius) has only a relatively modest oxidative capacity (measured by citrate synthase activity, an enzyme of the TCA cycle indicative of oxidative capacity; ~14 μmol $\cdot$ min^{-1} $\cdot$ g^{-1} in spinotrapezius, Delp and Duan, 1996). Therefore, during treadmill exercise, where muscles with high oxidative capacities are recruited (e.g. red gastrocnemius; citrate synthase activity ~36 μmol $\cdot$ min^{-1} $\cdot$ g^{-1}; Delp and Duan, 1996), $\dot{V}O_2$ kinetics would be expected to be even more rapid than that demonstrated in the spinotrapezius, although this has yet to be documented. In the future, it would be important to be able to measure and understand the control of $\dot{V}O_2$ dynamics in the laboratory rat (and mouse) because many of the major chronic diseases that affect humans (e.g. diabetes and chronic heart failure) can be surgically or pharmacologically or even genetically induced in these animals.

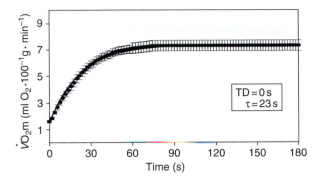

Figure 5.10 Muscle oxygen uptake ($\dot{V}O_{2m}$) profile across the rest to electrically-induced muscular contractions transition in rat spinotrapezius. Note that at stimulation onset (time zero) $\dot{V}O_2$ increases without discernible delay in a mono-exponential fashion to the steady state. Figure from Behnke *et al.* (2002).

Invertebrates and reptiles

As noted throughout this text, the majority of $\dot{V}O_2$ dynamics studies have been performed upon mammals. However, arthropods (e.g. insects and crustaceans) comprise the largest and most diverse group of animals on earth. Surprisingly, given their numerical superiority and capacity for harming mankind (locusts, mosquitoes, fruit flies) or helping mankind (bees, leeches, crabs) little is known about the aerobic responses to any form of locomotion within this phylum (i.e. *Arthropoda*). Nonetheless, novel and inventive experimental techniques have been developed to study the metabolic responses of a few select species, for example, the crab and cockroach. Specifically, the ghost crab (*Ocypode guadichaudii*; Figure 5.11), has a single-chambered heart, and relies upon gill chambers for O_2 extraction after inspiration (via openings on legs) of either water or air. Both of these structural adaptations could pose serious limitations to O_2 uptake ($\dot{V}O_2$) and delivery. Specifically, in humans O_2 is drawn into the lungs where it diffuses across an extremely thin (i.e. ~0.3 µm) blood–gas barrier into the circulation. However, in the crab, O_2 must diffuse through a chitin layer of the gills that has a diffusive conductance for O_2 that is much less (i.e. greater resistance to diffusion) than that of the human blood–gas interface. Indeed, McMahon (1981) proposed that it is this chitin layer which poses the major limitation to the rate of O_2 diffusion into the blood. Combined with the sluggish increase in heart rate at the onset of exercise (Herreid *et al.*, 1979), it is not surprising that $\dot{V}O_2$ kinetics at exercise onset are slow in this species. Nonetheless, ghost crabs do exhibit a $\dot{V}O_2$ response to treadmill exercise that is qualitatively similar to that of mammals, that is a mono-exponential increase to the steady state (Figure 5.11; Full and Herreid, 1983). However, the half time ($t_{1/2}$) of this response averages around 100 s, corresponding to a τ of ~144 s (i.e. $\tau = t_{1/2} \div 0.693$ for a first-order

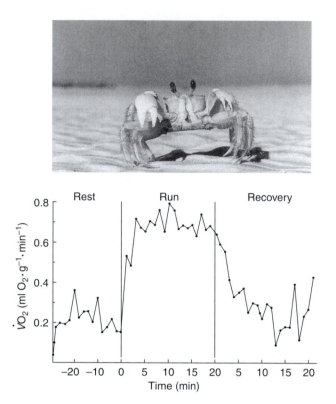

Figure 5.11 The Ghost crab (*Ocypode guadichaudii*), believed to be the fastest land crab exhibits a $\tau \dot{V}O_2$ of ~144 s during sideways treadmill running (from Full and Herreid, 1983, with permission). Time zero is the onset of exercise.

reaction) at a velocity of $0.28 \text{ km} \cdot \text{h}^{-1}$, running sideways. It should be mentioned that this particular crab species appears to be an exception amongst crabs, as the majority of these creatures that have been studied exhibit even slower $\dot{V}O_2$ dynamics (Herreid *et al.*, 1979; Full and Herreid, 1980).

Amongst those species in which $\dot{V}O_2$ dynamics and $\dot{V}O_{2\,max}$ have been studied, the lungless salamander (*Plethodin jordani*) possibly represents the lower extreme of aerobic function. These animals must rely on their skin for the exchange of respiratory gases. Indeed, the lungless salamander has been studied extensively as a model of diffusion limitation (Piiper *et al.*, 1976; Feder *et al.*, 1988). With respect to O_2 uptake, this reptile, which normally performs rapid, sprint-type exercise that is anaerobic in nature, demonstrates a disappearingly low $\dot{V}O_{2\,max}$ of ~7–8 ml $\cdot$ min$^{-1} \cdot$ kg^{-1} (Full, 1986). Given this low aerobic capacity, it should not be surprising that the $\dot{V}O_2$ on-kinetics for this animal are extremely slow, that is τ ~180 s (Full, 1986). From one perspective, the lungless salamander may be likened to the severe lung disease patient who exhibits a severe diffusion limitation to O_2 uptake.

Amphibians

Within the amphibian class, it has typically been the anuran order (frogs and toads that lack a tail) in which problems related to metabolic control have been studied. One particular challenge for measuring $\dot{V}O_2$ kinetics during locomotory activity in frogs and toads is that they move on land by means of saltatory movement which means that they hop rather than walk or run. Notwithstanding this impediment, Walton and Anderson (1988) measured the $\dot{V}O_2$ at the onset of hopping activity in Fowler's toad (*Bufo woodhousei fowleri*)(Figure 5.12). Fowler's toad has a $\dot{V}O_{2\,max}$ ~20 ml · min^{-1} · kg^{-1} and according to the relationship shown in Figure 5.2, very slow $\dot{V}O_2$ kinetics are to be expected. From the responses in Figure 5.12 we have calculated τ values of 4.24 and 6.72 min for transitions to hopping at 0.09 and 0.45 km · h^{-1}, respectively.

The amphibian cardiorespiratory system does not appear to have been designed to support either rapid or substantial increases in oxidative phosphorylation ($\dot{V}O_2$). However, key features within amphibian skeletal muscle makes it excellent for the study of metabolic control. First, individual muscle fibres are relatively large compared with human or rodent muscle cells, individual myocytes can easily be separated into distinct fibre types and amphibian muscle can possess quite high mitochondrial volume densities. Second, anuran muscle lacks myoglobin and thus, in accordance with Fick's law of diffusion, the fall in muscle intracellular PO_2 is a direct measure of $\dot{V}O_2$. (Fick's law of diffusion applied to the single myocyte preparation: $\dot{V}O_2 = DO_2 * P_eO_2 - P_iO_2$ where DO_2 is the muscle O_2 diffusion constant and P_iO_2 and P_eO_2 represent intracellular and extracellular PO_2, respectively.) These advantages, plus the overall robustness of anuran muscle and single muscle fibres have made these animals the model of choice for many early as well as current studies of muscle function and metabolic control.

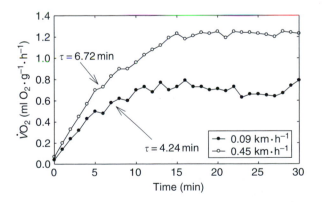

Figure 5.12 Pulmonary $\dot{V}O_2$ of Fowler's toad (*Bufo woodhousei fowleri*) during 30 min of treadmill hopping at 0.09 km · h^{-1} (closed symbols) and 0.45 km · h^{-1} (open symbols). Note that mean response times (τ or MRT) are extremely slow.

Whole muscle

Some of the first skeletal muscle $\dot{V}O_2$ kinetics data was collected over 75 years ago. Fenn (1927) measured the rise and fall in $\dot{V}O_2$ following 5–10 s tetanic contractions in isolated semitendinosus of the English frog (*Rana pipiens*). $\dot{V}O_2$ was calculated by measuring the fall in O_2 in a stirred and sealed chamber. Given that the chamber volume was large and the response time of the O_2 measuring device long, Fenn described the rise in $\dot{V}O_2$ following the contraction as 'immediate'. A similar technique was used by Hill (1940) to measure $\dot{V}O_2$ in whole sartorius muscle (at 0°C) isolated from *Rana temporia*. Following an extended tetanic contraction, Hill demonstrated that the rate of rise of $\dot{V}O_2$ and increased heat production followed a similar time course and further that lowering pH from 7.2 to 6.0 significantly slowed both of these responses. More recently, Mahler (1978) has utilized isolated frog muscles to demonstrate that the muscle $\dot{V}O_2$ control is a linear, first-order process. Specifically, he demonstrated that $\tau\dot{V}O_2$ during recovery from differing periods of tetanic contraction was invariant with the metabolic demand. See Chapter 7 for a more detailed discussion of this issue.

Single myocytes

The large, easily fibre-typed, robust frog myocytes can be isolated with tendons intact allowing for concomitant measurement of metabolic variables and force. Furthermore, studying the single myocyte removes many confounding factors associated with fibre (type) recruitment and O_2 delivery that are present when studying intact muscles. To our knowledge, Nagesser and colleagues (1993) performed the first measurements of $\dot{V}O_2$ in single frog (African clawed frog, *Xenopus laevis*) myocytes at the onset of contractions. While the kinetics *per se* were not formally characterized their measurements revealed that the $\dot{V}O_2$ response at the onset and offset of contractions were quite rapid in the highly oxidative type III and markedly slower in the least oxidative type I myocyte. Most recently, our laboratory has measured $\dot{V}O_2$ kinetics in single isolated *Xenopus laevis* lumbrical muscle myocytes during a series of repetitive isometric tetanic contractions (Hogan, 1999; Kindig *et al.*, 2003b). Using phosphorescence quenching to measure PO_2 essentially instantaneously and keeping the chamber dead space to a minimum, these studies revealed that $\dot{V}O_2$ increased at the onset of contractions with no discernible delay. The kinetics were rapid and fit well by a mono-exponential model with a τ of ~12 s (Figure 5.13).

Whilst it is obviously challenging to measure $\dot{V}O_2$ kinetics in single myocytes, this technique is proving to be valuable in the study of the key issues associated with metabolic control at exercise onset. Specifically, the heated contention regarding whether $\dot{V}O_2$ kinetics are limited by O_2 delivery to the muscle or metabolic inertia within the myocytes themselves (discussed in Chapters 8, 9 and 12) can be addressed in single myocytes: (1) Kindig and colleagues (2003a) demonstrated that progressively increasing the extracellular PO_2 from 20 to 60 Torr did not alter the initial speed of the fall in P_iO_2 at contractions onset suggesting that

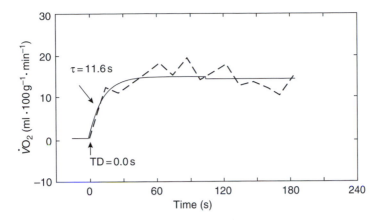

Figure 5.13 V̇O₂ (jagged line) and single mono-exponential + time delay fit (smooth line) measured in a representative single myocyte isolated from *Xenopus laevis* lumbrical muscle in response to a 3-min bout of isometric tetanic contractions (frequency: 1 every 3 s). Kinetic parameters reveal no time delay prior to the rise in V̇O₂ and a rapid primary component time constant (τ). Figure adapted from Kindig *et al.* (2003a).

an extracellular PO_2 of 20 mmHg provides a sufficient driving force to facilitate V̇O₂ kinetics; (2) Hogan (2001) showed that, at contractions onset, the time prior to a detectable fall in intramyocyte PO_2 was ~13 s during the first contraction bout and this was reduced significantly to ~5 s with the second contraction bout. This is important in that it demonstrated that 'priming exercise' can speed V̇O₂ kinetics under identical ambient conditions and in the absence of alterations in fibre (type) recruitment or elevated muscle blood flow; (3) The creatine kinase-catalysed breakdown of phosphocreatine is believed to play an important role in maintaining sufficient energy for contraction at the onset of work and we tested the hypothesis that this reaction contributes to the metabolic inertia evidenced at exercise onset. When creatine kinase was acutely inhibited pharmaceutically, the fall in P_iO_2 at contractions onset was markedly speeded compared with matched control trials (Figure 5.14). This finding demonstrates that the creatine kinase reaction contributes to the 'metabolic inertia' seen at exercise onset; (4) V̇O₂ kinetics are faster in highly oxidative myocytes than in their low oxidative counterparts at equivalent extracellular PO_2 values.

What clearly remains to be resolved in amphibian muscle is the anomaly between findings at the single isolated myocyte vs those of the whole exercising animal. Specifically, single myocytes evidence rapid V̇O₂ kinetics whereas those for the whole animal are exorbitantly slow (compare Figures 5.12 and 5.13). These findings are certainly not consistent with amphibian V̇O₂ kinetics being limited by an oxidative enzyme inertia within the exercising muscles (Chapters 9 and 12). It is possible, however, that akin to disease conditions that limit muscle O_2 delivery in humans and other mammals, the amphibian pulmonary and

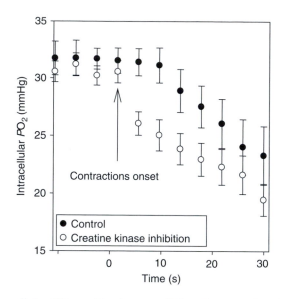

Figure 5.14 Intracellular PO_2 profiles (mean ± SE) under control and acute creatine kinase inhibition conditions in single myocytes isolated from the lumbrical muscle of *Xenopus laevis*. In this figure, the fall in intracellular PO_2 is only shown over the initial 30 s of the 2-min isometric tetanic contraction bout. Whereas there was no discernible fall in mean intracellular PO_2 under control conditions for ~8 s, there was an immediate and profound fall in intracellular PO_2 under creatine kinase inhibition conditions indicative of a faster increase in $\dot{V}O_2$. Adapted from Kindig *et al.* (2005).

cardiovascular systems operate so sluggishly that their whole body $\dot{V}O_2$ kinetics are limited by an inability to deliver O_2 in sufficient quantity to utilize the inherently rapid myocyte $\dot{V}O_2$ kinetics potential.

Conclusions

Within the animal kingdom, the relationship between $\dot{V}O_2$ kinetics and $\dot{V}O_{2\,max}$ demonstrated in humans is found across a range of $\dot{V}O_{2\,max}$ values approaching two orders of magnitude from the aerobically pedestrian lungless salamander to the fleet Thoroughbred racehorse. Judicious selection of animal models within this range has provided compelling evidence that, within healthy mammals, muscle and pulmonary $\dot{V}O_2$ kinetics are limited by processes within the myocyte. Thus, removal of NO inhibition of mitochondrial function (and also creatine kinase inhibition) both speed $\dot{V}O_2$ kinetics. The amphibian may constitute an exception in that isolated frog myocytes exhibit markedly faster $\dot{V}O_2$ kinetics than found in the intact, hopping animal. As with other lines of enquiry, it is evident that comparative physiological approaches can yield important original information regarding the control of $\dot{V}O_2$ kinetics. As the incomparable Knut Schmidt-Nielsen was fond of saying, 'for every physiological question, there is an animal model designed specifically to answer it'.

Glossary of terms

HR	heart rate
L-NAME	L-nitro arginine methyl ester (inhibits nitric oxide synthase)
MRT	mean response time (time delay + time constant, τ or tau, denotes time to 63% of final response)
PO_2	partial pressure of O_2, P_iO_2 is intracellular, P_eO_2 is extracellular
PO_2m	microvascular PO_2
$\dot{Q}O_2$	perfusive O_2 conductance (i.e. blood flow, $\dot{Q}$ × arterial O_2 content)
DO_2	diffusive O_2 conductance
Phase I	initial increase in $\dot{V}O_2$ at exercise onset caused by elevated pulmonary blood flow (also called the cardiodynamic phase)
Phase II	the exponential increase in $\dot{V}O_2$ that is initiated when venous blood from the exercising muscles arrives at the lungs. Corresponds closely with muscle $\dot{V}O_2$ dynamics.
RBC	red blood cell
τ or tau	denotes time to 63% of final response (please note that, with the exception of the horse, kinetics data on the species presented in this chapter have not been partitioned into time delay and exponential components. Consequently, τ of the overall response is synonymous with the MRT.
$t_{1/2}$	time to reach 50% of the final response
$\dot{V}O_2$	oxygen uptake
$\dot{V}O_{2\,max}$	maximal oxygen uptake (achieved under conditions of large muscle mass exercise unless otherwise specified)

References

Andersen, P. and Saltin, B. (1985). Maximal perfusion of skeletal muscle in man. *Journal of Physiology*, **366**, 233–49.

Armstrong, R.B., Essen-Gustavsson, B., Hoppeler, H., Jones, J.H., Kayar, S.R., Laughlin, M.H., Lindhom, A., Longworth, K.W., Taylor, C.R. and Weibel, E.R. (1992). O_2 delivery at $\dot{V}O_{2\,max}$ and oxidative capacity in muscles of Standardbred horses. *Journal of Applied Physiology*, **73**, 2274–82.

Barstow, T.J. and Mole, P.A. (1991). Linear and nonlinear characteristics of oxygen uptake kinetics during heavy exercise. *Journal of Applied Physiology*, **71**, 2099–106.

Barstow, T.J., Casaburi, R. and Wasserman, K. (1993). O_2 uptake kinetics and the O_2 deficit as related to exercise intensity and blood lactate. *Journal of Applied Physiology*, **75**, 755–62.

Behnke, B.J., Barstow, T.J., Kindig, C.A., McDonough, P., Musch, T.I. and Poole, D.C. (2002). Dynamics of oxygen uptake following exercise onset in rat skeletal muscle. *Respiration Physiology and Neurobiology*, **133**, 229–39.

Butler, P.J., Woakes, A.J., Smale, K., Roberts, C.A., Hillidge, C.J., Snow, D.H. and Marlin, D.J. (1993). Respiratory and cardiovascular adjustments during exercise of increasing exercise intensity and during recovery in Thoroughbred racehorses. *Journal of Experimental Biology*, **179**, 159–80.

Carter, H., Pringle, J.S.M., Jones, A.M. and Doust, J.H. (2002). Oxygen uptake kinetics during treadmill running across exercise intensity domains. *European Journal of Applied Physiology*, **86**, 347–54.

Casaburi, R., Weissman, M.L., Huntsman, D.J., Whipp, B.J. and Wasserman, K. (1979). Determinants of gas exchange kinetics during exercise in the dog. *Journal of Applied Physiology*, **46**, 1054–60.

Chappell, M.A. (1984). Maximum oxygen consumption during exercise and cold exposure in deer mice, peromyscus maniculatus. *Respiration Physiology*, **55**, 367–77.

Delp, M.D. and Duan, C. (1996). Composition and size of type I, IIA, IID/X, and IIB fibers and citrate synthase activity of rat muscle. *Journal of Applied Physiology*, **80**, 261–70.

Engelen, M., Porszasz, J., Riley, M., Wasserman, K., Maehara, K. and Barstow, T.J. (1996). Effects of hypoxic hypoxia on O_2 uptake and heart rate kinetics during heavy exercise. *Journal of Applied Physiology*, **81**, 2500–8.

Feder, M.E., Full, R.F. and Piiper, J. (1988). Elimination kinetics of acetylene and Freon 22 in resting and active lungless salamanders. *Respiration Physiology*, **72**, 229–40.

Fenn, W.O. (1927). The gas exchange of isolated muscles during stimulation and recovery. *American Journal of Physiology*, **83**, 309–22.

Forster, H.V., Pan, L.G., Bisgard, G.E., Dorsey, S.M. and Britton, M.S. (1984). Temporal pattern of pulmonary gas exchange during exercise in ponies. *Journal of Applied Physiology*, **57**, 760–7.

Full, R.J. (1986). Locomotion without lungs: energetics and performance of a lungless salamander. *American Journal of Physiology*, **251**, R775–80.

Full, R.J. and Herreid, C.F. (1980). Energetics of running sideways. *American Zoologist*, **20**, 909.

Full, R.J. and Herreid, C.F. (1983). Aerobic response to exercise of the fastest land crab. *American Journal of Physiology*, **244**, R530–6.

Geor, R.J., McCutcheon, L.J. and Hinchcliff, K.W. (2000). Effects of warm-up intensity on kinetics of oxygen consumption and carbon dioxide production during high-intensity exercise in horses. *American Journal of Vetinary Research*, **61**, 638–45.

Gerbino, A., Ward, S.A. and Whipp, B.J. (1996). Effects of prior exercise on pulmonary gas-exchange kinetics during high-intensity exercise in humans. *Journal of Applied Physiology*, **80**, 99–107.

Gleeson, T.T. and Baldwin, K.M. (1981). Cardiovascular response to treadmill exercise in untrained rats. *Journal of Applied Physiology*, **50**, 1206–11.

Grassi, B., Poole, D.C., Richardson, R.S., Knight, D.R., Erickson, B.K. and Wagner, P.D. (1996). Muscle O_2 uptake kinetics in humans: implications for metabolic control. *Journal of Applied Physiology*, **80**, 988–98.

Grassi, B., Gladden, L.B., Samaja, M., Stary, C.M. and Hogan, M.C. (1998a). Faster adjustment of O_2 delivery does not affect $\dot{V}O_2$ on-kinetics in isolated in situ canine muscle. *Journal of Applied Physiology*, **85**, 1394–403.

Grassi, B. Gladden, L.B., Stary, C.M., Wagner, P.D. and Hogan, M.C. (1998b). Peripheral O_2 diffusion does not affect $\dot{V}O_2$ on-kinetics in isolated in situ canine muscle. *Journal of Applied Physiology*, **85**, 1404–12.

Grassi, B., Hogan, M.C., Kelley, K.M., Aschenbach, W.G., Hamann, J.J., Evans, R.K., Patillo, R.E. and Gladden, L.B. (2000). Role of convective O_2 delivery in determining $\dot{V}O_2$ on-kinetics in canine muscle contracting at peak $\dot{V}O_2$. *Journal of Applied Physiology*, **89**, 1293–301.

Grassi, B., Hogan, M.C., Greenhaff, P.L., Hamann, J.J., Kelley, K.M., Aschenbach, W.G., Constantin-Teodosiu, D. and Gladden, L.B. (2002). Oxygen uptake on-kinetics in dog gastrocnemius in situ following activation of pyruvate dehydrogenase by dichloroacetate. *Journal of Physiology*, **538**, 195–207.

Herreid, C.F., Lee, L.W. and Shah, G.M. (1979). Respiration and heart rate in exercising land crabs. *Respiration Physiology*, **36**, 109–20.

Hill, D.K. (1940). The time course of the oxygen consumption of the stimulated frog's muscle. *Journal of Physiology*, **98**, 207–27.

Hodgson, D.R., Rose, R.J., Kelso, T.B., McCutcheon, Bayly, W.M. and Gollnick, P.D. (1990). Respiratory and metabolic responses in the horse during moderate and heavy exercise. *Pflugers Archives*, **417**, 73–8.

Hogan, M.C. (1999). Phosphorescence quenching method for measurement of intracellular PO_2 in isolated skeletal muscle fibers. *Journal of Applied Physiology*, **86**, 720–4.

Hogan, M.C. (2001). Fall in intracellular PO_2 at the onset of contractions in Xenopus single skeletal muscle fibers. *Journal of Applied Physiology*, **90**, 1871–6.

Hoppeler, H., Jones, J.H., Lindstedt, S.L., Claassen, H., Longworth, K.E., Taylor, C.R., Straub, R. and Lindholm, A. (1987). Relating maximal oxygen consumption to skeletal muscle mitochondria in horses. In J.R. Gillespie and N.E. Robinson (Eds) *Equine Exercise Physiology 2*. ICEEP, Davis, CA. pp. 278–89.

Hughson, R.L. and Morrissey, M.A. (1982). Delayed kinetics of respiratory gas exchange in the transition from prior exercise. *Journal of Applied Physiology*, **52**, 921–9.

Katz, L.M., Bayly, W.M., Roeder, M.J., Kingston, J.K. and Hines, M.T. (2000). Effects of training on maximum oxygen consumption of ponies. *American Journal of Vetinary Research*, **61**, 986–91.

Kindig, C.A., Gallatin, L.L., Erickson, H.H., Fedde, M.R. and Poole, D.C. (2000). Cardiorespiratory impact of the nitric oxide synthase inhibitor L-NAME in the exercising horse. *Respiration Physiology and Neurobiology*, **120**, 151–66.

Kindig, C.A., McDonough, P., Erickson, H.H. and Poole, D.C. (2001). Effect of L-NAME on oxygen uptake kinetics during heavy-intensity exercise in the horse. *Journal of Applied Physiology*, **91**, 891–6.

Kindig, C.A., McDonough, P., Erickson, H.H. and Poole, D.C. (2002). Nitric oxide synthase inhibition speeds oxygen uptake kinetics in horses during moderate domain running. *Respiration Physiology and Neurobiology*, **132**, 169–78.

Kindig, C.A., Howlett, R.A. and Hogan, M.C. (2003a). Effect of extracellular PO_2 on the fall in intracellular PO_2 in contracting single myocytes. *Journal of Applied Physiology*, **94**, 1964–70.

Kindig, C.A., Kelley, K.M., Howlett, R.A., Stary, C.M. and Hogan, M.C. (2003b). Assessment of oxygen uptake dynamics in isolated single myocytes. *Journal of Applied Physiology*, **94**, 353–7.

Kindig, C.A., Howlett, R.A., Stary, C.M., Walsh, B. and Hogan, M.C. (2005). Effects of acute creatine kinase inhibition on metabolism and tension development in isolated single myocytes. *Journal of Applied Physiology*, **98** (published online 27 August 2004).

Koga, S., Shiojiri, T., Shibasaki, M., Kondo, N., Fukuba, Y. and Barstow, T.J. (1999). Kinetics of oxygen uptake during supine and upright heavy exercise. *Journal of Applied Physiology*, **87**, 253–60.

Kramer, K. and Quensel, W. (1938). Untersuchungen über den Muskelstoffwechsel des Warmblüters. *Pflugers Archives*, **239**, 620–43.

Langsetmo, I., Weigle, G.E., Fedde, M.R., Erickson, H.H., Barstow, T.J. and Poole, D.C. (1997). $\dot{V}O_2$ kinetics in the horse during moderate and heavy exercise. *Journal of Applied Physiology*, **83**, 1231–41.

MacDonald, M.J., Pedersen, P.K. and Hughson, R.L. (1997). Acceleration of $\dot{V}O_2$ kinetics in heavy submaximal exercise by hyperoxia and prior to high-intensity exercise. *Journal of Applied Physiology*, **83**, 1318–25.

McMahon, B.R. (1981). Oxygen uptake and acid–base balance during activity in decapod crustaceans. In C.F. Herreid and C.R. Fourtner (Eds) *Locomotion and Energetics in Arthropods*. Plenum, New York.

Mahler, M. (1978). Kinetics of oxygen consumption after a single isometric tetanus of frog sartorius muscle at 20°C. *Journal of General Physiology*, **71**, 559–80.

Marconi, C., Pendergast, D., Krasney, J.A., Rennie, D.W. and Cerretelli, P. (1982). Dynamic and steady-state metabolic changes in running dogs. *Respiration Physiology*, **50**, 93–110.

Musch, T.I., Friedman, D.B., Haidet, G.C., Stray-Gundersen, J., Waldrop, T.G. and Ordway, G.A. (1986). Arterial blood gases and acid–base status of dogs during graded dynamic exercise. *Journal of Applied Physiology*, **61**, 1914–19.

Musch, T.I., Bruno, A., Bradford, G.E., Vayonis, A. and Moore, R.L. (1988). Measurement of metabolic rate in rats: a comparison of techniques. *Journal of Applied Physiology*, **65**, 964–70.

Mahler, M. (1978). Kinetics of oxygen consumption after a single isometric tetanus of frog sartorius muscle at 20°C. *Journal of General Physiology*, **71**, 559–80.

Nagesser, A.S., van der Laarse, W.J. and Elzinga, G. (1993). ATP formation and ATP hydrolysis during fatiguing, intermittent stimulation of different types of single muscle fibres from *Xenopus laevis*. *Journal of Muscle Research and Cell Motility*, **14**, 608–18.

Ozyener, F., Rossiter, H.B., Ward, S.A. and Whipp, B.J. (2001). Influence of exercise intensity on the on- and off-transient kinetics of pulmonary oxygen uptake in humans. *Journal of Physiology*, **533**, 891–902.

Parsons, D., Musch, T.I., Moore, R.L., Haidet, G.C. and Ordway, G.A. (1985). Dynamic exercise training in foxhounds. II. Analysis of skeletal muscle. *Journal of Applied Physiology*, **59**, 190–7.

Paterson, D.H. and Whipp, B.J. (1991). Asymmetries of oxygen uptake transients at the on- and offset of heavy exercise in humans. *Journal of Physiology*, **443**, 575–86.

Persson, S.G.B., Ekmon, L., Lydin, G. and Tufvesson, G. (1973). Circulatory effects of splenectomy in the horse. II. Effect of plasma volume and total and circulatory red-cell volume. *Zentralbl. Veterinaermed*, **20**, 456–68.

Piiper, J., di Pampero, P.E. and Cerretelli, P. (1968). Oxygen debt and high-energy phosphates in gastrocnemius muscle of the dog. *American Journal of Physiology*, **215**, 523–31.

Piiper, J., Gatz, R.N. and Crawford, E.C. (1976). Gas transport characteristics in an exclusively skin-breathing salamander, Desmognathus fuscus (Plethodontidae). In G.M. Hughes (Ed.) *Respiration of Amphibious Vertebrates*. Academic Press, London, pp. 339–56.

Powers, S.K., Beadle, R.E., Lawler, J. and Thompson, D. (1987). Respiratory gas exchange kinetics in transition from rest or prior exercise in ponies. In J.R. Gillespie and N.E. Robinson (Eds) *Equine Exercise Physiology 2*. ICEEP, Davis, Ca, pp. 148–60.

Richardson, R.S., Knight, D.R., Poole, D.C., Kurdak, S.S., Hogan, M.C., Grassi, B. and Wagner, P.D. (1995). Determinants of maximal exercise $\dot{V}O_2$ during single leg knee-extensor exercise in humans. *American Journal of Physiology*, **266**, H1453–61.

Rose, R.J., Hodgson, D.R., Bayly, W.M. and Gollnick, P.D. (1989). Kinetics of $\dot{V}O_2$ and $\dot{V}O_2$ in the horse and comparison of five methods for determination of maximum oxygen uptake. *Equine Veterinary Journal*, **9**, 39–42.

Rossiter, H.B., Ward, S.A., Kowalchuk, J.M., Howe, F.A., Griffiths, J.R. and Whipp, B.J. (2002). Dynamic asymmetry of phosphocreatine concentration and O_2 uptake between the on- and off-transients of moderate and high-intensity exercise in humans. *Journal of Physiology*, **541**, 991–1002.

Schefer, V. and Talan, M.I. (1996). Oxygen consumption in adult and aged C57BL/6J mice during acute treadmill exercise of different intensity. *Experimental Gerontology*, **31**, 387–92.

Stainsby, W.M. and Welch, H.G. (1966). Lactate metabolism of contracting dog skeletal muscle in situ. *American Journal of Physiology*, **211**, 177–83.

Walton, M. and Anderson, B.D. (1988). The aerobic cost of saltatory locomotion in the Fowler's Toad (*Bufo woodhousei fowleri*). *Journal of Experimental Biology*, **136**, 273–88.

Young, L.E., Marlin, D.J., Deaton, C., Brown-Feltner, H., Roberts, C.A. and Wood, J.L. (2002). Heart size estimated by echocardiography correlates with maximal oxygen uptake. *Equine Vetinary Journal*, **34**, 467–71.

Part III

Mechanistic bases of $\dot{V}O_2$ kinetics

6 Relationship between $\dot{V}O_2$ responses at the mouth and across the exercising muscles

Brad J. Behnke, Thomas J. Barstow and David C. Poole

Introduction

Oxygen uptake ($\dot{V}O_2$) is measured most conveniently across the mouth which permits characterization of pulmonary $\dot{V}O_2$ ($p\dot{V}O_2$) kinetics during transitions in metabolic rate such as following the onset of exercise. However, as $p\dot{V}O_2$ reflects the culmination of muscle $\dot{V}O_2$ ($m\dot{V}O_2$) and $\dot{V}O_2$ from the rest of the body as well as convective O_2 transport and changes in lung gas stores (Barstow and Molé, 1987), inferences to processes occurring within specific systems, for example muscle are indirect and interpretations regarding $m\dot{V}O_2$ must be made with caution. Because of transit time delays and the interposition of O_2 stores between the sites of O_2 exchange and measurement, determination of $m\dot{V}O_2$ directly at the site of capillary–myocyte O_2 exchange is likely to be a closer representation of 'true' muscle O_2 utilization than that made at more remote sites. Therefore, to validate $p\dot{V}O_2$ measurements as a true reflection of muscle metabolism, it is crucial to understand the fidelity with which $p\dot{V}O_2$ dynamics reflect those actually occurring within the muscle. Ultimately, the muscle itself or the mitochondrial matrix needs to be studied directly to justify statements regarding $m\dot{V}O_2$. Whereas it has been possible to determine $\dot{V}O_2$ across the exercising limbs (Grassi *et al.*, 1996; Bangsbo *et al.*, 2000), single muscles (Behnke *et al.*, 2002a; Kindig *et al.*, 2002) and even individual muscle fibres (Kindig *et al.*, 2003), technical limitations have so far precluded *in vivo* measurements at the mitochondria. It is also pertinent that the invasive steps required to determine $m\dot{V}O_2$ run the risk of altering the $\dot{V}O_2$ response itself. Moreover, when electrically-induced muscle contractions are utilized which is usually necessary to elicit muscle contractions in anaesthetized animals or individual muscles/muscle fibres, the intact cardiovascular responses as well as the physiological fibre recruitment patterns are altered. Thus, whereas measurements made in such preparations can provide useful insights into metabolic control, it must be accepted that a certain 'ecological validity' is lost when compared to the intact individual performing voluntary muscular exercise.

The purpose of this chapter is to examine the relationship between $p\dot{V}O_2$ and $m\dot{V}O_2$ kinetics, with emphasis placed upon recent experimental advances that either extend or alter conventional standpoints.

Pulmonary V̇O₂ on-kinetics

At the onset of moderate-intensity exercise, work rate and therefore ATP demand increases in a square-wave fashion, whereas V̇O₂ follows a finite kinetic response (Barstow *et al.*, 1994; Figure 6.1). Specifically, following the onset of dynamic moderate-intensity exercise, pV̇O₂ increases immediately (within the first breath) due principally to the rapid elevation of cardiac output that drives mixed venous blood through the lungs (Phase I, Whipp and Wasserman, 1972; Whipp *et al.*, 1982; Figure 6.2). Following a transit delay from the exercising

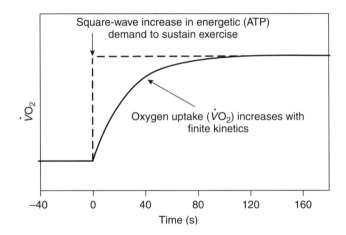

Figure 6.1 At the onset of exercise (time zero), energetic demand (dashed line) increases immediately in a square-wave or step-wise fashion whereas O₂ uptake (V̇O₂; solid line) increases more slowly with finite kinetics.

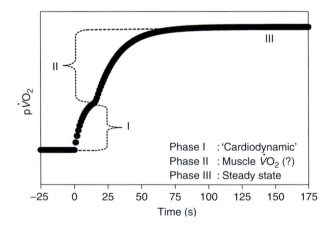

Figure 6.2 Three phases of the pulmonary V̇O₂ (pV̇O₂) response to dynamic, moderate-intensity exercise. Phase II has been considered to closely approximate muscle O₂ uptake (mV̇O₂). See text for discussion.

muscles, arrival of venous blood with a lower O_2 content signals the initiation of Phase II and raises $p\dot{V}O_2$ to the steady state (Phase III; Figure 6.2).

Until recently, the dynamics of $p\dot{V}O_2$ Phase II (i.e. time constant, τ, determined from the model fitting) had been assumed to reflect $\tau m\dot{V}O_2$. Specifically, at a time when very few measurements of $m\dot{V}O_2$ had been made (and these were restricted principally to amphibian (Mahler, 1985) and canine (Piiper *et al.*, 1968) muscle), Barstow and coworkers (Barstow and Molé, 1987; Barstow *et al.*, 1990) utilized elaborate simulations, to predict that in healthy individuals during Phase II, $p\dot{V}O_2$ kinetics matched closely the response occurring within or across the muscle, that is $m\dot{V}O_2$. However, these researchers also demonstrated that the profiles of $p\dot{V}O_2$ in Phases I and II were dependent upon venous blood volume as well as the dynamics of cardiac output and thus pathological conditions that alter cardiovascular function may change the different phases of the $p\dot{V}O_2$ response in a complex manner. For example, if a CHF patient had blunted muscle $\dot{V}O_2$ kinetics due to a sluggish increase in cardiac output, the Phase II $p\dot{V}O_2$ kinetics might appear to be faster than those actually occurring within the muscles (Figure 6.3; Barstow and Molé, 1987). This could lead one to conclude erroneously that the patient who demonstrated somewhat 'normal' Phase II $p\dot{V}O_2$ kinetics had preserved muscle oxidative function. If the entire oxygen deficit were calculated, however, it would be noticed that the patient had an unusually large total lag in $\dot{V}O_2$ as the steady state was approached. Thus, in this case, the presence of a 'normal' Phase II $p\dot{V}O_2$ response concomitant with a prolonged Phase I may be indicative of dysfunctional gas exchange within the exercising muscle (see Chapter 13).

Mouth vs muscle

Barstow and coworkers (Barstow and Molé, 1987; Barstow *et al.*, 1990) provided an understanding of the theoretical relationship between $p\dot{V}O_2$ and $m\dot{V}O_2$ kinetics. They modelled the contracting leg muscles, venous circulation and pulmonary gas exchange, which allowed them to examine independently changes in the venous volume separating the muscle from pulmonary gas exchange sites, the kinetics of adjustment of the circulation, and the kinetics of $m\dot{V}O_2$, on $p\dot{V}O_2$. They found that the size of the venous volume affected the duration of Phase I, but did not affect the fidelity with which Phase II $p\dot{V}O_2$ kinetics resembled those of $m\dot{V}O_2$. Further, within physiological limits for the kinetics of the circulation and of $m\dot{V}O_2$, the kinetics of $p\dot{V}O_2$ during Phase II matched closely those of $m\dot{V}O_2$. However, there was a lack of empirical evidence that the Phase II response at the mouth actually resembled that at the muscle. Poole and colleagues (1992) demonstrated that for incremental style exercise, $p\dot{V}O_2$ (primary phase only, slow component omitted) and $\dot{V}O_2$ leg (considered to be a close approximation of $m\dot{V}O_2$) increased in a quantitatively proportional fashion across the span of work rates from moderate to severe domain exercise (Figure 6.4). However, at that time, the kinetics of $\dot{V}O_2$ leg remained unresolved. To address this issue, Grassi and colleagues (Grassi *et al.*, 1996) used constant-infusion thermodilution

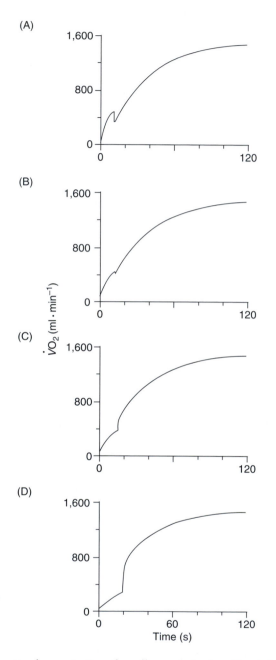

Figure 6.3 Schematic demonstrating the effects of slowing blood flow kinetics on pulmonary $\dot{V}O_2$ ($p\dot{V}O_2$) kinetics at the onset of exercise. Note that as the time constant for the increase of blood flow was increased from 5 s (A) to 8 s (B), 15 s (C) and 30 s (D), Phase I becomes lengthened and Phase II becomes progressively more rapid. From Barstow and Molé (1987) with permission.

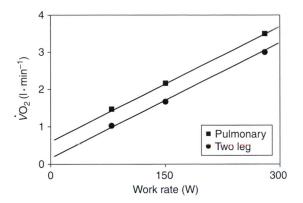

Figure 6.4 Pulmonary and leg $\dot{V}O_2$ vs work rate. Note the similarity of the close to linear relationship between O_2 uptake measured at the mouth ($p\dot{V}O_2$) and $\dot{V}O_2$ across the leg musculature to a given work rate. Figure from the data of Poole *et al.* (1992).

techniques in combination with arterial and femoral venous blood sampling to measure leg blood flow and compare directly $\dot{V}O_2$ leg with that of $p\dot{V}O_2$ at the onset of moderate-intensity exercise. In that investigation, $p\dot{V}O_2$ measurements were corrected for breath-to-breath changes in lung gas stores in order to derive alveolar $\dot{V}O_2$ ($\dot{V}O_2$ alv.) (Beaver *et al.*, 1981; Grassi *et al.*, 1996, see Chapter 2). Thus, $\dot{V}O_2$ leg was determined via the Fick principle ($\dot{V}O_2$ leg = $\dot{Q}$ × [a-vO_2]) where $\dot{Q}$ is leg blood flow measured in the femoral vein and 'a' and 'v' denote arterial and femoral venous O_2 contents. These investigators demonstrated that the profile for $\dot{V}O_2$ leg was similar to that measured at the mouth, that is a delay phase (Phase I) followed by a mono-exponential increase to the steady state with no statistical differences in the Phase II time constant between $p\dot{V}O_2$ and $\dot{V}O_2$ leg (Grassi *et al.*, 1996; Figure 6.5). Whereas Grassi and colleagues (1996) had examined moderate-intensity exercise, Bangsbo *et al.* (2000) found qualitatively similar responses for the extremely technically challenging conditions of severe-intensity exercise. Specifically, there was a lag or delay evident in the $\dot{V}O_2$ leg increase at the onset of contractions as found earlier by Grassi *et al.* (1996) (Figure 6.6). One intriguing observation made in both these studies was that $p\dot{V}O_2$ actually increased faster than $\dot{V}O_2$ leg during Phase I (see Figure 6.5). As noted earlier, this likely reflects both the spatial and temporal misalignment of $p\dot{V}O_2$ relative to $m\dot{V}O_2$. Finally, Rossiter *et al.* (1999, 2001, 2002) compared the kinetics of the fall in phosphocreatine (PCr), using ^{31}P NMR, with the rise in pulmonary $\dot{V}O_2$ determined simultaneously. After correcting the $p\dot{V}O_2$ for the venous transport delay between muscle and lungs (Phase I), the temporal profiles of the fall in PCr and rise in $p\dot{V}O_2$ were indistinguishable, providing further evidence that the Phase II $p\dot{V}O_2$ kinetics in healthy subjects reflects the kinetics of $m\dot{V}O_2$.

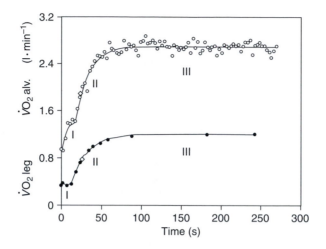

Figure 6.5 Comparison between alveolar ($\dot{V}O_2$ alv., i.e. p$\dot{V}O_2$ corrected for changes in lung gas stores) and leg $\dot{V}O_2$ ($\dot{V}O_2$ leg) kinetics. Note that in Phase II, $\dot{V}O_2$ legs increased with a similar time course to pulmonary $\dot{V}O_2$. It is interesting to note that in Phase I, $\dot{V}O_2$ alv. increases substantially whereas $\dot{V}O_2$ leg does not. From Grassi *et al.* (1996) with permission.

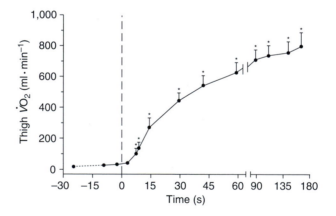

Figure 6.6 $\dot{V}O_2$ kinetics across the human thigh at the onset of severe exercise. Note the short time delay followed by a near-exponential increase in thigh $\dot{V}O_2$. From Bangsbo *et al.* (2000) with permission.

With respect to the $\dot{V}O_2$ slow component manifested in the heavy- and severe-intensity domains (see Chapter 12), Poole *et al.* (1991) utilized similar methodology as Grassi *et al.* (1996) described earlier, to investigate the relationship between p$\dot{V}O_2$ and leg $\dot{V}O_2$ during severe-intensity cycle ergometry. Beyond three minutes of constant-load exercise, the temporal profiles of p$\dot{V}O_2$ and leg

$\dot{V}O_2$ were remarkably similar. Indeed, the increase in leg $\dot{V}O_2$ could account for over 80% of the 700 ml·min^{-1} p$\dot{V}O_2$ increase observed from 3 min to fatigue (~20 min) in these subjects.

Muscle $\dot{V}O_2$

There exists substantial controversy regarding the mechanistic bases for the kinetic profile of p$\dot{V}O_2$ at the onset of exercise (i.e. duration of Phase I; kinetics of Phase II). Therefore, resolution of the precise temporal characteristics of m$\dot{V}O_2$ constitutes a crucial step in addressing the important question: what limits $\dot{V}O_2$ kinetics at the onset of exercise in healthy individuals? In addition, chronic disease conditions (e.g. diabetes, chronic heart failure (CHF)) that alter the relationship between muscle O_2 delivery (m$\dot{Q}O_2$) and $\dot{V}O_2$ are likely to alter m$\dot{V}O_2$ dynamics profoundly and this may contribute to the elevated O_2 deficit incurred in diabetic (Regensteiner et al., 1998) and CHF (Grassi et al., 1997) patients following exercise onset. For instance, a pathological slowing of m$\dot{Q}O_2$ dynamics relative to that of m$\dot{V}O_2$ such as has been demonstrated in Type I diabetes will lower the microvascular O_2 pressure (PO_2m) and this will impair blood–tissue O_2 transfer (Behnke et al., 2002b, Chapter 13). Resolution of the mechanism(s) of limitation of p$\dot{V}O_2$ kinetics in healthy individuals represents a necessary first step in providing the foundation upon which to determine the cause of slowed p$\dot{V}O_2$ kinetics in pathological conditions.

As mentioned in Chapter 12, at the onset of contractions, there is a delayed increase in m$\dot{V}O_2$ across the exercising muscles (Grassi et al., 1998a,b) or limb(s) (Grassi et al., 1996; Bangsbo et al., 2000, 2002). Whereas it is not possible to definitively apportion this delay between that due to transit delays (Bangsbo et al., 2000) between the site of gas exchange in the capillary and measurements made from effluent venous blood O_2 content, if real it has profound energetic implications. For example, the delayed increase in m$\dot{V}O_2$ (1) increases the size of the O_2 deficit; (2) is difficult to reconcile with the notion of a m$\dot{Q}O_2$ limitation to O_2 kinetics as it occurs concomitant with a sizeable and almost instantaneous increase of m$\dot{Q}O_2$; (3) challenges current models of metabolic control. Specifically, at exercise onset key metabolic controllers such as [PCr], [Pi], [Cr] and [ADP] are known to change without a discernible delay (Binzoni et al., 1992; Yoshida and Watari, 1993; Rossiter et al., 1999; 2001). Thus, we would expect m$\dot{V}O_2$ also to increase immediately. To address this issue, Behnke and colleagues (2002a) utilized a combination of phosphorescence quenching and intravital microscopy technologies to calculate the temporal profile of $\dot{V}O_2$ *within* a contracting muscle. Phosphorescence quenching is a relatively new technique (Rumsey et al., 1988) which allows quantification of PO_2m (Poole et al., 1995) which at any given time point will be determined by the relationship between muscle O_2 delivery and uptake (i.e. m$\dot{Q}O_2$-to-m$\dot{V}O_2$ relationship). Therefore, using this technique one can track the profile of changes in muscle PO_2m and therefore the dynamic balance between m$\dot{Q}O_2$ and m$\dot{V}O_2$ in response to conditions that alter muscle metabolism and/or m$\dot{Q}O_2$, for example, contractions

(Behnke *et al.*, 2001), metabolic blockade (Bailey *et al.*, 2000) and hypoxic/hyperoxic challenges (Poole *et al.*, 1995). In healthy muscles in response to contractions, muscle PO_2m demonstrates a pronounced delay followed by an exponential fall to the steady state (Figure 6.7).

The initial delay in PO_2m fall that is observed at the onset of contractions (Figure 6.7) can, in theory, result from either (1) no increase in either $m\dot{Q}O_2$ or $m\dot{V}O_2$ (which would seem unlikely) or alternatively, (2) if the increase in $m\dot{Q}O_2$ is being matched by that of $m\dot{V}O_2$ such that PO_2m remains unaltered across the time delay. Kindig *et al.* (2002) measured the increase in red blood cell (RBC) flux, velocity and haematocrit across the rest–contractions transition within individual capillaries of the rat spinotrapezius muscle and demonstrated an immediate increase in O_2 delivery within the first contraction cycle (Figure 6.8). These data in combination with the PO_2m profile permits estimation of $m\dot{V}O_2$ using the following version of the Fick principle:

$$m\dot{V}O_2\,(t) \propto \dot{Q}\,m(t) * (CaO_2 - CmO_2)$$

where $m\dot{V}O_2\,(t)$ is the $\dot{V}O_2$ of the muscle at time t, $\dot{Q}\,m(t)$ is muscle blood flow at time t, and CaO_2 and CmO_2 are the oxygen contents of the arterial and microvascular blood, respectively. CaO_2 is measured from arterial blood samples and CmO_2 is calculated from the PO_2m measurements using the appropriate O_2 dissociation curve. While strictly speaking, the Fick equation is based on venous,

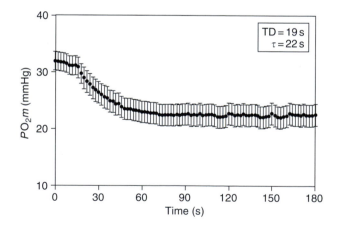

Figure 6.7 Dynamic profile of microvascular PO_2 (PO_2m; determined by the $m\dot{Q}O_2$-to-$m\dot{V}O_2$ relationship) within the spinotrapezius muscle in response to contractions. Note the presence of a time delay before PO_2m begins to decline. This delay can arise only if (1) both $m\dot{Q}O_2$ and $m\dot{V}O_2$ are not increasing above resting values, or (2) $m\dot{Q}O_2$ and $m\dot{V}O_2$ are increasing in concert such that PO_2m is unaltered for 10–20 s. Simultaneous measurements of O_2 delivery ($m\dot{Q}O_2$) indicate that the latter explanation is valid. From the data of Behnke *et al.* (2001). Please see text for additional details.

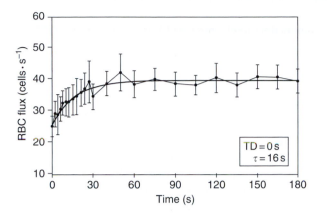

Figure 6.8 Profile of the increase in capillary RBC flux (measurement of m$\dot{Q}O_2$) across the rest–contractions transient. RBC flux (and therefore, m$\dot{Q}O_2$) increases immediately after the first contraction (1 Hz, twitch). From the data of Kindig *et al.* (2002).

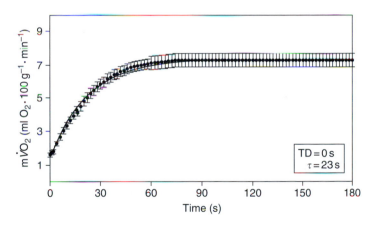

Figure 6.9 Calculated kinetic profile of spinotrapezius muscle $\dot{V}O_2$ (m$\dot{V}O_2$) in response to light- to moderate-intensity contractions. Note the immediate increase (<2 s) in m$\dot{V}O_2$ followed by a mono-exponential increase to the steady state. From Behnke *et al.* (2002a,b) with permission.

not microvascular, content of O_2, it is reasonable to assume that the time course (kinetics) of changes in microvascular O_2 content will be similar to those in the muscle venous blood. From this approach, Behnke and colleagues demonstrated that muscle $\dot{V}O_2$ increases without a discernible delay (i.e. <2 s) across the rest–contractions transient (Figure 6.9). Measurements made within single muscle fibres (Xenopus frog) have corroborated that $\dot{V}O_2$ increases essentially immediately in response to contractions (Kindig *et al.*, see Chapter 5). In combination, these data provide compelling evidence that $m\dot{Q}O_2$ increases within the first contraction cycle following exercise onset and within individual muscles this increase is matched by an elevated $m\dot{V}O_2$ that serves to maintain PO_2m constant for up to 20 s. Beyond this point, fractional O_2 extraction is increased and PO_2m decreases exponentially to the steady state. It is interesting to note that this pattern of change, i.e. a time delay of ~10–20 s followed by an exponential fall to a new exercise steady-state level, has recently been reported for tissue oxygenation using non-invasive near infrared spectroscopy (NIRS) (DeLorey *et al.*, 2003; Grassi *et al.*, 2003). The lack of a precipitous fall in PO_2m at the onset of contractions or any subsequent reduction in PO_2m below that found in the steady state suggests that $m\dot{Q}O_2$ is not limiting $m\dot{V}O_2$ kinetics (at least in healthy muscle). Moreover, evidence that increases in $m\dot{V}O_2$ and altered concentrations of mediators of mitochondrial phosphorylation (i.e. [PCr], [Pi], [Cr] and [ADP$_{free}$]) occur with a similar temporal profile is consistent with current models of mitochondrial control (Whipp and Mahler, 1980; Meyer, 1988; Rossiter *et al.*, 1999, 2001, 2002; Saks *et al.*, 2000; Behnke *et al.*, 2002a).

Conclusions

In healthy subjects measurements of $p\dot{V}O_2$ provide a quantitatively close representation of $m\dot{V}O_2$ that has a high temporal fidelity. This is true for the primary phase of $\dot{V}O_2$ (Phase II) and also the $\dot{V}O_2$ slow component. What remains to be reconciled is the relationship between $p\dot{V}O_2$ and $m\dot{V}O_2$ across the first few seconds of exercise (Phase I). Those measurements made in humans reveal a delay of up to 20 s in the $m\dot{V}O_2$ that occurs concomitant with a rapid Phase I increase in $p\dot{V}O_2$. Current models of metabolic control and the observation that the phosphorylation potential changes within the first second or so of contractions are not consistent with such a delayed increase $m\dot{V}O_2$. Moreover, direct measurement of $m\dot{V}O_2$ in the electrically stimulated rat spinotrapezius, dog gastrocnemius and single muscle fibres of the frog indicate an immediate increase in $m\dot{V}O_2$ with no delay. Consequently, the possibility must be acknowledged that some technical limitation may have artefactually induced the delayed increase in $m\dot{V}O_2$ found in humans.

With respect to interpreting muscle metabolic function from measurements of $p\dot{V}O_2$ in patient populations, it is evident that Phase I and Phase II are not independent of one another. Specifically, prolongation of Phase I in cardiac myopathy, for example, will cause a speeding of Phase II $p\dot{V}O_2$ that may obscure pathological slowing of $m\dot{V}O_2$ kinetics. This issue is addressed in greater detail in Chapter 14.

Glossary of terms

ADP	adenosine diphosphate (ADP$_{free}$, the metabolically important fraction of intracellular ADP)
ATP	adenosine triphosphate

CaO_2, CmO_2	arterial and microvascular blood O_2 contents
CHF	chronic heart failure
Cr	creatine
HR	heart rate
PCr	phosphocreatine
Pi	inorganic phosphate
Phase I	initial increase in $\dot{V}O_2$ at exercise onset caused by elevated pulmonary blood flow (also called the cardiodynamic phase)
Phase II	the exponential increase in $\dot{V}O_2$ that is initiated when venous blood from the exercising muscles arrives at the lungs. Corresponds closely with muscle $\dot{V}O_2$ dynamics as demonstrated in this chapter
PO_2	partial pressure of O_2; PO_2m, microvascular PO_2
$\dot{Q}$ m	muscle blood flow
$\dot{Q}O_2$	perfusive O_2 conductance (i.e. blood flow, $\dot{Q}$ × arterial O_2 content)
τ or tau	denotes time to 63% of final response
TD	time delay
$\dot{V}O_2$	oxygen uptake ($p\dot{V}O_2$, pulmonary; $m\dot{V}O_2$, muscle; $\dot{V}O_2$ alv., calculated alveolar; $\dot{V}O_2$ leg, across the exercising leg)

References

Bangsbo, J., Krustrup, P., Gonzalez-Alonso, J., Boushel, R. and Saltin, B. (2000). Muscle oxygen kinetics at onset of intense dynamic exercise in humans. *American Journal of Physiology*, **279**, R899–906.

Bangsbo, J., Gibala, M.J., Krustrup, P., Gonzalez-Alonso, J. and Saltin, B. (2002). Enhanced pyruvate dehydrogenase activity does not affect muscle O_2 uptake at onset of intense exercise in humans. *American Journal of Physiology*, **282**, R273–80.

Bailey, J.K., Kindig, C.A., Behnke, B.J., Musch, T.I., Schmid-Schoenbein, G.W. and Poole, D.C. (2000). Spinotrapezius muscle microcirculatory function: effects of surgical exteriorization. *American Journal of Physiology*, **279**, H3131–7.

Barstow, T.J. and Molé, P.A. (1987). Simulation of pulmonary O_2 uptake during exercise transients in humans. *Journal of Applied Physiology*, **63**, 2253–61.

Barstow, T.J., Lamarra, N. and Whipp, B.J. (1990). Modulation of muscle and pulmonary O_2 uptakes by circulatory dynamics during exercise. *Journal of Applied Physiology*, **68**, 979–89.

Barstow, T.J., Buchtal, S., Zanconato, S. and Cooper, D.M. (1994). Muscle energetics and pulmonary oxygen uptake kinetics during moderate exercise. *Journal of Applied Physiology*, **77**, 1742–9.

Beaver, W.L., Lamarra, N. and Wasserman, K. (1981). Breath-by-breath measurement of true alveolar gas exchange. *Journal of Applied Physiology*, **51**, 1662–75.

Behnke, B.J., Kindig, C.A., Musch, T.I., Koga, S. and Poole, D.C. (2001). Dynamics of microvascular oxygen pressure across the rest–exercise transition in rat skeletal muscle. *Respiration Physiology and Neurobiology*, **126**, 53–63.

Behnke, B.J., Barstow, T.J., Kindig, C.A., McDonough, P., Musch, T.I. and Poole, D.C. (2002a). Dynamics of oxygen uptake following exercise onset in rat skeletal muscle. *Respiration Physiology and Neurobiology*, **133**, 229–39.

Behnke, B.J., Kindig, C.A., McDonough, P., Poole, D.C. and Sexton, W.L. (2002b). Dynamics of microvascular oxygen pressure during rest–contraction transition in skeletal muscle of diabetic rats. *American Journal of Physiology*, **283**, H926–32.

Binzoni, T., Ferretti, G., Schenker, K. and Cerretelli, P. (1992). Phosphocreatine hydrolysis by 31P-NMR at the onset of constant-load exercise in humans. *Journal of Applied Physiology*, **73**, 1644–9.

DeLorey, D.S., Kowalchuk, J.M. and Paterson, D.H. (2003). Relationship between pulmonary O_2 uptake kinetics and muscle deoxygenation during moderate-intensity exercise. *Journal of Applied Physiology*, **95**, 113–20.

Grassi, B., Poole, D.C., Richardson, R.S., Knight, D.R., Erickson, B.K. and Wagner, P.D. (1996). Muscle O_2 uptake kinetics in humans: implications for metabolic control. *Journal of Applied Physiology*, **80**, 988–98.

Grassi, B., Marconi, C., Meyer, M., Rieu, M. and Cerretelli, P. (1997). Gas exchange and cardiovascular kinetics with different protocols in heart transplant recipients. *Journal of Applied Physiology*, **82**, 1952–62.

Grassi, B., Gladden, L.B., Samaja, M., Stary, C.M. and Hogan, M.C. (1998a). Faster adjustment of O_2 delivery does not affect $\dot{V}O_2$ on-kinetics in isolated in situ canine muscle. *Journal of Applied Physiology*, **84**, 1398–403.

Grassi, B., Gladden, L.B., Stary, C.M., Wagner, P.D. and Hogan, M.C. (1998b). Peripheral O_2 diffusion does not affect $\dot{V}O_2$ on-kinetics in isolated in situ canine muscle. *Journal of Applied Physiology*, **85**, 1404–12.

Grassi, B., Pogliaghi, S., Rampichini, S., Quaresima, V., Ferrari, M., Marconi, C. and Cerretelli, P. (2003). Muscle oxygenation and pulmonary gas exchange kinetics during cycling exercise on-transitions in humans. *Journal of Applied Physiology*, **95**, 149–58.

Kindig, C.A., Richardson, T.E. and Poole, D.C. (2002). Skeletal muscle capillary hemo-dynamics from rest to contractions: implications for oxygen transfer. *Journal of Applied Physiology*, **92**, 2513–20.

Kindig, C.A., Kelley, K.M., Howlett, R.A., Stary, C.M. and Hogan, M.C. (2003). Assessment of O_2 uptake dynamics in isolated single skeletal myocytes. *Journal of Applied Physiology*, **94**, 353–7.

Mahler, M. (1985). First-order kinetics of muscle oxygen consumption, and an equivalent proportionality between $\dot{Q}O_2$ and phosphocreatine level. *Journal of General Physiology*, **86**, 135–65.

Meyer, R.A. (1988). A linear model of muscle respiration explains monoexponential phosphocreatine changes. *American Journal of Physiology*, **254**, C548–53.

Piiper, J., Di Prampero, P.E. and Cerretelli, P. (1968). Oxygen debt and high-energy phosphates in gastrocnemius muscle of the dog. *American Journal of Physiology*, **215**, 523–31.

Poole, D.C., Schaffartzik, W., Knight, D.R., Derion, T., Kennedy, B., Guy, H.J., Prediletto, R. and Wagner, P.D. (1991). Contribution of excising legs to the slow com-ponent of oxygen uptake kinetics in humans. *Journal of Applied Physiology*, **71**, 1245–60.

Poole, D.C., Gaesser, G.A., Hogan, M.C., Knight, D.R. and Wagner, P.D. (1992). Pulmonary and leg $\dot{V}O_2$ during submaximal exercise: implications for muscular efficiency. *Journal of Applied Physiology*, **72**, 805–10.

Poole, D.C., Wagner, P.D. and Wilson, D.F. (1995). Diaphragm microvascular plasma PO_2 measured in vivo. *Journal of Applied Physiology*, **79**, 2050–7.

Regensteiner, J.G., Bauer, T.A., Reusch, J.E., Brandenburg, S.L., Sippel, J.M., Vogelsong, A.M., Smith, S., Wolfel, E.E., Eckel, R.H. and Hiatt, W.R. (1998). Abnormal oxygen uptake kinetic responses in women with type II diabetes mellitus. *Journal of Applied Physiology*, **85**, 310–17.

Rossiter, H.B., Ward, S.A., Doyle, V.L., Howe, F.A., Griffiths, J.R. and Whipp, B.J. (1999). Inferences from pulmonary O_2 uptake with respect to intramuscular [phospho-creatine] kinetics during moderate exercise in humans. *Journal of Physiology*, **518**, 921–32.

Rossiter, H.B., Ward, S.A., Kowalchuk, J.M., Howe, F.A., Griffiths, J.R. and Whipp, B.J. (2001). Effects of prior exercise on oxygen uptake and phosphocreatine kinetics during high-intensity knee-extension exercise in humans. *Journal of Physiology*, **537**, 291–303.

Rossiter, H.B., Ward, S.A., Kowalchuk, J.M., Howe, F.A., Griffiths, J.R. and Whipp, B.J. (2002). Dynamic asymmetry of phosphocreatine concentration and O_2 uptake between the on- and off-transients of moderate- and high-intensity exercise in humans. *Journal of Physiology*, **541**, 991–1002.

Rumsey, W.L., Vanderkooi, J.M. and Wilson, D.F. (1988). Imaging of phosphorescence: a novel method for measuring oxygen distribution in perfused tissue. *Science*, **241**, 1649–51.

Saks, V.A., Kongas, O., Vendelin, M. and Kay, L. (2000). Role of the creatine/phosphocreatine system in the regulation of mitochondrial respiration. *Acta Physiologica Scandinavica*, **168**, 635–41.

Whipp, B.J. and Mahler, M. (1980). Dynamics of pulmonary gas exchange during exercise. In J.B. West (Ed.) *Pulmonary Gas Exchange*, Vol. 2. Academic, New York, pp. 33–96.

Whipp, B.J. and Wasserman, K. (1972). Oxygen uptake kinetics for various intensities of constant-load work. *Journal of Applied Physiology*, **33**, 351–6.

Whipp, B.J., Ward, S.A., Lamarra, N., Davis, J.A. and Wasserman, K. (1982). Parameters of ventilatory and gas exchange dynamics during exercise. *Journal of Applied Physiology*, **52**, 1506–13.

Yoshida, T. and Watari, H. (1993). 31P-nuclear magnetic resonance spectroscopy study of the time course of energy metabolism during exercise and recovery. *European Journal of Applied Physiology*, **66**, 494–9.

7 Intramuscular phosphate and pulmonary $\dot{V}O_2$ kinetics during exercise

Implications for control of skeletal muscle oxygen consumption

Harry B. Rossiter, Franklyn A. Howe and Susan A. Ward

Introduction

Measurement of pulmonary oxygen uptake ($\dot{V}O_2$) profiles during exercise provides a relatively simple, non-invasive and commonly employed strategy for assessing the integration of pulmonary, cardiovascular, neural and muscle-energetic systems in health and disease. However, the determinants of $\dot{V}O_2$ response dynamics are less simple to localize and thus remain the source of much debate. Indeed these are not new issues; Krogh and Lindhard (1913), Hill and Lupton (1923) and later Hill (1926) recognized the importance of the dynamic phase of $\dot{V}O_2$ and its role in determining the oxygen deficit at exercise onset (Krogh and Lindhard, 1913) and the oxygen debt (Hill, 1926) following cessation; that is the deficit being 're-paid' as a debt at the cessation of exercise (Hill, 1926). Note that the term 'O_2 debt' suggested by Hill has been largely displaced by 'excess post-exercise O_2 consumption' (EPOC; Gaesser and Brooks, 1984). The term 'EPOC' has the advantage that its name does not suppose a mechanistic, and potentially erroneous, origin of the increased O_2 consumption post-exercise.

What Hill was actually describing was a linear and symmetrical system, where the controlling variables for $\dot{V}O_2$ exert their influence in the same way at the onset and cessation of exercise, through predictable mechanisms. Since this pioneering work, these models of Hill and Krogh have been adapted and updated; however, the central tenets of this hypothesis remain intact. Later work by di Prampero *et al.* (1970) and Whipp (1970), among others, largely corroborated the suggestions of these pioneers; namely, that the responses of $\dot{V}O_2$ to square-wave exercise are generally well described by a simple exponential function. More recent investigations have concentrated on particular kinetic features of the $\dot{V}O_2$ profile, in order to characterize the pulmonary response in detail and subsequently identify systemic or intramuscular events that share these characteristics, thereby identifying potential control mediators. For example, most investigators would agree that $\dot{V}O_2$ kinetics are intensity-dependent, with profiles that conform to first-order behaviour (i.e. are dynamically linear) below the lactate threshold (LT) (e.g. Linnarsson, 1974; Hughson and Morrisey, 1982;

Whipp *et al.*, 1982) and that manifest temporal- and amplitude-based non-linearities at high (supra-LT) intensities (e.g. Linnarsson, 1974; Barstow and Molé, 1991; Paterson and Whipp, 1991) (see Chapter 12 for specific discussion of these points).

In order to appropriately characterize a system and its controlling determinants, it is necessary to determine the dynamic responses of its key components to specific input forcing functions. Both 'deterministic' (e.g. step, ramp, sinusoid, impulse) and 'stochastic' (e.g. pseudo-random binary sequence (PRBS)) work rate ($\dot{W}$) functions have been used to 'force' the $\dot{V}O_2$ control system in order to extract its response characteristics in the form of a transfer function ($H_{(s)}$). These $\dot{W}$ forcings differ in the appropriateness of their application, depending on factors such as the desired range of stimulating frequencies (i.e. system components having rapid response kinetics are best excited by high rather than low frequencies), the time for which they can be applied, and the likely 'order' of the component(s) of the control system under study (e.g. Fujihara *et al.*, 1973). As a general principle, combinations of work-rate forcings and $\dot{V}O_2$ measurement strategies that produce the most dynamic information with optimal signal-to-noise characteristics are the most useful for such investigative purposes.

The simplest, first-order configuration can be characterized by a transfer function of the general form:

$$H_{(s)} = Ae^{-sTD}/(1 + s\tau) \tag{7.1}$$

where s is the Laplace notation of the complex frequency variable, A is the steady-state (zero-frequency) response amplitude, and TD and τ are delay and time-constant terms, respectively.

A first-order system is one whose input–output relationship (e.g. $\dot{W} - \dot{V}O_2$) can be fully described by equations whose operators are a series of linear differential equations (e.g. with mono-exponential response characteristics for square-wave exercise). Thus, on–off symmetry of response to repeating functions, such as the square-wave, sinusoid and PRBS, should prevail. Dynamic linearity demands that G (the system gain, related to A), τ and TD are independent both of the baseline $\dot{W}$ and of the actual forcing function amplitude and frequency characteristics (thus satisfying the Boltzmann principle of 'superposition': e.g. Milsum, 1966; Fujihara *et al.*, 1973; Riggs, 1976; Lamarra *et al.*, 1983, 1987). The principle of superposition states that the system response to two separate inputs can be calculated by simply adding the response to each input, considered as if the other input were not present (Riggs, 1976).

In the particular context of the control of $\dot{V}O_2$ and thence muscle O_2 consumption ($m\dot{V}O_2$), it is reasonable to assume that

(1) the power-related rate of muscular ATP hydrolysis ($d[ATP]/dt$ or $[\dot{ATP}]$) is the system 'input', and
(2) the rate of mitochondrial oxidative phosphorylation (i.e. $d(m\dot{V}O_2)/dt$ or $m\dot{V}O_2$) in the involved musculature is the system 'output'.

The control of $m\dot{V}O_2$ can therefore be considered to lie among the reactants and products (or some combination thereof) within the sequence of steps that link [ATP] to $m\dot{V}O_2$.

Identification of the $m\dot{V}O_2$ transfer function requires further inference. [ATP] is a difficult quantity to accurately determine in exercising humans, although it may be possible to infer from the initial rate of PCr hydrolysis (see section on 'Spatial considerations'). Nonetheless, it is often assumed that a 'square-wave' increase in $\dot{W}$ (i.e. the abrupt imposition of a constant work rate, typically from a baseline of rest or light exercise) will give rise to an increment in ATP turnover rate which bears a constant proportionality to the imposed $\dot{W}$ increment (i.e. remaining unchanged for the duration of the exercise bout) and which is reflected in the magnitude of the steady-state increment in $m\dot{V}O_2$ and consequently $\dot{V}O_2$. While this notion is commonly held (and, under most conditions, is probably correct; e.g. Crow and Kushmerick, 1982; but also see Gonzalez-Alonso et al., 2000 for discussion), some exceptions have been reported. Most notably, during high-intensity constant-load knee-extension exercise, Bangsbo et al. (2001) reported that the total ATP turnover rate actually increased over the three-minute duration of the bout.

In addition, accurate measurement of intramuscular $m\dot{V}O_2$ and its kinetic features in humans (assumption (2)) is also challenging, not the least because of its invasive nature (e.g. Andersen and Saltin, 1985). A major source of concern, for example, is the appropriate temporal alignment of the rapidly changing blood flow and venous O_2 content profiles at a sampling site downstream of the working muscles (for discussion, see Bangsbo et al., 2000). Consequently, the kinetics of $m\dot{V}O_2$ are often inferred from the more readily (and non-invasively) measured pulmonary $\dot{V}O_2$ response. It is important to recognize, however, that this expedient also requires special consideration during the transient phase and is likely to be rigorous only under certain conditions. That is, increases in $m\dot{V}O_2$ occurring at the mitochondrion are separated from the lung by volume- and time-dependent processes. The venous return (and thence cardiac output ($\dot{Q}_T$)) and the 'effective' venous volume (V_V) between the capillary exchange interfaces in working muscle and lung are the two major variables that influence the accuracy with which the $m\dot{V}O_2$ response kinetics can be estimated from those of $\dot{V}O_2$ (Barstow et al., 1990). Using the reasonable assumption that the exponential increase in $m\dot{V}O_2$ begins essentially instantaneously at the onset of square-wave exercise (e.g. Behnke et al., 2002; also see Chapter 6 for discussion), the $m\dot{V}O_2$ response profile is then expressed at the lung after a delay related to the corresponding kinetics of $\dot{Q}_T$ and V_V change (Barstow et al., 1990). That is, the first ~15–20 s of the $\dot{V}O_2$ response (Phase I) occur in effective isolation from the increased metabolic rate in the working muscles, rather reflecting any concomitant increase in pulmonary blood flow (Krogh and Lindhard, 1913; Whipp et al., 1982). It is the subsequent phase of the $\dot{V}O_2$ response ('Phase II', or the 'fundamental' phase) that reflects the increasing $m\dot{V}O_2$. For example, using a modelling approach, Barstow et al. (1990) predicted that the Phase II $\tau\dot{V}O_2$ should closely reflect that of $m\dot{V}O_2$ (i.e. to within 10%) when reasonable assumptions regarding the values of τ m$\dot{V}O_2$, $\tau \dot{Q}_T$, V_V and the utilization of stored O_2 were used. (These authors emphasized, however, that this kinetic 'association' might not continue to hold if abnormalities in the dynamics of blood flow and/or muscle or pulmonary O_2 exchange were present). This model prediction was subsequently corroborated by direct m$\dot{V}O_2$ measurements in healthy young humans by Grassi *et al.* (1996), who reported that τ m$\dot{V}O_2$ and the Phase II $\tau \dot{V}O_2$ did indeed cohere to within ~10% during moderate-intensity cycle ergometry. It is important to note, however, that this issue has not yet been systematically addressed during higher intensities of exercise.

Variables of interest

The control of m$\dot{V}O_2$ during exercise has been investigated in a range of animal preparations (isolated mitochondria *in vitro*, muscle preparations *in vitro* and *in situ*) – as well as in humans using invasive (i.e. biopsy) and non-invasive (magnetic resonance spectroscopy (MRS) and near infra-red spectroscopy (NIRS)) techniques (e.g. Chance and Williams, 1955; Piiper *et al.*, 1968; Kushmerick and Paul, 1976; Mahler, 1978; Whipp and Mahler, 1980; Bessman and Gieger, 1981; Crow and Kushmerick, 1982; Andersen and Saltin, 1985; Chance *et al.*, 1985; Meyer, 1988; Connett and Honig, 1989; McCully *et al.*, 1994; Grassi *et al.*, 1996, 1998). It is useful to consider the several resulting control models in the context of the primary chemical moieties that link the system 'output' (m$\dot{V}O_2$) to its 'input' (the $\dot{W}$-related [ATP]), that is (a) ADP and/or inorganic phosphate (Pi) from the power-generating sites to the mitochondrion, (b) O_2 and (c) oxidizable substrate in the form of NADH (Figure 7.1). These reactants are linked by the general approximate equation:

$$3ADP + 3Pi + NADH + H^+ + \tfrac{1}{2}O_2 \rightarrow 3ATP + NAD^+ + H_2O \qquad (7.2)$$

The control of oxidative phosphorylation may be thought to be particularly 'effective', in the sense that intramuscular [ATP] is consistently maintained, certainly during volitional dynamic exercise; a declining [ATP] appears to be confined to conditions for which muscle perfusion is highly compromised, such as intense isometric exercise or experimentally induced vascular occlusion paradigms. Chance *et al.*(1985) have suggested that, as the rate of oxidative phosphorylation during exercise appears to be so tightly controlled (and hence [ATP] homeostasis protected), the transfer function is likely to lie with one or more of the reactants that are (very) closely associated with ATP hydrolysis (Figure 7.1 and Eqn (7.2)). Indeed, in such a system, the reduction in [ATP] itself might be expected to be the most potent controller of all (Chance *et al.*, 1985).

The availability of O_2 has been argued by some to exert a limiting influence on m$\dot{V}O_2$ and, thence, $\dot{V}O_2$ kinetics (e.g. Hughson and Morrisey, 1982; Tschakovsky and Hughson, 1999). And while most investigators agree that

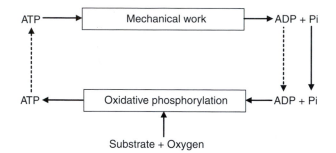

Figure 7.1 Schematic representation of the variables immediately involved in oxidative phosphorylation. The diagram represents the orientation of the intramuscular reactants given in Eqn (7.2). Putative control mechanisms have been suggested to occur within one or more of the reactants feeding into the mitochondrion, for example ADP or Pi, oxidizable substrate (NADH), and oxygen. ADP and ATP are 'shuttled' between the site of power production and oxidative phosphorylation (depicted by the dashed arrows) via exchange of high-energy phosphate with Cr or PCr and catalysed by the creatine kinase reaction (Eqn(7.4)).

a perfusion-related limitation is unlikely to contribute appreciably to the control of $m\dot{V}O_2$ kinetics in the moderate-intensity domain (e.g. Whipp and Mahler, 1980; Grassi *et al.*, 1998; Tschakovsky and Hughson, 1999; Whipp *et al.*, 2002; also see Chapter 12), this may not be the case above LT (e.g. Tschakovsky and Hughson, 1999; Whipp *et al.*, 2002). Furthermore, as intramitochondrial PO_2 could reasonably be viewed as a feedforward determinant of $m\dot{V}O_2$, a step in the 'O$_2$ cascade' located downstream of the muscle capillary bed also has the potential to influence $m\dot{V}O_2$ control. Interestingly, too, considerations of O$_2$ limitation do not necessarily preclude the involvement of intramuscular feedback processes (ADP-mediated feedback control, for instance, as discussed later), whereby the actual $m\dot{V}O_2$ transfer function (i.e. the 'controller') could involve a system not immediately related to O$_2$ availability although its actions may be limited by it.

An alternative form of feedforward control proposes that substrate delivery to the electron transport chain (in the form of NADH) determines the rate of oxidative phosphorylation, with pyruvate dehydrogenase (PDH) imposing a 'stenosis' at the level of pyruvate processing (Timmons *et al.*, 1996). Timmons and co-workers (1996, 1998) have demonstrated a reduction in the components of the O$_2$ deficit (i.e. PCr hydrolysis and blood [lactate] accumulation) with prior PDH activation using dichloroacetate (DCA) administration. As a result, they suggested that $m\dot{V}O_2$ kinetics at exercise onset should be speeded (i.e. by removing/alleviating the stenosis at PDH), and, indeed, Greenhaff and colleagues (2002) have shown that an acetyl group deficit is evident at exercise onset. However, DCA administration has, thus far, failed to demonstrate any discernible speeding of $\tau\ m\dot{V}O_2$ or $\tau\ \dot{V}O_2$ in animals

(Grassi *et al.*, 2002) or humans (Bangsbo *et al.*, 2002; Rossiter *et al.*, 2003b; Jones *et al.*, 2004). In a similar context, the process that signals increased cytoplasmic ATP hydrolysis (e.g. Ca^{2+} release from the sarcoplasmic reticulum) could theoretically exert a feedforward control of $m\dot{V}O_2$ (see Hansford, 1994, for review; and Chapter 9).

The other main category of $m\dot{V}O_2$ control involves feedback, with control being exerted from the products of ATP hydrolysis via the biochemical system transfer function linking ATP hydrolysis to oxidative phosphorylation (Figure 7.1). For example, intracellular increases in both free (or un-bound) [ADP] ($[ADP]_{free}$) and [Pi] have been shown to increase the rate of mitochondrial respiration in isolated preparations (Chance and Williams, 1955). During exercise, therefore, increases in intracellular $[ADP]_{free}$ and/or [Pi] have been proposed to exert feedback control, increasing $m\dot{V}O_2$ via traditional Michaelis–Menten enzyme dynamics (e.g. Chance and Williams, 1955; Chance *et al.*, 1981). These proposals are discussed in greater detail later in the context of whole-body exercise in humans (see 'Simultaneous determination of intramuscular phosphates and $\dot{V}O_2$').

Spatial considerations

The pertinent sites of bioenergetic concern in skeletal muscle cells are separated not only by the mitochondrial membrane itself, but also by the distance between the force-producing cross-bridge and the mitochondrion. It is necessary, therefore, to consider the significance of the creatine kinase (CK) reaction which catalyses the reversible exchange of high-energy phosphate between creatine (Cr) and ADP, both at the mitochondrion (the Mi isoform) and close to the contractile machinery (the MM isoform). Thus, ADP produced at the cross-bridge:

$$ATP \rightarrow ADP + Pi + \alpha H^+ \qquad (7.3)$$

(where α is a stoichiometric coefficient) is functionally cycled between the cross-bridge and the mitochondrion by exchange with PCr:

$$ADP + PCr + H^+ \leftrightarrow ATP + Cr \qquad (7.4)$$

The net outcome of these reactions can, therefore, be considered to be

$$PCr + \beta H^+ \rightarrow Cr + Pi \qquad (7.5)$$

where β is a stoichiometric coefficient, which is pH-dependent and ranges from approximately 0.4 to 0.8 at pH 7.0 and 6.0, respectively (e.g. LeMasters, 1984). The PCr system has consequently been suggested to provide an important spatial buffer between sites of energy production and utilization (Figure 7.2). But, possibly as importantly, is the growing recognition that the PCr system may also play a crucial role in the control of $m\dot{V}O_2$ kinetics (e.g. Bessman and Geiger, 1981;

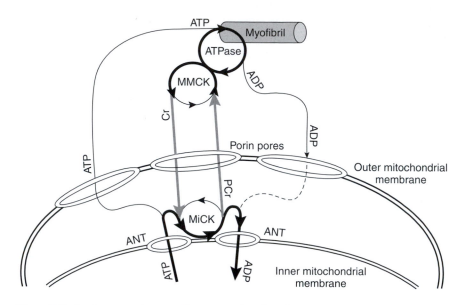

Figure 7.2 A schematic diagram illustrating the phosphocreatine (PCr), creatine kinase (CK) and adenine nucleotide translocase (ANT) systems. Phosphate exchange occurs between creatine (Cr) and PCr via CK and is 'shuttled' between sites of CK at the mechanical machinery (MMCK) and the mitochondria (MiCK). PCr and Cr entry to the mitochondrial intermembrane space is relatively uninhibited, compared to ADP, where entry to the mitochondrion is restricted (dotted line). This restriction is thought to be fibre-type dependent – see text. High-energy phosphates are primarily transferred between the mitochondrion and myofibrils by the exchange of PCr/Cr rather than ATP/ADP: this is the basis for the 'creatine shuttle' hypothesis of $m\dot{V}O_2$ control. The weighting of the arrows indicates the relative flux of each pathway during exercise, that is ATP is thought to be quickly hydrolysed on exiting the inner space via MiCK, producing PCr. The rates of entry and exit of both ATP and ADP to the cytosol (via porin pores) are likely to be limited, compared to Cr and PCr flux. Pi has been excluded from the diagram for clarity; for a more complete picture see Saks *et al.* (2001). (The authors would like to thank Brandon Walsh, 2002 for this figure).

Mahler, 1985; Wallimann *et al.*, 1992; Van Deursen *et al.*, 1993; Greenhaff, 2003; Saks *et al.*, 2001; Walsh *et al*; 2001; Roman *et al.*, 2002).

Similarly, the adenine nucleotide translocase (ANT) and porin systems are a key energetic link between the mitochondrial and cytosolic compartments of muscle (Figure 7.2). ANT catalyses the transmembrane exchange between ATP (generated intramitochondrially by oxidative phosphorylation) and intermembrane ADP. The rate of the ANT translocase reaction is determined, in part, by [ATP] (i.e. ATP being a competitive inhibitor). Thus, the extramitochondrial [ATP]/[ADP] ratio has been proposed as a potential controller of $m\dot{V}O_2$ by determining the rate of ADP delivery to the mitochondrion. This hypothesis was expanded by Owen and Wilson (1974) and Holian *et al.* (1977) who, having demonstrated that the apparent Km for ADP was dependent on both [ATP] and [Pi], suggested that the rate of oxidative phosphorylation may be dependent on [ATP]/[ADP]·[Pi] or the 'phosphorylation potential' (see Wilson, 1994 for review).

While access to the inter-membrane space is restricted for ADP (but this may be fibre type dependent, e.g. Saks *et al.*, 2001), both Cr and Pi can move relatively freely between the cytoplasm and the inter-mitochondrial membrane space. Thus, they have the potential to more directly influence $m\dot{V}O_2$. Indeed, the premise of the 'Cr shuttle' hypothesis of oxidative phosphorylation control (Bessman and Geiger, 1981) utilizes this property of 'free' movement (relative to ADP) in order to transduce a feedback signal to where it is required; that is local increases in [Cr] resulting from energy buffering at the cross-bridge (Eqn(7.3)) being transduced to the inter-mitochondrial membrane space where Cr can accept a high-energy phosphate from a newly formed ATP, in turn increasing [ADP] to provide an increase in substrate for oxidative phosphorylation (i.e. Michaelis–Menten feedback control; Figure 7.2). Therefore, the rate of delivery of Cr to the mitochondrion and the consequent rate of PCr hydrolysis has the potential to provide an appropriate feedback signal for $m\dot{V}O_2$ control, rather than direct feedback from [ADP]$_{free}$. Meyer (1988) reported, for rat *gastrocnemius* muscle, that the rate of PCr hydrolysis was proportional to stimulation frequency and τ[PCr] remained essentially constant both over a wide range of stimulation frequencies and also between the on- and off-transients (i.e. on–off symmetry). This finding is consistent with the proposal of a dynamically linear $m\dot{V}O_2$ control system related to [PCr]. Furthermore, Mahler (1985) demonstrated that, for isolated frog *sartorius* muscle (at 20°C), [PCr] and $m\dot{V}O_2$ kinetics were essentially indistinguishable from each other. These findings thus corroborate the earlier proposals of Bessman and Geiger (1981), implicating Cr (or PCr) as a crucial factor in $m\dot{V}O_2$ feedback control.

More recently it has been suggested that the [PCr]/[Cr] may be of crucial importance with regard to the creatine shuttle system (e.g. Saks *et al.*, 2001; Walsh *et al.*, 2001). Walsh *et al.* (2001) found that a low [PCr]/[Cr] caused [ADP]-stimulated mitochondrial respiration to become sensitized (i.e. flux at a greater rate than predicted), compared to when the [PCr]/[Cr] was high. This suggests that local (i.e. inter-membrane) alterations in [PCr] and/or [Cr] may facilitate [ADP] access or provision to the respiratory sites that increase $m\dot{V}O_2$. Interestingly, this concept is compatible with the development of a $\dot{V}O_2$ slow component only at exercise intensities that reduce [PCr]/[Cr] sufficiently (i.e. high-intensity) and not during moderate reductions in [PCr]/[Cr] as seen during moderate-intensity exercise (see below for discussion on the $\dot{V}O_2$ slow component).

The energetic buffering provided by PCr also allows the ATP requirement to be estimated, at least for square-wave exercise. As PCr is the sole buffer of ATP hydrolysis at the initial instant (t_i) of exercise onset, the initial rate of change of [PCr] (dPCr/dt$_i$)is thought to reflect the rate of ATP hydrolysis at exercise onset (e.g. Kemp *et al.*, 2001). As discussed earlier, the rate of ATP hydrolysis is thought to be constant throughout constant-load exercise (at least for those work-rates where $\dot{V}O_2$ can attain a steady-state). Therefore, for a particular imposed work-rate, the initial rate of ATP hydrolysis, reflected in $dPCr/dt_i$, is often used to estimate the associated ATP requirement (e.g. Conley *et al.*, 1998, 2001; Kemp *et al.*, 2001).

Simultaneous determination of intramuscular phosphates and $\dot{V}O_2$

Most of the control models proposed earlier have been developed in 'reduced', well-controlled preparations, which range from isolated mitochondria to isolated muscle (e.g. Chance and Williams, 1955, 1956; Owen and Wilson, 1974; Kushmerick and Paul, 1976; Mahler, 1985). However, while such conditions are necessary to examine the intricacies of enzyme-catalysed reaction kinetics, they are necessarily simplistic when considering the integrative and systemic nature of whole-body exercise.

Many of the key biochemical moieties implicated in the control of $m\dot{V}O_2$ during exercise are accessible by [31]phosphorus magnetic resonance spectroscopy (^{31}P-MRS). ^{31}P-MRS provides the opportunity to measure *in vivo*, non-invasively and with high temporal resolution phosphorous-containing molecules whose concentrations are maintained above ~1–2 mM. Importantly, the technique is selectively sensitive to the unbound forms of the metabolites of interest (i.e. the thermodynamically relevant concentrations).

In addition, intramuscular pH can be estimated via the pH-sensitive property of the chemical shift of Pi. As the chemical shift of PCr within the MR spectrum is not pH-sensitive (at least over the physiological range), the relationship:

$$pH = 6.75 + \log\left[\frac{\delta_c - 3.27}{5.69 - \delta_c}\right] \tag{7.6}$$

(where δ_c is the chemical shift of Pi relative to PCr; Moon and Richards, 1973) allows determination of intramuscular pH with the same temporal frequency as other ^{31}P metabolites.

However, because $[ADP]_{free}$ is normally maintained at sub-micromolar levels in skeletal muscle, it cannot be estimated directly by MRS; rather requiring calculation based on the equilibrium of the CK reaction and assumptions regarding total intramuscular Cr (TCr) content. As [Cr] cannot be measured by ^{31}P MRS, its estimation relies on the assumption of a constant value for [TCr] (commonly ~36.9 mM, based on biochemical assay of human muscle biopsy samples (e.g. Sahlin *et al.*, 1987)). And as the calculated $[ADP]_{free}$ value can be very sensitive to the value of [TCr], interpretation of the calculated $[ADP]_{free}$ should be made with caution. The assumptions inherent in the $[ADP]_{free}$ calculation are numerous and, while reasonable, may affect the confidence with which this calculation can be applied. Importantly, however, as the [TCr] assumption affects the baseline and amplitude of the exercise-induced $[ADP]_{free}$ response in essentially the same proportion, the $[ADP]_{free}$ time course may be more confidently estimated (see Kushmerick, 1998, for discussion).

Previous studies to investigate putative intramuscular $m\dot{V}O_2$ control theories in terms of $\dot{V}O_2$ kinetics have been constrained by the technical challenges of determining $\dot{V}O_2$ kinetics within the magnetic environment of a super-conducting magnet. For example, in the studies both of Barstow *et al.* (1994a,b) and of McCreary *et al.* (1996), subjects performed exercise: (a) on separate days for the ^{31}P and $\dot{V}O_2$ determinations and (b) using either different muscle groups (Barstow *et al.*, 1994a,b) or small muscle groups (McCreary *et al.*, 1996). A greater degree of interpretational robustness is conferred when the ^{31}P and $\dot{V}O_2$ measurements are made simultaneously and from the same muscle groups (i.e. input and output functions being measured under precisely the same conditions) and also with signal-to-noise characteristics appropriate for statistically confident kinetic estimation. The methods employed for simultaneous pulmonary gas exchange and ^{31}P-MRS kinetic measurements have been previously described (Rossiter *et al.*, 1999; Whipp *et al.*, 1999). Briefly, the ^{31}P-MR free induction decay can be determined approximately every 2 s from a ~12 cm hemisphere of *quadriceps* muscle. Pulmonary gas exchange is determined breath-by-breath using a volume (turbine) and gas concentration (mass spectrometer) analysis system, custom-designed to allow rigorous measurement within the restrictions of the magnetic environment (Whipp *et al.*, 1999). In this way, a range of work rates (and, therefore, associated [ATP] values) can be imposed, with ^{31}P and $\dot{V}O_2$ variables being determined simultaneously from recruitment of the same muscles with the same fibre profile, allowing the putative control theories to be investigated with greater rigour than previously (cf. Barstow *et al.*, 1994a,b; McCreary *et al.*, 1996).

Kinetic profiles

The Phase II or fundamental $\dot{V}O_2$ kinetics for moderate-intensity (i.e. sub-LT) exercise (most commonly determined from cycle ergometry) are generally agreed to conform well to a first-order system (e.g. Casaburi *et al.*, 1978; Whipp *et al.*, 1982; Lamarra *et al.*, 1983, 1987; Swanson and Hughson, 1988; Hughson *et al.*, 1990; Haouzi *et al.*, 1993; Fukuba *et al.*, 2000). For example, in response to a square-wave increase in work rate, $\dot{V}O_2$ is well described by an exponential with the general form:

$$\tau \cdot d\dot{V}O_2/dt + \Delta\dot{V}O_{2(t)} = \Delta\dot{V}O_{2(ss)} \tag{7.7}$$

where the product of the instantaneous rate of change of $\dot{V}O_2$ ($d\dot{V}O_2/dt$) and τ determines the value of $\dot{V}O_2$ at time t after exercise onset ($\Delta\dot{V}O_{2(t)}$), which asymptotes at a value $\Delta\dot{V}O_{2(ss)}$. And, indeed, the 'functional' system gain ('functional' in the sense that the gain is unconventional in not being a dimensionless quantity, that is equal to $\Delta\dot{V}O_{2(ss)}/\Delta\dot{W}$) for moderate-intensity exercise is generally accepted not to significantly differ across gender or with training status or age (e.g. Hagberg *et al.*, 1980; Babcock *et al.*, 1994; although see Mallory *et al.*, 2002 for a different view; see also Chapters 13 and 15). The Phase II $\tau\dot{V}O_2$ has been reported to be essentially the same for the on- and off-transients, at least for cycle ergometry (e.g. Özyener *et al.*, 2001). τ typically ranges between 20 and 40 s in healthy young adults (e.g. Whipp *et al.*, 1982; Barstow and Molé, 1991; Paterson and Whipp, 1991), tending to be shorter in trained subjects (Hagberg *et al.*, 1980) and appreciably longer in elderly sedentary subjects (Babcock *et al.*, 1994).

Above LT, it has been consistently demonstrated that $\dot{V}O_2$ manifests a secondary kinetic component that supplements the fundamental component (e.g. Whipp and Wasserman, 1972; Linnarsson, 1974; Barstow and Molé, 1991; Paterson and Whipp, 1991; Burnley *et al.*, 2000; Özyener *et al.*, 2001; Carter *et al.*, 2002). This secondary component has been demonstrated for many different modes of exercise, including cycle ergometry (e.g. Barstow and Molé, 1991; Paterson and Whipp, 1991), treadmill running (e.g. Langsetmo *et al.*, 1997; Carter *et al.*, 2002), swimming (e.g. Demarie *et al.*, 2001) and knee-extensor exercise (e.g. Rossiter *et al.*, 2001). This secondary component develops slowly, becoming discernible from the fundamental component only after a relatively long delay of ~2–3 min. When a steady state is attainable (i.e. below 'critical power', the asymptote of the power–duration relationship for high-intensity exercise (Moritani *et al.*, 1981)), the resulting $\dot{V}O_2$ is greater than that predicted from the sub-LT $\dot{V}O_2 - \dot{W}$ relationship, with values as much as 13 ml$\cdot$min$^{-1}\cdot$W^{-1} not being uncommon for cycle ergometry. For these reasons, this kinetic component has been termed both the '$\dot{V}O_2$ slow component' and the 'excess $\dot{V}O_2$ component'. In contrast to moderate exercise, on–off symmetry of the $\dot{V}O_2$ kinetics is not retained above LT (Barstow and Molé, 1991; Paterson and Whipp, 1991; Özyener *et al.*, 2001).

The response kinetics of $\dot{V}O_2$ and their intensity-dependence have provided important clues to the control of $m\dot{V}O_2$, not least because of the ability to explore dynamic co-relationships between $\dot{V}O_2$ and putative feedback controllers of the kind discussed in the previous section. The kinetics of many of the variables involved in the various control hypotheses can be discerned in the examples of the ^{31}P spectra in response to rest–exercise–rest transitions in both the moderate- and high-intensity domains in Figure 7.3 (Rossiter *et al.*, 2002a). The area under the PCr peak (at a relative chemical shift of 0 ppm) is proportional to the volume-weighted average [PCr] within the field of view of the MR probe. It is evident that PCr essentially buffers any tendency for [ATP] to fall, not only at exercise onset but also subsequently in the transient of both moderate and heavy 6-min exercise bouts. The three resonances of ATP (only two of which can be easily visualized in Figure 7.3) reflect the effects of chemical bond and molecular structure, which are subtly different for each of the three ^{31}P metabolites (γ-ATP at ~2 ppm; α-ATP at ~8 ppm and β-ATP at ~16 ppm). During the phase of PCr hydrolysis, a corresponding increase in [Pi] is also observed (via the net CK reaction; Eqn (7.5)). While [Cr] is not measured directly in the spectrum, it can be simply inferred from

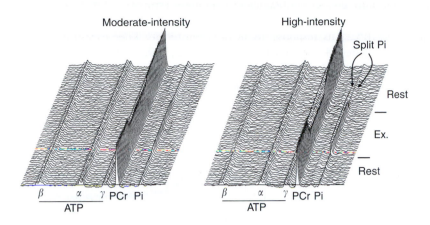

Figure 7.3 Two examples of ^{31}P spectra from the same subject during moderate- (sub-LT)
and high- (supra-LT) intensity square-wave knee-extensor exercise (a rest–
exercise–rest square-wave bout of 4–6–6 minutes, respectively). The subject was
lying prone in the bore of a whole-body 1.5 T, super-conducting magnet. The
area under the PCr peak (at a relative chemical shift of 0 ppm) is proportional
to [PCr] within the field of view of the MR probe (a ~12 cm hemisphere of the
quadriceps muscle). Note that PCr buffers any potential fall in [ATP] at exercise
onset and throughout the later stages of the transient. The three resonances of
ATP are at ~2 ppm (γ-ATP), ~8 ppm (α-ATP) and ~16 ppm (β-ATP). During
the period in which PCr is hydrolysed, an increase in [Pi] (at ~−5 ppm) can be
seen (via the net CK reaction; Eqn(7.5)). Note that during high-intensity exercise, a secondary Pi peak emerges (from behind the original) representing Pi that
is resonating in a low pH environment. (Figures reproduced, with permission,
from Rossiter *et al.*, 2002a).

the [PCr] response (i.e. [Cr] = [TCr] − [PCr], recalling that [TCr] can be assumed
to remain constant throughout the exercise).

It is important to emphasize that the relatively large MR probe effectively
'homogenizes' the muscle, so that any differences between the metabolic profiles
in different fibre types (e.g. baseline values and subsequent kinetics) cannot be
identified. While this homogenised signal is the relevant one for comparison
with pulmonary $\dot{V}O_2$, whole-body MRS is as yet not sufficiently sensitive to
allow single-fibre spectroscopy. Techniques such as chemical-shift imaging
(see Whipp *et al.*, 2002 for an example) have adequate spatial resolution to
elucidate differences between individual muscles in a large limb, and insight into
regional heterogeneities of muscle function may be evident in the specific
characteristics of the ^{31}P spectrum (see 'Heterogeneity of Pi kinetics'). However,
as yet, the specifics of cellular energetics in different fibre types are difficult to
elucidate in humans using this technique.

The larger muscle mass provided by the knee-extensor exercise model,
coupled with the ability to monitor ^{31}P variables and $\dot{V}O_2$ simultaneously and at
high temporal sampling rates (relative to the underlying kinetics), introduces

a substantially greater confidence of parameter estimation (cf. McCreary *et al.*, 1996). A representative example of the time-aligned kinetic profiles for $\dot{V}O_2$ and *quadriceps* [PCr] in response to moderate-intensity knee-extensor exercise is shown in Figure 7.4 (adapted from Rossiter *et al.*, 2002a). It is clear that the [PCr]

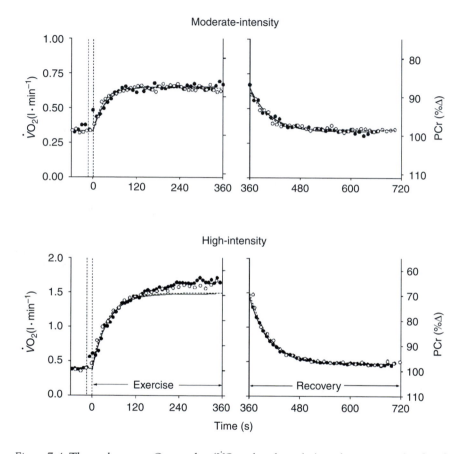

Figure 7.4 The pulmonary O_2 uptake ($\dot{V}O_2$; closed circles) and intramuscular [PCr] (expressed as a relative change from a baseline of 100%; open circles) kinetic responses during moderate- and high-intensity square-wave exercise transitions (rest–exercise–rest: also see Figure 7.3). The responses are phase-aligned, that is the Phase II or fundamental $\dot{V}O_2$ response is shifted in time so that it overlies the [PCr] response, thereby accounting for the limb-to-lung transit delay. All responses (PCr and $\dot{V}O_2$ on- and off-transients) are fitted with mono-exponential curves; for moderate exercise, the entire response (following Phase I) is modelled, whereas for high-intensity exercise only that portion of the response that conforms to an exponential is modelled. Note that during high-intensity exercise both time- and amplitude-based non-linearities are apparent in the $\dot{V}O_2$ response ($\dot{V}O_2$ slow component), and that these are reflected, almost entirely, in the intramuscular [PCr] kinetics. Also note that no deviation from mono-exponentiality is discernible in the high-intensity off-transients of either $\dot{V}O_2$ or [PCr]. Redrawn from Rossiter *et al.* (2002a).

profile bears a close temporal relationship to the Phase II $\dot{V}O_2$ component. The on- and off-transient [PCr] and Phase II $\dot{V}O_2$ responses are well described by a mono-exponential function (Eqn (7.7)). Of particular interest is that these $\dot{V}O_2$ and [PCr] responses are essentially indistinguishable from each other. For example, for the on-transient, within each subject the $\tau \dot{V}O_2$ and τ [PCr] were similar, averaging 35 and 34 s respectively (based on subjects in Rossiter *et al.*, 1999, 2002a). A similar kinetic association was also evident within subjects during the off-transient. In contrast to moderate-intensity cycle ergometry, however, the off-transient kinetics were appreciably slower than for the on-transient, with $\tau \dot{V}O_2$ averaging 50 s, τ [PCr] 51 s (Rossiter *et al.*, 2002a).

There is much debate as to whether [PCr] kinetics during moderate exercise are consequent to those of $m\dot{V}O_2$ or *vice versa* (e.g. Whipp and Mahler, 1980; Tschakovsky and Hughson, 1999). This uncertainty arises because it is not straightforward to separate PCr into its discrete contributions as an energy buffer (see above) and as a putative control-linked metabolite (i.e. whereby a fall in [PCr] or increase in [Cr] and/or [ADP]$_{free}$ could be the necessary signal transducer for increasing $m\dot{V}O_2$). At present, support for the latter (control) function derives largely from demonstrations of the close dynamic correlation between [PCr] and $m\dot{V}O_2$ (e.g. Piiper *et al.*, 1968; Crow and Kushmerick, 1982; Mahler, 1985) or its proxy, $\dot{V}O_2$ (Barstow *et al.*, 1994b; McCreary *et al.*, 1996; Rossiter *et al.*, 1999). This proposal is strengthened by the observations of Rossiter *et al.* (1999) that the similarity between τ [PCr] and $\tau \dot{V}O_2$ for knee-extensor exercise was preserved, despite $\tau \dot{V}O_2$ varying substantially between their subjects (range: 20–68 s). Further support is provided by the demonstration that, again for knee-extensor exercise, the off-transient $\dot{V}O_2$ kinetics are slow (relative to the on-transient) (Rossiter *et al.*, 2002a); that is despite $\dot{V}O_2$ at any point in the recovery phase being higher than expected (from the on-transient), [PCr] is not replenished any more rapidly (τ [PCr] and $\tau \dot{V}O_2$ being essentially the same) (Figure 7.4). This does raise a more fundamental question: why are the recovery kinetics of [PCr] slower than those for the on-transient? Finally, during the steady-state of moderate-intensity exercise, when O_2 delivery is sufficient [PCr] is not replenished until exercise is ceased or $\dot{W}$ reduced. During exercise, net [PCr] is only reduced, not increased – even though this would only require a very small (and transient) increase in $\dot{V}O_2$ (e.g. Crow and Kushmerick, 1982; Meyer, 1988; Conley *et al.*, 1998; Rossiter *et al.*, 1999; Kemp *et al.*, 2001; among others). This scenario contrasts with the transient lactate (and presumably metabolic H^+) production that has been reported for work rates in the upper reaches of the moderate-intensity domain (e.g. Cerretelli *et al.*, 1979). This is presumably reflective of an increased transient glycolytic contribution to ATP resynthesis, which supplements the PCr contribution prior to oxidative phosphorylation reaching a flux plateau; with the ensuing lactate yield subsequently being metabolized oxidatively at the expense of $\dot{V}O_2$ (e.g. Cerretelli *et al.*, 1979). However, Haseler *et al.* (1999) have suggested that [PCr] recovery is indeed dependent on O_2 availability, as they were able to elicit a speeding of τ [PCr] with high fractions of inspired O_2 in exercise-trained subjects. As such, the debate regarding the role of [PCr] in determining $m\dot{V}O_2$ kinetics continues.

It is appropriate at this juncture to revisit the broad assumption that the Phase II $\dot{V}O_2$ kinetics are dynamically linear and first-order in the moderate-intensity domain. For example, on–off symmetry of responses to repeating functions, such as the square-wave, sinusoid and PRBS, should prevail for first-order kinetics to be manifest. Symmetry (i.e. similar τ $\dot{V}O_2$ values for both the on- and off-transition) has been reported for the Phase II $\dot{V}O_2$ response to square-wave exercise (Griffiths et al., 1986; Barstow and Molé, 1991; Özyener et al., 2001). However, during sinusoidal and PRBS exercise it is conventional practice to assume linearity and thence analyse the on- and off-transients together to yield 'lumped' response parameters (usually by frequency analysis techniques) (Casaburi et al., 1978; Essfeld et al., 1987; Hughson et al., 1990; Hoffman et al., 1992; Fukuoka et al., 1997). It is of some interest, therefore, that on–off $\dot{V}O_2$ symmetry during cycle ergometry has not been unequivocally demonstrated.

There are some reports of asymmetrical on- and off-transient $\dot{V}O_2$ responses to moderate-intensity square-wave cycle-ergometry (e.g. Fukuoka et al., 1997; Brittain et al., 2001). One explanation for these observations may lie in the use of highly fit subjects with a consequently extended work rate range for moderate exercise: this would serve to 'amplify' the expression of system non-linearities that might not be readily discriminated with smaller work rate increments (e.g. Brittain et al., 2001). The cause of such non-linearities is unclear, although one possible influence might derive from the transient blood [lactate] increase seen at exercise onset for higher work-rates in the moderate-intensity domain (Cerretelli et al., 1979). Although evident at some $\dot{W}$ values in the study of Brittain et al. (2001), the on–off asymmetry described for square-wave prone knee-extensor exercise is particularly striking; in this instance the [PCr] response is similarly asymmetrical (Rossiter et al., 2002a) (Figure 7.4); the corresponding arterial [lactate] response was not measured in these studies, however. Furthermore, while the requirement that $\tau\dot{V}O_2$ should be independent of the $\dot{W}$ amplitude for square-wave forcings has not been investigated extensively, there is evidence in the work of Lamarra et al. (1983, 1987) and Brittain et al. (2001) of departures from linearity in this regard, also. Finally, according to the principle of superposition, the Phase II τ should not be influenced by the form of the work-rate forcing function. This is not true of a non-linear system, where the outputs may be dependent on domains of one or more of its operators. And, thus, while the Phase II $\dot{V}O_2$ response has been widely reported to be well described by a first-order function over a wide range of $\dot{W}$ values and intensity domains (square-wave (Griffiths et al., 1986; Barstow and Molé, 1991; Özyener et al., 2001); ramp (Whipp et al., 1981; Swanson and Hughson, 1988); impulse (Lamarra et al., 1987; Hughson et al., 1990)), it is perhaps surprising that a formal and comprehensive investigation of response superposition has not yet been undertaken (although see Lamarra et al., 1983). Based on the foregoing discussion, it seems apparent that the superposition criterion might not be entirely satisfied. These instances are clear when high-intensity exercise is considered, but may also be the case even in the moderate-intensity domain. Indeed, it is of interest to recall that Milsum (1966) has invoked evolutionary pressures as a means of explaining non-linear biological system behaviour: as such systems only rarely encounter inputs resembling steps and impulses (the differential of a step) in nature, this ameliorates the evolutionary pressure to develop linear system responses. 'Consequently the step response may not represent an important evolutionary performance criterion of the system' (Milsum, 1966), and thus it may develop a non-linear behaviour.

But it is above LT that non-linearities in $\dot{V}O_2$ dynamics really emerge, largely as a reflection of the $\dot{V}O_2$ slow component. This time- and intensity-dependent increase in $\dot{V}O_2$ is a useful characteristic that has become vital to understanding the control of $m\dot{V}O_2$. Poole *et al.* (1991) were the first to demonstrate that much, if not all, of the $\dot{V}O_2$ slow component (i.e. ~86%) was likely to originate in the exercising musculature, using cycle ergometer exercise and arterial and venous catheterization techniques. As can be seen in the example of Figure 7.4, the $\dot{V}O_2$ slow component is accompanied by a component of intramuscular [PCr] hydrolysis having a very similar profile. This recent finding, that a similarly slow phase is manifest in the responses of one of the key components common to many of the control hypotheses, would seem to rule out an appreciable contribution to the $\dot{V}O_2$ slow component from muscles that do not contribute to the measured work (i.e. respiratory, cardiac or stabilizing musculature; see Whipp *et al.*, 2002, for review).

A $m\dot{V}O_2$ slow component could theoretically be manifest either by a decrease in P:O_2 ratio (i.e. a less O_2-efficient ATP production) or by an increase in ATP requirement (i.e. a less ATP-efficient force production). We, and others, have reported that the fundamental $\tau \dot{V}O_2$ for supra-LT exercise was not discernibly different than for moderate exercise (e.g. Barstow and Molé, 1991; Özyener *et al.*, 2001; Rossiter *et al.*, 2002a). Rossiter *et al.* (2002a) reported that, by 6 min of constant-load knee-extensor exercise, the $\dot{V}O_2$ slow component had elicited an additional average increase in $\dot{V}O_2$ of ~14% (i.e. normalized to the amplitude of the fundamental component); this $\dot{V}O_2$ slow component that was accompanied by a ~12% increase in [PCr] hydrolysis; that is ~88% of the $\dot{V}O_2$ slow component being manifest in the exercising muscle in the profile of [PCr] hydrolysis (based on data from Rossiter *et al.*, 2001, 2002a,b). This is indicative of the slow component being due to a high ATP-cost of force production, rather than a high O_2-cost of ATP production. For example, if there were a progressive reduction in the P:O_2 ratio leading to expression of the $\dot{V}O_2$ slow component, it would be likely that an increase in $\dot{V}O_2$ would occur without a concomitant fall in [PCr], because the substrates for oxidative phosphorylation should be in good supply at these sub-maximal work rates (see Figures 7.1 and 7.2): that is [ADP]$_{free}$ and [Pi] are raised above baseline values (e.g. Figures 7.5 and 7.6); O_2 is available, as $\dot{V}O_2$ still has the potential to increase (e.g. Figure 7.4); and acetyl-groups appear to accumulate (e.g. Greenhaff *et al.*, 2002). An increased ATP requirement leading to an increased requirement for oxidative ATP production, however, would give rise to a demand for increased energy buffering (by PCr) at the cross-bridge and thus cause [PCr] to fall.

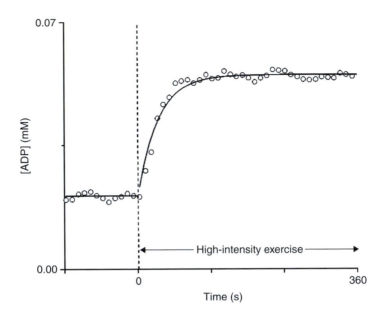

Figure 7.5 The calculated intramuscular [ADP]$_{free}$ response to high-intensity square-wave knee-extensor exercise. The calculation of [ADP]$_{free}$ requires assumptions of total creatine content and equilibrium of the creatine kinase reaction. Note that the [ADP]$_{free}$ response does not manifest a slow-component-like phase, unlike $\dot{V}O_2$ and [PCr] (see Figure 7.4 for examples).

As discussed earlier (see 'Variables of interest' and Figures 7.1 and 7.2), one of the prime candidates for m$\dot{V}O_2$ control is [ADP]$_{free}$ (Chance *et al.*, 1955, 1985). It is interesting therefore, that during high-intensity knee-extensor exercise, the kinetics of calculated [ADP]$_{free}$ do not correspond closely to those of $\dot{V}O_2$ (Figure 7.5). That is, while the Phase II components of [ADP]$_{free}$ and $\dot{V}O_2$ response are similar, there is a tendency for τ [ADP]$_{free}$ to be slightly faster than τ $\dot{V}O_2$ (i.e. ~38 s vs ~45 s, respectively; Rossiter *et al.*, 2003a). This might well be explained by the alkalinizing effect of PCr hydrolysis at exercise onset speeding the rate of ADP accumulation via the CK reaction. It should be emphasized, however, that the difference between these τ values approaches the region of uncertainty induced by circulatory modulation between the muscle and the lung (Barstow *et al.*, 1990). In contrast, during the slow component region of high-intensity exercise, [ADP]$_{free}$ is maintained, rather than continually increasing. That is, only a trivially small ADP slow component could actually be discerned (averaging only ~2% of the Phase II amplitude after 8 min of exercise, compared to ~16% in $\dot{V}O_2$ from the same subjects) (Rossiter *et al.*, 2002c). It could be argued that the falling intramuscular pH during supra-LT exercise drives the CK reaction in the direction of PCr breakdown, thereby generating a [PCr] slow component and maintaining a constant ADP provision to the mitochondrion (see Conley *et al.*, 2001, for example). Based on these observations, it is clear that $\dot{V}O_2$

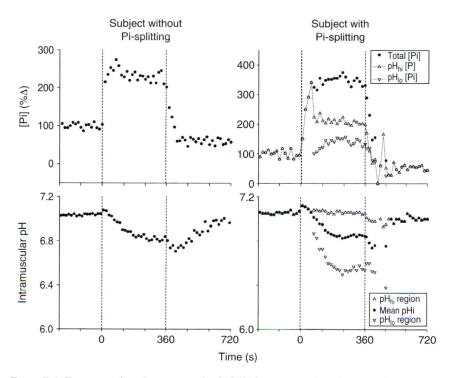

Figure 7.6 Two examples of intramuscular [Pi] ([Pi] is expressed as changes relative to the
baseline of 100%) and pH kinetics during high-intensity exercise. While [Pi]
is not consistently well characterized by an exponential response, the intramuscular pH determined from the chemical shift of Pi (Eqn (7.6)) is a rigorous
estimate. Pi-peak splitting only occurs during high-intensity exercise
(i.e. when a slow component of $\dot{V}O_2$ is manifest), and reflects 'regions' of
muscle that express two pH values. For pH, the mean intramuscular pH
(closed circles) can be seen to be composed of a heterogeneous range of pH
values from normal (~7.05; up-triangles) to very low (~6.5 in this example;
down triangles). Redrawn, in part, from Rossiter *et al.* (2002b).

does not track calculated $[ADP]_{free}$, but rather the [PCr] (or [Cr]) dynamics
(Figures 7.4 and 7.5). Interestingly, however, Walsh *et al.* (2001) recently suggested that the rate of [ADP]-stimulated $m\dot{V}O_2$ may be dependent on both [PCr]
and [Cr]. As [PCr] is reduced during the slow component region, this could
therefore sensitize the mitochondrion to the $[ADP]_{free}$ present. Hence, the
absence of an $[ADP]_{free}$ slow component does not rule out direct [ADP] feedback
control. However, these several observations do favour the creatine shuttle
hypothesis of $m\dot{V}O_2$ control (Bessman and Geiger *et al.*, 1981).

One of the candidate mechanisms of the $\dot{V}O_2$ slow component is the muscle
fibre-type recruitment profile, recognizing that fast-twitch fibres have a low
oxidative efficiency (Crow and Kushmerick, 1982; see Chapters 11 and 12).

For example, the $\dot{V}O_2$ slow component for cycle-ergometry has been reported to be more marked in subjects with a high proportion of fast-twitch fibres in the power generating muscles (e.g. Barstow *et al.*, 1996; Pringle *et al.*, 2003). In addition, the amplitudes of the integrated electromyogram (iEMG) and of the $\dot{V}O_2$ slow component during high-intensity cycle ergometry have been reported to be correlated (Shinohara and Moritani, 1992; Saunders *et al.*, 2000; Borrani *et al.*, 2001; Burnley *et al.*, 2002). In contrast, Scheuermann *et al.* (2001) and Lucia *et al.* (2000) were unable to discern any increase in iEMG in association with the $\dot{V}O_2$ slow component; it being suggested that conventional surface EMG techniques may not have the necessary power to discriminate reliably between the recruitment of type I and type II fibre populations (Scheuermann *et al.*, 2001).

Regardless, there are certain necessary consequences for muscle metabolism that derive from the fibre-type recruitment hypothesis. For instance, regions of the exercising muscle should manifest evidence of fatigue during the slow component period. A $m\dot{V}O_2$ slow component should therefore not necessarily be discernible within each individual muscle fibre recruited, but rather only in the sum of the recruited musculature. Thus far, studies in the single fibre of the frog *sartorius* muscle by Hogan and colleagues have not been able to demonstrate a progressive reduction in intracellular PO_2 of delayed onset during prolonged stimulations (e.g. Kindig *et al.*, 2003a,b). Such findings are not consistent with these fibres manifesting a slow component. However, while developing muscle fatigue is almost certainly a factor during exercise of this intensity (e.g. Shinohara and Moritani, 1992), muscular fatigue has yet to be conclusively demonstrated to occur in unison with the $\dot{V}O_2$ slow component. Furthermore, recruitment of less oxidatively efficient fibres *per se* is not a pre-requisite for the 'recruitment' hypothesis, if the $P:O_2$ falls in the fatigued (or fatiguing) fibres. Recruitment of a fresh fibre (even a type I fibre), when the initially recruited fibre pool cannot sustain the required power output, could result in a $\dot{V}O_2$ slow component if the $P:O_2$ were reduced in the fatigued fibres (i.e. if $P:O_2$ is altered by fatigue). The data herein suggest that $P:O_2$ is unlikely to be changed; however, this awaits conclusive demonstration. These issues are discussed further in Chapter 12.

The MRS approach allows determination of the kinetics of two of the key variables implicated in fatigue, namely [Pi] and pH (using Eqn(7.6)). Figure 7.6 shows examples from two subjects of the kinetics of [Pi] and pH during high-intensity knee-extensor exercise. The kinetics of total free [Pi] do not consistently correlate well with those of $\dot{V}O_2$ (unlike [PCr]) and are highly variable between subjects, as shown in the two examples in Figure 7.6 (see Rossiter *et al.*, 2002b for discussion). The consistent features of the [Pi] and pH responses within this intensity are that [Pi] is high (and in some instances continually increasing) and pH is low (and in some cases continuously falling). These features indicate dynamics that are intensity-dependent, these features not being evident in the moderate-intensity domain. The complex features of these fatigue indices may prove important in understanding the intensity-dependent dynamics of $m\dot{V}O_2$.

Heterogeneity of Pi kinetics

Interpretation of the relative concentration of [Pi], as determined by MRS, is complex. One of the factors affecting the area under the peaks in the ^{31}P spectrum is the longitudinal (T_1) relaxation time of the relevant ^{31}P nuclei. It is important to know the extent to which the T_1 time may change during the course of an experiment, in order to provide an expression of confidence with respect to determination of metabolite concentrations. If T_1 changes during an experiment, it can give the misleading impression of a change in metabolite concentrations in the field of interest, without any change having actually occurred. While it is thought that the T_1 of PCr is constant during the types of experiment detailed herein, whether the T_1 of Pi remains constant is not clear. Nonetheless, while [Pi] determination is potentially complicated by T_1 issues, the ability to determine pH from the frequency of the Pi resonance is maintained as long as Pi is clearly discernible in the spectrum.

An interesting feature, introduced earlier, is the splitting of the Pi peak in the MR spectrum. This splitting appears to be intensity-dependent, only occurring when $\dot{V}O_2$ and [PCr] slow components are manifest (e.g. Rossiter *et al.*, 1999, 2002b). While Pi-peak splitting is not a consistent feature of high-intensity exercise in all subjects (apparent in about half of the subjects we have studied to date; see Figure 7.6 for an example of each), when it is not apparent, a broadening of the Pi peak is clearly discernible (Figure 7.7; Rossiter *et al.*, 2002b). This suggests that there are 'regions' of muscle (only during high-intensity exercise), which can be characterized by either one or two 'compartments' that each expresses a range of different pH values. This progressive broadening within the exercising muscle is compatible with the recruitment of fibres having a greater reliance on glycolytic metabolism (and hence H^+ production). Thus, it has been suggested that the splitting of the Pi peak (Figures 7.3 and 7.8) is a manifestation of fast-twitch fibre recruitment (Yoshida and Watare, 1994). While this proposal has not yet been conclusively verified, the Pi-peak splitting does reflect portions of the exercising muscle that express a 'normal' pH (i.e. ~7.05) despite the high exercise intensity, and portions that express a low pH (i.e. below ~6.95, and as low as ~6.2). It is likely, therefore, that those regions of muscle at low pH (Figure 7.6; see Rossiter *et al.*, 2002b) are, at least, closely associated to fast-twitch fibres having a high capacity for anaerobic metabolism and metabolic H^+ production. These Pi responses are consistent with either progressive or developing fatigue and recruitment of regions of muscle that have the capacity to express a low pH – and only occur when a $\dot{V}O_2$ slow component is evident.

Of the experimental impositions that have been shown to reduce the $\dot{V}O_2$ slow component, two are of note with regard to MRS-derived inferences for m$\dot{V}O_2$. These are during repeated high-intensity exercise (e.g. Gerbino *et al.*, 1996; MacDonald *et al.*, 1997; Burnley *et al.*, 2000; Rossiter *et al.*, 2001) and following DCA administration (Rossiter *et al.*, 2003b). Interestingly, in both conditions, the splitting of the Pi peak is concurrently reduced (Rossiter *et al.*, 2001, 2003b).

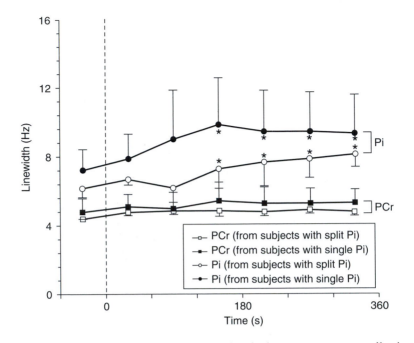

Figure 7.7 When a split Pi peak is not observed in high-intensity exercise, all subjects manifest a broadening of Pi line-width (i.e. the 'spread' in Hz of the Pi peak at half height) after ~3 min of exercise, unlike PCr. This suggests a heterogeneous intramuscular pH profile during high-intensity exercise in all subjects, which may be below the resolution of MRS to detect an actual splitting of the Pi peak. Redrawn, in part, from Rossiter *et al.* (2002b).

DCA can activate the pyruvate dehydrogenase complex, thus allowing pyruvate to enter the mitochondrion more rapidly at exercise onset and alleviating any early lactate accumulation. Using MRS, we have found that DCA administration was associated with a reduction in the intramuscular acidosis, the extent of Pi-peak splitting and the $\dot{V}O_2$ slow component magnitude – in some cases, the slow component being eliminated entirely (Rossiter *et al.*, 2003b). Similarly, following 'priming' high-intensity exercise, the $\dot{V}O_2$ slow component magnitude is reduced, both for cycle ergometry (e.g. Gerbino *et al.*, 1996; McDonald *et al.*, 1997; Burnley *et al.*, 2000) and for knee-extensor exercise (Rossiter *et al.*, 2001). Figure 7.8 shows an example of an MRS spectrum (vertically aligned to more easily observe the Pi peak) during repeated high-intensity knee-extensor exercise in a subject who demonstrated a large degree of Pi-peak splitting. It demonstrates that the Pi-peak splitting was reduced during the second exercise bout, where there was also an apparent reduction in the reliance on anaerobic metabolism (i.e. the magnitudes of intramuscular pH and [PCr] decline were also reduced, and the fundamental $\tau\dot{V}O_2$ was speeded (Rossiter *et al.*, 2001) – although this

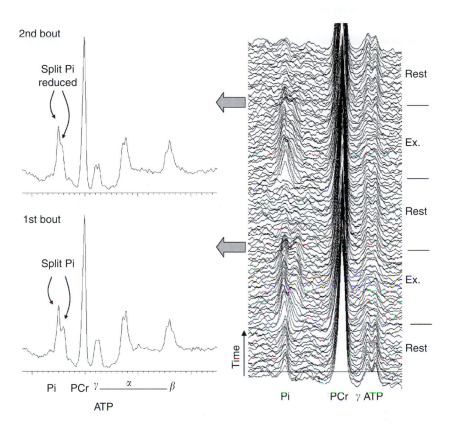

Figure 7.8 A stacked series of spectra showing the splitting of the Pi peak (at ~5 ppm) during repeated high-intensity square-wave knee-extensor exercise. The single spectra (to the left) show the average of the last minute of two exercise bouts. The spectra are vertically aligned to more easily observe the frequency of the Pi resonance (expressed in relation to PCr at 0 ppm). The degree (i.e. the negative frequency shift, towards the right) of the splitting of the Pi peak is reduced during the second exercise bout, indicating a lesser reduction in pH during the second bout. This is manifest concurrently with a reduction in the magnitude of the V̇O₂ slow component. These data suggest that both the absolute intramuscular pH fall during the second bout and the [Pi] in a low pH environment are reduced. Both these have been suggested to contribute to muscle fatigue, which is one of the suggested mechanisms by which a V̇O₂ slow component is manifest (see Chapter 12).

latter finding is not consistently the case for other modes of exercise; for example see Burnley *et al.* (2000) and Chapters 10 and 12 herein.

Interpreting control

In this chapter, we have discussed the predominant theories of control of skeletal muscle oxidative phosphorylation *in vivo* in exercising humans. Figure 7.1

summarizes the three main classes of theory: phosphate feedback, O_2 delivery and substrate delivery. Traditional concepts of control analysis imply that the flux of a particular system (i.e. the rate of oxidative phosphorylation) is controlled by a single enzyme within the pathway. Fell (1997) has recently challenged this approach by suggesting that for a system in flux, metabolic control analysis allows a better understanding of the kinetic implications of each enzyme within the 'fluxing' system. This approach assigns a flux control coefficient to each enzyme in the chain of events in such a system. Assignment of a flux control co-efficient can be achieved by altering the activities of one or more of these enzymes within the system (with knowledge of the flux, the concentrations of the key metabolites and the changes in both brought about by experimental intervention). While it is still not straightforward to apply these rules to *in vivo* systems, the basic tenets may nonetheless be applied (qualitatively at least) to the three examples discussed here (Eqn (7.2)). Oxygen delivery would be expected to have a low flux control co-efficient, as increasing delivery (e.g. via blood flow) to exercising muscle does not appear to substantially increase the system flux (i.e. reduce $\tau m\dot{V}O_2$). For example, increasing O_2 delivery to near maximal levels does not increase $m\dot{V}O_2$ flux (i.e. reduce $\tau m\dot{V}O_2$) in canine muscle, except for work rates requiring $m\dot{V}O_{2\,max}$ (Grassi *et al.*, 1998). Likewise, activating the PDH complex prior to exercise onset (with DCA) to increase the availability of NADH does not lead to a speeding of $\tau m\,\dot{V}O_2$ or $\tau\dot{V}O_2$ (Bangsbo *et al.*, 2002; Grassi *et al.*, 2002; Rossiter *et al.*, 2003b; Jones *et al.*, 2004), again suggesting a low flux control co-efficient for this enzyme in oxidative phosphorylation. Strikingly, however, muscle CK 'knockout' (Wallimann *et al.*, 1992; Van Deursen *et al.*, 1993; Roman *et al.*, 2002) has been suggested to markedly increase the rate of oxidative phosphorylation at the onset of muscle stimulation. However, as this knockout model may be 'contaminated' by compensatory adaptations (mitochondrial volume density is dramatically increased, for instance), the most compelling evidence is perhaps that of Kindig *et al.* (2005), who inhibited CK in a single frog myocyte with pharmacological interventions. They found that the fall in intracellular PO_2 was markedly speeded at the onset of contractions (indicative of a more rapid $\tau m\dot{V}O_2$). This would imply a high flux control co-efficient for CK in oxidative phosphorylation. However, Kindig *et al.* (2005) also found that force production was dramatically attenuated, even following the first contraction. This was possibly due to a reduction in [ATP] (in the absence of the PCr system to buffer a fall) which might be expected to act as the most potent respiratory stimulus of all (Chance *et al.*, 1985).

These demonstrations are in accordance with suggestions that the PCr system acts as a metabolic 'damper', preventing sudden swings in ATP requirement being transduced throughout the many systems feeding into oxidative phosphorylation. The PCr system (regulated by CK), therefore, may conceptually be viewed as slowing the rate of increase of $m\dot{V}O_2$ thus determining its kinetics. This damping action appears to be crucial in order to maintain ATP supply (and therefore force production; e.g. Kindig *et al.*, 2005) during sudden increases in requirement. These findings, as well as those discussed in this chapter, emphasize the important role of CK in shaping the kinetics of $m\dot{V}O_2$ and $\dot{V}O_2$.

Summary

The investigation of the putative phosphate-related controllers of oxidative phosphorylation in conjunction with pulmonary $\dot{V}O_2$ allow investigation of the potential transfer function controlling $\dot{V}O_2$ (and by inference $m\dot{V}O_2$). These studies demonstrate that the dynamic features of intramuscular metabolism that most consistently correlate to pulmonary $\dot{V}O_2$ are the kinetics of [PCr]. However, $\dot{V}O_2$ kinetics are intensity-dependent and, therefore, reflect non-linear system behaviour. It is interesting, therefore, that investigations spanning a range of exercise intensities have also revealed similar non-linear [PCr] kinetics. For supra-LT intensities, where non-linear behaviour is most obvious (i.e. when slow components are manifest), [PCr] and $\dot{V}O_2$ maintain their tight kinetic coupling. [ADP]$_{free}$, [Pi] and pH kinetics, on the other hand, are more variable between subjects in this high-intensity region. The causes of this non-linear behaviour are presently unclear, but have been suggested to reflect increased recruitment of muscle fibres that have a greater propensity for glycolytic metabolism consequent to failing force production in early-recruited fibres. Interestingly, the behaviour of Pi-peak splitting in the MR spectrum under different experimental conditions is consistent with an increase in the heterogeneity of force production and H^+-generating processes, which could reflect an increased reliance on fast-twitch muscle fibre recruitment. Manipulations to alleviate metabolic H^+ production, such as prior high-intensity exercise or DCA administration, also 'relieve' the heterogeneity of muscle metabolism during exercise and return the kinetics of $\dot{V}O_2$ and PCr towards dynamics that are more clearly first-order (e.g. mono-exponential). These studies strongly implicate a crucial role of PCr and, therefore, the CK reaction in determining $\dot{V}O_2$ kinetics during exercise in humans.

Glossary of terms

A	amplitude of the exponential
ADP	adenosine diphosphate
ANT	adenine nucleotide translocase
ATP	adenosine triphosphate
[ÅTP]	rate of ATP hydrolysis
Cr	creatine
CK	creatine kinase
DCA	dichloroacetate
δ_c	chemical shift of Pi relative to PCr
EPOC	excess post-exercise O_2 consumption
G	functional system gain (e.g. $\Delta\dot{V}O_{2(ss)}/\Delta\dot{W}$)
$H_{(s)}$	transfer function
iEMG	integrated electromyogram
Km	Michaelis constant
LT	lactate threshold
MRS	magnetic resonance spectroscopy
$m\dot{V}O_2$	muscle oxygen consumption

NADH   nicotinamide adenine dinucleotide
NIRS   near infra-red spectroscopy
^{31}P phosphorus
PCr   phosphocreatine
PDH   pyruvate dehydrogenase
Pi   inorganic phosphate
ppm   chemical shift in parts per million
PRBS   pseudo-random binary sequence
$\dot{Q}_T$ cardiac output
T_1 longitudinal relaxation time (of nuclei under magnetization)
τ time constant (i.e. time taken to reach 63% of the final amplitude in an exponential function)
TCr   total creatine
TD   time delay
$\dot{V}O_2$ pulmonary oxygen uptake
V_V venous volume
$\dot{W}$ work rate
Δ denotes 'change'
Subscript i   indicates 'initial'
Subscript(s)   complex frequency variable
Subscript (ss) indicates 'steady-state'
Subscript t   indicates 'with respect to time'
[ ]   denotes concentration

References

Andersen, P. and Saltin, B. (1985). Maximal perfusion of skeletal muscle in man. *Journal of Physiology*, **366**, 233–49.

Babcock, M.A., Paterson, D.H., Cunningham, D.A. and Dickenson, J.R. (1994). Exercise on-transient gas exchange kinetics are slowed as a function of age. *Medicine and Science in Sports and Exercise*, **26**, 440–6.

Bangsbo, J., Krustrup, P., Gonzalez-Alonso, J., Boushel, R. and Saltin, B. (2000). Muscle oxygen kinetics at onset of intense dynamic exercise in humans. *American Journal of Physiology*, **279**, R899–906.

Bangsbo, J., Krustrup, P., Gonzalez-Alonso, J. and Saltin, B. (2001). ATP production and efficiency of human skeletal muscle during intense exercise: effect of previous exercise. *American Journal of Physiology*, **280**, E956–64.

Bangsbo, J., Gibala, M.J., Krustrup, P., Gonzalez-Alonso, J. and Saltin, B. (2002). Enhanced pyruvate dehydrogenase activity does not affect muscle O_2 uptake at onset of intense exercise in humans. *American Journal of Physiology*, **282**, R273–80.

Barstow, T.J. and Molé, P.A. (1991). Linear and non-linear characteristics of oxygen uptake kinetics during heavy exercise. *Journal of Applied Physiology*, **71**, 2099–106.

Barstow, T.J., Lamarra, N. and Whipp, B.J. (1990). Modulation of muscle and pulmonary O_2 uptakes by circulatory dynamics during exercise. *Journal of Applied Physiology*, **68**, 979–89.

Barstow, T.J., Buchthal, S., Zanconato, S. and Cooper, D.M. (1994a). Muscle energetics and pulmonary oxygen uptake kinetics during moderate exercise. *Journal of Applied Physiology*, **77**, 1742–9.

Barstow, T.J., Buchthal, S., Zanconato, S. and Cooper, D.M. (1994b). Changes in the potential controllers of human skeletal muscle respiration during incremental calf exercise. *Journal of Applied Physiology*, **77**, 2169–76.

Barstow, T.J., Jones, A.M., Nguyen, P.H. and Casaburi, R. (1996). Influence of muscle fiber type and pedal frequency on oxygen uptake kinetics of heavy exercise. *Journal of Applied Physiology*, **81**, 1642–50.

Behnke, B.J., Barstow, T.J., Kindig, C.A., McDonough, P., Musch, T.I. and Poole, D.C. (2002). Dynamics of oxygen uptake following exercise onset in rat skeletal muscle. *Respiration Physiology and Neurobiology*, **133**, 229–39.

Bessman, S.P. and Geiger, P.J. (1981). Transport of energy in muscle: the phosphorylcreatine shuttle. *Science*, **211**, 448–52.

Borrani, F., Candau, R., Millet, G.Y., Perrey, S., Fuchslocher, J. and Rouillon, J.D. (2001). Is the $\dot{V}O_2$ slow component dependent on progressive recruitment of fast-twitch fibers in trained runners? *Journal of Applied Physiology*, **90**, 2212–20.

Brittain, C.J., Rossiter, H.B., Kowalchuk, J.M. and Whipp, B.J. (2001). Effect of prior metabolic rate on the kinetics of oxygen uptake during moderate-intensity exercise. *European Journal of Applied Physiology*, **86**, 125–34.

Burnley, M., Jones, A.M., Carter, H. and Doust, J.H. (2000). Effects of prior heavy exercise on phase II pulmonary oxygen uptake kinetics during heavy exercise. *Journal of Applied Physiology*, **89**, 1387–96.

Burnley, M., Doust, J.H., Ball, D. and Jones, A.M. (2002). Effects of prior heavy exercise on $\dot{V}O_2$ kinetics during heavy exercise are related to changes in muscle activity. *Journal of Applied Physiology*, **93**, 167–74.

Carter, H., Pringle, J.S., Jones, A.M. and Doust, J.H. (2002). Oxygen uptake kinetics during treadmill running across exercise intensity domains. *European Journal of Applied Physiology*, **86**, 347–54.

Casaburi, R., Whipp, B.J., Wasserman, K. and Koyal, S.N. (1978). Ventilatory and gas exchange responses to cycling with sinusoidally varying pedal rate. *Journal of Applied Physiology*, **44**, 97–103.

Cerretelli, P., Pendergast, D., Paganelli, W.C. and Rennie, D.W. (1979). Effects of specific muscle training on $\dot{V}O_2$ on-response and early blood lactate. *Journal of Applied Physiology*, **47**, 761–9.

Chance, B. and Williams, C.M. (1955). Respiratory enzymes in oxidative phosphorylation. I. Kinetics of oxygen utilisation. *Journal of Biological Chemistry*, **217**, 383–93.

Chance, B. and Williams, C.M. (1956). The respiratory chain and oxidative phosphorylation. *Advances in Enzymology*, **17**, 65–134.

Chance, B., Eleff, S., Leigh, J.S. Jr, Sokolow, D. and Sapega, A. (1981). Mitochondrial regulation of phosphocreatine/inorganic phosphate ratios in exercising human muscle: a gated ^{31}P NMR study. *Proceedings of the National Academy of Science, USA*, **78**, 6714–18.

Chance, B., Leigh, J.S. Jr, Clark, B.J., Marvis, J., Kent, J., Nioka, S. and Smith, D. (1985). Control of oxidative metabolism and oxygen delivery in human skeletal muscle: A steady-state analysis of the work/energy cost transfer function. *Proceedings of the National Academy of Science, USA*, **82**, 8384–8.

Conley, K.E., Kushmerick, M.J. and Jubrias, S.A. (1998). Glycolysis is independent of oxygenation state in stimulated human skeletal muscle in vivo. *Journal of Physiology*, **511**, 935–45.

Conley, K.E., Kemper, W.F. and Crowther, G.J. (2001). Limits to sustainable muscle performance: interaction between glycolysis and oxidative phosphorylation. *Journal of Experimental Biology*, **204**, 3189–94.

Connett, R.J. and Honig, C.R. (1989). Regulation of $\dot{V}O_2$ in red muscle: do current biochemical hypotheses fit in vivo data? *American Journal of Physiology*, **256**, R898–906.

Crow, M.T. and Kushmerick, M.J. (1982). Chemical energetics of slow- and fast-twitch muscles of the mouse. *Journal of General Physiology*, **79**, 147–66.

Demarie, S., Sardella, F., Billat, V., Magini, W. and Faina, M. (2001). The $\dot{V}O_2$ slow component in swimming. *European Journal of Applied Physiology*, **84**, 95–9.

Di Prampero, P.E., Davies, C.T.M., Cerretelli, P. and Margaria, R. (1970). An analysis of O_2 debt contracted in submaximal exercise. *Journal of Applied Physiology*, **29**, 547–51.

Essfeld, D., Hoffmann, U. and Stegemann, J. (1987). $\dot{V}O_2$ kinetics in subjects differing in aerobic capacity: investigation by spectral analysis. *European Journal of Applied Physiology*, **56**, 508–15.

Fell, D. (1997). *Understanding the Control of Metabolism*. Portland Press, London, UK.

Fujihara, Y., Hilderbrandt, J.R. and Hilderbrandt, J. (1973). Cardiorespiratory transients in exercising man. I. Tests of superposition. *Journal of Applied Physiology*, **35**, 58–67.

Fukuba, Y., Hara, K., Kimura, Y., Takahashi, A., Ward, S.A. and Whipp, B.J. (2000). Estimating the parameters of aerobic function during exercise using an exponentially increasing work-rate protocol. *Medical and Biological Engineering and Computing*, **38**, 433–7.

Fukuoka, Y., Shigematsu, M., Fukuba, Y., Koga, S. and Ikegami, H. (1997). Dynamics of respiratory response to sinusoidal work load in humans. *International Journal of Sports Medicine*, **18**, 264–9.

Gaesser, G.A. and Brooks, G.A. (1984). Metabolic bases of excess post-exercise oxygen consumption: a review. *Medicine and Science in Sports and Exercise*, **16**, 29–43.

Gerbino, A., Ward, S.A. and Whipp, B.J. (1996). Effects of prior exercise on pulmonary gas-exchange kinetics during high-intensity exercise in humans. *Journal of Applied Physiology*, **80**, 99–107.

Gonzalez-Alonso, J., Quistorff, B., Krustrup, P., Bangsbo, J. and Saltin, B. (2000). Heat production in human skeletal muscle at the onset of intense dynamic exercise. *Journal of Physiology*, **524**, 603–15.

Grassi, B., Poole, D.C., Richardson, R.S., Knight, D.R., Erickson, B.K. and Wagner, P.D. (1996). Muscle O_2 uptake kinetics in humans: implications for metabolic control. *Journal of Applied Physiology*, **80**, 988–98.

Grassi, B., Gladden, L.B., Samaja, M., Stary, C.M. and Hogan, M.C. (1998). Faster adjustment of O_2 delivery does not affect $\dot{V}O_2$ on-kinetics in isolated in situ canine muscle. *Journal of Applied Physiology*, **85**, 1394–403.

Grassi, B., Hogan, M.C., Greenhaff, P.L., Hamann, J.J., Kelley, K.M., Aschenbach, W.G., Constantin-Teodosiu, D. and Gladden, L.B. (2002). Oxygen uptake on-kinetics in dog gastrocnemius in situ following activation of pyruvate dehydrogenase by dichloroacetate. *Journal of Physiology*, **538**, 195–207.

Greenhaff, P.L. (2003). The creatine–phosphocreatine system: there's more than one song in its repertoire. *Journal of Physiology*, **537**, 657.

Greenhaff, P.L., Campbell-O'Sullivan, S.P., Constantin-Teodosiu, D., Poucher, S.M., Roberts, P.A. and Timmons, J.A. (2002). An acetyl group deficit limits mitochondrial ATP production at the onset of exercise. *Biochemical Society Transactions*, **30**, 275–80.

Griffiths, T.L., Henson, L.C. and Whipp, B.J. (1986). Influence of inspired oxygen concentration on the dynamics of the exercise hyperpnoea in man. *Journal of Physiology*, **380**, 387–403.

Hagberg, J.M., Hickson, R.C., Ehsani, A.A. and Holloszy, J.O. (1980). Faster adjustment to and from recovery from submaximal exercise in the trained state. *Journal of Applied Physiology*, **48**, 218–24.

Hansford, R.G. (1994). Role of calcium in respiratory control. *Medicine and Science in Sports and Exercise*, **26**, 44–51.

Haouzi, P., Fukuba, Y., Casaburi, R., Stringer, W. and Wasserman, K. (1993). O_2 uptake kinetics above and below the lactic acidosis threshold during sinusoidal exercise. *Journal of Applied Physiology*, **75**, 1683–90.

Haseler, L.J., Hogan, M.C. and Richardson, R.S. (1999). Skeletal muscle phosphocreatine recovery in exercise-trained humans is dependent on O_2 availability. *Journal of Applied Physiology*, **86**, 2013–18.

Hill, A.V. (1926). *Muscular Activity: The Herter Lectures for 1924*. Williams & Wilkins Co., Baltimore, USA. Chs III–IV, pp. 87–111.

Hill, A.V. and Lupton, H. (1923). Muscular exercise, lactic acid and the supply and utilisation of oxygen. *Quarterly Journal of Medicine*, **16**, 135–71.

Hoffmann, U., Essfeld, D., Wunderlich, H.G. and Stegemann, J. (1992). Dynamic linearity of $\dot{V}O_2$ responses during aerobic exercise. *European Journal of Applied Physiology*, **64**, 139–44.

Holian, A., Owen, C.S. and Wilson, D.F. (1977). Control of respiration in isolated mitochondria: quantitative evaluation of the dependence of respiratory rates on [ATP], [ADP] and [Pi]. *Archives of Biochemistry and Biophyisics*, **181**, 164–71.

Hughson, R.L. and Morrisey, M. (1982). Delayed kinetics of respiratory gas exchange in the transition from prior exercise. *Journal of Applied Physiology*, **52**, 921–9.

Hughson, R.L., Winter, D.A., Patla, A.E., Swanson, G.D. and Cuervo, L.A. (1990). Investigation of $\dot{V}O_2$ kinetics in humans with pseudorandom binary sequence work rate change. *Journal of Applied Physiology*, **68**, 796–801.

Jones, A.M., Koppo, K., Wilkerson, D.P., Wilmshurst, S. and Campbell, I.T. (2004). Dichloroacetate does not speed phase-II pulmonary $\dot{V}O_2$ kinetics following the onset of heavy intensity cycle exercise. *Pflugers Archives*, **447**(6), 867–74.

Kemp, G.J., Roussel, M., Bendahan, D., Le Fur, Y. and Cozzone, P.J. (2001). Interrelations of ATP synthesis and proton handling in ischaemically exercising human forearm muscle studied by 31P magnetic resonance spectroscopy. *Journal of Physiology*, **535**, 901–28.

Kindig, C.A., Howlett, R.A. and Hogan, M.C. (2003a). Effect of extracellular PO_2 on the fall in intracellular PO_2 in contracting single myocytes. *Journal of Applied Physiology*, **94**, 1964–70.

Kindig, C.A., Kelley, K.M., Howlett, R.A., Stary, C.M. and Hogan, M.C. (2003b). Assessment of O_2 uptake dynamics in isolated single skeletal myocytes. *Journal of Applied Physiology*, **94**, 353–7.

Kindig, C.A., Howlett, R.A., Stary, C.M., Walsh, B. and Hogan, M.C. (2005). Effects of acute creatine kinase inhibition on metabolism and tension development in isolated single myocytes. *Journal of Applied Physiology*, **98** (published online 27 August 2004).

Krogh, A. and Lindhard, J. (1913). The regulation of respiration and circulation during the initial stages of muscular work. *Journal of Physiology*, **47**, 112–36.

Kushmerick, M.J. (1998). Energy balance in muscle activity: simulations of ATPase coupled to oxidative phosphorylation and to creatine kinase. *Comparitive Biochemistry and Physiology*, **120**, 109–23.

Kushmerick, M.J. and Paul, J.R. (1976). Aerobic recovery metabolism following a single isometric tetanus in frog sartorius muscle at $0°$ C. *Journal of Physiology*, **254**, 693–709.

Lamarra, N., Whipp, B.J., Blumenberg, M. and Wasserman, K. (1983). Model-order estimation of cardiorespiratory dynamics during moderate exercise. In: B.J. Whipp and D.M. Wiberg (Eds) *Modelling and Control of Breathing*. Elsevier Biomedical, Oxford, UK.

Lamarra, N., Whipp, B.J., Ward, S.A. and Wasserman, K. (1987). The effect of hyperoxia on the coupling of ventilatory and gas-exchange dynamics in response to impulse exercise testing. In G. Benchetrit, P. Baconnier and J. Demongeot (Eds) *Concepts and Formalizations in the Control of Breathing*. Manchester University Press, pp. 87–100.

Langsetmo, I., Weigle, G.E., Fedde, M.R., Erickson, H.H., Barstow, T.J. and Poole, D.C. (1997). $\dot{V}O_2$ kinetics in the horse during moderate and heavy exercise. *Journal of Applied Physiology*, **83**, 1235–41.

LeMasters, J.J. (1984). The ATP-to-oxygen stoichiometries of oxidative phosphorylation by rat liver mitochondria. An analysis of ADP-induced oxygen jumps by linear nonequilibrium thermodynamics. *Journal of Biological Chemistry*, **259**, 13123–30.

Linnarsson, D. (1974). Dynamics of pulmonary gas exchange and heart rate changes at the start and end of exercise. *Acta Physiologica Scandanavica* (Suppl.), **415**, 1–68.

Lucia, A., Hoyos, J. and Chicharro, J.L. (2000). The slow component of $\dot{V}O_2$ in professional cyclists. *British Journal of Sports Medicine*, **34**, 367–74.

McCreary, C.R., Chilibeck, P.D., Marsh, G.D., Paterson, D.H. Cunningham, D.A. and Thompson, R.T. (1996). Kinetics of pulmonary oxygen uptake and muscle phosphates during moderate-intensity calf-exercise. *Journal of Applied Physiology*, **81**, 1331–8.

McCully, K.K., Iotti, S., Kendrick, K., Wang, Z., Posner, J.D., Leigh, J.S. Jr and Chance, B. (1994). Simultaneous in vivo measurements of HbO_2 saturation and PCr kinetics after exercise in normal humans. *Journal of Applied Physiology*, **77**, 5–10.

MacDonald, M., Pedersen, P.K. and Hughson, R.L. (1997). Acceleration of $\dot{V}O_2$ kinetics in heavy submaximal exercise by hyperoxia and prior high-intensity exercise. *Journal of Applied Physiology*, **83**, 1318–25.

Mahler, M. (1978). Kinetics of oxygen consumption after a single isometric tetanus of the frog sartorius muscle at 20° C. *Journal of General Physiology*, **73**, 159–74.

Mahler, M. (1985). First order kinetics of muscle oxygen consumption, and equivalent proportionality between $\dot{Q}O_2$ and phosphorylcreatine level. Implications for the control of respiration. *Journal of Applied Physiology*, **86**, 135–65.

Mallory, L.A., Scheuermann, B.W., Hoelting, B.D., Weiss, M.L., McAllister, R.M. and Barstow, T.J. (2002). Influence of peak $\dot{V}O_2$ and muscle fiber type on the efficiency of moderate exercise. *Medicine and Science in Sports and Exercise*, **34**, 1279–87.

Meyer, R.A. (1988). A linear model of muscle respiration explains mono-exponential phosphocreatine changes. *American Journal of Physiology*, **254**, C548–53.

Milsum, J.H. (1966). *Biological Control Systems Analysis*. McGraw-Hill, New York.

Moon, R.B. and Richards, J.H. (1973). Determination of intracellular pH by ^{31}P magnetic resonance. *Journal of Biological Chemistry*, **248**, 7276–8.

Moritani, T., Nagata, A., deVries, H.A. and Muro, M. (1981). Critical power as a measure of physical work capacity and anaerobic threshold. *Ergonomics*, **24**, 339–50.

Owen, C.S. and Wilson, D.F. (1974). Control of respiration by the mitochondrial phosphorylation state. *Archives of Biochemistry and Biophysics*, **161**, 581–91.

Özyener, F., Rossiter, H.B., Ward, S.A. and Whipp, B.J. (2001). Influence of exercise intensity on the on- and off-transient kinetics of pulmonary oxygen uptake in humans. *Journal of Physiology*, **533**, 891–902.

Paterson, D.H. and Whipp, B.J. (1991). Asymmetries of oxygen uptake transients at the on- and offset of heavy exercise in humans. *Journal of Physiology*, **443**, 575–86.

Piiper, J., Di Prampero, P.E. and Cerretelli, P. (1968). Oxygen debt and high-energy phosphates in gastrocnemius muscle in the dog. *American Journal of Physiology*, **215**, 523–31.

Poole, D.C., Schaffartzik, W., Knight, D.R., Derion, T., Kennedy, B., Guy, H.J., Prediletto, R. and Wagner, P.D. (1991). Contribution of exercising legs to the slow component of oxygen uptake kinetics in humans. *Journal of Applied Physiology*, **71**, 1245–53.

Pringle, J.S., Doust, J.H., Carter, H., Tolfrey, K., Campbell, I.T. and Jones, A.M. (2003). Oxygen uptake kinetics during moderate, heavy and severe intensity 'submaximal' exercise in humans: the influence of muscle fibre type and capillarisation. *European Journal of Applied Physiology*, **89**, 289–300.

Riggs, D.S. (1976). *Control Theory and Physiological Feedback Mechanisms*. Krieger, Huntingdon, New York.

Roman, B.B., Meyer, R.A. and Wiseman, R.W. (2002). Phosphocreatine kinetics at the onset of contractions in skeletal muscle of MM creatine kinase knockout mice. *American Journal of Physiology*, **283**, C1776–83.

Rossiter, H.B., Ward, S.A., Doyle, V.L., Howe, F.A., Griffiths, J.R. and Whipp, B.J. (1999). Inferences from pulmonary O_2 uptake with respect to intramuscular [PCr] kinetics during moderate exercise in humans. *Journal of Physiology*, **518**, 921–32.

Rossiter, H.B., Ward, S.A., Kowalchuk, J.M., Howe, F.A., Griffiths, J.R. and Whipp, B.J. (2001). Effects of prior exercise on oxygen uptake and phosphocreatine kinetics during high-intensity knee-extension exercise in humans. *Journal of Physiology*, **537**, 291–303.

Rossiter, H.B., Ward, S.A., Kowalchuk, J.M., Howe, F.A., Griffiths, J.R. and Whipp, B.J. (2002a). Dynamic asymmetry of phosphocreatine concentration and O_2 uptake between the on- and off-transients of moderate- and high-intensity exercise in humans. *Journal of Physiology*, **541**, 991–1002.

Rossiter, H.B., Ward, S.A., Howe, F.A., Kowalchuk, J.M., Griffiths, J.R. and Whipp, B.J. (2002b). Dynamics of intramuscular ^{31}P-MRS Pi peak splitting and the slow components of PCr and O_2 uptake during exercise. *Journal of Applied Physiology*, **93**, 2059–69.

Rossiter, H.B., Ward, S.A., Howe, F.A., Kowalchuk, J.M., Griffiths, J.R. and Whipp, B.J. (2002c). The slow component of pulmonary oxygen uptake ($\dot{V}O_2$) and the calculated intramuscular [ADP] during high-intensity exercise in humans. *Proceedings of the International Society for Magnetic Resonance in Medicine (Hawaii)*, **10**, 1877.

Rossiter, H.B., Ward, S.A., Howe, F.A., Wood, D.M., Kowalchuk, J.M., Griffiths, J.R. and Whipp, B.J. (2003a). The effects of dichloroacetate on the kinetics of intramuscular [ADP] and pulmonary oxygen uptake ($\dot{V}O_2$) during high-intensity exercise in humans. *Proceedings of the International Society for Magnetic Resonance in Medicine (Toronto)*, **11**, 1537.

Rossiter, H.B., Ward, S.A., Howe, F.A., Wood, D.M., Kowalchuk, J.M., Griffiths, J.R. and Whipp, B.J. (2003b). Effects of dichloroacetate on $\dot{V}O_2$ and intramuscular ^{31}P metabolite kinetics during high-intensity exercise in humans. *Journal of Applied Physiology*, **95**, 1105–15.

Sahlin, K., Katz, A. and Henriksson, J. (1987). Redox state and lactate accumulation in human skeletal muscle during dynamic exercise. *Biochemistry Journal*, **245**, 551–6.

Saks, V.A., Kaambre, T., Sikk, P., Eimre, M., Orlova, E., Paju, K., Piirsoo, A., Appaix, F., Kay, L., Regitz-Zagrosek, V., Fleck, E. and Seppet, E. (2001). Intracellular energetic units in red muscle cells. *Biochemistry Journal*, **356**, 643–57.

Saunders, M.J., Evans, E.M., Arngrimsson, S.A., Allison, J.D., Warren, G.L. and Cureton, K.J. (2000). Muscle activation and the slow component rise in oxygen uptake during cycling. *Medicine and Science in Sports and Exercise*, **32**, 2040–5.

Scheuermann, B.W., Hoelting, B.D., Noble, M.L. and Barstow, T.J. (2001). The slow component of O_2 uptake is not accompanied by changes in muscle EMG during repeated bouts of heavy exercise in humans. *Journal of Physiology*, **531**, 245–56.

Shinohara, M. and Moritani, T. (1992). Increase in neuromuscular activity and oxygen uptake during heavy exercise. *Annals of Physiological Anthropology*, **11**, 257–62.

Swanson, G.D. and Hughson, R.L. (1988). On the modeling and interpretation of oxygen uptake kinetics from ramp work rate tests. *Journal of Applied Physiology*, **65**, 2453–8.

Timmons, J.A., Poucher, S.M., Constantin-Teodosiu, D., Worrall, V., Macdonald, I.A. and Greenhaff, P.L. (1996). Increased acetyl group availability enhances contractile function of canine skeletal muscle during ischemia. *Journal of Clinical Investigation*, **97**, 879–83.

Timmons, J.A., Gustafsson, T., Sundberg, C.J., Jansson, E. and Greenhaff, P.L. (1998). Muscle acetyl group availability is a major determinant of oxygen defect in humans during submaximal exercise. *American Journal of Physiology*, **274**(2 Pt 1), E377–80.

Tschakovsky, M.E. and Hughson, R.L. (1999). Interaction of factors determining oxygen uptake at the onset of exercise. *Journal of Applied Physiology*, **86**, 1101–13.

Van Deursen, J., Heerschap, A., Oerlemans, F., Ruitenbeek, W., Jap, P., ter Laak, H. and Wieringa, B. (1993). Skeletal muscles of mice deficient in muscle creatine kinase lack burst activity. *Cell*, **74**, 621–31.

Wallimann, T., Wyss, M., Brdiczka, D., Nicolay, K. and Eppenberger, H.M. (1992). Intracellular compartmentation, structure and function of creatine kinase isoenzymes in tissues with high and fluctuating energy demands: the phosphocreatine circuit for cellular energy homeostasis. *Biochemistry Journal*, **281**, 21–40.

Walsh, B. (2002). The role of exercise and exercise-related factors in the control of mitochondrial oxidative function. PhD Thesis, Karolinska Insitute, Stockholm.

Walsh, B., Tonkonogi, M., Söderlund, K., Hultman, E., Saks, V. and Sahlin, K. (2001). The role of phosphorylcreatine and creatine in the regulation of mitochondrial respiration in human skeletal muscle. *Journal of Physiology*, **537**, 971–8.

Whipp, B.J. (1970). The rate constant for the kinetics of oxygen uptake during light exercise. *Journal of Applied Physiology*, **86**, 261–3.

Whipp, B.J. and Mahler, M. (1980). Dynamics of pulmonary gas exchange during exercise. In J.B. West (Ed.) *Pulmonary Gas Exchange Vol. II: Organism and Environment*. Academic Press Inc, NY, pp. 33–96.

Whipp, B.J. and Wasserman, K. (1972). Oxygen uptake kinetics for various intensities of constant load work. *Journal of Applied Physiology*, **33**, 351–6.

Whipp, B.J., Davis, J.A., Torres, F. and Wasserman, K. (1981). A test to determine the parameters of aerobic function during exercise. *Journal of Applied Physiology*, **50**, 217–21.

Whipp, B.J., Ward, S.A., Lamarra, N., Davis, J.A. and Wasserman, K. (1982). Parameters of ventilatory and gas exchange dynamics during exercise. *Journal of Applied Physiology*, **52**, 1506–13.

Whipp, B.J., Rossiter, H.B., Ward, S.A., Avery, D., Doyle, V.L., Howe, F.A. and Griffiths, J.R. (1999). Simultaneous determination of muscle [31]phosphate and O_2 uptake kinetics during whole-body NMR spectroscopy. *Journal of Applied Physiology*, **86**, 742–7.

Whipp, B.J., Rossiter, H.B. and Ward, S.A. (2002). Exertional oxygen uptake kinetics: a stamen of stamina? *Biochemical Society Transactions*, **30**, 237–47.

Wilson, D.F. (1994). Factors affecting the rate and energetics of mitochondrial oxidative phosphorylation. *Medicine and Science in Sports and Exercise*, **26**, 37–43.

Yoshida, T. and Watari, H. (1994). Exercise-induced splitting of the inorganic phosphate peak: investigation by time-resolved ^{31}P-nuclear magnetic resonance spectroscopy. *European Journal of Applied Physiology*, **69**, 465–73.

8 Regulation of $\dot{V}O_2$ on-kinetics by O_2 delivery

Richard L. Hughson

Introduction

Daily life is full of challenges in which the energy demands of the working muscles might quickly go from rest to substantial loads. It is critical, therefore, to understand the factors that regulate how quickly aerobic metabolic pathways adapt to these challenges. This knowledge will then provide a key to exploring the consequences of impaired function due to disease or environment. However, there are many controversies over the specific factors that regulate the rate of increase in oxygen uptake ($\dot{V}O_2$) at the onset of different intensities of exercise. Recent reviews (Tschakovsky and Hughson, 1999a; Grassi, 2001; Hughson *et al.*, 2001) have highlighted some of the factors to consider in exploring debates that have persisted for over twenty years (Whipp and Mahler, 1980; Hughson and Morrissey, 1983). It is also critical to explore reviews that have focused on regulation of blood flow especially at the onset of exercise (Laughlin *et al.*, 1996; Saltin *et al.*, 1998; Delp, 1999; Hughson and Tschakovsky, 1999; Shoemaker and Hughson, 1999) and muscle metabolism (Di Prampero, 1981; Wilson and Rumsey, 1988; Tschakovsky and Hughson, 1999a; Greenhaff *et al.*, 2002).

The complex topic of adaptation of oxidative metabolism at the onset of exercise depends on interpretation and application of some specific principles of physiology. This review will examine the evidence for how different factors can interact to regulate the rapidity with which $\dot{V}O_2$ increases at the onset of different intensities of exercise. A key section examines the physiological basis for the integration of O_2 transport with the interactive biochemical processes that determine O_2 utilization at the onset of exercise. Principles of control theory will be examined with specific application to studying $\dot{V}O_2$ kinetics. The ability to resolve differences in measured $\dot{V}O_2$ kinetics will be considered along with the resulting limitations in identifying rate-limiting steps in the adaptation of aerobic energy supply to meet the demands of constant load exercise.

As a starting point, it is necessary to delineate the various domains over which to consider the kinetics of $\dot{V}O_2$ as well as the appropriate descriptors of the kinetic phases (Figure 8.1). The simplest classification is into three exercise-intensity domains. For each domain, there is an early 'Phase I' response that reflects the rapid return to the lungs of blood due to the action of the muscle pump. This

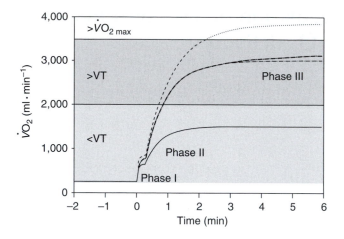

Figure 8.1 Schematic representation of $\dot{V}O_2$ kinetic responses in different work-rate regions: below ventilatory threshold (<VT, moderate exercise), above ventilatory threshold but below $\dot{V}O_{2\,max}$ (>VT, heavy and severe exercise) and above $\dot{V}O_{2\,max}$ (>$\dot{V}O_{2\,max}$, severe exercise). Each curve has a Phase I and a Phase II and in addition the >VT figure has a discernible 'slow component' (Phase III). The thin dash-dot line in the >VT domain is an extension of the Phase II response. For the >$\dot{V}O_{2\,max}$ exercise, the dotted line represents the theoretical value of $\dot{V}O_2$ if it could extend beyond this upper limit to meet all of the metabolic demands through aerobic metabolism under the assumption that it would continue along its apparent exponential path. It is common in the >$\dot{V}O_{2\,max}$ exercise for $\dot{V}O_2$ to have an end-exercise value less than $\dot{V}O_{2\,max}$ due to fatigue in which case, the exercise would be termed 'extreme' (see Chapter 1 for full discussion of exercise intensity domains) (see figure 2 in Hughson *et al.* (2000)).

early return of blood does not reflect an increase in metabolism; rather, after a delay of ~15–20 s there is a more rapid increase in $\dot{V}O_2$ referred to as 'Phase II' or sometimes as the primary phase that corresponds to the increase in $\dot{V}O_2$ at the working muscles. The first region (i.e. moderate domain, <VT in Figure 8.1) includes exercise intensities from just above rest to a work rate just below the ventilatory threshold (referred to by some researchers as the 'anaerobic threshold' (Wasserman *et al.*, 1973) or the 'aerobic threshold' (Luhtanen *et al.*, 1990) although there is considerable controversy regarding these terms and implied mechanisms (Brooks, 1985; Davis, 1985)). The work-rate at the ventilatory threshold typically occurs at ~50–60% of $\dot{V}O_{2\,max}$. Within this 'so-called' moderate intensity domain, the 'Phase II' response normally approaches the required steady-state $\dot{V}O_2$ in an apparently mono-exponential manner. The second region of exercise intensities (>VT in Figure 8.1) spans from the ventilatory threshold to just below the work rate associated with $\dot{V}O_{2\,max}$ and incorporates both heavy- and severe-intensity domains (see Chapter 1 for definitions). These domains typically include, in addition to the Phase II, a discernible slow component response that can begin 1–2 min after the start of exercise. The third intensity domain includes work rates above $\dot{V}O_{2\,max}$ ($> \dot{V}O_{2\,max}$ in Figure 8.1). By definition, this domain includes obligatory energy supply from anaerobic metabolism for at least the portion of demand above the upper limit of oxidative energy supply as shown by the hypothetical extrapolation of the $\dot{V}O_2$ curve. The three hypothetical responses shown in Figure 8.1 are ideal representations of the $\dot{V}O_2$ responses. The simplicity of the ideal curves masks the complex mechanisms that govern how rapidly oxidative metabolism adapts at the onset of exercise.

Evidence for slower $\dot{V}O_2$ kinetics in moderate exercise

Experimental evidence for changes in $\dot{V}O_2$ kinetics due to manipulations of the O_2 transport system with either increased or decreased inspired partial pressure of O_2 came from the classical experiments of Linnarrson working in Stockholm in the early 1970s (Linnarsson 1974; Linnarsson *et al.*, 1974). The work rates utilized in these experiments probably spanned the ventilatory threshold so it was not clear if sub-ventilatory threshold $\dot{V}O_2$ kinetics were altered by changes in O_2 delivery. The first experiments to clearly show slowing of $\dot{V}O_2$ kinetics at the onset of exercise below ventilatory threshold came from experiments by Hughson and Morrissey in 1982 (Hughson and Morrissey, 1982). The rate of increase in $\dot{V}O_2$ was determined to be faster for a step transition in work-rate from rest to 80% ventilatory threshold than a transition from 40% to 80% ventilatory threshold. Parallel changes in the kinetics of heart rate (i.e. slower adaptation of heart rate in the 40–80% transition) suggested that slower adaptation of O_2 transport was the mechanism responsible for the slower increase in $\dot{V}O_2$. The observations of slower $\dot{V}O_2$ kinetics have subsequently been confirmed and suggest non-linear characteristics of energy supply at the onset of moderate exercise (Di Prampero *et al.*, 1989; Brittain *et al.*, 2001).

Additional evidence for the effect of O_2 delivery on $\dot{V}O_2$ kinetics comes from experiments that impaired O_2 transport by different methods. Beta-adrenergic receptor blockade causes a reduction in heart rate and O_2 delivery, and slows $\dot{V}O_2$ kinetics during exercise maintained below ventilatory threshold (Hughson, 1984). Several different research groups slowed $\dot{V}O_2$ kinetics with hypoxia across a wide range of work rates (Linnarsson, 1974; Murphy *et al.*, 1989; Engelen *et al.*, 1996). As considered later, hypoxia also has important effects on muscle metabolism that influence $\dot{V}O_2$ kinetics (Linnarsson *et al.*, 1974; Richardson *et al.*, 1995; Haseler *et al.*, 1998). A change in O_2 delivery at the onset of exercise also accompanies a change in body position (Hughson *et al.*, 1993; MacDonald *et al.*, 1998). In the supine posture, slower $\dot{V}O_2$ kinetics probably result from the reduced perfusion pressure in this posture. That is, in the upright position, the effect of gravity adds about 50 mmHg increased driving pressure for arterial blood to perfuse the working leg quadriceps muscles during cycling. This can be especially important at the onset of exercise when vascular conductance is increasing to meet the blood flow demands of the exercising muscle. Evidence to support the hypothesis that a reduced perfusion pressure gradient contributed to slower $\dot{V}O_2$ kinetics was provided by experiments that increased the perfusion pressure gradient in the supine posture by applying lower body negative pressure during the cycling exercise (Hughson *et al.*, 1993).

Evidence for faster $\dot{V}O_2$ kinetics

The manipulations described just above reduced O_2 transport causing slower $\dot{V}O_2$ kinetics. These experiments do not provide sufficient evidence for stating that O_2 availability has a regulatory effect on the rate of increase in oxidative metabolism at the onset of normal exercise (e.g. upright cycling or running at sea level). Some experiments designed to increase O_2 transport at the onset of exercise to acceler-ate $\dot{V}O_2$ kinetics have yielded uncertain conclusions. The first experiments with hyperoxia did show a reduction in O_2 deficit that would indicate faster $\dot{V}O_2$ kinetics (Linnarsson, 1974). These experiments, that were subsequently corrob-orated (MacDonald *et al.*, 1997), were conducted at a work rate that was probably above ventilatory threshold so they do not provide evidence for moderate-intensity exercise. Attempts to study the effects of hyperoxia on $\dot{V}O_2$ kinetics below the ventilatory threshold found slightly but not significantly faster $\dot{V}O_2$ kinetics in one study (MacDonald *et al.*, 1997) but no effect in another (Hughson and Kowalchuk, 1995). The absence of a large effect should not necessarily be taken as evidence that O_2 did not contribute to the rate of increase in $\dot{V}O_2$ because it is uncertain whether there actually was increased O_2 delivery. Hyperoxia causes vasoconstriction so that blood flow is adjusted to maintain essentially constant total O_2 delivery (Welch *et al.*, 1977; MacDonald *et al.*, 2000). Two important considerations in the interpretation of these results are first whether the methods of analysing gas exchange kinetics are sufficiently sensitive to be able to detect a change if it exists, and second whether there are alternative methods of assessing whether elevated inspired PO_2 had an impact on muscle metabolism consistent with altered kinetics. The latter factor will be considered in this chapter by examining data obtained by muscle biopsy and magnetic resonance spectroscopy during inspiration of various O_2 concentrations in 'Physiological basis for O_2 transport and utilization limitations'. The ability to resolve differences will be considered in the final section on 'Limitations of current experimental techniques to extract information'.

An alternative method to achieve increased O_2 availability at the onset of exercise is to increase muscle blood flow. In a pump-perfused dog muscle prepara-tion, Grassi *et al.* (1998) elevated muscle blood flow to the required end-exercise level for electrically stimulated exercise prior to the onset of the contractions. They found that the time to reach 63% increase of $\dot{V}O_2$ from baseline to con-tracting levels was 23.8 s for spontaneous flow conditions and 21.8 s for previously elevated blood flow. This difference of just under 10% was not significantly differ-ent and the authors concluded that a metabolic inertia regulated the rate at which $\dot{V}O_2$ increased at the onset of exercise. In contrast to these experiments with dog muscle, a recent study with human forearm found faster $\dot{V}O_2$ kinetics when blood

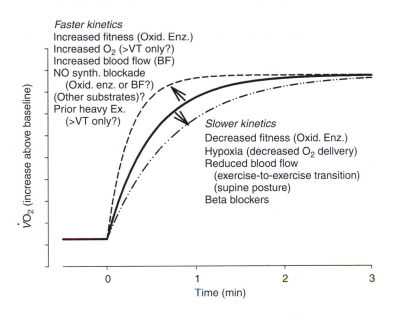

Faster kinetics
Increased fitness (Oxid. Enz.)
Increased O_2 (>VT only?)
Increased blood flow (BF)
NO synth. blockade
   (Oxid. enz. or BF?)
(Other substrates)?
Prior heavy Ex.
   (>VT only?)

Slower kinetics
Decreased fitness (Oxid. Enz.)
Hypoxia (decreased O_2 delivery)
Reduced blood flow
   (exercise-to-exercise transition)
   (supine posture)
Beta blockers

$\dot{V}O_2$ (increase above baseline)

0   1   2   3

Time (min)

Figure 8.2 Summary of factors that might cause faster or slower $\dot{V}O_2$ kinetics. See text for more details.

flow was elevated during the onset of exercise (Perrey *et al.*, 2001). In these experiments with human subjects, blood flow was increased at the start of exercise by elevating arterial blood pressure through activating the muscle chemoreflex in ischemic leg muscles. Even though there was not the full step increase in blood flow as achieved with the dog model, muscle $\dot{V}O_2$ was significantly elevated through the first minutes of rhythmic handgrip exercise. It is worth noting that the forearm was positioned at heart level so perfusion pressure in the control condition was equivalent to mean arterial pressure and not the higher pressures that normally accompany upright leg exercise. However, the small muscle mass involved in this type of exercise should not be expected to challenge cardiovascular supply limits. Rather, for a given change in vascular conductance consistent with the metabolic demand (Tschakovsky and Hughson, 1999b) there was increased perfusion because of the elevated arterial pressure during activation of the muscle chemoreflex. Thus, there are situations where the kinetics of $\dot{V}O_2$ are accelerated during the onset of moderate-intensity exercise by supplying more O_2 during the rest to exercise transition at least for exercise performed with the forearm muscles. The factors that appear to alter $\dot{V}O_2$ kinetics are summarized in Figure 8.2.

$\dot{V}O_2$ kinetics with heavy submaximal exercise

Elevated $\dot{V}O_2$ values at the onset of exercise have been observed consistently when exercise above ventilatory threshold is preceded by a 'warm up bout' of similar-intensity exercise. Whether this represents faster $\dot{V}O_2$ kinetics has been debated (see Chapter 10). Gerbino *et al.* (1996) and later MacDonald *et al.* (1997) demonstrated faster overall kinetics of $\dot{V}O_2$ in the second bout of exercise but did not specifically identify faster kinetics of the Phase II response. Gerbino *et al.* first hypothesized that the prior heavy exercise caused a more rapid increase in muscle blood flow and O_2 delivery in the second bout of exercise and that there was a right shift of the O_2–haemoglobin dissociation curve allowing for greater drop-off of O_2. Data supportive of this hypothesis were obtained from experiments examining two consecutive bouts of heavy exercise in human forearm muscles (MacDonald *et al.*, 2001). In the second bout of forearm exercise, blood flow was higher in the early adaptive phase and the arterial–venous O_2 content difference was greater (MacDonald *et al.*, 2001). Recent experiments that examined leg blood flow and whole body $\dot{V}O_2$ during repeated bouts of heavy leg kicking exercise also found data consistent with elevated leg blood flow and a faster $\dot{V}O_2$ response in the second bout of exercise (Hughson *et al.*, 2003). Figure 8.3 shows this pattern for a single subject. Across all subjects in these experiments, there was a small non-significant reduction in the Phase II time constant (from 32.8 ± 4.0 s to 27.4 ± 2.2 s) but the mean response time (MRT) was substantially and significantly reduced (from 124.0 ± 14.3 s to 88.3 ± 5.5 s) (Hughson *et al.*, 2003). Consistent with the faster MRT, the $\dot{V}O_2$ at 3 min of exercise was significantly elevated and the

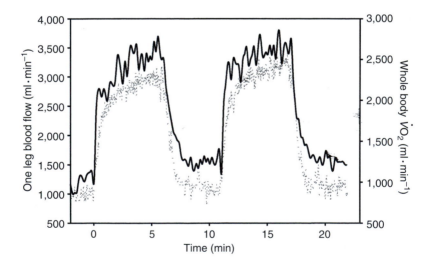

Figure 8.3 $\dot{V}O_2$ measured at the mouth (dotted line) and leg blood flow measured by Doppler ultrasound from the femoral artery (solid line) are shown for two consecutive bouts of heavy knee-extension and flexion exercise for a single fit subject. Note that prior to the second bout of exercise leg blood flow is elevated and it remains higher than the first bout of exercise especially in the first two minutes. It is also evident that $\dot{V}O_2$ is elevated in the second bout of exercise. Figure redrawn and modified from Hughson *et al.* (2003).

increase in $\dot{V}O_2$ between 3 and 6 min was significantly reduced in the second bout of exercise.

Additional information comes from the experiments of MacDonald *et al.* (1997) who studied consecutive bouts of exercise above the ventilatory threshold while breathing a hyperoxic gas mixture. They observed faster overall kinetics (as MRT) for $\dot{V}O_2$ in the first bout of heavy exercise while breathing high inspired O_2. They also observed in the second bout that both prior exercise and high inspired O_2 combined to yield the fastest kinetics response in these experiments. The finding of faster $\dot{V}O_2$ kinetics while breathing high inspired O_2 in the first bout of exercise above the ventilatory threshold is quite important for interpretation of subsequent experiments that have considered rate limiting steps in this exercise domain. Several investigators have concluded, from experiments that did not include hyperoxia, that kinetics for $\dot{V}O_2$ were not limited by O_2 availability for work rates between ventilatory threshold and $\dot{V}O_{2\,max}$ (Paterson and Whipp, 1991; Barstow 1994; Burnley *et al.*, 2000) or even for work rates above peak $\dot{V}O_2$ of single leg exercise (Bangsbo *et al.*, 2000). The results from the experiments of MacDonald *et al.* (1997) as well as the early work of Linnarsson and colleagues (Linnarsson *et al.*, 1974) demonstrate clearly that in the heavier exercise domains that high inspired O_2 must be included in the experimental design if one is going to eliminate O_2 transport as a limiting step regulating the adaptation of aerobic energy supply.

Tordi *et al.* (2003) have recently demonstrated a faster Phase II time constant during heavy (above ventilatory threshold) exercise when the exercise was preceded by three repeated all-out 30 s sprints (Figure 8.4). These sprints, followed

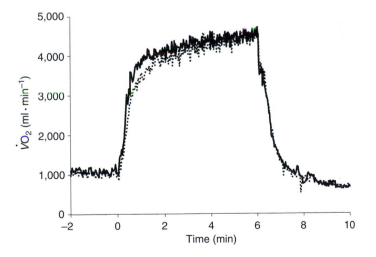

Figure 8.4 $\dot{V}O_2$ responses of a single subject are shown for two bouts of exercise at ~85% $\dot{V}O_{2\,peak}$ with no prior exercise (dotted line) and 10 min after 3 bouts of all-out 30 s sprint cycling (solid line). The Phase II time constant was reduced from 20.6 s for the no prior exercise condition to 16.4 s after the repeated sprint cycling. Figure redrawn and modified from Tordi *et al.* (2003).

by 6 min of passive recovery and 4 min baseline cycling at 25 W were probably associated with a marked alteration in muscle acid–base and metabolic condition prior to the heavy exercise. These conditions were consistent with the hypothesis of Gerbino *et al.* (1996) and the results of MacDonald *et al.* (2001) that local metabolic acidosis could promote faster increases in muscle blood flow and greater off-loading of O_2 at the working muscles. It would be interesting to obtain muscle biopsy samples under the conditions studied by Tordi *et al.* (2003) because intracellular metabolism must have been altered increasing active enzyme and substrate concentration and this probably also contributed to the faster kinetics for $\dot{V}O_2$ in the bout of heavy exercise after the repeated sprints.

Physiological basis for O_2 transport and utilization limitations

At the onset of exercise, there is an immediate increase in the rate of ATP splitting to provide the energy for muscular contraction. In the very first contractions, stores of ATP and phosphocreatine (PCr) can meet the demands. However, muscular contraction with release of calcium ions along with splitting of the high-energy phosphate compounds starts to provide necessary activating factors and substrates to stimulate the metabolic pathways so that ATP can be regenerated by glycolysis and oxidative phosphorylation. Certainly there is a lag in the accumulation of the metabolic substrates and oxidative phosphorylation cannot instantaneously achieve the steady-state requirement. Coincident with the processes that increase intramuscular substrate concentrations, there is a rapid response within the cardiovascular system to achieve O_2 delivery to meet the metabolic demands. The cardiovascular response is initiated by 'cortical irradiation' as proposed almost 100 years ago by Krogh and Lindhard (1913), or alternatively a 'central command' (Rowell, 1993) by which signals from the motor cortex to the muscles send parallel signals to the autonomic nervous system that cause rapid removal of parasympathetic activity to the heart. Thus, heart rate accelerates within the next cardiac cycle after the onset of exercise. But this mechanism is limited to increasing heart rate to $\sim 100 \; \mathrm{b \cdot min^{-1}}$ and further increases are achieved by activation of the sympathetic nervous system. Also at the onset of exercise, muscle contraction compresses the veins which have valves to force the blood to return to the heart via the 'muscle pump'. Again, this mechanism is limited because it does not direct blood to the muscle fibres that are active. This critical phase of adaptation is accomplished by local mechanisms that allow for selective distribution of blood flow to the active fibres (Laughlin *et al.*, 1996; Murrant and Sarelius, 2000).

Delivery of blood flow to muscle at the very onset of exercise is rapid and it has been observed in many situations to exceed the immediate demand as evidenced by no increase in O_2 extraction in the first ~ 15 s after the start of exercise (Grassi *et al.*, 1996; Hughson *et al.*, 1996; Bangsbo *et al.*, 2000; Krustrup *et al.*, 2001; van Beekvelt *et al.*, 2001). The reader is cautioned in the interpretation of these data. Figure 8.5 shows the clear two-phase adaptive response of blood flow as identified in many studies (Rådegran and Saltin, 1998; Shoemaker and

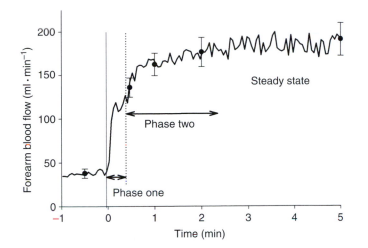

Figure 8.5 Forearm blood flow is shown for the rest to exercise transition to highlight the clear two-phase adaptive response. Phase one indicates the increase in flow attributed to the actions of the muscle pump while phase two reflects the increase in vascular conductance due to dilation associated with release of vasoactive dilator substances from the exercising muscles. The steady state is achieved when balance exists between O_2 supply and removal of metabolic by-products.

Hughson, 1999). The increase in blood flow in phase one is related to the muscle pump and for larger muscle mass exercise also to the increase in heart rate and cardiac output. The fact that this adaptation of blood flow was not sufficient to meet the metabolic demands is shown clearly by the further increase in phase two where blood flow continues to increase until 2–3 min of exercise. The pattern of increase in phase two is characteristic of a feedback control system just as one would expect if blood flow were adapting to meet the metabolic demand (Laughlin *et al.*, 1996; Murrant and Sarelius, 2000) where muscle metabolites continue to change over a similar time period (Green *et al.*, 1995a; Haseler *et al.*, 1998). Further evidence that the flow is increasing to meet the metabolic demand can be discerned from the pattern of change in O_2 extraction. For example in moderate or heavy rhythmic forearm exercise, arterial–venous O_2 content difference was essentially unchanged in the first 10 s after the start of exercise and began to increase by 20 s (Figure 8.6) (van Beekvelt *et al.*, 2001). O_2 extraction continued to increase for approximately the first minute of exercise and then remain relatively constant or even decreased slightly in very heavy exercise (Figure 8.6). The fact that arterial–venous O_2 content difference reached an upper limit and blood flow continued to adapt allowed $V̇O_2$ to reach its highest values during exercise. These observations from forearm exercise are consistent with the pattern seen for blood flow and $V̇O_2$ with leg exercise (Grassi *et al.*, 1996; Bangsbo *et al.*, 2000; MacDonald *et al.*, 2000; Krustrup *et al.*, 2001).

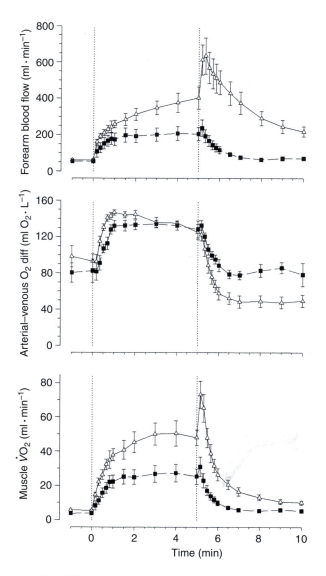

Figure 8.6 Forearm blood flow, arterial–venous O_2 content difference and muscle $\dot{V}O_2$ are shown for two different intensities (■25% and △75% peak work rate) of rhythmic hand-grip exercise and the first 5 min of recovery. Values are mean ± SE, $n = 6$. Figure redrawn and modified from van Beekvelt *et al.* (2001).

Collectively, the data summarized here provide strong evidence that muscle blood flow adapts to meet a metabolic demand, it does not adapt to the steady state or required level prior to the demand of moderate or higher intensities of exercise. Thus, delivery of O_2 to the working muscles is the regulated variable within a feedback control system. The balance between O_2 delivery and O_2 utilization will determine the intracellular PO_2. The following section will consider the interactions between the intracellular PO_2 and the metabolic state that determine the rate of oxidative production of ATP.

Muscle metabolism at the onset of exercise

Based on the pioneering work of Wilson and colleagues (Wilson and Rumsey, 1988) that was concerned with steady-state ATP production, Tschakovsky and Hughson (1999a) have proposed that intracellular PO_2 interacts with metabolic enzymes and substrates to yield the appropriate conditions to support the progressively increasing level of oxidative metabolism at the onset of exercise. Metabolic control is complex and requires a multidimensional perspective to understand how various factors combine to determine the rate of ATP production. Figure 8.7 portrays this complex interaction by presenting a surface upon which the rate of ATP production is the same at any point. Initially we will consider only the first plane defined by 'Intracellular PO_2' on the x-axis and 'Increasing energetic state' on the y-axis. This is based on key concepts developed by Wilson (Wilson and Rumsey, 1988) and demonstrated in a dog muscle preparation (Hogan et al., 1992) as described by Arthur et al. (1992). The 'Energetic state' is determined by the relative concentration of high-energy phosphates (Connett et al., 1990; Arthur et al., 1992) such that a high-energetic state has a relatively high concentration of PCr, and low concentrations of ADP, AMP and P_i. Thus, to achieve a given rate of ATP flux through the oxidative metabolic pathways in the face of lower intracellular PO_2 the energetic state must be adjusted as represented in Figure 8.7 by moving from point 'A' to 'B'. That is, there will be a reduction in the concentration of PCr and an increase in ADP, AMP and P_i to support the required rate of oxidative metabolism. (See also figure 4 in Hughson et al. (2001) for schematic representation of interaction between PO_2 and phosphorylation and redox potentials to achieve a given ATP flux.)

The range of PO_2 presented in Figure 8.7 was measured in exercising human muscle by magnetic resonance spectroscopy (Richardson et al., 1995; Tran et al., 1999). Richardson, Haseler and colleagues (Richardson et al., 1995; Richardson et al., 2002) have shown that intracellular PO_2 is ~4–5 mmHg across a wide range of work rates when breathing normal room air and that intracellular PO_2 decreases during exercise in hypoxia and increases with hyperoxia. A consequence of this alteration in intracellular PO_2 is that muscle PCr concentration (that can be taken as a surrogate marker for energetic state) decreases in hypoxia and increases in hyperoxia. This latter observation is extremely important to providing experimental evidence that the 'normal' level of intracellular PO_2 requires an adjustment of energetic state to achieve the steady-state ATP flux through oxidative pathways.

The third dimension shown as 'Increasing [enzyme or substrate]' in the z-axis of Figure 8.7 has not received a lot of attention. However, it is extremely important in understanding several recent experimental models that manipulated $\dot{V}O_2$ kinetics. Enzymes in this presentation could be considered as an increase in

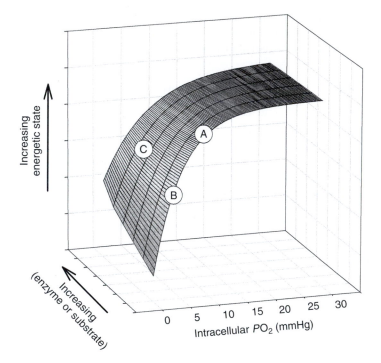

Figure 8.7 This figure portrays the hypothesized interaction of several key factors that can determine the rate of ATP production from oxidative metabolism. The surface represents a constant ATP flux under different conditions as affected by intracellular PO_2, the energetic state and muscle enzyme or substrate concentration changes. Here, the energetic state (Arthur *et al.*, 1992; Connett *et al.*, 1990) is higher when there is less breakdown of phosphocreatine and relatively lower concentrations of ADP and AMP. Thus, for conditions moving from 'A' to 'B' as intracellular PO_2 declines within a range observed in human muscle (Richardson *et al.*, 1995), the energetic state must also decline (less phosphocreatine and increased creatine, ADP and P_i) to sustain a given rate of oxidative ATP production. The third dimension in this figure is a theoretical increase in oxidative enzymes (such as with increased physical fitness) or increased substrate (see text for potential mechanisms) that could allow a given ATP flux at either or both improved energetic state or intracellular PO_2. See text for more complete development.

mitochondrial oxidative enzyme concentration such as would occur with increased physical fitness (training) (Green *et al.*, 1995b). Certainly, faster $\dot{V}O_2$ kinetics have been observed following training that might be attributed to increased oxidative enzymes and/or improved O_2 transport (Hickson *et al.*, 1978; Phillips *et al.*, 1995; see Chapter 15). Movement from points 'B' to 'C' in Figure 8.7 could describe these manipulations. At present, it is not known what happens to intracellular PO_2 at a given metabolic rate after training but it is reasonable to propose that it would be increased as suggested by the move to a higher PO_2 at point 'C'. The overall reduction in sympathetic vasoconstrictor tone (in the gut and resting muscle, for example) with improved fitness (Rowell, 1993) might lead to reduced muscle blood flow at the same metabolic demand (Proctor et al., 1998) but the increased capillarization (Green et al., 1995b) might enhance blood–myocyte O_2 delivery. In any case, it is well established that PCr depletion is reduced at any work rate after endurance training (Green et al., 1995a) and this is consistent with a higher energetic state indicated by point 'C' relative to point 'B'.

Recent experiments have found that inhibition of nitric oxide synthase with L-NAME is associated with faster $\dot{V}O_2$ kinetics in the horse (Kindig et al., 2000, 2001) and also the human (Jones et al., 2003, 2004). As nitric oxide interacts with cytochrome oxidase to downregulate mitochondrial O_2 consumption it was hypothesized that L-NAME would reduce nitric oxide production and therefore decrease its interaction with cytochrome oxidase allowing a faster increase in $\dot{V}O_2$ at the onset of exercise (Kindig et al., 2000, 2001; Jones et al., 2003, 2004). Just as considered with increased oxidative enzyme concentration with physical training L-NAME might alter the 'effective' enzyme concentration such that the same rate of ATP flux (point 'C' in Figure 8.7) could be achieved at a relatively greater energetic state (less depletion of phosphocreatine) and/or a greater intracellular PO_2. At present, it is uncertain whether other effects of L-NAME related to O_2 supply mechanisms might have affected the kinetics of $\dot{V}O_2$. Inhibition of nitric oxide synthase causes vasoconstriction in arterioles of resting muscle. In a model of human forearm exercise, Shoemaker et al. (1997) found no difference in the kinetics of blood flow adaptation due to local inhibition of nitric oxide synthase. In the presence of whole body L-NAME the pattern of distribution of blood flow might be markedly altered due to the general vasoconstrictor response with the superimposed increase in vascular conductance in working muscles. Mean arterial blood pressure is elevated and heart rate is reduced by L-NAME while blood flow through the exercising legs of humans is not different (Frandsen et al., 2001) suggesting that blood flow might be preferentially distributed to the legs with increased vasoconstriction in other vascular beds. These observations in humans suggest important species differences where a reduction in whole body conductance was found in the horse (Kindig et al., 2000) and blood flow was reduced in some muscles of exercising rat (Hirai et al., 1994). The pattern of distribution in the rest to exercise transition during L-NAME studies is not known but it is conceivable that the elevated arterial pressure might have facilitated a more rapid increase in exercising muscle blood flow as observed in recent experiments where the muscle chemoreflex elevated blood pressure prior to submaximal arm exercise (Perrey et al., 2001). In addition, it is important to consider that the time course for return of venous blood from the working muscles will be altered by the L-NAME induced pattern of blood flow distribution and that this can alter the apparent dynamics of $\dot{V}O_2$ at the lungs (Essfeld et al., 1991).

The inclusion in the model of 'substrates' demonstrates that other factors can modify the availability of substrate for oxidative phosphorylation with an impact on redox and phosphorylation potentials (Wilson and Rumsey, 1988). Greenhaff and colleagues (Greenhaff *et al.*, 2002) hypothesized that an acetyl group deficit limits mitochondrial ATP production at the onset of exercise. They further hypothesized that increased activation of the pyruvate dehydrogenase enzyme complex by dichloroacetate would increase the concentration of acetylcarnitine to facilitate entry of metabolic substrate into the citric acid cycle. Recent experiments using dichloroacetate to activate pyruvate dehydrogenase have not found faster $\dot{V}O_2$ kinetics in humans (Bangsbo *et al.*, 2002) or dogs (Grassi *et al.*, 1998). Thus even though activation of pyruvate dehydrogenase is a critical step for increasing oxidative phosphorylation, there is no evidence that it is the primary rate limiting step nor that it is independent of O_2 availability. In any case, Figure 8.7 shows that it is not necessary to propose that L-NAME, dichloroacetate or other manipulations of the metabolic components take oxidative metabolism out of the domain of interaction between O_2 supply and utilization because the constant ATP flux surface shows the wide range of interaction of multiple variables.

Figure 8.7 can also be used to help understand the current controversy about whether $\dot{V}O_2$ kinetics at the onset of sub-ventilatory threshold exercise are limited solely by an inertia in a metabolic pathway or whether O_2 plays a role in regulating the increase in $\dot{V}O_2$. If point 'A', which is close to the normal intracellular PO_2 during moderate exercise (Richardson *et al.*, 1995), is taken as the reference point then any increase in PO_2, for example breathing a hyperoxic gas mixture, might cause a relatively small increase in energetic state. Thus, the relative difference in steady-state phosphocreatine concentration would be small and the time course of change in phosphocreatine and the increase in $\dot{V}O_2$ might not be 'detectably' different from the normoxic control. That is, statistically insignificant differences in $\dot{V}O_2$ kinetics between normoxic and hyperoxic test conditions should not in isolation be taken as evidence that O_2 does not play a role in regulating the adaptation of oxidative phosphorylation under normal conditions of light to moderate exercise. The real question that must be asked is whether PO_2 at the level of the electron transport chain of the mitochondria remains above the level at which changes in phosphorylation and redox potentials are required to maintain a given rate of respiration? Many researchers have mistakenly taken the extremely low value of the Km for mitochondrial respiration of ~0.03–0.1 mmHg to suggest that O_2 will not become rate limiting. However, there is evidence that the phosphorylation potential and redox potential must change even for PO_2 above 30 mmHg (Erecinska and Wilson, 1982). Here, it is appropriate to quote from Erecinska and Wilson (p. 6 in Erecinska and Wilson, 1982) where they conclude that the effect of O_2 up to 30 mmHg is

> evidence that oxidative phosphorylation is, in fact, dependent on oxygen concentrations at values much higher than those which affect the respiratory activity. ... Thus although a fall in oxygen tension does cause a decrease in the rate of ATP synthesis, it does not affect the rate of ATP utilization. However, such a situation leads to an immediate decline in the [ATP]/[ADP][Pi] which induces, through the near equilibrium relations in the first two sites of oxidative phosphorylation, an increase in reduction of cytochrome c and activation of cytochrome c oxidase. The consequent

enhancement of respiration proceeds to the point at which the rate of ATP synthesis again matches the rate of ATP utilization.

The scheme described by Erecinska and Wilson (1982) was set out for a steady-state condition in which a transient change in PO_2 occurred. At the onset of exercise, the situation is slightly more complex as the rate of oxidative phosphorylation is increasing at the same time that PO_2 is decreasing. However, the argument is the same, there is an interaction between O_2 and the build up of appropriate metabolic substrates, phosphorylation and redox potentials as the steady-state $\dot{V}O_2$ is attained over the first minutes of exercise. A simplified framework of the hypothetical ATP flux during the rest to exercise transition for a work rate of about 50–60% $\dot{V}O_2$ peak is presented in the two-dimensions of energetic state and intracellular PO_2 in Figure 8.8. The point marked as '~20 s' is based on two measured events. First, intracellular PO_2 has been reported to decrease to 4–5 mmHg within the first 20 s of knee-extensor exercise in a group of competitive cyclists (Richardson *et al.*, 1995). Second, given a time constant for the increase in $\dot{V}O_2$ of ~30 s the ATP flux rate would be about half-way between rest and steady-state values. Even if one assumed a very fast time constant of 20 s then the response would still be only 63% of the way between rest and steady state. Thus, further increases in ATP flux are associated primarily

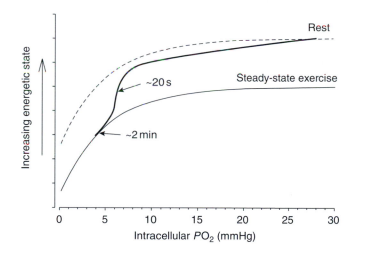

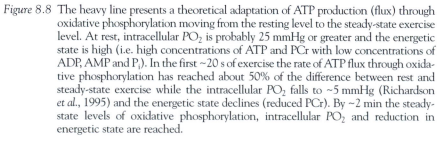

Figure 8.8 The heavy line presents a theoretical adaptation of ATP production (flux) through oxidative phosphorylation moving from the resting level to the steady-state exercise level. At rest, intracellular PO_2 is probably 25 mmHg or greater and the energetic state is high (i.e. high concentrations of ATP and PCr with low concentrations of ADP, AMP and P_i). In the first ~20 s of exercise the rate of ATP flux through oxidative phosphorylation has reached about 50% of the difference between rest and steady-state exercise while the intracellular PO_2 falls to ~5 mmHg (Richardson *et al.*, 1995) and the energetic state declines (reduced PCr). By ~2 min the steady-state levels of oxidative phosphorylation, intracellular PO_2 and reduction in energetic state are reached.

with the change in energetic state indicating greater breakdown of PCr and increased concentrations of ADP, AMP and Pi.

Information about the kinetics of muscle metabolism at the onset of exercise has come from recent experiments with nuclear magnetic resonance spectroscopy measurements of muscle PCr and P_i. The similarity of the kinetics of PCr hydrolysis and $\dot{V}O_2$ kinetics suggested that the dynamic response of PCr might serve as a surrogate for exercising muscle oxidative phosphorylation (Barstow et al., 1994; Whipp and Mahler, 1980). While recent evidence from heavier exercise questions this link (Rossiter et al., 2001), it is informative to examine differences in PCr kinetics as a function of various experimental manipulations. The time constant for PCr recovery after plantar flexion exercise depends on arterial PO_2 with significant slowing in hypoxia (33.5 ± 4.1 s) and acceleration in hyperoxia (20.0 ± 1.8 s) compared to normoxia (25.0 ± 2.7 s) (Haseler et al., 1999). Haseler et al. (1999) observed that the end-exercise values for [PCr] were slightly but not significantly different, ranging from 64% to 70% of resting levels for hypoxia to hyperoxia respectively. Importantly, however they found that muscle pH was not significantly changed from resting values for any gas breathing condition supporting the notion that this was relatively low-intensity exercise. The same research group observed the PCr responses at the onset of plantar flexion exercise and found different steady-state values (Haseler et al., 1998). They did not characterize the time constant for these onset of exercise tests but there was an indication from the data presented that a longer time was required to achieve steady state in the hypoxia than hyperoxia condition implying differences in kinetics (Haseler et al., 1998). Observations from repeated bouts of heavy knee-extension exercise made Rossiter et al. (2001) question the link between $\dot{V}O_2$ and PCr kinetics. They observed that $\dot{V}O_2$ Phase II time constant was reduced from 46.6 ± 6.0 s in the first bout to 40.7 ± 8.4 s in the second bout of heavy exercise, consistent with several (Gerbino et al., 1996; Tordi et al., 2003) but not all (Burnley et al., 2000) studies of repeated heavy cycling exercise. In contrast, PCr time constant was not significantly affected changing from 34.86 ± 4.64 s in bout one to 32.13 ± 10.96 s in bout two. What did occur though was a significantly smaller reduction in [PCr] from rest to exercise indicating dynamic nonlinearities in the metabolic control with heavy exercise.

Control theory and $\dot{V}O_2$ kinetics

By studying $\dot{V}O_2$ kinetics we desire to better understand the physiological regulatory mechanisms that control the rate at which the oxidative energy supply system adapts to the challenges of changing metabolic demand. Pioneering research on $\dot{V}O_2$ kinetics published in 1933 by Margaria et al. (1933) and in the 1950s by Henry (1951) had already incorporated concepts of control theory in the application of exponential models to describe the data. An exponential model implies some form of feedback regulation in which the difference between the current $\dot{V}O_2$ and the required steady-state $\dot{V}O_2$ is progressively reduced at a rate that is proportional to the intensity of the 'error signal' (Figure 8.9).

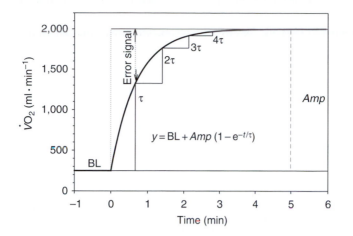

Figure 8.9 This single component exponential response for $\dot{V}O_2$ portrays two key concepts. First, the rate of increase in $\dot{V}O_2$ is quantified by the time constant (τ) of the exponential equation where y is the $\dot{V}O_2$, BL is the baseline $\dot{V}O_2$, and Amp (dashed line) is the amplitude of increase in $\dot{V}O_2$ above baseline. Note that for each multiple of τ, $\dot{V}O_2$ has increased (thin solid vertical lines) by ~63% of the difference between the value at the previous τ and the required steady state as indicated by the Amp. By the completion of 4τ the $\dot{V}O_2$ has reached ~98% of the total Amp. The second concept on this figure is that of the metabolic error signal (dotted lines above the $\dot{V}O_2$ response). At each increment in τ the magnitude of the error signal decreases.

There are two key components of the kinetic response that are of interest. These are the amplitude and the time course. Over a wide range of work rates the amplitude has been taken to be predictable because there is an approximately linear increase in $\dot{V}O_2$ as a function of the work rate (Whipp *et al.*, 1981). For each increment in work rate expressed in Watts, there is ~10 ml · min^{-1} increase in $\dot{V}O_2$ but there are examples of deviations from this, even during moderate-intensity exercise (Brittain *et al.*, 2001). In general, it is acceptable to state that physiological responses to moderate intensities of exercise obey the principle of superposition such that any increase in work rate is matched by the appropriate increase in output $\dot{V}O_2$. For work rates above ventilatory threshold but below $\dot{V}O_2$ peak, $\dot{V}O_2$ might appear to increase less per increment in work rate during Phase II (e.g. Pringle *et al.*, 2003) but with time $\dot{V}O_2$ increases above the predicted value. For work rates that have an energy demand above $\dot{V}O_2$ peak the amplitude must be less than the requirement. Thus at these higher work rates description of the amplitude component of kinetics becomes more complicated (Hughson *et al.*, 2000). As considered next, the description of the time course is considerably more complex.

Kinetic analysis of the time course of increase in $\dot{V}O_2$ measured in expired gases has focused primarily on Phase II under the assumption that this reflects the time course of change in muscle $\dot{V}O_2$ (Barstow *et al.*, 1994; see Chapter 6). It is normal to fit a single exponential curve (or equivalent such as a semi-logarithmic fit) to these data to achieve an estimate of the rate of increase given by the time constant (τ). The τ really expresses the curvature of an exponential response. A small value of τ indicates a rapid increase. The following equation describes a progressive increase in a variable such as $\dot{V}O_2$ as a function of time. From this equation, we determine the amplitude of the response 'Amp' and the time constant 'τ'.

$$y = Amp * \left(1 - exp\left(\frac{-t}{\tau}\right)\right)$$

In this equation, the value of y progressively approaches the value 'Amp' because the term $exp(-t / \tau)$ approaches 0 with increasing time. It is of interest that at the specific time that $t = \tau$ the exponent term becomes $exp(-1)$ which is 0.3679. That is, $1 - 0.3679 = 0.6321$ so that at one τ the response has risen to 63.21% of the final amplitude. This occurs progressively with each increment in τ as shown in Figure 8.9 and it introduces the concept of dynamic linearity. That is, the rate of change is constant over the entire response between baseline and steady-state plateau. A system with dynamic linearity has the same τ independent of the amplitude.

There is considerable controversy in the literature concerning the presence or absence of dynamic linearity in the τ for $\dot{V}O_2$ across a wide range of work rates (Whipp and Wasserman, 1972; Hughson and Morrissey, 1982; Paterson and Whipp, 1991; Brittain *et al.*, 2001; Özyener *et al.*, 2001). Some researchers have reported that τ stays constant from moderate through to severe work rates, where the latter implies a work rate with an energy demand that may exceed $\dot{V}O_2$ peak (Özyener *et al.*, 2001). One study reported that τ was 20.4 ± 10.5 s for work rates below ventilatory threshold and 28.2 ± 13.1 s for work rates above ventilatory threshold yet these mean values that were 40% different were not statistically significant (Scheuermann *et al.*, 2001). In contrast, it has been observed that τ for $\dot{V}O_2$ can differ between sub-ventilatory threshold work-rates, especially when the condition of prior exercise is modified (Hughson and Morrissey, 1982; Brittain *et al.*, 2001). The method of fitting data for heavy to severe intensities requires some additional consideration. In the study of Özyener *et al.* (2001) where Phase II τ was reported to be constant (i.e. consistent with dynamic system linearity), the amplitude of this phase was not constant across work rates decreasing from 11.52 to 9.99 ml·min^{-1}·W^{-1} on going from moderate to severe work intensities. There are two important consequences of this finding. The first from a physiological perspective is that there is no known reason for muscles to become 'more efficient' (i.e. use less O_2 per W external work rate) at these higher intensities as detailed in the next paragraph. The second from a modelling perspective is that this indicates failure to conform to system linearity. Even in moderate-intensity exercise, the amplitude might not be constant perhaps due to differences in recruitment patterns and metabolic efficiency (Brittain *et al.*, 2001) although here the amplitude is increased rather than decreased. Thus, there have been reports of non-linearity of both the amplitude and the τ for the $\dot{V}O_2$ response to a range of step increases in work-rate (Hughson and Morrissey, 1982; Brittain *et al.*, 2001; Hughson *et al.*, 2001; Rossiter *et al.*, 2001; Pringle *et al.*, 2003). It is therefore very important that interpretation of models fitted to $\dot{V}O_2$ kinetics data be made with extreme caution. If either of amplitude (in $ml \cdot min^{-1} \cdot W^{-1}$) or τ should change, then it should not be assumed that constancy of the other parameter can be taken as evidence for consistent physiological regulation.

An alternative interpretation of the kinetics in heavy to severe exercise has been provided by Hughson *et al.* (2000). In their study, when the data obtained at exercise intensities of 57%, 96% or 125% of $\dot{V}O_2$ peak were fit by the least-squares best-fit approach, the value of τ for the Phase II response decreased from 29.4 to 22.1 to 16.3 s, respectively. As in the study of Özyener *et al.* (2001) the amplitude of the Phase II response did not correspond to the increase in work rate. Indeed the amplitude at the end of Phase II extrapolated to ~82% and 85% $\dot{V}O_2$ peak rather than the required 96% and 125% for these work rates. Based on these observations, Hughson *et al.* (2000) concluded that the amplitude in the 96% work-rate was limited by O_2 availability. It is not necessary for the meta-bolic demand to exceed $\dot{V}O_{2\,max}$ for O_2 availability to be limiting the rate of oxidative phosphorylation. Clear support for this statement comes from examin-ing the heart rate (Linnarsson, 1974; Hughson *et al.*, 2000) and leg blood flow responses (Rådegran and Saltin, 1998; Bangsbo *et al.*, 2000; Hughson *et al.*, 2003) which do not achieve the required end-exercise value within the duration of the Phase II. Indeed, Hughson *et al.* (2000) noted the similarity of the time course of change in $\dot{V}O_2$ and heart rate. As O_2 extraction reaches its greatest value by approximately 60 s during intense exercise (Bangsbo *et al.*, 2000; Krustrup *et al.*, 2001; van Beekvelt *et al.*, 2001) the further increase in $\dot{V}O_2$ that is observed beyond this time is entirely a function of increased O_2 delivery by greater mus-cle blood flow. Given this argument, it is not appropriate to estimate τ, that is, the rate at which $\dot{V}O_2$ increases toward the plateau, when the plateau value does not represent the true metabolic error signal. Instead, Hughson *et al.* (2000) pro-posed that the $\dot{V}O_2$ response should be referenced to the theoretical 'predicted' metabolic demand as estimated from a linear extrapolation of the energy cost to work-rate relationship. When the data were re-evaluated by forcing the ampli-tude to be that of the predicted $\dot{V}O_2$ for each work rate, the estimated τ for Phase II increased considerably to 49.7 and 40.2 s for the 96% and 125% work rates, respectively. Given the possibility that predicted $\dot{V}O_2$ might deviate due to sys-tem non-linearities (Whipp *et al.*, 1981; Brittain *et al.*, 2001), Hughson *et al.* (2000) determined τ when the amplitude was increased or decreased by 5% but this did not change the main message that τ was slower at higher work rates. In using the predicted $\dot{V}O_2$ as the amplitude, it is assumed that just as for mod-erate exercise, the error signal that drives the O_2 transport – utilization system is determined by the difference between the required and the current values of $\dot{V}O_2$ as shown in Figure 8.9. These data provide further evidence of dynamic non-linearity in the $\dot{V}O_2$ response suggesting that the relative contribution of potential rate-limiting steps might change with exercise intensity or other conditions.

Limitations of current experimental techniques to extract information

Breath-by-breath variability impacts the ability to resolve differences between curve-fitting parameters that describe $\dot{V}O_2$ kinetics (Lamarra et al., 1987). The variability between tests can be due to methodological limitations, human variability in response, or true physiological differences. The question becomes one of the ability to resolve real differences when they exist. As noted above, a 40% difference in the τ values for below versus above ventilatory threshold were not considered significantly different (Scheuermann et al., 2001). Rossiter et al. (2001) found that a 14% difference in τ was significant for $\dot{V}O_2$ kinetics but a 7.8% difference in τ for PCr kinetics was not different. Other examples of non-significant differences include an 8.4% faster response of muscle $\dot{V}O_2$ in a dog muscle preparation with faster adaptation of muscle blood flow (Grassi et al., 1998).

Even within a single test, it is not clear that a mono-exponential response pattern is the appropriate model choice. Given the evidence that blood flow adapts with two very distinct mechanisms (the muscle pump and regulatory feedback) it might not be surprising that availability of O_2 as an important regulatory substrate could have a clearly different impact on metabolism at different times in the adaptive process. This concept is shown hypothetically in Figure 8.8 as PO_2 declines over the first 20 s of exercise. The consequence of this is that $\dot{V}O_2$ kinetics might be dictated more by a 'metabolic inertia' in the first ~20 s of exercise but that the reduction in PO_2 to <5 mmHg requires metabolic adaptations in the phosphorylation and redox potentials to support oxidative metabolism after this (Hughson et al., 2001) so that the rate of increase in $\dot{V}O_2$ would be modulated by availability of O_2 (Tschakovsky and Hughson, 1999a). Given the possibility that O_2 might have a different impact on metabolism at different times after the onset of exercise, Hughson et al. (2001) simulated $\dot{V}O_2$ kinetics data with two different τ values, $\tau = 30$ s for the first 0.5 min of exercise and $\tau = 36$ s from 0.5 to 5 min then fit the data by a least-squares approach. When they fitted the data by a least-squares method, they found an estimate of $\tau = 30.7$ s with no clear justification from the fitting for rejecting the mono-exponential model. That is, even though a large component of the adaptive response had a τ for $\dot{V}O_2$ that was almost 17% different, it could not be detected in this simulated data set.

Conclusions

Evidence has been presented that the study of $\dot{V}O_2$ kinetics is complex. It is complex because of uncertainty about the physiological mechanisms that regulate the increase in $\dot{V}O_2$. Biochemical evidence supports a role for O_2 in adjusting the phosphorylation and redox potentials required to drive oxidative metabolism while independent changes in muscle enzymes or substrates can interact with both O_2 and phosphorylation and redox potentials to establish the rate of oxidative phosphorylation. The study of $\dot{V}O_2$ kinetics is also complex because there is strong evidence that the relative contribution of different physiological mechanisms probably changes according to work rate, environmental conditions and factors such as prior exercise. Finally, the study of $\dot{V}O_2$ kinetics is complex because small but physiologically significant alterations in the interaction of O_2 transport and utilization mechanisms are frequently impossible to detect by normal statistical procedures.

In this review, the belief has been presented that across a wide range of metabolic demands the kinetics of $\dot{V}O_2$ are best considered to be non-linear. Linear models with one, two or three exponential components have been employed for convenience of giving approximate descriptions of the time course of the increase in oxidative metabolism but we should recognize that there are truly complex control systems interacting under this simple explanation. If it is true that intracellular PO_2 reaches a level of <5 mmHg during even moderate exercise (Richardson *et al.*, 1995; Vanderthommen *et al.*, 2003) and that it is only slightly higher even with hyperoxic gas breathing (Richardson *et al.*, 1999), then it is necessary that biochemical adaptations in the phosphorylation and redox potentials take place to permit the appropriate ATP flux rate.

At the onset of exercise, there must be some form of 'metabolic inertia' as the substrates increase to drive the oxidative production of ATP toward the steady-state demand. However, the real question is whether the adaptation toward the new steady-state metabolic rate is independent of O_2 availability and entirely dependent on 'metabolic inertia' under physiological conditions as suggested by some scientists (Yoshida and Whipp, 1994; Burnley *et al.*, 2000; Grassi, 2001). An alternative way of thinking of this situation is that the 'metabolic inertia' could be independent of O_2 if the intracellular PO_2 remained above 20–30 mmHg (Wilson and Rumsey, 1988) but there is compelling evidence from many research labs based on estimates of PO_2 (Connett *et al.*, 1990; Richardson *et al.*, 1995; Tran *et al.*, 1999; Vanderthommen *et al.*, 2003) or the measurement of metabolites associated with redox and phosphorylation potentials (Hogan *et al.*, 1992; Haseler *et al.*, 1998, 1999) against such a proposal. Therefore, as intracellular PO_2 drops, it is obligatory that interplay between intracellular PO_2 and the phosphorylation and redox potentials modify the 'metabolic inertia' during the adaptation of oxidative phosphorylation so that the interaction between O_2 transport and O_2 utilization mechanisms determine $\dot{V}O_2$ kinetics (Tschakovsky and Hughson, 1999a; Hughson *et al.*, 2001). (See Chapter 12 for additional discussion on this topic.)

Glossary of terms

A	amplitude of a response, for example, of the increase in $\dot{V}O_2$ above baseline
ADP	adenosine diphosphate

AMP	adenosine monophosphate
Amp	amplitude
ATP	adenosine triphosphate
L-NAME	nitro-L-arginine methyl ester
MRT	mean response time
O_2	oxygen
O_2 deficit	difference between energy required for the work rate and energy supplied through oxidative metabolism
PCr	phosphocreatine
P_i	inorganic phosphate
PO_2	partial pressure of oxygen
τ	time constant (time taken to reach 63% of the final amplitude in an exponential function)
t	time
$\dot{V}O_2$	oxygen uptake
$\dot{V}O_{2\,max/peak}$	the maximum $\dot{V}O_2$ attained during for example an incremental exercise test to exhaustion
VT	ventilatory threshold
[ ]	denotes concentration

References

Arthur, P.G., Hogan, M.C., Bebout, D.E., Wagner, P.D. and Hochachka, P.W. (1992). Modeling the effects of hypoxia on ATP turnover in exercising muscle. *Journal of Applied Physiology*, **73**, 737–42.

Bangsbo, J., Krustrup, P., González-Alonso, J., Boushel, R. and Saltin, B. (2000). Muscle oxygen kinetics at onset of intense dynamic exercise in humans. *American Journal of Physiology*, **279**, R899–906.

Bangsbo, J., Gibala, M.J., Krustrup, P., González-Alonso, J. and Saltin, B. (2002). Enhanced pyruvate dehydrogenase activity does not affect muscle O_2 uptake at onset of intense exercise in humans, *American Journal of Physiology*, **282**, R273–80.

Barstow, T.J. (1994). Characterization of $\dot{V}O_2$ kinetics during heavy exercise. *Medicine and Science in Sports and Exercise*, **26**, 1327–34.

Barstow, T.J., Buchthal, S., Zanconato, S. and Cooper, D.M. (1994). Muscle energetics and pulmonary oxygen uptake kinetics during moderate exercise. *Journal of Applied Physiology*, **77**, 1742–9.

Brittain, C.J., Rossiter, H.B., Kowalchuk, J.M. and Whipp, B.J. (2001). Effect of prior metabolic rate on the kinetics of oxygen uptake during moderate-intensity exercise. *European Journal of Applied Physiology*, **86**, 125–34.

Brooks, G.A. (1985). Response to Davis' manuscript. *Medicine and Science in Sports*, **17**, 19–21.

Burnley, M., Jones, A.M., Carter, H. and Doust, J.H. (2000). Effects of prior heavy exercise on phase II pulmonary oxygen uptake kinetics during heavy exercise. *Journal of Applied Physiology*, **89**, 1387–96.

Connett, R.J., Honig, C.R., Gayeski, T.E.J. and Brooks, G.A. (1990). Defining hypoxia: a systems view of $\dot{V}O_2$, glycolysis, energetics, and intracellular PO_2. *Journal of Applied Physiology*, **68**, 833–42.

Davis, J.A. (1985). Anaerobic threshold: review of the concept and directions for future research. *Medicine and Science in Sports and Exercise*, **17**, 6–18.

Delp, M.D. (1999). Control of skeletal muscle perfusion at the onset of dynamic exercise. *Medicine and Science in Sports and Exercise*, **31**, 1011–18.

Di Prampero, P.E. (1981). Energetics of muscular exercise. *Review of Physiology, Biochemistry and Pharmacology*, **89**, 143–222.

Di Prampero, P.E., Mahler, P., Giezendanner, D. and Cerretelli, P. (1989). The effects of priming exercise on $\dot{V}O_2$ kinetics and O_2 deficit at the onset of stepping and cycling. *Journal of Applied Physiology*, **66**, 2023–31.

Engelen, M., Porszasz, J., Riley, M., Wasserman, K., Maehara, K. and Barstow, T.J. (1996). Effects of hypoxic hypoxia on O_2 uptake and heart rate kinetics during heavy exercise. *Journal of Applied Physiology*, **81**, 2500–8.

Erecinska, M. and Wilson, D.F. (1982). Regulation of cellular energy metabolism, *Journal of Membrane Biology*, **70**, 1–14.

Essfeld, D., Hoffmann, U. and Stegemann, J. (1991). A model for studying the distortion of muscle oxygen-uptake patterns by circulation parameters. *European Journal of Applied Physiology*, **62**, 83–90.

Frandsen, U., Bangsbo, J., Sander, M., Hoffner, L., Betak, A., Saltin, B. and Hellsten, Y. (2001). Exercise-induced hyperaemia and leg oxygen uptake are not altered during effective inhibition of nitric oxide synthase with N-G-nitro-L-arginine methyl ester in humans. *Journal of Physiology*, **531**, 257–64.

Gerbino, A., Ward, S.A. and Whipp, B.J. (1996). Effects of prior exercise on pulmonary gas-exchange kinetics during high-intensity exercise in humans. *Journal of Applied Physiology*, **80**, 99–107.

Grassi, B. (2001). Regulation of oxygen consumption at the onset of exercise. Is it really controversial? *Exercise and Sports Science Reviews*, **29**, 134–8.

Grassi, B., Poole, D.C., Richardson, R.S., Knight, D.R., Erickson, B.K. and Wagner, P.D. (1996). Muscle O_2 uptake kinetics in humans: implications for metabolic control. *Journal of Applied Physiology*, **80**, 988–98.

Grassi, B., Gladden, L.B., Samaja, M., Stary, C.M. and Hogan, M.C. (1998). Faster adjustment of O_2 delivery does not affect $\dot{V}O_2$ on-kinetics in isolated in situ canine muscle. *Journal of Applied Physiology*, **85**, 1394–403.

Green, H.J., Cadefau, J., Cussó, R., Ball-Burnett, M. and Jamieson, G. (1995a). Metabolic adaptations to short-term training are expressed early in submaximal exercise. *Canadian Journal of Physiology and Pharmacology*, **73**, 474–82.

Green, H.J., Jones, S., Ball-Burnett, M., Farrance, B. and Ranney, D. (1995b). Adaptations in muscle metabolism to prolonged voluntary exercise and training. *Journal of Applied Physiology*, **78**, 138–45.

Greenhaff, P.L., Campbell-O'Sullivan, S.P., Constantin-Teodosiu, D., Poucher, S.M., Roberts, P.A. and Timmons, J.A. (2002). An acetyl group deficit limits mitochondrial ATP production at the onset of exercise. *Biochemical Society Transactions*, **30**, 275–80.

Haseler, L.J., Richardson, R.S., Videen, J.S. and Hogan, M.C. (1998). Phosphocreatine hydrolysis during submaximal exercise: the effect of FI_{O2}. *Journal of Applied Physiology*, **85**, 1457–63.

Haseler, L.J., Hogan, M.C. and Richardson, R.S. (1999). Skeletal muscle phosphocreatine recovery in exercise-trained humans is dependent on O_2 availability. *Journal of Applied Physiology*, **86**, 2013–18.

Henry, F.M. (1951). Aerobic oxygen consumption and alactic debt in muscular work. *Journal of Applied Physiology*, **3**, 427–38.

Hickson, R.C., Bomze, H.A. and Holloszy, J.O. (1978). Faster adjustment of O_2 uptake to the energy requirement of exercise in the trained state. *Journal of Applied Physiology*, **44**, 877–81.

Hirai, T., Visnski, M.D., Kearns, K.J., Zelis, R. and Musch, T.I. (1994). Effects of NO synthase inhibition on the muscular blood flow response to treadmill exercise in rats. *Journal of Applied Physiology*, **77**, 1288–93.

Hogan, M.C., Arthur, P.G., Bebout, D.E., Hochachka, P.W. and Wagner, P.D. (1992). Role of O_2 in regulating tissue respiration in dog muscle working in situ. *Journal of Applied Physiology*, **73**, 728–36.

Hughson, R.L. (1984). Alterations in the oxygen deficit-oxygen debt relationships with beta-adrenergic receptor blockade in man. *Journal of Physiology*, **349**, 375–87.

Hughson, R.L. and Kowalchuk, J.M. (1995). Kinetics of oxygen uptake for submaximal exercise in hyperoxia, normoxia, and hypoxia. *Canadian Journal of Applied Physiology*, **20**, 198–210.

Hughson, R.L. and Morrissey, M.A. (1982). Delayed kinetics of respiratory gas exchange in the transition from prior exercise. *Journal of Applied Physiology*, **52**, 921–9.

Hughson, R.L. and Morrissey, M.A. (1983). Delayed kinetics of $\dot{V}O_2$ in the transition from prior exercise. Evidence for O_2 transport limitation of $\dot{V}O_2$ kinetics. A review, *International Journal of Sports Medicine*, **11**, 94–105.

Hughson, R.L. and Tschakovsky, M.E. (1999). Cardiovascular dynamics at the onset of exercise. *Medicine and Science in Sports and Exercise*, **31**, 1005–10.

Hughson, R.L., Cochrane, J.E. and Butler G.C. (1993). Faster O_2 uptake kinetics at onset of supine exercise with than without lower body negative pressure. *Journal of Applied Physiology*, **75**, 1962–7.

Hughson, R.L., Shoemaker, J.K., Tschakovsky, M. and Kowalchuk, J.M. (1996). Dependence of muscle $\dot{V}O_2$ on blood flow dynamics at the onset of forearm exercise. *Journal of Applied Physiology*, **81**, 1619–26.

Hughson, R.L., O'Leary, D.D., Betik, A.C. and Hebestreit, H. (2000). Kinetics of oxygen uptake at the onset of exercise near or above peak oxygen uptake. *Journal of Applied Physiology*, **88**, 1812–19.

Hughson, R.L., Tschakovsky, M.E. and Houston, M.E. (2001). Regulation of oxygen consumption at the onset of exercise. *Exercise and Sports Science Reviews*, **29**, 129–33.

Hughson, R.L., Schijvens, H., Burrows, S., Devitt, D., Betik, A.C. and Hopman, M.T.E. (2003). Blood flow and metabolic control at the onset of heavy exercise. *International Journal of Sport and Health Science*, **1**, 1–9.

Jones, A.M., Wilkerson, D.P., Koppo, K., Wilmshurst, S. and Campbell, I.T. (2003). Inhibition of nitric oxide synthase by L-NAME speeds phase II pulmonary $\dot{V}O_2$ kinetics in the transition to moderate-intensity exercise in man. *Journal of Physiology*, **552**, 265–72.

Jones, A.M., Wilkerson, D.P., Wilmshurst, S. and Campbell, I.T. (2004). Influence of L-NAME on pulmonary O_2 uptake kinetics during heavy-intensity cycle exercise. *Journal of Applied Physiology*, **96**, 1033–8.

Kindig, C.A., Gallatin, L.L., Erickson, H.H., Fedde, M.R. and Poole, D.C. (2000). Cardiorespiratory impact of the nitric oxide synthase inhibitor L-NAME in the exercising horse. *Respiration Physiology and Neurobiology*, **120**, 151–66.

Kindig, C.A., McDonough, P., Erickson, H.H. and Poole, D.C. (2001). Effect of L-NAME on oxygen uptake kinetics during heavy-intensity exercise in the horse. *Journal of Applied Physiology*, **91**, 891–6.

Krogh, A. and Lindhard, J. (1913). The regulation of respiration and circulation during the initial stages of muscular work. *Journal of Physiology*, **47**, 112–36.

Krustrup, P., González-Alonso, J., Quistorff, B. and Bangsbo, J. (2001). Muscle heat production and anaerobic energy turnover during repeated intense dynamic exercise in humans. *Journal of Physiology*, **536**, 947–56.

Lamarra, N., Whipp, B.J., Ward, S.A. and Wasserman, K. (1987). Effect of interbreath fluctuations on characterizing exercise gas exchange kinetics. *Journal of Applied Physiology*, **62**, 2003–12.

Laughlin, M.H., Korthuis, R.J., Duncker, D.J. and Bache, R.J. (1996). Control of blood flow to cardiac and skeletal muscle during exercise. In L.B. Rowell and J.T. Shepherd (Eds) *Handbook of Physiology. Exercise: Regulation and Integration of Multiple Systems.* Oxford University Press, New York, pp. 705–69.

Linnarsson, D. (1974). Dynamics of pulmonary gas exchange and heart rate changes at start and end of exercise. *Acta Physiologica Scandinavica*, **415**, 1–68.

Linnarsson, D., Karlsson, J., Fagraeus, L. and Saltin, B. (1974). Muscle metabolites and oxygen deficit with exercise in hypoxia and hyperoxia. *Journal of Applied Physiology*, **36**, 399–402.

Luhtanen, P., Rahkila, P., Rusko, H. and Viitasalo, J.T. (1990). Mechanical work and efficiency in treadmill running at aerobic and anaerobic thresholds. *Acta Physiologica Scandinavica*, **139**, 153–9.

MacDonald, M.J., Pedersen, P.K. and Hughson, R.L. (1997). Acceleration of $\dot{V}O_2$ kinetics in heavy submaximal exercise by hyperoxia and prior high-intensity exercise. *Journal of Applied Physiology*, **83**, 1318–25.

MacDonald, M.J., Shoemaker, J.K., Tschakovsky, M.E. and Hughson, R.L. (1998). Alveolar oxygen uptake and femoral artery blood flow dynamics in upright and supine leg exercise in humans. *Journal of Applied Physiology*, **85**, 1622–8.

MacDonald, M.J., Tarnopolsky, M.A. and Hughson, R.L. (2000). Effect of hyperoxia and hypoxia on leg blood flow and pulmonary and leg oxygen uptake at the onset of kicking exercise. *Canadian Journal of Physiology and Pharmacology*, **78**, 67–74.

MacDonald, M.J., Naylor, H.L., Tschakovsky, M.E. and Hughson, R.L. (2001). Evidence that peripheral circulatory factors limit the rate of increase in muscle O_2 uptake at the onset of heavy exercise. *Journal of Applied Physiology*, **90**, 83–9.

Margaria, R., Edwards, H.T. and Dill, D.B. (1933). The possible mechanisms of contracting and paying the oxygen debt and the role of lactic acid in muscular contraction. *American Journal of Physiology*, **106**, 689–715.

Murphy, P.C., Cuervo, L.A. and Hughson, R.L (1989). Comparison of ramp and step exercise protocols during hypoxic exercise in man. *Cardiovascular Research*, **23**, 825–32.

Murrant, C.L. and Sarelius, I.H. (2000). Coupling of muscle metabolism and muscle blood flow in capillary units during contraction. *Acta Physiologica Scandinavica*, **168**, 531–41.

Özyener, F., Rossiter, H.B., Ward, S.A. and Whipp, B.J. (2001). Influence of exercise intensity on the on- and off-transient kinetics of pulmonary oxygen uptake in humans. *Journal of Physiology*, **533**, 891–902.

Paterson, D.H. and Whipp, B.J. (1991). Asymmetries of oxygen uptake transients at the on- and offset of heavy exercise in humans. *Journal of Physiology*, **443**, 575–86.

Perrey, S., Tschakovsky, M.E. and Hughson, R.L. (2001). Muscle chemoreflex elevates muscle blood flow and O_2 uptake at exercise onset in nonischemic human forearm. *Journal of Applied Physiology*, **91**, 2010–16.

Phillips, S.M., Green, H.J., MacDonald, M.J. and Hughson, R.L. (1995). Progressive effect of endurance training on $\dot{V}O_2$ kinetics at the onset of submaximal exercise. *Journal of Applied Physiology*, **79**, 1914–20.

Pringle, J.S., Doust, J.H., Carter, H., Tolfrey, K., Campbell, I.T. and Jones, A.M. (2003). Oxygen uptake kinetics during moderate, heavy and severe intensity 'submaximal' exercise in humans: the influence of muscle fibre type and capillarisation. *European Journal of Applied Physiology*, **89**, 289–300.

Proctor, D.N., Shen, P.H., Dietz, N.M., Eickhoff, T.J., Lawler, L.A., Ebersold, E.J., Loeffler, D.L. and Joyner, M.J. (1998). Reduced leg blood flow during dynamic exercise in older endurance-trained men. *Journal of Applied Physiology*, **85**, 68–75.

Rådegran, G. and Saltin, B. (1998). Muscle blood flow at onset of dynamic exercise in humans. *American Journal of Physiology*, **274**, H314–22.

Richardson, R.S., Noyszewski, E.A., Kendrick, K.F., Leigh, J.S. and Wagner, P.D. (1995). Myoglobin O_2 desaturation during exercise – evidence of limited O_2 transport. *Journal of Clinical Investigation*, **96**, 1916–26.

Richardson, R.S., Leigh, J.S., Wagner, P.D. and Noyszewski, E.A. (1999). Cellular PO_2 as a determinant of maximal mitochondrial O_2 consumption in trained human skeletal muscle. *Journal of Applied Physiology*, **87**, 325–31.

Richardson, R.S., Noyszewski, E.A., Haseler, L.J., Bluml, S. and Frank, L.R. (2002). Evolving techniques for the investigation of muscle bioenergetics and oxygenation. *Biochemical Society Transactions*, **30**, 232–7.

Rossiter, H.B., Ward, S.A., Kowalchuk, J.M., Howe, F.A., Griffiths, J.R. and Whipp, B.J. (2001). Effects of prior exercise on oxygen uptake and phosphocreatine kinetics during high-intensity knee-extension exercise in humans. *Journal of Physiology*, **537**, 291–303.

Rowell, L.B. (1993). *Human Cardiovascular Control*. Oxford University Press, New York.

Saltin, B., Rådegran, G., Koskolou, M.D. and Roach, R.C. (1998). Skeletal muscle blood flow in humans and its regulation during exercise. *Acta Physiologica Scandinavica*, **162**, 421–36.

Scheuermann, B.W., Hoetling, B.D., Noble, M.L. and Barstow, T.J. (2001). The slow component of O_2 uptake is not accompanied by changes in muscle EMG during repeated bouts of heavy exercise in humans. *Journal of Physiology*, **531**, 245–56.

Shoemaker, J.K. and Hughson, R.L. (1999). Adaptation of blood flow during the rest to work transition in humans. *Medicine and Science in Sports and Exercise*, **31**, 1019–26.

Shoemaker, J.K., Halliwill, J.R., Hughson, R.L. and Joyner, M.J. (1997). Contributions of acetylcholine and nitric oxide to forearm blood flow at exercise onset and recovery. *American Journal of Physiology*, **273**, H2388–95.

Tordi, N., Perrey, S., Harvey, A. and Hughson, R.L. (2003). Oxygen uptake kinetics during two bouts of heavy cycling separated by fatiguing sprint exercise in humans. *Journal of Applied Physiology*, **94**, 533–41.

Tran, T.K., Sailasuta, N., Kreutzer, U., Hurd, R., Chung, Y.R., Mole, P., Kuno, S. and Jue, T. (1999). Comparative analysis of NMR and NIRS measurements of intracellular PO_2 in human skeletal muscle. *American Journal of Physiology*, **276**, R1682–90.

Tschakovsky, M.E. and Hughson, R.L. (1999a). Interaction of factors determining oxygen uptake at the onset of exercise. *Journal of Applied Physiology*, **86**, 1101–13.

Tschakovsky, M.E. and Hughson, R.L. (1999b). Ischemic muscle chemoreflex response elevates blood flow in non-ischemic exercising human forearm muscle. *American Journal of Physiology*, **277**, H635–42.

van Beekvelt, M.C.P., Shoemaker, J.K., Tschakovsky, M.E., Hopman, M.T.E. and Hughson, R.L. (2001). Blood flow and muscle oxygen uptake at the onset and end of moderate and heavy dynamic forearm exercise. *American Journal of Physiology*, **280**, R1741–7.

Vanderthommen, M., Duteil, S., Wary, C., Raynaud, J.S., Leroy-Willig, A., Crielaard, J.M. and Carlier, P.G. (2003). A comparison of voluntary and electrically induced contractions by interleaved H-1- and P-31-NMRS in humans. *Journal of Applied Physiology*, **94**, 1012–24.

Wasserman, K., Whipp, B.J., Koyal, S.N. and Beaver, W.L. (1973). Anaerobic threshold and respiratory gas exchange during exercise. *Journal of Applied Physiology*, **35**, 236–43.

Welch, H.G., Bonde-Petersen, F., Graham, T., Klausen, K. and Secher, N. (1977). Effects of hyperoxia on leg blood flow and metabolism during exercise. *Journal of Applied Physiology*, **42**, 385–90.

Whipp, B.J. and Mahler, M. (1980). Dynamics of pulmonary gas exchange during exercise. In J.B. West (Ed.) *Pulmonary Gas Exchange*, Vol. II. Academic Press, Inc., New York, pp. 33–96.

Whipp, B.J. and Wasserman, K. (1972). Oxygen uptake kinetics for various intensities of constant-load work. *Journal of Applied Physiology*, **33**, 351–6.

Whipp, B.J., Davis, J.A., Torres, F. and Wasserman, K. (1981). A test to determine parameters of aerobic function during exercise. *Journal of Applied Physiology*, **50**, 217–22.

Wilson, D.F. and Rumsey, W.L. (1988). Factors modulating the oxygen dependence of mitochondrial oxidative phosphorylation. *Advances in Experimental Biology and Medicine*, **222**, 121–31.

Yoshida, T. and Whipp, B.J. (1994). Dynamic asymmetries of cardiac output transients in response to muscular exercise in man. *Journal of Physiology*, **480**, 355–9.

9 Limitation of skeletal muscle $\dot{V}O_2$ kinetics by inertia of cellular respiration

Bruno Grassi

Metabolic transitions and oxidative phosphorylation

Chapter 8 presents evidence that changing the conditions of O_2 delivery can adjust the phosphorylation and redox potentials necessary to achieve a given $\dot{V}O_2$. Thus, decreasing muscle microvascular and intracellular partial pressures (PO_2) slows $\dot{V}O_2$ kinetics and results in a greater perturbation of the intracellular milieu ($\Delta[PCr]$, $\Delta[H^+]$, for example) across the rest–exercise transition. However, to establish that O_2 supply limits the speed of $\dot{V}O_2$ kinetics in healthy muscle under normal circumstances it must be demonstrated that increasing muscle microvascular and intracellular PO_2 and contents speed $\dot{V}O_2$ kinetics. This chapter focuses on carefully controlled experiments that evaluate specifically whether conditions that substantially increase mitochondrial O_2 availability can speed $\dot{V}O_2$ kinetics. One central theme developed in this book is that the rate at which skeletal muscle oxidative metabolism ($\dot{V}O_2$) adjusts to a new metabolic requirement is one of the factors that determines exercise tolerance.

Pulmonary $\dot{V}O_2$ kinetics in health and disease

In exercising humans, analysis of $\dot{V}O_2$ kinetics is usually performed on the basis of breath-by-breath pulmonary $\dot{V}O_2$ measurements. Inferences on muscle $\dot{V}O_2$ kinetics from pulmonary $\dot{V}O_2$ kinetics are made complex by transit delays and interposition of O_2 stores from the sites of gas exchange at the muscle level and those in the lungs (di Prampero, 1981; Whipp *et al.*, 1982; Cerretelli and di Prampero, 1987), not to mention changes in O_2 stores within the lungs (e.g. Capelli *et al.*, 2001, see also Chapters 2 and 3). In any case, the 'Phase II', or 'primary component' (see Whipp *et al.*, 1982, see Chapter 1) of pulmonary $\dot{V}O_2$ kinetics is usually considered to reflect rather closely gas exchange kinetics occurring at the muscle level (Whipp *et al.*, 1982, see Chapter 6). This concept has been confirmed both by modelling (Barstow *et al.*, 1990) and experimental studies (Grassi *et al.*, 1996; Rossiter *et al.*, 1999). Pulmonary $\dot{V}O_2$ on-kinetics is known to be faster in trained than in untrained individuals (Cerretelli *et al.*, 1979, see Chapter 15), slower after bed-rest deconditioning (Convertino *et al.*, 1984), faster during exercise that recruits predominantly slow twitch (Type I) versus fast twitch (Type II) muscles or muscle fibres (Barstow *et al.*, 1996; Pringle *et al.*, 2003) and slower in old subjects compared to young controls (Babcock *et al.*, 1994, see Chapter 13). The notion that determination of pulmonary $\dot{V}O_2$ kinetics represents a valuable tool for the functional evaluation of oxidative metabolism is strengthened by the observation that both in young (Phillips *et al.*, 1995) and in middle-aged subjects (Fukuoka *et al.*, 2002) this kinetics seems more sensitive than other indices of 'aerobic fitness' (such as $\dot{V}O_{2\,max}$, or $\dot{V}O_{2\,peak}$) to perturbations such as exercise training.

The important question that emerges is how to interpret, mechanistically, a slower (or a faster) $\dot{V}O_2$ kinetics, in a subject or in a group of subjects. Is the capacity to deliver O_2 to muscle fibres, or the capacity by muscle fibres to utilize the O_2 they receive, the factor responsible for setting (or changing) $\dot{V}O_2$ kinetics? This same question can be posed for pathological conditions. In this case, a few examples are straightforward: patients with metabolic myopathies directly affecting muscle oxidative metabolism (such as mitochondrial myopathies or McArdle's disease) show an exaggerated cardiocirculatory response (i.e. an enhanced O_2 delivery) but, according to preliminary data gathered by our laboratory, a slower than normal $\dot{V}O_2$ kinetics (Grassi *et al.*, 2002b). In these patients, the latter seems to be attributable to a skeletal muscle limitation. For other pathological conditions, however, the situation is less clear. It is well known, for example, that patients affected by diseases or conditions presumably associated with limitations in the capacity to deliver O_2 to exercising muscles present slower than normal $\dot{V}O_2$ kinetics. This is true for congestive heart failure (Sietsema *et al.*, 1994), chronic respiratory diseases (Nery *et al.*, 1982), peripheral vascular disease (Bauer *et al.*, 1999), type II diabetes (Regensteiner *et al.*, 1998), heart transplant recipients (Cerretelli *et al.*, 1988; Grassi *et al.*, 1997; Marconi *et al.*, 2002; Borrelli *et al.*, 2003), and heart and lung transplant recipients (Grassi *et al.*, 1993, see Chapter 14). At first sight, the slower than normal $\dot{V}O_2$ kinetics in these patients could be attributed to a limitation in the capacity to deliver O_2 to working muscles. In heart transplant recipients, however, attempts to acutely increase the rate of adjustment of O_2 delivery during transitions did not significantly speed the $\dot{V}O_2$ kinetics (Grassi *et al.*, 1997). According to a recent paper (Marconi *et al.*, 2002) a substantially restored chronotropic competence in some paediatric heart transplant recipients did not significantly affect $\dot{V}O_2$ kinetics and $\dot{V}O_{2\,peak}$, which remained significantly impaired. Moreover, in all pathological conditions mentioned earlier, associated defects of skeletal muscle oxidative metabolism are described (Brass, 1996; Palange and Wagner, 2000; Marconi *et al.*, 2002; Ventura-Clapier *et al.*, 2002; Borrelli *et al.*, 2003; Scheuermann-Freestone *et al.*, 2003), suggesting a compromised capacity by skeletal muscles to utilize the O_2 they receive, which would be superimposed on any limitation in O_2 delivery. This fascinating topic is the subject of Chapter 14.

The relevance of determining the limiting factor(s) for $\dot{V}O_2$ kinetics

What can slower (or faster) $\dot{V}O_2$ kinetics tell us? Besides pointing to a functional impairment (or improvement) of the integrated function of the pulmonary, cardiovascular and muscular systems (which would represent interesting information by itself), does it allow any inference to be made regarding the site(s) of the impairment (or improvement)? An answer to this question would require a precise knowledge of the limiting, or regulating, factor(s) of $\dot{V}O_2$ kinetics. This aspect has been a matter of debate and controversy for many years, mainly between those in favour of the concept that the finite kinetics of $\dot{V}O_2$ adjustment to an increase in work rate is attributable to an intrinsic slowness of intracellular oxidative metabolism to adjust to the new metabolic requirement (oxidative 'metabolic *inertia*' hypothesis) (see e.g. Margaria *et al.*, 1965; di Prampero and Margaria, 1968; Cerretelli *et al.*, 1980; Whipp and Mahler, 1980), and those who suggest that an important limiting factor resides in the finite kinetics of O_2 delivery to muscle fibres ('O_2 delivery limitation' hypothesis) (e.g. Hughson, 1990; Tschakovsky and Hughson, 1999; Hughson *et al.*, 2001, see Chapter 8). It is well established that, upon a step increase in work rate, variables related to O_2 delivery (e.g. HR, $\dot{Q}$, $\dot{Q}m$) adjust to the new requirement according to a finite kinetic profile that is slower than the increase in metabolic demand but almost always faster than the achieved $\dot{V}O_2$ kinetics (rev. Delp, 1999). Thus, in theory, the kinetics of O_2 delivery could influence the rate of adjustment of $\dot{V}O_2$.

Interest in the factors regulating $\dot{V}O_2$ kinetics derives also from the fact that such research can yield valuable insights into basic mechanisms of metabolic control during muscular contraction. Whereas metabolic steady-states provide a stable scenario to gather data, it is within the transient responses that the best insights into systems control can be derived.

Experimental approaches

For some time the approach to the 'O_2 delivery' versus oxidative 'metabolic inertia' problem has been to define whether the adjustment of O_2 delivery (usually estimated on the basis of HR or $\dot{Q}$) was indeed faster than that of O_2 utilization (usually inferred from the kinetics of pulmonary $\dot{V}O_2$) (e.g. Cerretelli *et al.*, 1980; Hughson, 1990). This approach, besides providing only indirect evidence in favour or against the hypotheses outlined earlier, was confounded by the fact that, in humans, for methodological reasons, the investigated variables (HR, $\dot{Q}$, pulmonary $\dot{V}O_2$) were quite 'distant' from the relevant ones, that is muscle blood flow and muscle $\dot{V}O_2$. This problem has been at least partially overcome by recent studies which determined the kinetics of $\dot{Q} \cdot CaO_2$ and $\dot{V}O_2$ in humans at the level of the exercising limbs (e.g. Grassi *et al.*, 1996; Hughson *et al.*, 1996; Bangsbo *et al.*, 2000). A common finding from all these studies is that, during the first seconds of exercise, increases in $\dot{Q} \cdot CaO_2$ exceed increases in $\dot{V}O_2$, whereas for the ensuing part of the transition the results are more equivocal and have led to different interpretations. In these studies, moreover, measurements were carried out across exercising limbs, so that transit delays from the sites of gas exchange to the measurement sites may have confounded the overall picture, as demonstrated by Bangsbo *et al.* (2000), who estimated such delays by dye injection into the arterial circulation.

Recently, another series of studies 'got inside the muscle', during metabolic transitions, by utilizing different techniques, such as the intravascular phosphorescence quenching technique for the determination of microvascular PO_2 (Behnke *et al.*, 2002) or NIRS for the determination of tissue oxygenation (DeLorey *et al.*, 2003; Grassi *et al.*, 2003a). A common denominator, among these different techniques, lies in the fact that the measured variables permit evaluation of the balance (or lack thereof) between $\dot{Q} \cdot CaO_2$ and $\dot{V}O_2$ in the area of interest, being therefore conceptually similar to O_2 extraction but without any capillary-to-venous sampling delays. An increased microvascular PO_2, or an increased oxygenation, following an increase in work, would indicate a faster adjustment of $\dot{Q} \cdot CaO_2$ vs that of $\dot{V}O_2$, thereby providing indirect evidence in favour of the 'metabolic inertia' hypothesis. The results of these studies, conducted either by the phosphorescence quenching technique (Behnke *et al.*, 2002) in rats, or by NIRS in humans (DeLorey *et al.*, 2003; Grassi *et al.*, 2003a) suggest unchanged (or slightly decreased) fractional O_2 extraction for several seconds after an increase in work rate, reflecting a tight coupling between $\dot{Q} \cdot CaO_2$ and $\dot{V}O_2$ during that period. The immediate and pronounced increase in muscle blood flow (associated with the action of the muscle pump and active vasodilation) at the onset of exercise is well known (e.g. Laughlin *et al.*, 1996). The above-mentioned studies (Behnke *et al.*, 2002; DeLorey *et al.*, 2003; Grassi *et al.*, 2003a) suggest that such rapid and pronounced increase in $\dot{Q} \cdot CaO_2$ at the transition allows $\dot{V}O_2$ to increase even in the presence of an unchanged (or slightly decreased) fractional O_2 extraction (see Chapter 6). Only after this initial delay is completed does an increased O_2 extraction at the muscle level contribute, together with the ongoing $\dot{Q} \cdot CaO_2$ increase, to the further increase in $\dot{V}O_2$. The O_2 extraction pattern suggested by these studies (Behnke *et al.*, 2002; DeLorey *et al.*, 2003; Grassi *et al.*, 2003a) is similar to that suggested by the a-vO_2 diff. data obtained across exercising legs in humans (Grassi *et al.*, 1996, see also fig. 2 in Grassi, 2000) and across the isolated *in situ* dog gastrocnemius preparation (Grassi *et al.*, 2002a). (Note that an increased O_2 extraction is reflected by an *increased* muscle deoxygenation by NIRS, by an *increased* a-vO_2 diff., but by a *decreased* microvascular or intracellular [see later] PO_2).

A similar time-course was also described by Hogan (2001) for intracellular PO_2 (determined by phosphorescence quenching) in an isolated amphibian muscle fibre model (Chapter 5). In this model, O_2 is uniformly made available in the medium surrounding the cell, and PO_2 is the result of the balance between O_2 availability and O_2 utilization at the intracellular level. At contraction onset, a mono-exponential decrease in intracellular PO_2 is preceded by about 10 s or so in which the PO_2 remains constant (Hogan, 2001). Considering that, in the same experimental model, $\dot{V}O_2$ increases with a very short time delay (less than 2 s) at contraction onset (Kindig *et al.*, 2003), the finding of a 10 s delay before the start of PO_2 decrease within the cell suggests that there is plenty of O_2 available at the mitochondrial level during the first few seconds of contractions in these myocytes. Thus, upon a step increase in metabolic demand, skeletal muscle O_2 fractional extraction elicits a 'biphasic' response (i.e. no change for a few seconds, followed by a mono-exponential increase to reach a new steady state). This profile is evident across experimental models ranging from exercising humans to single amphibian fibres (Grassi et al., 1996, 2002a, 2003a; Hogan, 2001; Behnke et al., 2002; DeLorey et al., 2003) (see Figure 9.1).

Returning to the principal focus of this chapter, the absence of an increased O_2 extraction, during the first few seconds of the transition represents indirect evidence against a lack of O_2 limiting $\dot{V}O_2$ kinetics during that period. However, the tight coupling between the increased $\dot{Q} \cdot CaO_2$ and the increased $\dot{V}O_2$ does not allow absolute rejection of the notion that O_2 delivery ($\dot{Q} \cdot CaO_2$) is limiting the $\dot{V}O_2$ kinetics. Thus, the possibility has to be acknowledged that an enhanced rate of $\dot{Q} \cdot CaO_2$ could lead to a faster $\dot{V}O_2$ response. Moreover, the experiments mentioned earlier do not allow us to make iron-clad conclusions regarding the role of O_2 delivery in limiting $\dot{V}O_2$ kinetics over the ensuing phases of the $\dot{V}O_2$ transition (i.e. beyond the initial few seconds). To demonstrate whether $\dot{Q} \cdot CaO_2$ does (or does not) represent a significant limiting factor for $\dot{V}O_2$ kinetics, experiments showing that a significantly faster than normal or an enhanced $\dot{Q} \cdot CaO_2$ is (or is not) associated with faster than normal $\dot{V}O_2$ kinetics were needed. A crucial feature of such investigations is that $\dot{Q} \cdot CaO_2$ is either actually set by the investigators or at least measured. Previous experiments (particularly those using elevated inspired O_2 fractions) have presumed that increasing CaO_2 necessarily increases $\dot{Q} \cdot CaO_2$. However, altering CaO_2 often causes a reciprocal change in $\dot{Q}$ such that $\dot{Q} \cdot CaO_2$ is maintained constant.

Experiments using the isolated *in situ* dog gastrocnemius preparation

To test the hypothesis that augmented muscle O_2 delivery would (or would not) alter $\dot{V}O_2$ kinetics, our group resorted to the classical isolated *in situ* dog gastrocnemius preparation (see Kramer et al., 1939), utilized previously to study muscle $\dot{V}O_2$ kinetics by Piiper et al. (1968) and by di Prampero and Margaria (1968). Whereas Piiper et al. (1968) observed a faster $\dot{Q} \cdot CaO_2$ kinetics compared to that of $\dot{V}O_2$, these authors did not experimentally manipulate $\dot{Q} \cdot CaO_2$ to see whether $\dot{V}O_2$ kinetics could be speeded or not. Our experiments were carried out in the laboratories of Drs Michael C. Hogan, Peter D. Wagner (University of California, San Diego) and L. Bruce Gladden (Auburn University), who have been utilizing the isolated *in situ* dog gastrocnemius preparation for many years. The main idea behind the first series of experiments was to enhance O_2 delivery to the muscle, and to see if this enhancement produced faster muscle $\dot{V}O_2$ kinetics or not, thereby providing direct evidence in favour (or against) the 'O_2 delivery hypothesis'.

In a separate series of studies, we decided to evaluate the potential role of convective and diffusive O_2 delivery to muscle in limiting $\dot{V}O_2$ kinetics across the transition to different intensities of contraction. It is pertinent that the role

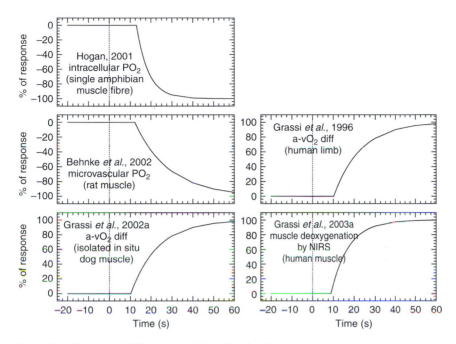

Figure 9.1 Kinetics of different variables related to O_2 extraction, upon a step increase in metabolic demand, as determined in studies conducted by utilizing different techniques and experimental models (Grassi *et al.*, 1996, 2002a, 2003a; Hogan, 2001; Behnke *et al.*, 2002). The equation representing a mono-exponential increase of the variables was the following:

$$y(t) = y_{BL} + A\,[1 - e^{-(t - TD)/\tau}]$$

whereas the equation representing a mono-exponential decrease of the variables was the following:

$$y(t) = y_{BL} - A\,[1 - e^{-(t - TD)/\tau}]$$

In the equations, y_{BL} indicates the baseline value and A the amplitude between y_{BL} and the aymptotic value. In order to facilitate visual comparison of kinetics of variables which, in the original studies, were expressed by utilizing their respective units, data are presented as a percentage of the total response, that is to say, y_{BL} was set equal to 0, and A was set equal to 100 for the variables which increased during the transition [a-vO$_2$ diff., muscle deoxygenation], or to -100 for the variables which decreased during the transition (intracellular PO_2 and microvascular PO_2). The vertical broken lines (time = 0) indicate the time at which the metabolic demand was increased. All variables show a very similar 'biphasic' response, that is an early phase, lasting about 10 s, in which no significant change vs the baseline value is observed, followed by the mono-exponential increase (or decrease) to the asymptotic value. See text for further details. (The original data from Grassi *et al.* (1996) were 'corrected' to take into account the estimated 'dead space' volume of blood from venules to the site of blood gas sampling.)

of convective and diffusive O_2 delivery in limiting $\dot{V}O_{2\,max}$ has been the focus of considerable scientific investigation (e.g. di Prampero and Ferretti, 1990; Wagner, 2000).

Convective O_2 delivery

The first hypothesis tested was whether convective O_2 delivery to muscle represented a limiting factor for muscle $\dot{V}O_2$ kinetics. In these experiments, all delays in the adjustment of convective O_2 delivery from rest to electrically induced isometric tetanic contractions at ~60% (Grassi *et al.*, 1998a) or 100% (Grassi *et al.*, 2000) $\dot{V}O_{2\,max}$ were eliminated by pump-perfusing the muscle and keeping $\dot{Q}m$ constantly elevated. In order to prevent vasoconstriction, a vasodilatory drug (adenosine) was infused intra-arterially in association with the constantly elevated $\dot{Q}m$. Elimination of all delays in convective O_2 delivery during the transition did not affect muscle $\dot{V}O_2$ kinetics at the lower contraction intensity (Grassi *et al.*, 1998a), whereas the kinetics was slightly but significantly faster (vs the control condition) at the higher intensity, leading to ~25% reduction in the calculated O_2 deficit (Grassi *et al.*, 2000) (Figure 9.2).(The 'O_2 deficit' indicates the amount of energy deriving from non-oxidative energy sources during the transition, as a consequence of the finite $\dot{V}O_2$ kinetics; see di Prampero, 1981.) These results suggest that, for transitions from rest to submaximal $\dot{V}O_2$, $\dot{V}O_2$ kinetics is not limited by convective O_2 delivery to muscle, whereas for transitions to peak $\dot{V}O_2$ convective O_2 delivery plays a relatively minor (although significant) role as a limiting factor. It is noteworthy that in the study dealing with transitions to 100% of peak $\dot{V}O_2$ (Grassi *et al.*, 2000), in the 'treatment' condition, the faster $\dot{V}O_2$ kinetics and, as a consequence, the lower O_2 deficit, were associated with significantly less muscle fatigue, directly confirming the important role of $\dot{V}O_2$ kinetics and O_2 deficit in determining muscle fatigue and exercise tolerance.

Peripheral O_2 diffusion

A second series of experiments were performed to determine whether or not peripheral O_2 diffusion might constitute a limiting factor for muscle $\dot{V}O_2$ kinetics. In the previously described experimental intervention (see Figure 9.2), we eliminated all delays in convective O_2 delivery to muscle capillaries, that is to say, we managed to get a lot of O_2 (bound to Hb) in muscle capillaries from the very onset of contractions. However, from the muscle capillary to mitochondria (Figure 9.3) O_2 still has a rather long path to cover, and resistances to overcome. Specifically, O_2 has to be released from haemoglobin, and cross the red blood cell membrane, the capillary wall, the interstitial space, the sarcolemma, and the cytoplasm of the muscle fibre before entering the mitochondria, where it is eventually consumed. This process of 'peripheral O_2 diffusion' is driven (according to Fick's law of diffusion), by the difference in PO_2 between the capillaries ($PcapO_2$) and mitochondria ($PmitO_2$) in relation to the O_2 diffusive properties of the structures and spaces along the pathway (Figure 9.3). It is pertinent that

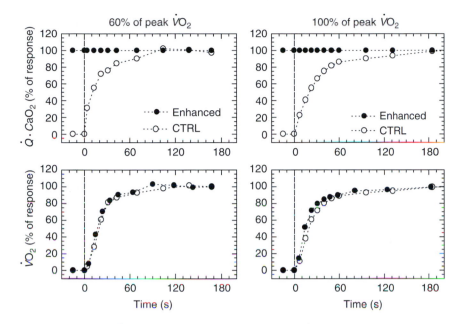

Figure 9.2 Muscle $\dot{Q} \cdot CaO_2$ (top panels) and muscle $\dot{V}O_2$ (bottom panels) during transitions from rest to contractions corresponding to about 60% (left-hand panels) and 100% (right-hand panels) of the muscle peak $\dot{V}O_2$. Two conditions were compared: (a) control (CTRL), characterized by spontaneous adjustment of $\dot{Q} \cdot CaO_2$; (b) enhanced convective O_2 delivery (Enhanced), in which the muscle was pump-perfused, $\dot{Q} \cdot CaO_2$ was kept constantly elevated and a vasodilatory drug was administered. After enhancing convective O_2 delivery, no difference in $\dot{V}O_2$ kinetics was observed for transitions to 60% of peak $\dot{V}O_2$ (lower-left panel), whereas a slightly faster $\dot{V}O_2$ kinetics was observed for transitions to about 100% of peak $\dot{V}O_2$ (lower-right panel). Data are expressed as a percentage of the total response. The data are taken from the studies by Grassi *et al.* (1998a, 2000). See text for further details. Reproduced, with permission, from Grassi, B. (2003).

peripheral O_2 diffusion is considered one of the principal factors limiting $\dot{V}O_{2\,max}$ in healthy humans (e.g. Wagner, 2000). Thus, peripheral O_2 diffusion will be enhanced by an increased driving pressure for O_2, that is defined by the difference between $PcapO_2$ and $PmitO_2$. To accomplish this elevated O_2, we experimentally increased $PcapO_2$ by having dogs breathe a hyperoxic gas mixture ($FIO_2 = 1.00$) and administered RSR 13. RSR 13 is an allosteric inhibitor of O_2 binding to haemoglobin that causes a rightward shift of the haemoglobin–O_2 dissociation curve which reduces the affinity of haemoglobin for O_2. Both in the control and in the 'treatment' condition, $\dot{Q}m$ was kept constantly elevated through the transition and adenosine was infused to prevent any hyperoxic vasoconstriction. For the same $\dot{Q}m$, $\dot{V}O_2$ and a-vO_2 diff. determined across the contracting muscle, a rightward shift of the haemoglobin–O_2 dissociation curve

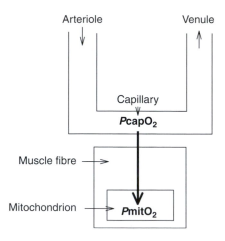

Figure 9.3 Schematic representation of the path for peripheral O_2 diffusion. According to Fick's law of diffusion, the 'driving pressure' for O_2, that is defined by the difference between $PcapO_2$ and $PmitO_2$ is one of the main determinants of peripheral O_2 diffusion. See text for further details.

increased the measured venous PO_2 and the mean $PcapO_2$ (calculated by the Bohr integration method). Both interventions (hyperoxic breathing, right-shifted haemoglobin–O_2 dissociation curve) induced a significant increase in mean $PcapO_2$ and $\dot{V}O_2$ kinetics were determined during contractions at 60% (Grassi *et al.*, 1998b) and 100% (Grassi *et al.*, 2001) of $\dot{V}O_{2\,max}$. At neither exercise intensity did the elevated $PcapO_2$ significantly affect muscle $\dot{V}O_2$ kinetics.

Role of exercise intensity

Considered together, these investigations provide compelling evidence in favour of the hypothesis that an oxidative metabolic *inertia* within the muscle is the limiting factor for muscle $\dot{V}O_2$ kinetics during transitions to contractions of relatively low metabolic intensity. On the other hand, during transitions to contractions of relatively high metabolic intensity, convective O_2 delivery could play a relatively minor but significant role as a limiting factor.

In humans, the VT (considered synonymous with the gas exchange threshold, GET, for present purposes) is thought to discriminate between work intensities at which O_2 delivery is not (those below VT) or is (those above VT) a limiting factor for pulmonary $\dot{V}O_2$ kinetics (Gaesser and Poole, 1996). For example, data by MacDonald *et al.* (1997), obtained in humans during constant-load exercise above VT, describe a faster overall pulmonary $\dot{V}O_2$ kinetics (as shown by the lower MRT) when the exercise was preceded by a high-intensity 'warm up' exercise, that was presumed to enhance O_2 delivery during the subsequent bout, and/or when the subjects were inspiring a hyperoxic mixture. On the other hand, the same procedures did not affect pulmonary $\dot{V}O_2$ on-kinetics during constant-load exercise below VT. In that study (MacDonald *et al.*, 1997), the lower MRT during transitions above VT were essentially due to a reduced amplitude of the slow component of the $\dot{V}O_2$ kinetics, whereas the time constant of the primary component was not affected. Similar findings, as far as the effects of a 'warm up' exercise, have been reported by several other authors (e.g. Burnley *et al.*, 2000), and they would fit in the previously-described *scenario* if the slow component itself is considered, at least in part, an expression of relatively inadequate O_2 delivery to muscle. In the heavy and severe intensity exercise domains, then, muscle would be recruiting a larger number of the presumably less efficient (in oxidative terms) fast-twitch fibres, which are usually considered responsible for the slow component (Gaesser and Poole, 1996). Following the 'warm up' exercise, an improved O_2 delivery would reduce the need for recruiting fast-twitch fibres, thereby reducing the amplitude of the slow component and determining a faster overall $\dot{V}O_2$ kinetics. This topic is explored in greater detail in Chapters 10 and 12.

Possible site(s) of inertia of oxidative metabolism

Within the metabolic *inertia* hypothesis, the rate of adjustment of oxidative phosphorylation during metabolic transitions would be mainly determined by the levels of cellular metabolic controllers and/or enzyme activation.

Pyruvate dehydrogenase

There are several possible rate-limiting reactions within the complex oxidative pathways. Recent research pointed, as a possible limiting step, to acetyl group availability within mitochondria and to the activation of the PDH enzyme. It has been demonstrated that activation of PDH by pharmacological intervention results in a 'sparing' of PCr during the rest–exercise transition in both canine and human muscle. This finding suggests the generation of a lower O_2 deficit and therefore a faster adjustment of muscle $\dot{V}O_2$ kinetics (e.g. Timmons *et al.*, 1998). We tested this hypothesis in the isolated dog gastrocnemius *in situ* preparation. Activation of PDH was increased by administration of the drug DCA. The transition investigated was from rest to electrically stimulated contractions corresponding to ~60–70% of the muscle $\dot{V}O_{2\,max}$. DCA infusion elevated PDH activation significantly, resulting in a marked stockpiling of acetylcarnitine at rest. During contractions, less muscle fatigue was observed but there was no alteration of 'anaerobic' energy provision or $\dot{V}O_2$ kinetics (Grassi *et al.*, 2002a). Thus, in this experimental model, PDH activation status did not seem to be responsible for the metabolic *inertia* of oxidative phosphorylation. Similar conclusions arose from studies in humans (Bangsbo *et al.*, 2002; Jones *et al.*, 2004). In another study, Rossiter *et al.* (2003) confirmed that PDH activation by DCA does not determine, in humans, faster pulmonary $\dot{V}O_2$ kinetics, nor a faster kinetics of PCr hydrolysis even in the presence of a reduced O_2 deficit (as reflected by less

PCr hydrolysis and lower blood lactate accumulation), which might be partially attributed to a reduced amplitude of the $\dot{V}O_2$ response and to an improved metabolic efficiency. An increased metabolic efficiency after DCA was also observed by our group (Grassi et al., 2002a) in the dog gastrocnemius in situ. In the presence of less muscle fatigue (i.e. higher force production) after DCA, we observed unchanged $\dot{V}O_2$ and no significant differences in the calculated substrate level phosphorylation. 'Closing the circle', then, the increased metabolic efficiency after DCA could explain, at least in part, the PCr 'sparing' described by Timmons et al. (1998), with no need to hypothesize a faster $\dot{V}O_2$ kinetics, which is clearly not found experimentally.

Inhibition of mitochondrial respiration by NO

The metabolic inertia of skeletal muscle oxidative metabolism might be related, at least in part, to a regulatory role of NO on mitochondrial respiration. Amongst a myriad of functions, which includes arterial vasodilation, NO competitively inhibits $\dot{V}O_2$ in the electron transport chain, specifically at the cytochrome c oxidase level (Brown, 2000). Through its combined effects of vasodilation and $\dot{V}O_2$ inhibition, NO may serve as part of a feedback mechanism aimed at reducing the reliance on O_2 extraction to meet tissue O_2 needs, thereby maintaining higher intramyocyte PO_2 levels during exercise (rev. in Kindig et al., 2001). Inhibition of NO synthase by the administration of the arginine analogue L-NAME to exercising horses produced a significantly faster pulmonary $\dot{V}O_2$ kinetics, both during heavy (Kindig et al., 2001) and moderate intensity exercise (Kindig et al., 2002). Significantly faster pulmonary $\dot{V}O_2$ kinetics after L-NAME treatment were also described by Jones et al. in humans during transitions to moderate (2003) and heavy (2004) intensity exercise. A faster muscle $\dot{V}O_2$ kinetics after L-NAME administration, on the other hand, was not observed in a recent study conducted by our group in the isolated dog gastrocnemius in situ preparation (see preliminary data in Grassi et al., 2003b). Thus, although inhibition of mitochondrial respiration by NO could be responsible, in part, for the metabolic inertia of oxidative metabolism, the issue needs clarification and warrants further investigations.

Functional coupling between PCr hydrolysis and oxidative phosphorylation

One crucial question is 'What is the source of the metabolic inertia seen at exercise onset?' One putative answer was provided 30–40 years ago by the work of the 'Margaria group' at the University of Milano. Both the papers by Piiper et al. (1968) and by di Prampero and Margaria (1968) described an inverse linear relationship between [PCr] (squared brackets denote concentrations) and muscle $\dot{V}O_2$ in steady-state conditions, thereby suggesting some link between the two variables. A regulatory role of PCr hydrolysis on $\dot{V}O_2$ kinetics was clearly hypothesized by Margaria et al. (1965): '...the oxidative processes in muscles are dictated by the concentration at a given time of the high energy compounds when split'. Many years later, technological advancements in the field of nuclear magnetic resonance spectroscopy allowed the observation of a close correlation between the Phase II pulmonary V̇O₂ kinetics and those of [PCr] in humans performing constant-load quadriceps exercise. This relationship is evident both in the absence (Rossiter *et al.*, 1999) and in the presence (Rossiter *et al.*, 2001) of the V̇O₂ slow component. The close kinetic coupling between V̇O₂ and [PCr] is also maintained when the amplitudes of responses of both variables are acutely reduced by pharmacological interventions (Rossiter *et al.*, 2003). Thus, PCr hydrolysis may not be considered just as an ATP buffer, but it could represent (through changes in concentration of [Cr], or of other variables related to this) one of the main controllers of oxidative phosphorylation (e.g. Mahler, 1980, 1985; Whipp and Mahler, 1980; Cerretelli and di Prampero, 1987; Meyer, 1988, see Chapter 7).

How could a phenomenon occurring in the cytoplasm (PCr hydrolysis) be functionally related to oxidative phosphorylation, occurring in mitochondria? The answer was delineated in the original work by Mahler (1980) (see Figure 9.4), and the concept seems valid also today (e.g. Kaasik *et al.*, 1999). During muscle contraction, [ATP] changes in the cytosol are prevented by the activity of the extramitochondrial isoform of CK (e-CK), which permits the energy contained in the high-energy phosphate bond of PCr to be utilized to resynthesize ATP. The outer mitochondrial membrane is permeable to Cr, which enters the mitochondrion. The resulting increase in [Cr] in the mitochondrial intermembrane space leads to ADP production through the

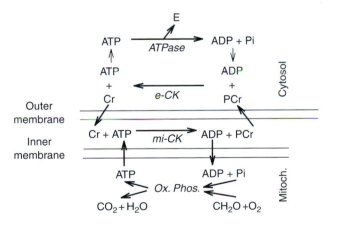

Figure 9.4 Schematic representation of the mechanism through which PCr hydrolysis in the cytoplasm could be functionally coupled to oxidative phosphorylation in the mitochondrion (modified from Mahler, 1980). See text for further details. E = free energy; e-CK = extramitochondrial isoform of CK; mi-CK = mitochondrial isoform of CK. Reproduced with permission from Grassi, B. (2003).

activity of the mitochondrial isoform of CK (mi-CK), which is functionally coupled to oxidative phosphorylation through its close proximity to an ATP–ADP translocator on the inner mitochondrial membrane. The nascent ADP reaches the mitochondrial matrix to be reconverted to ATP using the energy derived from oxidative phosphorylation. Then, closing the circle, the ATP produced by oxidative phosphorylation is transported to the mitochondrial intermembrane space by the translocase, and reacts with Cr, thereby resynthesizing PCr, which can leave the mitochondrion and reconstitute cytoplasmic PCr levels. This rather complex series of reactions should couple $\dot{V}O_2$, which occurs in mitochondria, with PCr hydrolysis occurring in the cytoplasm. Teleologically, it makes sense to couple an energetic mechanism (PCr hydrolysis) which is fast enough to meet sudden increases in metabolic demand, to the regulation of oxidative phosphorylation through the levels of its metabolites. The constancy of intracellular [ATP] across a broad spectrum of metabolic transients spanning 2 or 3 orders of magnitude bears testimony to the effectiveness of mitochondrial oxidative control.

Conclusions

Among the various mechanisms responsible for ATP resynthesis, oxidative phosphorylation is relatively slow to increase in response to an increased metabolic demand. The rate of adjustment of skeletal muscle oxidative metabolism during metabolic transitions, which can be evaluated on the basis of the analysis of $\dot{V}O_2$ kinetics, has implications for exercise tolerance and muscle fatigue. Analysis of this kinetics represents a valid and powerful tool for functional evaluation of healthy subjects, athletes and patients. Experiments conducted on an isolated canine muscle preparations *in situ* provide insights into several key aspects of skeletal muscle $\dot{V}O_2$ kinetics. At moderate work intensities, the principal factors limiting these kinetics reside in an intrinsic slowness of intracellular oxidative metabolism to adjust to the augmented metabolic needs. In contrast, at heavy or severe work intensities (i.e. above the lactate or ventilatory thresholds), O_2 delivery to the mitochondria may play a minor role in limiting $\dot{V}O_2$ kinetics. The rate of adjustment of oxidative phosphorylation in mitochondria could be functionally related with PCr hydrolysis occuring in the cytoplasm.

Acknowledgements

The experiments on the isolated *in situ* dog gastrocnemius preparation were carried out in the laboratories of Drs Peter Wagner, Michael C. Hogan and L. Bruce Gladden, with whom I also had the privilege to discuss most of the topics presented in this chapter. Constructive criticism by Drs Pado Cerretelli and Jerzy A. Zoladz is also acknowledged. Financial support by EC Contract QLK6-CT-2001-00323, by NATO Collaborative Linkage Grant LST.CLG.979220, by Telethon – UILDM Project GUP030534 and by institutional funds (FIRST) by the University of Milano is acknowledged.

Glossary of terms

ADP	adenosine diphosphate
ATP	adenosine triphosphate
BL	baseline
CaO_2	arterial O_2 concentration
a-vO_2 diff.	arterio-venous O_2 concentration difference
Cr	creatine
CK	creatine kinase
DCA	dichloroacetate
FIO_2	fraction of O_2 in inspired air
H^+	hydrogen ion
Hb	haemoglobin
HR	heart rate
L-NAME	N^{ω}-nitro-L-arginine-methyl ester
MRT	mean response time
NIRS	near-infrared spectroscopy
NO	nitric oxide
PO_2	partial pressure of O_2
$PcapO_2$	mean partial pressure of O_2 in capillaries
PDH	pyruvate dehydrogenase
$PmitO_2$	mean partial pressure of O_2 in mitochondria
O_2	oxygen
PCr	phosphocreatine
$\dot{Q}$	cardiac output
$\dot{Q} \cdot CaO_2$	O_2 delivery (blood flow multiplied by arterial O_2 concentration)
$\dot{Q}$m	muscle blood flow
RSR 13	2-(4-{[(3,5-dimethylanilino) carbonyl]methyl}phenoxy)-2-methylpropionic acid
TD	time delay
τ	time constant
$\dot{V}O_2$	O_2 consumption
$\dot{V}O_{2\,max}$	maximal O_2 consumption
$\dot{V}O_{2\,peak}$	peak O_2 consumption
VT	ventilatory threshold

References

Babcock, M.A. Paterson, D.H., Cunningham, D.A. and Dickinson, J.R. (1994). Exercise on-transient gas exchange kinetics are slowed as a function of age. *Medicine and Science in Sports and Exercise*, **26**, 440–6.

Bangsbo, J., Krustrup, P., Gonzalez-Alonso, J., Boushel, R. and Saltin, B. (2000). Muscle oxygen kinetics at onset of intense dynamic exercise in humans. *American Journal of Physiology*, **279**, R899–906.

Bangsbo, J., Gibala, M.J., Krustrup, P., Gonzalez-Alonso, J. and Saltin, B. (2002). Enhanced pyruvate dehydrogenase activity does not affect muscle O_2 uptake at onset of intense exercise in humans. *American Journal of Physiology*, **282**, R273–80.

Barstow, T.J., Lamarra, N. and Whipp, B.J. (1990). Modulation of muscle and pulmonary O_2 uptakes by circulatory dynamics during exercise. *Journal of Applied Physiology*, **68**, 979–89.

Barstow, T.J., Jones, A.M., Nguyen, P.H. and Casaburi, R. (1996). Influence of muscle fiber type and pedal frequency on oxygen uptake kinetics of heavy exercise. *Journal of Applied Physiology*, **81**, 1642–50.

Bauer, T.A., Regensteiner, J.G., Brass, E.P. and Hiatt, W.R. (1999). Oxygen uptake kinetics are slowed in patients with peripheral arterial disease. *Journal of Applied Physiology*, **87**, 809–19.

Behnke, B.J., Kindig, C.A., Musch, T.I., Sexton, W.L. and Poole, D.C. (2002). Effects of prior contractions on muscle microvascular oxygen pressure at onset of subsequent contractions. *Journal of Physiology*, **593**, 927–34.

Borrelli, E., Pogliaghi, S., Molinello, A., Diciolla, F., Maccherini, M. and Grassi, B. (2003). Serial assessment of peak $\dot{V}O_2$ and $\dot{V}O_2$ kinetics early after heart transplantation. *Medicine and Science in Sports and Exercise*, **35**, 1798–804.

Brass, E.P. (1996). Skeletal muscle metabolism as a target for drug therapy in peripheral arterial disease. *Vascular Medicine*, **1**, 55–9.

Brown, G.C. (2000). Nitric oxide as a competitive inhibitor of oxygen consumption in the mitochondrial respiratory chain. *Acta Physiologica Scandinavica*, **168**, 667–74.

Burnley, M., Jones, A.M., Carter, H. and Doust, J.H. (2000). Effects of prior heavy exercise on phase II pulmonary oxygen uptake kinetics during heavy exercise. *Journal of Applied Physiology*, **89**, 1387–96.

Capelli, C., Cautero, M. and di Prampero, P.E. (2001). New perspectives in breath-by-breath determination of alveolar gas exchange in humans. *Pflügers Archives*, **441**, 566–77.

Cerretelli, P. and di Prampero, P.E. (1987). Gas exchange in exercise. In L.E. Fahri and S.M. Tenney (Eds) *Handbook of Physiology*, Section 3, The Respiratory System, Vol. IV, Gas Exchange. American Physiological Society, Bethesda, pp. 297–339.

Cerretelli, P., Pendergast, D.R., Paganelli, W.C. and Rennie, D.W. (1979). Effects of specific muscle training on $\dot{V}O_2$ on-response and early blood lactate. *Journal of Applied Physiology*, **47**, 761–69.

Cerretelli, P., Rennie, D.W. and Pendergast, D.R. (1980). Kinetics of metabolic transients during exercise. In P. Cerretelli and B.J. Whipp (Eds) *Exercise Bioenergetics and Gas Exchange*. Elsevier, Amsterdam, pp. 187–209.

Cerretelli, P., Grassi, B., Colombini, A., Carù, B. and Marconi, C. (1988). Gas exchange and metabolic transients in heart transplant recipients. *Respiration Physiology*, **74**, 355–71.

Convertino, D.A., Goldwater, D.J. and Sandler, H. (1984). $\dot{V}O_2$ kinetics of constant load exercise following bed-rest induced deconditioning. *Journal of Applied Physiology*, **57**, 1545–50.

DeLorey, D.S., Kowalchuck, J.W. and Paterson, D.H. (2003). Relationship between pulmonary O_2 uptake kinetics and muscle deoxygenation during moderate-intensity exercise. *Journal of Applied Physiology*, **95**, 113–20.

di Prampero, P.E. (1981). Energetics of muscular exercise. *Reviews of Physiology, Biochemistry and Pharmacology*, **89**, 143–222.

di Prampero, P.E. and Ferretti, G. (1990). Factors limiting maximal oxygen consumption in humans. *Respiration Physiology*, **80**, 113–28.

di Prampero, P.E. and Margaria, R. (1968). Relationship between O_2 consumption, high energy phosphates and the kinetics of the O_2 debt in exercise. *Pflügers Archives*, **304**, 11–19.

Fukuoka, Y., Grassi, B., Conti, M., Guiducci, D., Sutti, M., Marconi, C. and Cerretelli, P. (2002). Early effects of exercise training on $\dot{V}O_2$ on- and off-kinetics in 50 yr old subjects. *Pflügers Archives*, **443**, 690–7.

Gaesser, G.A. and Poole, D.C. (1996). The slow component of oxygen uptake kinetics in humans. In J.O. Holloszy (Ed.) *Exercise and Sport Sciences Reviews*, Vol. 24. Williams & Wilkins, Baltimore, pp. 35–71.

Grassi, B. (2000). Skeletal muscle $\dot{V}O_2$ on-kinetics: set by O_2 delivery or by O_2 utilization? New insights into an old issue. *Medicine and Science in Sports and Exercise*, **32**, 108–16.

Grassi, B. (2003). Oxygen uptake Kinetics: old and recent lessons from experiments on isolated muscle in situ. *European Journal of Applied Physiology*, **90** (3–4), 242–9.

Grassi, B., Ferretti, G., Xi, L., Rieu, M., Meyer, M., Marconi, C. and Cerretelli, P. (1993). Ventilatory response to exercise after heart and lung denervation in humans. *Respiration Physiology*, **92**, 289–304.

Grassi, B., Poole, D.C., Richardson, R.S., Knight, D.R., Erickson, B.K. and Wagner, P.D. (1996). Muscle O_2 uptake kinetics in humans: implications for metabolic control. *Journal of Applied Physiology*, **80**, 988–98.

Grassi, B., Marconi, C., Meyer, M., Rieu, M. and Cerretelli, P. (1997). Gas exchange and cardiovascular kinetics upon different exercise protocols in heart transplant recipients. *Journal of Applied Physiology*, **82**, 1952–62.

Grassi, B., Gladden, L.B., Samaja, M., Stary, C.M. and Hogan, M.C. (1998a). Faster adjustment of O_2 delivery does not affect $\dot{V}O_2$ on-kinetics in isolated in situ canine muscle. *Journal of Applied Physiology*, **85**, 1394–403.

Grassi, B., Gladden, L.B., Stary, C.M., Wagner, P.D. and Hogan, M.C. (1998b). Peripheral O_2 diffusion does not affect $\dot{V}O_2$ on-kinetics in isolated in situ canine muscle. *Journal of Applied Physiology*, **85**, 1404–12.

Grassi, B., Hogan, M.C., Kelley, K.M., Aschenbach, W.G., Hamann, J.J., Evans, R.K., Pattillo, R.E. and Gladden, L.B. (2000). Role of convective O_2 delivery in determining $\dot{V}O_2$ on-kinetics in canine muscle contracting at peak $\dot{V}O_2$. *Journal of Applied Physiology*, **89**, 1293–301.

Grassi, B., Hogan, M.C., Kelley, K.M., Hamann, J.J., Aschenbach, W.G., Rampichini, S. and Gladden, L.B. (2001). Peripheral O_2 diffusion and $\dot{V}O_2$ on-kinetics in canine muscle at peak $\dot{V}O_2$ (abstract). *Medicine and Science in Sports and Exercise*, **33**, S329.

Grassi, B., Hogan, M.C., Greenhaff, P.L., Hamann, J.J., Kelley, K.M., Aschenbach, W.G., Constantin-Teodosiu, D. and Gladden, L.B. (2002a). $\dot{V}O_2$ on-kinetics in dog gastrocnemius in situ following activation of pyruvate dehydrogenase by dichloroacetate. *Journal of Physiology*, **538**, 195–207.

Grassi, B., Morandi, L., Pogliaghi, S., Rampichini, S., Marconi, C. and Cerretelli, P. (2002b). Functional evaluation of patients with metabolic myopathies during exercise (abstract). *Medicine and Science in Sports and Exercise*, **34**, S78.

Grassi, B., Pogliaghi, S., Rampichini, S., Quaresima, V., Ferrari, M., Marconi, C. and Cerretelli, P. (2003a). Muscle oxygenation and gas exchange kinetics during cycling exercise on-transition in humans. *Journal of Applied Physiology* **95**, 149–58.

Grassi, B., Hogan, M.C., Kelley, K.M., Howlett, R.A., Pattillo, R.E. and Gladden, L.B. (2003b). Effects of L-NAME during metabolic transitions in isolated canine muscle (abstract). *Medicine and Science in Sports and Exercise*, **35**, S227.

Hogan, M.C. (2001). Fall in intracellular PO_2 at the onset of contractions in *Xenopus* single skeletal muscle fibers. *Journal of Applied Physiology*, **90**, 1871–6.

Hughson, R.L. (1990). Exploring cardiorespiratory control mechanisms through gas exchange dynamics. *Medicine and Science in Sports and Exercise*, **22**, 72–9.

Hughson, R.L., Shoemaker, J.K., Tschakovsky, M.E. and Kowalchuck, J.M. (1996). Dependence of muscle $\dot{V}O_2$ on blood flow dynamics at the onset of forearm exercise. *Journal of Applied Physiology*, **81**, 1619–26.

Hughson, R.L., Tschakowsky, M.E. and Houston, M.E. (2001). Regulation of oxygen consumption at the onset of exercise. *Exercise and Sport Sciences Reviews*, **29**, 129–33.

Jones, A.M., Wilkerson, D.P., Koppo, K., Wilmshurst, S. and Campbell, I.T. (2003). Inhibition of nitric oxide synthase by L-NAME speeds phase II pulmonary $\dot{V}O_2$ kinetics in the transition to moderate intensity exercise in man. *Journal of Physiology*, **552**, 265–72.

Jones, A.M., Koppo, K., Wilkerson, D.P., Wilmshurst, S. and Campbell, I.T. (2004a). Dichloroacetate does not speed phase II pulmonary $\dot{V}O_2$ kinetics following the onset of heavy intensity cycle exercise. *Pflugers Archives*, **447**, 867–74.

Jones, A.M., Wilkerson, D.P., Wilmshurst, S. and Campbell, I.T. (2004b). Influence of L-NAME on pulmonary O_2 kinetics during heavy-intensity cycle exercise. *Journal of Applied Physiology*, **96**, 1033–8.

Kaasik, A., Minajeva, A., De Sousa, E., Ventura-Clapier, R. and Veksler, V. (1999). Nitric oxide inhibits cardiac energy production via inhibition of mitochondrial creatine kinase. *FEBS Letters*, **444**, 75–7.

Kindig, C.A., McDonough, P., Erickson, H.H. and Poole, D.C. (2001). Effect of L-NAME on oxygen uptake kinetics during heavy-intensity exercise in the horse. *Journal of Applied Physiology*, **91**, 891–6.

Kindig, C.A., McDonough, P., Erickson, H.H. and Poole, D.C. (2002). Nitric oxide synthase inhibition speeds oxygen uptake kinetics in horses during moderate domain running. *Respiratory Physiology & Neurobiology*, **132**, 169–78.

Kindig, C.A., Kelley, K.M., Howlett, R.A., Stary, C.M. and Hogan, M.C. (2003). Assessment of O_2 uptake dynamics in isolated single skeletal myocytes. *Journal of Applied Physiology*, **94**, 353–7.

Kramer, K., Obal, F. and Quensel, W. (1939). Untershungen über den Müskelstoffwechsel des Warmblüters. III Mitteilung. Die Sauerstoffaufnahme des Muskels während rhythmischer Tätigkeit. *Pflügers Archives*, **241**, 730–40.

Laughlin, M.H., Korthuis, R.J., Duncker, D.J. and Bache, R.J. (1996). Control of blood flow to cardiac and skeletal muscle during exercise. In L.B. Rowell and J.T. Shephard (Eds) *Handbook of Physiology*, Section 12: Exercise: Regulation and Integration of Multiple Systems. Oxford University Press, New York and Oxford, pp. 705–69.

MacDonald, M., Pedersen, P.K. and Hughson, R.L. (1997). Acceleration of $\dot{V}O_2$ kinetics in heavy submaximal exercise by hyperoxia and prior high-intensity exercise. *Journal of Applied Physiology*, **83**, 1318–25.

Mahler, M. (1980). Kinetics and control of oxygen consumption in skeletal muscle. In P. Cerretelli and B.J Whipp (Eds) *Exercise Bioenergetics and Gas Exchange*. Elsevier, Amsterdam, pp. 53–66.

Mahler, M. (1985). First-order kinetics of muscle oxygen consumption, and equivalent proportionality between $\dot{Q}O_2$ and phosphorylcreatine level. Implications for the control of respiration. *Journal of General Physiology*, **86**, 135–65.

Marconi, C., Marzorati, M., Fiocchi, R., Mamprin, F., Ferrazzi, P., Ferretti, G. and Cerretelli, P. (2002). Age-related heart rate response to exercise in heart transplant recipients. Functional significance. *Pflügers Archives*, **443**, 698–706.

Margaria, R., Mangili, F., Cuttica, F. and Cerretelli, P. (1965). The kinetics of the oxygen consumption at the onset of muscular exercise in man. *Ergonomics*, **8**, 49–54.

Meyer, R.A. (1988). A linear model of muscle respiration explains monoexponential phosphocreatine changes. *American Journal of Physiology*, **254**, C548–53.

Nery, L.E., Wasserman, K., Andrews, J.D., Huntsman, D.J., Hansen, J.E. and Whipp, B.J. (1982). Ventilatory and gas exchange kinetics during exercise in chronic obstructive pulmonary disease. *Journal of Applied Physiology*, **53**, 1594–602.

Palange, P. and Wagner, P.D. (2000). The skeletal muscle in chronic respiratory diseases, Summary of the ERS research seminar in Rome, Italy, February 11–12, 1999. *European Respiratory Journal*, 15, 807–15.

Phillips, S.M., Green, H.J., MacDonald, M.J. and Hughson, R.L. (1995). Progressive effect of endurance training on $\dot{V}O_2$ kinetics at onset of submaximal exercise. *Journal of Applied Physiology*, **79**, 1914–20.

Piiper, J., di Prampero, P.E. and Cerretelli, P. (1968). Oxygen debt and high-energy phosphates in gastrocnemius muscle of the dog. *American Journal of Physiology*, **215**, 523–31.

Pringle, J.S.M., Doust, J.H., Carter, H., Tolfrey, K., Campbell, I.T. and Jones, A.M. (2003). Oxygen uptake kinetics in humans: the influence of muscle fiber type and capillarisation. *European Journal of Applied Physiology*, **89**, 289–300.

Regensteiner, J.G., Bauer, T.A., Reusch, J.E.B., Brandenburg, S.L., Sippel, J.M., Vogelsong, A.M., Smith, S., Wolfel, E.E., Eckel, R.H. and Hiatt, W.R. (1998). Abnormal oxygen uptake kinetics in women with type II diabetes mellitus. *Journal of Applied Physiology*, **85**, 310–17.

Rossiter, H.B., Ward, S.A., Doyle, V.L., Howe, F.A., Griffiths, J.R. and Whipp, B.J. (1999). Inferences from pulmonary O_2 uptake with respect to intramuscular [phosphocreatine] kinetics during moderate exercise in humans. *Journal of Physiology*, **518**, 921–32.

Rossiter, H.B., Ward, S.A., Kowalchuck, J.M., Howe, F.A., Griffiths, J.R. and Whipp, B.J. (2001). Effects of prior exercise on oxygen uptake and phosphocreatine kinetics during high-intensity knee-extension exercise in humans. *Journal of Physiology*, **537**, 291–303.

Rossiter, H.B., Ward, S.A., Howe, F.A., Wood, D.M., Kowalchuck, J.M., Griffiths, J.R. and Whipp, B.J. (2003). Effects of dichloroacetate on $\dot{V}O_2$ and intramuscular ^{31}P metabolite kinetics during high-intensity exercise in humans. *Journal of Applied Physiology*, **95**, 1105–15.

Scheuermann-Freestone, M., Madsen, P.L., Manners, D., Blamire, A.M., Buckingham, R.E., Styles, P., Radda, G.K., Neubauer, S. and Clarke, K. (2003). Abnormal cardiac and skeletal muscle energy metabolism in patients with type 2 diabetes. *Circulation*, **107**, 3040–6.

Sietsema, K.E., Ben-Dov, I., Zhang, Y.Y., Sullivan, C. and Wasserman, K. (1994). Dynamics of oxygen uptake for submaximal exercise and recovery in patients with chronic heart failure. *Chest*, **105**, 1693–700.

Timmons, J.A., Gustafsson, T., Sundberg, C.J., Jansson, E. and Greenhaff, P.L. (1998). Muscle acetyl group availability is a major determinant of oxygen deficit in humans during submaximal exercise. *American Journal of Physiology*, **274**, E377–80.

Tschakovsky, M.E. and Hughson, R.L. (1999). Interaction of factors determining oxygen uptake at the onset of exercise. *Journal of Applied Physiology*, **86**, 1101–13.

Ventura-Clapier, V., De Sousa, E. and Veksler, V. (2002). Metabolic myopathy in heart failure. *News in Physiological Sciences*, **17**, 191–6.

Wagner, P.D. (2000). New ideas on limitations to $\dot{V}O_{2\,max}$. *Exercise and Sport Sciences Reviews*, **28**, 10–14.

Whipp, B.J. and Mahler, M. (1980). Dynamics of pulmonary gas exchange during exercise. In J.B. West (Ed.) *Pulmonary Gas Exchange*, Vol. II. Academic Press, New York, pp. 33–96.

Whipp, B.J., Ward, S.A., Lamarra, N., Davis, J.A. and Wasserman, K. (1982). Parameters of ventilatory and gas exchange dynamics during exercise. *Journal of Applied Physiology*, **52**, 1506–13.

10 'Priming exercise' and $\dot{V}O_2$ kinetics

Mark Burnley, Katrien Koppo and Andrew M. Jones

Introduction

The aphorism used by Peter Mitchell in his Nobel Prize lecture describing experimental progress on the chemiosmotic theory of bioenergetics, that 'the obscure we see eventually, the completely apparent takes longer' (Mitchell, 1978) will have resonance with anyone who has traced the origins and progress of studies investigating the character and control of the on-transient $\dot{V}O_2$ kinetics. It is clear that when O_2 delivery is not rate limiting, the kinetics of muscle oxygen consumption follow a mono-exponential time course (Mahler, 1980; Whipp and Mahler, 1980). However, it is not clear to what extent these kinetics are regulated by O_2 delivery or O_2 utilization and this has been a key focus of research into $\dot{V}O_2$ kinetics in the last twenty years. If O_2 delivery is a critical determinant of the $\dot{V}O_2$ kinetics, then interventions that increase O_2 delivery should speed the $\dot{V}O_2$ kinetics beyond the control condition (which we operationally define as upright cycle exercise breathing room air at sea level). In contrast, experiments that return null results support the opposite position, that O_2 utilization sets the kinetic time course, as demonstrated in isolated muscle preparations (Mahler, 1980).

An intervention that has received particularly detailed attention in relation to the determinants of the $\dot{V}O_2$ response is that of prior 'priming' or 'warm-up' exercise. This intervention is of importance because it has been demonstrated that prior heavy exercise increases bulk O_2 delivery to the exercising muscle and that it has dramatic effects on the response to subsequent exercise. This chapter will review the studies that have used prior exercise to examine the control of $\dot{V}O_2$ kinetics. The precise characteristics of the effect of prior exercise on the $\dot{V}O_2$ response will be considered in detail, as will the likely underlying mechanisms. The chapter will conclude with consideration of the implications of this topic for exercise tolerance in both health and disease, and with suggested directions for future research.

Investigations into the physiological effects of prior exercise

Prior exercise has been recognized for many years as an acute intervention that has profound effects on the metabolic, acid–base and cardiovascular responses to subsequent exercise. This interest has, of course, been due in large part to the near universal use of warm-up exercise in preparation for subsequent sport and exercise performance. A number of early studies monitored the effect of prior exercise on the $\dot{V}O_2$ response during subsequent exercise, although many of these studies lacked the temporal resolution required to describe its specific time course. For example, it was demonstrated that prior exercise performed at the work rate associated with $\dot{V}O_{2\,max}$, followed by 20–25 min of recovery pedalling, resulted in an elevated blood [lactate] at the onset of a subsequent exercise bout, an increase in the $\dot{V}O_2$ response in the first 2 min of exercise (Figure 10.1), and a blunting of the $\dot{V}CO_2$, blood [lactate] and pH responses (Weltman *et al.*, 1979; Buono and Roby, 1982). These results clearly demonstrated that prior exercise could serve to 'prime' the physiological response to exercise, resulting in an apparent increase in the aerobic contribution to subsequent exercise.

There are several other studies of note that investigated the effect of prior exercise on the physiological responses to subsequent exercise. Inbar and Bar-Or (1975) demonstrated that an intermittent warm-up (in which 30 s of exercise was alternated with 30 s rest for 15 min in order to elicit an average $\dot{V}O_2$ of ~60% $\dot{V}O_{2\,max}$) increased the peak $\dot{V}O_2$ achieved during an 'aerobic criterion task' lasting 4 min at a supra-maximal work rate in 7–9-year-old children. These authors also showed a trend for an increase in $\dot{V}O_2$ at all time points throughout exercise following the warm-up, although the O_2 deficit was unaltered. Interestingly, this study also demonstrated an improvement in exercise performance in the criterion task, as evidenced by an increase in the total pedal revolutions performed in

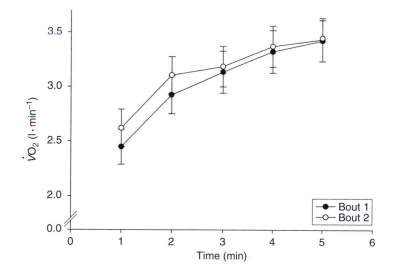

Figure 10.1 Superimposed $\dot{V}O_2$ responses to two 5 min bouts of cycle exercise separated by 25 min of unloaded pedalling. Values are mean ± SEM ($n = 10$). Note the increased $\dot{V}O_2$ response in the first 2 min of the second bout of exercise. The lack of temporal resolution in data such as these makes mechanistic inferences difficult. Data redrawn from Buono and Roby (1982).

4 min. In agreement with these data, Ingjer and Stromme (1979) observed an increase in $\dot{V}O_2$ during a 4 min run at 100% $\dot{V}O_{2\,max}$ following an active warm-up at 50–60% of $\dot{V}O_{2\,max}$. Interestingly, the warm-up did not result in a significant elevation of blood [lactate], but did result in a blunting of both the blood [lactate] and pH responses to the criterion exercise bout. An elevated $\dot{V}O_2$ response in the second of two supra-maximal exercise bouts has also been reported by Gutin *et al.* (1976). However, the criterion exercise bout in this study commenced only 30 s after the warm-up was completed. Consequently, separation of the $\dot{V}O_2$ responses to these two exercise bouts was not possible.

Several other studies have been unable to demonstrate an effect of prior warm-up exercise on the physiological response to subsequent exercise. For example, De Bruyn-Prevost (1980) found no clear effect of a number of different warm-up procedures on the responses to a standard sub-maximal exercise bout, although the most intense warm-up was designed to elicit a heart rate of 135 b·min^{-1}. Martin *et al.* (1975) reported that 15 min of running at 10 km·h^{-1} at a 2% grade had no effect on the $\dot{V}O_2$ or heart rate responses to subsequent exercise lasting 1.5 or 5 min. It is unlikely that the warm-ups used in these studies were performed at a sufficiently high intensity to result in disturbances in blood acid–base status. Collectively, investigations into the effects of warm-up exercise prior to 1982 suggest that intense bouts of exercise are likely to alter the physiological response during subsequent 'strenuous' exercise, chiefly by elevating $\dot{V}O_2$ and blunting the lactate, pH and $\dot{V}CO_2$ responses, whereas moderate-intensity prior exercise has no effect on the physiological responses to subsequent exercise.

The two major shortcomings of these studies in relation to the $\dot{V}O_2$ response are the lack of temporal resolution and the fact that the studies demonstrating an effect did so with criterion exercise tasks performed at work rates at or above those yielding $\dot{V}O_{2\,max}$. It is not clear what the appropriate method of characterizing the $\dot{V}O_2$ kinetics during peri-maximal exercise is (Whipp and Mahler, 1980; Whipp, 1994), due to the amplitude of the $\dot{V}O_2$ response being functionally constrained by the attainment of $\dot{V}O_{2\,max}$. As a result, to determine what effect prior exercise has on the kinetic features of the $\dot{V}O_2$ response requires exercise to be performed at work rates that are below $\dot{V}O_{2\,max}$ (i.e. in the heavy/severe domain; see Chapter 1). Investigations utilizing exercise of heavy intensity as the criterion bout have proved invaluable in elucidating the mechanisms underlying the effect of prior exercise and, as we will show, the mechanisms underlying the control of $\dot{V}O_2$ kinetics themselves.

The prior exercise effect

Renewed interest in the effect of prior exercise on the gas exchange responses to exercise was generated by the report of Gerbino *et al.* (1996) which built upon the previous exploratory work of the same group (Gausche *et al.*, 1989). Gerbino *et al.* (1996) demonstrated that prior heavy exercise could speed the overall $\dot{V}O_2$ kinetics during a second bout of heavy exercise performed 6 min after the first. Gerbino *et al.* (1996) also demonstrated that the heavy exercise $\dot{V}O_2$ kinetics were unaltered by a prior bout of moderate-intensity exercise. The implications of these findings were profound: no other study of the $\dot{V}O_2$ response in exercising humans during upright exercise at sea level had shown that the kinetics could be speeded by an acute, non-pharmacological intervention.

In the 1990s, the factors that limited or controlled the acceleration of oxidative metabolism following the onset of exercise continued to be debated. It was argued that during moderate-intensity exercise, the kinetics were limited predominantly by O_2 utilization, whereas during heavy-intensity exercise, O_2 availability also had the potential to influence $\dot{V}O_2$ kinetics (Whipp and Ward, 1990). Paterson and Whipp (1991) presented evidence consistent with this view: the primary $\dot{V}O_2$ kinetics of heavy exercise appeared to be slowed in comparison to those of moderate exercise. It was suggested that one possible cause of this was a perfusion inadequacy (Whipp and Ward, 1992), with the transient limitation to O_2 utilization also leading to increased lactate production (Paterson and Whipp, 1991). Investigations utilizing prior exercise models would subsequently prove pivotal in testing this hypothetical model of the $\dot{V}O_2$ response. Because a lactic acidosis was suggested to be associated with vasodilatation and a Bohr shift in the oxyhaemoglobin dissociation curve (Stringer et al., 1994), Gerbino et al. (1996) predicted that a metabolic acidosis caused by the performance of prior heavy-intensity exercise would speed the perfusion-limited kinetics during subsequent heavy-intensity exercise, whereas prior moderate-intensity exercise (which would not cause a sustained lactic acidosis) would have no such effect. Gerbino et al. (1996) further postulated that if the $\dot{V}O_2$ kinetics of moderate exercise were dictated by the kinetics of intramuscular energy transfer (thus consistent with the metabolic inertia hypothesis), then the metabolic acidosis resulting from the performance of prior heavy exercise should have no significant effect on the $\dot{V}O_2$ response to exercise below the lactate threshold.

In the study of Gerbino et al. (1996), the experimental design incorporated four separate double square-wave exercise tests: two bouts of moderate-intensity exercise; two bouts of heavy-intensity exercise; a bout of moderate exercise followed by a bout of heavy exercise; and a bout of heavy exercise followed by a bout of moderate exercise. The exercise bouts were each of 6 min duration and were separated by 6 min recovery in each of the conditions. The findings of the study clearly showed that the overall $\dot{V}O_2$ response to heavy exercise (i.e. the increase in $\dot{V}O_2$ from about 20 s to the end of exercise) was significantly slower than the response to moderate exercise, and that the performance of prior heavy exercise (which resulted in a residual lactacidosis) significantly speeded the $\dot{V}O_2$ kinetics during a subsequent heavy exercise bout (Figure 10.2). None of the other conditions were effective in altering the $\dot{V}O_2$ kinetics. Thus, it appeared that the overall $\dot{V}O_2$ kinetics in the first bout of heavy exercise might have been limited to some extent by inadequate muscle perfusion. The inability of the prior heavy exercise bout to speed the kinetics of moderate exercise was also consistent with the proposal that, in the moderate domain, the kinetics were mainly determined by a metabolic inertia. Therefore, the 'prior exercise effect' refers to a speeding of the overall $\dot{V}O_2$ kinetics during the second of two bouts of heavy-intensity exercise.

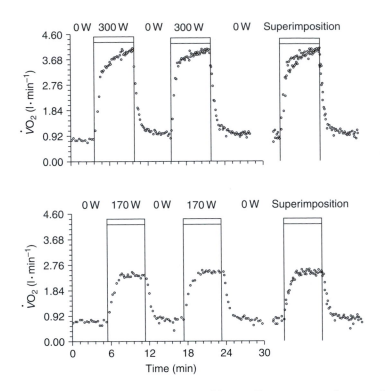

Figure 10.2 Oxygen uptake responses to repeated bouts of heavy exercise (top panel) and moderate exercise (bottom panel). Notice the speeded overall $\dot{V}O_2$ response in the second bout of heavy exercise compared to the similarity of the responses to repeated bouts of moderate exercise. Open symbols represent responses to first exercise bout and closed symbols represent responses to second exercise bout. Reproduced with permission from Gerbino *et al.* (1996).

The speeded heavy exercise $\dot{V}O_2$ kinetics observed by Gerbino *et al.* (1996) were associated with a significant reduction in blood lactate accumulation and an attenuated fall in blood pH, with an associated blunting of the $\dot{V}CO_2$ response. These findings were consistent with an increased aerobic contribution to energy turnover in the second heavy exercise bout that was associated with, and potentially consequent to, an improved O_2 delivery to muscle. Support for the concept that an O_2 transport limitation was the likely mechanism for the relatively sluggish heavy exercise $\dot{V}O_2$ kinetics was provided by the work of MacDonald *et al.* (1997). These investigators demonstrated that both prior heavy exercise and hyperoxia speeded the $\dot{V}O_2$ kinetics during heavy, but not moderate, intensity exercise. Importantly, the fastest overall kinetics were observed during the second bout of heavy exercise under hyperoxia, supporting the notion that if more O_2 were supplied to the muscle during the transient, then it could be utilized. The findings of Gerbino *et al.* (1996) and MacDonald *et al.* (1997) were therefore accepted as evidence that during exercise performed above the lactate threshold, O_2 delivery may become a critical determinant of the kinetics of $\dot{V}O_2$ (Tschakovsky and Hughson, 1999; Grassi, 2000).

In addition to the speeding of the overall $\dot{V}O_2$ kinetics, both Gerbino et al. (1996) and MacDonald et al. (1997) demonstrated that the performance of prior heavy exercise caused a significant reduction in the $\dot{V}O_2$ slow component amplitude during subsequent heavy exercise, although the potential mechanism(s) underpinning this change was/were not addressed. Gerbino et al. (1996) demonstrated that the off-transient $\dot{V}O_2$ kinetics were unaltered by prior heavy exercise. Subsequent work has shown that the character of the off-transient kinetics appears to depend simply upon the $\dot{V}O_2$ attained at the end of exercise, and does not appear to be related to how rapidly this amplitude is attained (Cunningham et al., 2000). It therefore appears that the effects of prior heavy exercise are confined to the on-transient (Gerbino et al., 1996; MacDonald et al., 1997; Scheuermann et al., 2001), a finding which may in itself provide important mechanistic insights.

The work of Gerbino et al. (1996) provided evidence that prior heavy exercise could markedly alter the $\dot{V}O_2$ response to subsequent heavy exercise. However, the response kinetics were not partitioned in this study due to the authors' concern that the signal-to-noise ratio would not allow parameters from the necessarily more complex characterization of the $\dot{V}O_2$ response to be estimated with sufficient statistical confidence to draw mechanistic inferences (see Chapter 3). Consequently, the data were characterized with a mono-exponential function applied from 25 s to the end of exercise (Figure 10.3A). The primary and slow components of the $\dot{V}O_2$ response are manifest in series (Whipp and Wasserman, 1972; Barstow and Molé, 1991; Paterson and Whipp, 1991), and as a result these components should ideally be treated as separate entities when breath-by-breath data are mathematically modelled (Figure 10.3B). Therefore, in using a mono-exponential function extended to the end of exercise, Gerbino et al. (1996) included both the primary and slow components in their fitting window (Figure 10.3A). The 'effective' time constant derived from this procedure may be speeded either as a consequence of a speeding of the primary kinetics, or of a reduction in the amplitude of the $\dot{V}O_2$ slow component: both will result in a reduction in the time taken to reach 63% of the end-exercise $\dot{V}O_2$ (Burnley et al., 2000; Koppo and Bouckaert, 2001). MacDonald et al. (1997) characterised their data with a three-component exponential function, but used the 'mean response time' to interpret the data; this parameter also reflects the rate at which the end-exercise $\dot{V}O_2$ is attained and cannot be used to discriminate between changes in the primary and slow component responses.

In light of the analyses of Gerbino et al. (1996) and MacDonald et al. (1997), we were therefore interested in characterizing the effect of prior heavy exercise on the primary and slow component responses using more complex modelling procedures in order to provide insights regarding the physiological mechanisms responsible for the overall speeding of the $\dot{V}O_2$ kinetics (Burnley et al., 2000; Koppo and Bouckaert, 2001). The results confirmed that there was a significant speeding of the overall $\dot{V}O_2$ kinetics when the response was described using the modelling approach of Gerbino et al. (1996) (Figure 10.4, top). However, when a modelling procedure that partitioned the primary and slow component responses was used,

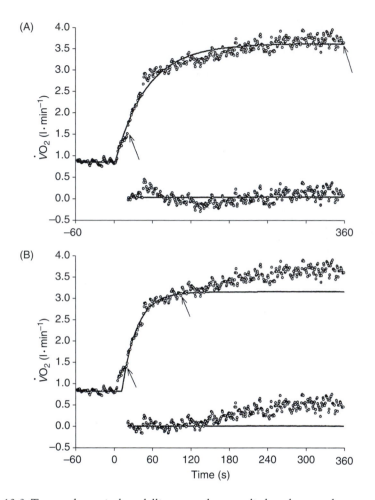

Figure 10.3 Two mathematical modelling procedures applied to the same heavy exercise
response. In panel A, a mono-exponential function was applied from 25 s to
the end of exercise. In panel B, the primary component was isolated using the
procedure detailed by Rossiter *et al.* (2001). Arrows indicate the fitting win-
dows used in each case. The residuals at the foot of each plot demonstrate a
clear trend throughout the response in panel A, whereas the residuals only
deviate from zero after ~120 s in panel B, demonstrating that the 'slow' kinetics in panel A ($\tau = 50.2$), compared to the primary kinetics ($\tau = 23$ s,
panel B), are largely a consequence of the emergence of the $\dot{V}O_2$ slow
component.

it was shown that this overall speeding was not a consequence of a speeding of
the primary kinetics (Figure 10.4, bottom), but was caused by a reduction in
the amplitude of the $\dot{V}O_2$ slow component (Burnley *et al.*, 2000; Koppo and
Bouckaert, 2001). These findings have subsequently been supported by our other

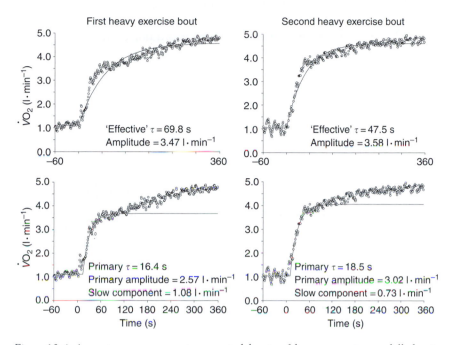

Figure 10.4 An extreme response to repeated bouts of heavy exercise modelled using mono-exponential curves fit from 25 s to the end of exercise (top panels) and mono-exponential fits isolating the primary phase (bottom panels). Included are the actual parameter estimates from these fitting procedures. Notice that the speeding of the overall $\dot{V}O_2$ kinetics (*top*) is related to an increase in the primary amplitude and a reduced slow component amplitude (*bottom*) whereas the kinetics of the primary response *per se* are unaltered. No change in the time constant is evident. Data redrawn from Burnley *et al.* (2002a).

experiments (Burnley *et al.*, 2001, 2002a,b; Koppo *et al.*, 2003) as well as by experiments conducted by other research groups (Bearden and Moffatt, 2001; Scheuermann *et al.*, 2001; Fukuba *et al.*, 2002; Perrey *et al.*, 2003; though see also Tordi *et al.*, 2003).

With the benefit of hindsight, the demonstration by MacDonald *et al.* (1997) that the overall $\dot{V}O_2$ kinetics of heavy exercise were speeded with hyperoxia should be interpreted cautiously. The data presented in that study show both no change in the time constant of the primary component (mean $\pm$ SEM: 18.8 ± 1.2 s (normoxia) vs 20.0 ± 2.7 s (hyperoxia); see their table 2) and a significantly longer time constant (17.6 ± 1.0 s (normoxia) vs 23.6 ± 2.0 s (hyperoxia); see their table 1) when breathing the hyperoxic inspirate. Furthermore, prior heavy exercise had no effect on the primary time constant during the second bout of heavy exercise either in normoxia (from 18.8 ± 1.2 to 18.6 ± 0.9 s) or in hyperoxia (from 20.0 ± 2.7 to 21.4 ± 1.9 s). Therefore, the speeding of the overall kinetics observed by MacDonald *et al.* (1997) were, in fact, largely attributable to a reduction in the amplitude of the $\dot{V}O_2$ slow component. As detailed later, further investigations into the character of the $\dot{V}O_2$ response during repeated bouts of heavy exercise revealed that the effects of prior exercise were largely seen in changes in the primary and slow component amplitudes, rather than in the kinetics of the response *per se*.

In addition to the lack of change in the time constant of the primary $\dot{V}O_2$ response, it was originally reported that the primary $\dot{V}O_2$ amplitude was unaltered by prior heavy exercise (Burnley *et al.*, 2000; Koppo and Bouckaert, 2001). However, this lack of change in the primary $\dot{V}O_2$ response may have been obscured by a significant increase in the baseline $\dot{V}O_2$ prior to the onset of the second bout of heavy exercise; that is, the absolute $\dot{V}O_2$ response was significantly higher at the end of the primary phase, but the increase in $\dot{V}O_2$ above baseline was unchanged. To eliminate the effect of the elevated baseline $\dot{V}O_2$, Burnley *et al.* (2001) performed another set of experiments wherein recovery duration was extended from 6 to 12 min to allow baseline $\dot{V}O_2$ to be restored. Because the recovery of blood [lactate] has a half-time of approximately 15–20 min (Weltman *et al.*, 1979), effects of the residual acidosis on $\dot{V}O_2$ kinetics should still have been demonstrable. The effects observed substantially confirmed the previous experiments, in that the primary component kinetics were unaltered and the amplitude of the $\dot{V}O_2$ slow component was reduced. Additionally, however, these data also showed that the primary component amplitude was increased by prior heavy exercise (Figure 10.4, bottom), an observation which was again confirmed by data from other laboratories (Bearden and Moffatt, 2001; Patel *et al.*, 2001; Fukuba *et al.*, 2002; Perrey *et al.*, 2003) as well as our own (Burnley *et al.*, 2002a).

Collectively, these studies can be used to describe the characteristic effect of prior heavy exercise on the heavy exercise $\dot{V}O_2$ response during upright cycle exercise. Figure 10.5 illustrates the essence of the effect. *In short, it appears that prior heavy exercise that normally results in a residual blood lactic acidosis speeds the overall $\dot{V}O_2$ response (Gerbino et al., 1996), as a result of an increased primary component amplitude and a reduced slow component amplitude, with no change in the primary component time constant* (Burnley *et al.*, 2000, 2001; Koppo and Bouckaert, 2001). To illustrate this latter point, when the $\dot{V}O_2$ response is normalized to account for the increased primary $\dot{V}O_2$ amplitude (Figure 10.5B), the difference between the two responses in this phase is eliminated, clearly demonstrating that the kinetics of the primary response are unaffected by prior heavy exercise. The increased primary component amplitude is only observed if the baseline $\dot{V}O_2$ is restored by extending recovery duration beyond the original 6 min (Bearden and Moffatt, 2001; Burnley *et al.*, 2001, 2002a). We consider these response profiles to represent the characteristic $\dot{V}O_2$ responses to repeated bouts of upright cycling exercise. However, the effect of prior exercise has also been investigated using other modes of exercise, and interesting additional inferences can be drawn from these data.

Another intervention that has received particular attention is prior exercise performed using a different muscle group to that used in the second exercise bout. This approach can discriminate between the effects of factors intrinsic to

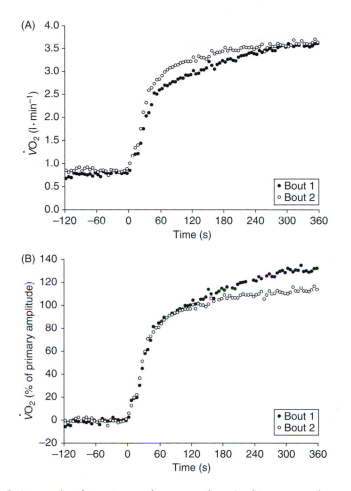

Figure 10.5 Averaged and superimposed responses from 8 subjects to two bouts of heavy exercise. Panel A shows the increased primary and reduced slow component amplitudes characteristic of the effect of prior heavy exercise. In panel B, these responses are normalized to the amplitude of the primary response. This normalization shows that the increase in the $\dot{V}O_2$ response in the first 2 min of exercise appears to be due only to the increased primary $\dot{V}O_2$ amplitude. This panel also demonstrates the significant reduction in the amplitude of the $\dot{V}O_2$ slow component following the performance of prior heavy exercise. Data redrawn from Burnley *et al.* (2002a).

the exercising muscle from systemic factors such as elevated blood [lactate]. Bohnert *et al.* (1998) were the first to investigate the effect of prior arm crank exercise on the $\dot{V}O_2$ response to heavy leg cycling. The authors reported that prior heavy arm crank exercise reduced both the $\dot{V}O_2$ slow component and the 'partial' O_2 deficit during the subsequent heavy leg cycle exercise. However, because the analysis in this study was based on single transitions and no complex modelling techniques were used, it was not possible to determine if the speeding of the overall $\dot{V}O_2$ kinetics (implied by the reduction in the partial O_2 deficit) following prior arm crank exercise was due to a true speeding of the $\dot{V}O_2$ primary component and/or the result of a reduction in the $\dot{V}O_2$ slow component. Two recent studies have re-examined the effect of prior arm cranking using a more complex modelling approach (Fukuba *et al.*, 2002; Koppo *et al.*, 2003). Both studies demonstrated that prior heavy exercise had no effect on the time constant of the primary $\dot{V}O_2$ response irrespective of whether the prior exercise was performed by the arms or the legs. Furthermore, both studies also showed that prior heavy exercise (either of the arms or the legs) led to an increased absolute $\dot{V}O_2$ at the end of the primary component phase (significant in both studies) and a reduced slow component amplitude (significant in the study of Koppo *et al.*, 2003) during subsequent heavy leg exercise. The effect of arm cranking on the $\dot{V}O_2$ response to leg exercise was qualitatively similar though quantitatively smaller than the effect of prior leg exercise (Figure 10.6). The mechanistic significance of these findings is considered later.

Alternative descriptions of the effect of prior exercise

Despite an increasing volume of data demonstrating that prior heavy exercise does not alter the primary $\dot{V}O_2$ kinetics, two recent studies (Rossiter *et al.*, 2001; Tordi *et al.*, 2003) have presented evidence that, in some situations, the primary component time constant may be reduced in the second heavy exercise bout.

Rossiter *et al.* (2001) reported that prior heavy exercise resulted in a speeding of the primary $\dot{V}O_2$ kinetics in a second bout of heavy exercise when subjects exercised in the prone position in a whole-body magnet for the measurement of muscle [PCr] responses by near-magnetic resonance spectroscopy. These investigators found that prior heavy exercise had no effect on the primary $\dot{V}O_2$ amplitude, but did reduce the amplitude of the $\dot{V}O_2$ slow component and significantly attenuated the decrement in muscle [PCr] at the onset of exercise, consistent with the speeded pulmonary $\dot{V}O_2$ kinetics. It is unclear why Rossiter *et al.* (2001) observed a speeding of the primary $\dot{V}O_2$ kinetics in their study, although differences in the exercise modality, intensity and muscle mass recruitment have been considered previously (Rossiter *et al.*, 2001). It is noteworthy that when the same research group investigated the effect of prior heavy exercise during upright cycling, they returned results consistent with those studies cited previously (Bearden and Moffatt, 2001; Burnley *et al.*, 2001; Fukuba *et al.*, 2002): Patel *et al.* (2001) showed no change in the primary $\dot{V}O_2$ time constant, an elevated primary $\dot{V}O_2$ amplitude and a reduced $\dot{V}O_2$ slow component. Since these authors used an identical modelling procedure to that of Rossiter *et al.* (2001), we believe that the speeding of the primary $\dot{V}O_2$ kinetics observed in that study may be peculiar to exercise in the prone position.

Exercise in the prone position provides the cardiovascular system with very similar control challenges to that faced in the supine position. Because the exercising

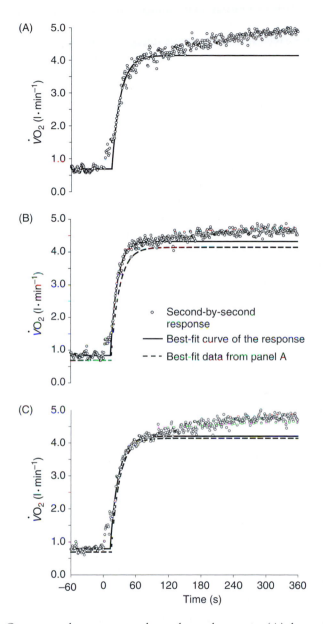

Figure 10.6 Oxygen uptake responses to heavy leg cycle exercise (A), heavy leg exercise after prior heavy leg exercise (B) and heavy leg exercise after prior heavy arm exercise (C). Solid lines indicate the best-fit mono-exponential description of the primary component. In panels B and C, the best fit of the response in panel A is given by the dashed line. Notice the reduced $\dot{V}O_2$ slow component after prior heavy exercise with the same muscle group (panel B), an effect that is appreciably smaller after prior arm cranking (panel C). Adapted from Koppo *et al.* (2002).

muscle is at a relative perfusion disadvantage compared to the upright condition, this may result in slowed primary kinetics (Hughson *et al.*, 1993). This being the case, the prior heavy exercise may have improved muscle perfusion, thus speeding the kinetics toward values that would be encountered during upright exercise. The time constant of the primary component in the study of Rossiter *et al.* (2001) was so slow in the control condition (~46.6 s, compared to typical values of 20–30 s during upright cycle exercise) that it does appear likely that there was a perfusion limitation in the control condition in this study. Consistent with this interpetation, Hughson *et al.* (1993) showed that the application of lower-body negative pressure during supine exercise speeded the moderate-intensity primary $\dot{V}O_2$ kinetics to the extent that they were not different from those measured during upright cycle exercise. The application of lower-body positive pressure during recumbent leg cycling, by contrast, has no effect on the pulmonary $\dot{V}O_2$ response (Williamson *et al.*, 1996), suggesting that muscle perfusion and therefore O_2 delivery is not rate limiting if exercise is performed with the exercising musculature below the level of the heart. Scheuermann *et al.* (2002) reported that prior heavy exercise speeded the $\dot{V}O_2$ kinetics during moderate-intensity upright exercise (from ~50 to ~27 s) in apparently healthy older subjects (~65 yrs). These investigators also attributed this effect to an improved muscle perfusion, since (1) no similar effect was observed in a control group of younger subjects, and (2) if factors related to a metabolic inertia had been responsible, prior moderate exercise should have had a similar effect when, in fact, it did not influence the $\dot{V}O_2$ response. *Thus, specific conditions exist whereby prior heavy exercise can speed the primary $\dot{V}O_2$ kinetics, possibly as a consequence of an improved muscle perfusion, in exactly the manner first proposed by Gerbino et al. (1996). These findings do not seem to be reflective of the responses observed in young healthy subjects performing upright cycle exercise, however.*

Tordi *et al.* (2003) have published what is so far the only study in which prior exercise has reduced the phase II time constant during subsequent heavy upright cycle exercise in young subjects. In this study, subjects performed three bouts of 30 s sprint exercise in order to maximize the metabolic acidosis. The authors reasoned that such a procedure would maximize any effect on muscle vasodilatation and therefore on any speeding of the primary $\dot{V}O_2$ kinetics. Their results are consistent with this proposal, although they did not measure blood [lactate], pH or vasodilatation. Whether the metabolic acidosis was greater in this study than in the study of Burnley *et al.* (2002b; whole blood [lactate] of 6.4 mM) is not clear. However, even if the metabolic acidosis were higher in the study of Tordi *et al.* (2003), a rationale for why there should be a 'threshold' for greater vasodilatation at higher acid loads is lacking. One possible explanation for the incongruity of the results of Tordi *et al.* (2003) with the rest of the literature is the training status of the subjects studied and the intensity of the criterion exercise bout. Tordi *et al.* (2003) studied trained cyclists ($\dot{V}O_{2\ peak}$ ~ 66 ml $\cdot$ kg^{-1} $\cdot$ min^{-1}) and tested them at a work-rate that resulted in the attainment of 97% $\dot{V}O_{2\ peak}$ at the end of exercise; in contrast, in those studies in which blood [lactate] was most significantly elevated by prior exercise (to 6–7 mM), the subjects were somewhat less fit

($\dot{V}O_{2\,peak}$ ~ 51–58 ml $\cdot$ kg^{-1} $\cdot$ min^{-1}) and they exercised at slightly lower intensities (87–93% $\dot{V}O_{2\,peak}$ at the end of exercise) (Burnley et al., 2001; Koppo et al., 2003). There is some evidence that $\dot{V}O_2$ peak is more sensitive to changes in O_2 availability in athletes compared to untrained subjects (Cardus et al., 1998), although whether this is also true for $\dot{V}O_2$ kinetics is presently unknown.

There is some evidence that a metabolic acidosis is not a necessary prerequisite to elicit changes in the $\dot{V}O_2$ kinetics following prior exercise. Although the majority of studies report that prior moderate exercise induced no significant changes in the $\dot{V}O_2$ kinetics to subsequent heavy exercise (e.g. Gerbino et al., 1996; MacDonald et al., 1997 Burnley et al., 2000;), others have shown that moderate exercise can influence the $\dot{V}O_2$ response during subsequent heavy exercise (Koppo and Bouckaert, 2000, 2002; Campbell-O'Sullivan et al., 2002). Specifically, Koppo and Bouckaert (2000) demonstrated that when the duration of prior moderate-intensity exercise was extended to equate the total work done to that during heavy exercise, the $\dot{V}O_2$ slow component was reduced during a subsequent heavy exercise bout. This finding was subsequently confirmed during exhaustive exercise (Koppo and Bouckaert, 2002). Burnley et al. (2001) reported that even prolonged prior moderate exercise had no significant effect on the $\dot{V}O_2$ slow component amplitude, although the relatively modest slow component amplitude observed in the control condition in this study (~270 ml $\cdot$ min^{-1} compared to ~570 ml $\cdot$ min^{-1} in that of Koppo and Bouckaert (2002)) may have precluded the detection of small differences between the conditions. Crucially, however, in all of these studies there was no elevation in the primary $\dot{V}O_2$ amplitude following prior moderate exercise. Therefore, it is possible that the reduction in the amplitude of the slow component observed by Koppo and Bouckaert (2000, 2002) reflects a phenomenon of subtly different mechanistic origin to that of the effect of prior heavy exercise.

Campbell-O'Sullivan et al. (2002) also observed changes in the $\dot{V}O_2$ response to heavy exercise following prior moderate-intensity cycling exercise. These authors demonstrated that the mean response time of pulmonary $\dot{V}O_2$ was significantly reduced (from 45.1 to 31.3 s) and PCr degradation was significantly reduced during a subsequent 10 min cycling exercise bout at 75% $\dot{V}O_{2max}$. Muscle acetylcarnitine concentration was increased at the onset of the heavy exercise bout leading the authors to suggest that a stockpiling of acetyl groups led to faster $\dot{V}O_2$ kinetics (Campbell-O'Sullivan et al., 2002). However, as mentioned earlier, a speeding of the overall $\dot{V}O_2$ kinetics may be either the result of a speeding of the primary kinetics, an elevation of the primary $\dot{V}O_2$ amplitude, and/or a reduction in the amplitude of the $\dot{V}O_2$ slow component. Since Campbell-O'Sullivan et al. (2002) did not characterize the $\dot{V}O_2$ response with due regard to its discrete kinetic components, it is difficult to draw inferences regarding underlying mechanisms from these data. However, the data of Koppo and Bouckaert (2000, 2002) demonstrate that the $\dot{V}O_2$ response to heavy exercise can be altered by prior exercise that does not elicit a metabolic acidosis, albeit not in the same way as shown in studies using repeated bouts of heavy exercise (see Koppo et al., 2002).

Mechanisms

Several different mechanisms might underlie the changes in $\dot{V}O_2$ kinetics observed following prior exercise. The mechanisms responsible for any changes will depend upon the experimental models employed. For example, experiments which place the exercising muscle at or above heart level are likely to result in different $\dot{V}O_2$ response profiles and hence different mechanistic inferences (Rossiter *et al.*, 2001; cf. Burnley *et al.*, 2000). We will therefore present evidence for and against four mechanisms that have been presented in the literature.

Increased activity of mitochondrial enzymes and/or increased availability of metabolic substrate

Some studies have suggested that the pyruvate dehydrogenase complex (PDC) provides a functional stenosis to substrate flux and is, therefore, a key component of the metabolic inertia that determines the $\dot{V}O_2$ kinetics in the transient phase of exercise (Greenhaff and Timmons, 1998; Greenhaff *et al.*, 2002). Several investigators have presented evidence consistent with this view: Timmons *et al.* (1998b) demonstrated that dichloroacetate infusion (which inhibits pyruvate dehydrogenase kinase and therefore increases PDC activity) decreased the reliance on substrate level phosphorylation during rest-to-exercise transitions in humans during exhaustive ischaemic muscle contractions. The same group also showed this effect during moderate-intensity non-ischaemic muscle contractions using the same exercise model (Timmons *et al.*, 1998a). Howlett *et al.* (1999) subsequently provided data that were similar to those of Timmons *et al.* (1998a). It was therefore hypothesised that substrate availability at least partly determines the rate at which aerobic ATP production accelerates at the onset of exercise. None of the aforementioned studies monitored pulmonary or muscle $\dot{V}O_2$ during the on-transient, but instead relied on the analysis of biopsy material before and during/after exercise.

As mentioned earlier, Campbell-O'Sullivan *et al.* (2002) reported that a 10 min cycling exercise at 55% $\dot{V}O_{2\,max}$ resulted in a stockpiling of acetyl groups prior to the onset of a second exercise bout. Since these authors observed a 'speeding' of the $\dot{V}O_2$ response during that second exercise bout, they proposed that there may be a lag in the activation of the PDC at the onset of exercise that prevents sufficient flux of acetyl groups into the tricarboxylic acid cycle, and that the performance of prior exercise might overcome this limitation by increasing metabolic substrate availability. However, recent studies that have measured both muscle metabolism and muscle $\dot{V}O_2$ kinetics in isolated dog gastrocnemius preparations (Grassi *et al.*, 2002) and in humans (Bangsbo *et al.*, 2002) demonstrated that the administration of dichloroacetate did not affect the primary $\dot{V}O_2$ time constant or the anaerobic energy provision during the initial phase of exercise. This indicates either that the effects of PDC activation on muscle $\dot{V}O_2$ might be too small to be measurable in whole muscle $\dot{V}O_2$, or that acetyl group availability is not a significant limitation to the acceleration of oxidative metabolism in the transition to a higher metabolic rate. Rossiter *et al.* (2003) have recently provided evidence that dichloroacetate does not alter either the primary $\dot{V}O_2$ or [PCr] time constant during heavy exercise, but rather *reduces* the amplitude of the primary $\dot{V}O_2$ (and [PCr]) response. *These responses are quite unlike those observed following prior heavy exercise, and it is therefore unlikely that increased mitochondrial substrate provision is responsible for the effect of prior heavy exercise.* Finally, increased PDC activation would also be expected to alter the $\dot{V}O_2$ response to moderate exercise, which has never been observed during repeated bouts of exercise in humans.

Muscle temperature

One of the features of prior exercise interventions is that, depending on the intensity and duration of the prior bout, muscle temperature will be elevated during the performance of the subsequent bout. It has been suggested that an increase in the temperature of the exercising musculature might contribute to the $\dot{V}O_2$ slow component by a Q_{10} effect on muscle metabolism and/or by a decrease in the phosphorylation efficiency (Brooks *et al.*, 1971; Willis and Jackman, 1994). Surprisingly, Koga *et al.* (1997) reported a small but statistically significant reduction in the $\dot{V}O_2$ slow component after raising leg muscle temperature by ~3°C by passive heating using hot-water-perfused pants. Although the authors contended that the increase in muscle temperature was probably not high enough to cause an increase in $\dot{V}O_2$, it remains unclear how an elevated muscle temperature may reduce, rather than increase, the magnitude of the $\dot{V}O_2$ slow component. The authors suggested that the mechanical efficiency was improved due to a reduction in muscle viscous resistance. This hypothesis might explain why prior exercise, irrespective of whether or not it induces a metabolic acidosis, reduces the $\dot{V}O_2$ slow component during the subsequent exercise bout.

Several recent studies have addressed the potential role of muscle temperature in the effect of prior exercise. To investigate whether it is the elevated muscle temperature, *per se*, that is responsible for the reduction in the $\dot{V}O_2$ slow component following prior exercise, Koppo *et al.* (2002) inserted an indwelling thermistor in the vastus lateralis of subjects and measured the muscle temperature and $\dot{V}O_2$ during two consecutive 6 min bouts of heavy exercise. On a different day, the subjects performed another 6 min bout of heavy exercise but this time the exercise was preceded by a passive heating of the upper legs until the same muscle temperature was reached as at the start of the second exercise bout recorded on the first test day. A reduction in the $\dot{V}O_2$ slow component was only observed in heavy exercise following prior heavy exercise and not following passive heating of the upper legs, and it was concluded that muscle temperature does not play a significant role in the reduction of the $\dot{V}O_2$ slow component following prior exercise. Identical results were presented in another paper that demonstrated that prior sprint exercise elicited the characteristic effects of prior heavy exercise (increased primary amplitude, reduced $\dot{V}O_2$ slow component), whereas prior heating in a hot bath had no significant impact on the $\dot{V}O_2$ responses

(Burnley *et al.*, 2002b). *Collectively, it would appear that prior 'warming up' alone, in the strictest sense of increased muscle or core temperature, is unlikely to account for the effect of prior heavy exercise on the $\dot{V}O_2$ response.*

Improved muscle perfusion

The original proposal that the effect of prior heavy exercise on heavy exercise $\dot{V}O_2$ kinetics could be largely attributed to an acidosis-mediated increase in O_2 delivery (Gausche *et al.*, 1989; Stringer *et al.*, 1994; Gerbino *et al.*, 1996) remains a plausible explanation for the finding of speeded $\dot{V}O_2$ kinetics (Rossiter *et al.*, 2001; Tordi *et al.*, 2003). The notion that prior exercise can result in muscle vasodilatation is consistent with feedback control of muscle blood flow (Hughson and Tschakovsky, 1999), as well as the suggestion that active muscle undergoes 'functional sympatholysis' during exercise (Hansen *et al.*, 2000). Specifically, exercise is associated with increased sympathetically mediated vasoconstrictor tone in most vascular beds, including the resting muscle, but vasodilatation in the active muscle (i.e. 'sympatholysis'). Because skeletal muscle blood flow has the potential to far outstrip the ability of the heart to raise cardiac output to supply O_2, this response serves to defend central blood pressure whilst adequately increasing muscle blood flow (Rowell and O'Leary, 1990). It is well established that metabolites produced during muscle contraction are vasoactive (Haddy and Scott, 1968; Hester and Choi, 2002). The attractiveness of the hypothesis that muscle perfusion is increased at the onset of the second of two bouts of heavy exercise stems from the fact that the lactacidosis associated with the performance of the first bout of heavy exercise is still present at the onset of the second bout (Gerbino *et al.*, 1996), even when recovery is extended to 12 min (Burnley *et al.*, 2001, 2002a), and therefore the sympatholysis may be more marked under these conditions. Furthermore, it is clear that the performance of prior (high intensity) exercise is associated with increased heart rate (Bearden and Moffatt, 2001; Burnley *et al.*, 2002a; Tordi *et al.*, 2003), estimated cardiac output (Tordi *et al.*, 2003), muscle oxygenation (Ward *et al.*, 1994; Burnley *et al.*, 2002a; Fukuba *et al.*, 2002) and muscle blood flow (Bangsbo *et al.*, 2001; Krustrup *et al.*, 2001 but see also Fukuba *et al.*, 2004). *Thus, there is evidence that O_2 delivery is increased at the onset of the second of two bouts of heavy exercise utilizing the same muscle group.*

Further apparent support for an O_2 delivery-related mechanism can be found in the prior arm cranking study of Bohnert *et al.* (1998). The similarity of the effect of prior arm cranking on the $\dot{V}O_2$ response, albeit smaller in magnitude, suggested that a systemic acidosis *per se* was capable of influencing O_2 delivery and thus the $\dot{V}O_2$ response of the exercising leg. More recent data casts doubt on the suggestion that an acidosis at a remote site can increase muscle perfusion (Fukuba *et al.*, 2004) or speed the primary $\dot{V}O_2$ kinetics during cycle exercise (Fukuba *et al.*, 2002; Koppo *et al.*, 2003). Fukuba *et al.* (2002) showed that prior arm cranking that resulted in a similar degree of metabolic acidosis to prior leg cycling increased the primary component amplitude but had no effect on the primary $\dot{V}O_2$ time constant. These responses were associated with no evidence of an enhanced leg muscle perfusion during subsequent heavy cycle exercise, in contrast to the increase in haemoglobin concentration in the vastus lateralis observed after prior leg exercise. Similarly, Koppo et al. (2003) showed no change in the primary $\dot{V}O_2$ time constant but a significantly greater absolute increase in the primary $\dot{V}O_2$ response during heavy leg exercise preceded by heavy arm exercise (Figure 10.6). In the absence of speeded primary $\dot{V}O_2$ kinetics and with limited evidence of improved leg muscle perfusion after prior arm exercise, the cause of these $\dot{V}O_2$ responses is unclear, although the similarity between these responses and those following prior leg exercise (Bohnert et al., 1998; Koppo et al., 2003) suggests a similar mechanistic basis.

Despite evidence that O_2 delivery may be increased at the onset of a second bout of heavy exercise, most studies have not observed a speeding of the primary $\dot{V}O_2$ kinetics, suggesting that factors probably intrinsic to the exercising muscle are the dominant mediators of the primary component time course even for exercise of heavy intensity (Whipp et al., 2002). In support of this suggestion, recent evidence from both amphibian (Hogan, 2000) and mammalian (Behnke et al., 2002) muscle preparations have shown that the kinetics of the fall in microvascular PO_2 (which reflects the dynamic relationship between O_2 delivery and O_2 utilization) are speeded in a second contraction period. That the speeded PO_2 kinetics were the result of a reduced time delay before the fall in PO_2 in both studies suggests that the foreshortened time delay had an intracellular origin. The suggestion of an intracellular origin for the speeded PO_2 kinetics is further supported by the fact that the baseline PO_2 values were identical between the two contraction periods (Hogan, 2000; Behnke et al., 2002). Further, Behnke et al. (2002) demonstrated no residual lactacidosis or improved muscle blood flow in the second bout of muscle contractions. Recently, Fukuba et al. (2004) reported faster $\dot{V}O_2$ kinetics despite no change in leg blood flow kinetics (as measured with Doppler) during repeated bouts of leg extension exercise. These results demonstrate that an improved blood flow is not a prerequisite for a 'priming' effect to be observed in contracting muscle.

The data of Hogan (2000) and Behnke et al. (2002) contrast with those collected in humans in some important respects, as noted by the authors. Since no change in blood acid–base status was observed following the first exercise bout (Behnke et al., 2002), the contractions were presumably of moderate intensity, which has generally been shown to be ineffective in yielding the characteristic effect of prior exercise outlined earlier. Second, although Behnke et al. (2002) measured no change in blood flow at the onset of the second contraction period, it should be noted that the microvascular PO_2 alone cannot discriminate between changes in O_2 delivery and utilization during the transient phase of exercise. Third, the use of electrical stimulation in these preparations contrasts with voluntary motor unit activation (De Luca, 1985; Hunter and Enoka, 2003) and the attendant changes in microvascular perfusion (Van Teeffelen and Segal, 2000) and cardiovascular function (Rowell and O'Leary, 1990) that occur in humans. Thus, while the work of Hogan (2000) and Behnke et al. (2002) provide important evidence in favour of an intracellular origin to the priming effect of exercise, the applicability of these data to exercise in humans is presently unclear and requires further work.

Although increased O_2 availability does not appear to alter the primary $\dot{V}O_2$ time constant, it is possible that the primary and slow component amplitudes are sensitive to muscle O_2 delivery. Koga *et al.* (1999) demonstrated that heavy exercise in the supine position led to a reduction in the amplitude of the $\dot{V}O_2$ primary component and an increase in the amplitude of the $\dot{V}O_2$ slow component. Furthermore, both hyperoxia (MacDonald *et al.*, 1997) and prior heavy exercise (Burnley *et al.*, 2001, 2002a) increase the primary amplitude and reduce the $\dot{V}O_2$ slow component. One possible explanation for these findings is that the primary amplitude is constrained by the amount of O_2 delivered to the exercising muscle during heavy exercise, a suggestion that would also be consistent with the observation that the primary gain ($ml \cdot min^{-1} \cdot W^{-1}$) tends to be lower during heavy and severe exercise compared to that observed during moderate exercise (Jones *et al.*, 2002; Pringle *et al.*, 2003).

However, there are data inconsistent with the view that the primary component gain is sensitive to O_2 availability. Grassi *et al.* (1998) showed no change in the steady-state $\dot{V}O_2$ response in the electrically stimulated canine gastrocnemius despite markedly increasing the driving pressure of O_2 from the capillary to the muscle by administration of hyperoxia and RSR-13. Furthermore, because the primary $\dot{V}O_2$ response appears to be principally under feedback control (Whipp and Mahler, 1980), the primary amplitude is only attained once the error signal has been corrected (i.e. the difference between the required and instantaneous $\dot{V}O_2$ has decayed to zero). Simply stated, a $\dot{V}O_2$ response constrained by O_2 availability would leave the error signal uncorrected. Despite these concerns, it is currently difficult to explain the effect of hyperoxia and supine exercise on the $\dot{V}O_2$ response amplitudes by any other mechanism than that presented here. There is, however, an alternative explanation for the effect of prior heavy exercise on these response amplitudes, as detailed below.

Motor unit recruitment

A well-established hypothesis for the emergence of the $\dot{V}O_2$ slow component during heavy exercise is that this phenomenon reflects the recruitment of additional motor units (Poole *et al.*, 1994; Whipp, 1994). If additional motor unit recruitment is indeed involved in the aetiology of the $\dot{V}O_2$ slow component (Shinohara and Moritani, 1992; Saunders *et al.*, 2000; Perrey *et al.*, 2001; Burnley *et al.*, 2002a and Krustrup *et al.*, 2004), the fact that the slow component is reduced by prior heavy exercise suggests that either motor unit recruitment has been altered or there has been a change in the metabolic characteristics of the recruited fibre population. We recently hypothesised, based on our findings that the primary $\dot{V}O_2$ amplitude was increased in the absence of a change in the primary time constant (Burnley *et al.*, 2001), that the increased primary amplitude itself may be caused by increased motor unit recruitment (Burnley *et al.*, 2002a). Consequently, the leg muscle integrated electromyogram (iEMG) should be increased in the first 2 min of a second bout of heavy cycling exercise. Our findings were consistent with this hypothesis: both the primary amplitude and iEMG

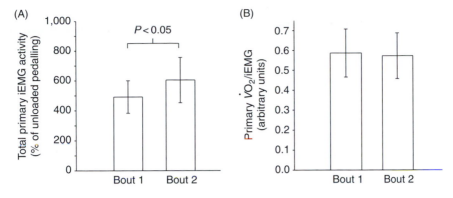

Figure 10.7 Averaged iEMG responses from three leg muscles in the first 2 min of two bouts of heavy exercise (panel A) and the primary $\dot{V}O_2$ response plotted as a function of the average muscle activity (panel B). The increase in muscle activity in panel A is approximately proportional to the change in the primary $\dot{V}O_2$ amplitude (panel B). Exercise bouts were separated by 12 min recovery. Reproduced with permission from Burnley *et al.* (2002a).

were increased in the second exercise bout, and these increases seemed to be proportional (Figure 10.7). Two other studies that have monitored muscle activity during repeated bouts of heavy cycle exercise did not detect significant changes in the leg muscle EMG (Scheuermann *et al.*, 2001; Tordi *et al.*, 2003), although the data of both groups showed a trend for higher iEMG values in the second heavy exercise bout. These findings do, however, reflect the limited sensitivity of surface EMG to subtle changes in motor unit recruitment during dynamic, multi-joint exercise such as cycling.

Figure 10.8 provides a hypothetical model of the effect of additional motor unit recruitment on the $\dot{V}O_2$ response to two bouts of heavy exercise separated by 12 min of recovery, based on a number of assumptions regarding motor unit recruitment during exercise. First, it is assumed that motor unit recruitment takes place in an orderly fashion from the smallest to the largest (the size principle; Henneman, 1985). Second, it is assumed that the recruitment of additional motor units mandates an O_2 cost independent of tension development (i.e. aerobic energy transfer utilized to maintain ionic homeostasis; Meyer and Foley, 1996). Third, the model assumes that the 'recruitment threshold' (the force or power output at which a motor unit is recruited) decreases as fatiguing exercise progresses, as recently demonstrated during ramped isometric contractions of the first dorsal interroseus by Carpentier *et al.* (2001) and by Adams and De Luca (2003) during isometric ramp-and-hold knee extension at 20% MVC. It is important to appreciate that the recruitment threshold occurs at a constant level of excitatory input from the central nervous system: the findings of Carpentier *et al.* (2001) and Adams and De Luca (2003) imply that this degree of excitation occurs at a lower level of tension development after prior fatiguing contractions.

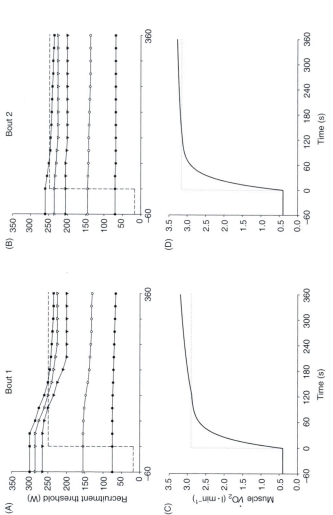

Figure 10.8 Hypothetical simulation of motor unit recruitment thresholds (panels A and B) and muscle $\dot{V}O_2$ (panels C and D) during repeated bouts of heavy exercise. Panels A and B show the recruitment threshold as a function of work-rate for five individual motor units. The dashed line represents the imposed work rate (panels A and B), the dotted line represents the primary O_2 demand (panels C and D). At the onset of the first bout of exercise, of those units monitored only the two 'low threshold' motor units are recruited (panel A), resulting in a 'normal' primary $\dot{V}O_2$ amplitude (panel C). As exercise continues, the recruitment thresholds of the three 'high threshold' motor units decline. These motor units are recruited as their thresholds drop under the work-rate curve. As this takes place, they too contribute to the $\dot{V}O_2$ response which results in the familiar slow component. In the second bout of exercise, the recruitment thresholds of the high threshold motor units remain depressed, resulting in the recruitment of two of them at the onset of exercise (panel B), which in turn results in an increased primary $\dot{V}O_2$ amplitude. Because fewer high threshold motor units are recruited as exercise progresses, the $\dot{V}O_2$ slow component is correspondingly reduced.

This model makes no assumptions about the mechanism responsible for the changes in recruitment threshold. Rather, it describes the effect of such an event on the $\dot{V}O_2$ response to heavy exercise. It is of interest, however, that Moritani et al. (1992) demonstrated that intermittent isometric contractions of the forearm following 1 min of suprasystolic occlusion were associated with an increased iEMG, suggesting that the metabolic state of the muscle may regulate voluntary motor unit recruitment. Furthermore, similar to the long latency of the effect of prior heavy exercise on the $\dot{V}O_2$ response, the depression of the recruitment threshold in high threshold motor units is also relatively long lasting (the recruitment thresholds were still depressed 15–30 min after the initial contractions; Carpentier et al., 2001), and this feature has been incorporated into the model. Thus, subsequent bouts of heavy exercise would likely recruit additional motor units at the onset of heavy exercise by virtue of the fact that motor units not normally recruited at that power output will discharge due to their recruitment thresholds being lowered. The effect, as shown in Figure 10.8, is an increased primary $\dot{V}O_2$ amplitude. Since more motor units share the power output, the rate of fatigue, lactate accumulation and rate of PCr degradation would all be reduced as a consequence, consistent with all recent experimental findings. Under these conditions, the effectiveness of the muscle pump may be increased and O_2 distribution within the muscle may be enhanced early in exercise. Further, since fewer motor units would need to be recruited as exercise progressed, the $\dot{V}O_2$ slow component would be correspondingly reduced. It is interesting to note that all of these factors would promote improved work-rate tolerance.

By far the biggest of the assumptions of the model is the applicability of the data of Carpentier et al. (2001) and Adams and De Luca (2003) to heavy dynamic cycle exercise. There are many potential problems in this regard. For example, it is not clear whether heavy cycle exercise is intense enough to alter the recruitment threshold of higher threshold motor units, given that Carpentier et al. (2001) used isometric contractions of a small muscle of the hand where force was ramped to 50% MVC; cycle exercise requires the coordination of most of the lower limb muscle mass to provide effective torque to the ergometer cranks. It has been estimated that high-intensity cycling requires no more than ~20% MVC shared across these muscles (Moritani and Yoshitake, 1998). It is of interest, therefore, that Adams and De Luca (2003) clearly observed additional motor unit recruitment during a series of sustained isometric contractions of the knee extensors at 20% MVC. Nevertheless, there is currently no experimental evidence from whole-body dynamic exercise in humans that corroborates the data of Adams and De Luca (2003) and until there is the model should be viewed as a plausible but speculative attempt to relate the changes in the $\dot{V}O_2$ primary and slow component amplitudes after prior heavy exercise with the increase in muscle activity observed by Burnley et al. (2002a). However, while this mechanism may explain the effects of prior heavy exercise when exercise is repeated using the same muscle group, it is more difficult to explain how this mechanism holds during cycling following prior arm exercise. Further work is clearly necessary to establish the precise role of motor unit recruitment in the $\dot{V}O_2$ response dynamics.

Conclusions and future directions

This chapter has reviewed the now relatively large body of work that has investigated the effect of prior heavy exercise on the pulmonary $\dot{V}O_2$ response to exercise. These investigations have highlighted the need to characterise the $\dot{V}O_2$ response with sufficient detail so that valid mechanistic inferences can be drawn from the observed response profiles. The original work of Gerbino *et al.* (1996) demonstrated that prior heavy exercise speeded the overall $\dot{V}O_2$ kinetics of heavy upright cycle exercise. Burnley *et al.* (2000), Koppo and Bouckaert (2001) and Scheuermann *et al.* (2001) subsequently showed that this speeding was the consequence of a reduction in the $\dot{V}O_2$ slow component. Further work by Burnley *et al.* (2001) and others (Burnley *et al.*, 2002a; Fukuba *et al.*, 2002; Koppo *et al.* 2003) showed that prior heavy exercise increased the size of the primary $\dot{V}O_2$ response and reduced the amplitude of the $\dot{V}O_2$ slow component without altering the primary time constant. Some evidence has been presented that prior moderate exercise, which does not elevate blood [lactate], may reduce the amplitude of the $\dot{V}O_2$ slow component (Koppo and Bouckaert, 2000, 2002), but in these studies the primary $\dot{V}O_2$ amplitude was unaltered. Two studies have presented evidence that the primary $\dot{V}O_2$ time constant is reduced by prior heavy exercise (Rossiter *et al.*, 2001; Tordi *et al.*, 2003). To what extent these results reflect differences in body position (Rossiter *et al.*, 2001) or experimental design (Tordi *et al.*, 2003) from those studies showing no change in the time constant awaits clarification.

In elucidating the mechanisms underpinning the effects of priming exercise, it is important to appreciate what the 'effect' is before generalizing to other exercise models (cf. Figure 10.9). *We suggest that the weight of evidence is in favour of the normal effect of prior heavy exercise being an increased primary $\dot{V}O_2$ amplitude, and a reduced $\dot{V}O_2$ slow component during subsequent heavy exercise, without a change in the primary $\dot{V}O_2$ time constant* (Figure 10.9B). The mechanism proposed must therefore be capable of yielding such a response profile. With this in mind, it would appear that muscle temperature, changes in mitochondrial enzyme activity and substrate flux, and altered blood flow cannot account completely or in all situations for the effect of prior heavy exercise. Muscle temperature changes typically seen during exercise do not alter the $\dot{V}O_2$ response appreciably during heavy exercise (Koga *et al.*, 1997; Koppo *et al.*, 2002). Neither changes in enzyme activity nor enhanced muscle blood flow seem to adequately explain the effects of prior heavy exercise. Improving the rate of substrate flux or O_2 delivery would be expected to speed the primary $\dot{V}O_2$ kinetics (a situation which has been rarely reported), and not to increase the primary $\dot{V}O_2$ amplitude. However, there are situations in which enhanced O_2 availability appears to influence the $\dot{V}O_2$ response amplitudes and not the primary $\dot{V}O_2$ kinetics (MacDonald *et al.*, 1997; Koga *et al.*, 1999). To what extent this may also explain the effect of prior heavy exercise has not been explored.

We have presented evidence that the increased primary $\dot{V}O_2$ amplitude observed after prior heavy exercise is associated with an increase in muscle activity measured

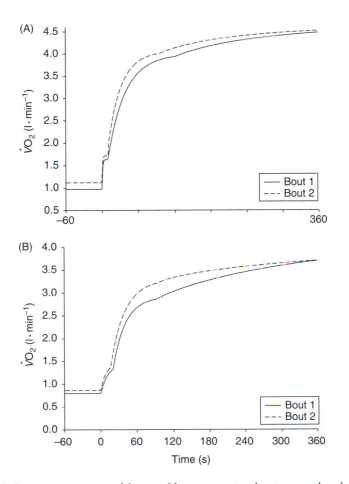

Figure 10.9 Responses to repeated bouts of heavy exercise showing a reduced primary time constant and an earlier emergence of the slow component (panel A) and increased primary amplitude and reduced slow component amplitude with no change in the primary time constant (panel B). Panel A is drawn from the parameter estimates of Tordi *et al.* (2003), and this response profile is consistent with enhanced O_2 delivery under conditions of O_2 delivery limited kinetics. Panel B is drawn from the parameter estimates of Burnley *et al.* (2002a), in which the authors suggest that an augmented motor unit recruitment at exercise onset was responsible for the increased primary $\dot{V}O_2$ amplitude. Notice that both panels show an increased $\Delta\dot{V}O_2/\Delta t$ in the second exercise bout, but the mechanisms proposed are completely different.

using electromyography (Burnley *et al.*, 2002a). This suggests that the recruitment of additional motor units at the onset of exercise may account for the altered $\dot{V}O_2$ response amplitudes in the absence of changes in the primary $\dot{V}O_2$ time constant. Though we believe that this is currently the most plausible hypothesis linking the observed $\dot{V}O_2$ responses to the underlying physiology, there remain many gaps in our mechanistic understanding of these responses. The observation of an effect of prior arm cranking on the primary and slow component $\dot{V}O_2$ amplitudes is not easily explained by the motor unit recruitment hypothesis, and there is no evidence that leg muscle activity is altered by prior arm cranking. The possibility that metabolites could be shuttled from remote sites to the legs and have a direct effect on metabolism or muscle function and thus the $\dot{V}O_2$ kinetics has not yet been explored in the present context. Crucial tests of the hypothesis presented here have yet to be conducted, and these will undoubtedly further our understanding of the physiological response to repeated bouts of exercise.

The implications of the effects of priming exercise on sport or exercise performance, though seemingly obvious, have been little explored. Two studies from our group have shown conflicting results in the effect of prior exercise on the time to exhaustion. Koppo and Bouckaert (2002) showed no change in the time to exhaustion at 90% $\dot{V}O_{2\ peak}$ following moderate or heavy exercise, whereas Jones *et al.* (2003) showed significant increases in cycling time at 100%, 110% and 120% $\dot{V}O_{2\ peak}$ following 6 min of heavy exercise and 10 min recovery. A striking feature of these two studies is that the blood [lactate] at exercise onset in the study of Jones *et al.* (2003) was less than half that observed at exercise onset in the data of Koppo and Bouckaert (2002), (~2.5 vs ~6.5 mM). *Further work is clearly needed to establish the optimal exercise intensity, duration and recovery periods required to improve exercise tolerance using prior exercise. The study of this intervention in athletic and particularly patient populations in the context of exercise tolerance clearly represents another important avenue for future experimental work.*

The 'prior exercise effect' has inspired a great many scientists to work towards an understanding of the physiological effect of priming exercise, and the $\dot{V}O_2$ response originally identified (Gerbino et al., 1996) is one of the most studied recent phenomena in this field of respiratory physiology. The theory Gerbino et al. (1996) originally advanced to explain the speeded $\dot{V}O_2$ kinetics has been thoroughly tested and has been significantly developed and extended recently, such that the mechanism responsible for the effect may differ significantly from that originally proposed. The hypotheses that enhanced O_2 availability or altered motor unit recruitment patterns increase the primary $\dot{V}O_2$ amplitude and reduce the $\dot{V}O_2$ slow component, currently stand as the two most likely to explain the prior exercise effect. It therefore seems appropriate to end this chapter as we began, with a quote from a Nobel Laureate that best summarizes our reflections on the original Gerbino hypothesis:

> So what happened to the old theory that I fell in love with as a youth? Well, I would say it's become an old lady, that has very little attractive left in her and the young today will not have their hearts pound when they look at her anymore. But, we can say the best we can for any old woman, that she has been a very good mother and she has given birth to some very good children.
>
> (Richard P. Feynman, 1965)

Glossary of terms

ATP	adenosine triphosphate
'effective' τ	effective time constant (time taken to reach 63% of end-exercise $\dot{V}O_2$ response)
EMG	electromyogram
iEMG	integrated electromyogram
MVC	maximal voluntary contraction
O_2	molecular oxygen
O_2 deficit	difference between energy required for work-rate and energy supplied though oxidative metabolism. The 'partial' O_2 deficit is calculated assuming the end-exercise $\dot{V}O_2$ is the energy requirement of exercise.
PCr	phosphocreatine
PDC	pyruvate dehydrogenase complex
Q_{10}	the increase in oxygen consumption caused by a 10°C increase in temperature (e.g. a Q_{10} of 2 would imply that oxygen consumption doubles for every 10°C increase in temperature)
RSR-13	a drug used to cause a rightward shift in the oxyhaemoglobin dissociation curve to facilitate peripheral O_2 diffusion
SEM	standard error of the mean
τ	time constant (time taken to reach 63% of the final amplitude in an exponential function)
$\dot{V}CO_2$	rate of pulmonary carbon dioxide output
$\dot{V}O_2$	rate of pulmonary oxygen uptake
$\dot{V}O_{2\ max/peak}$	maximum $\dot{V}O_2$ attained during, for example, an incremental exercise test to exhaustion
[]	denotes concentration

References

Adams, A. and De Luca, C.J. (2003). Recruitment order of motor units in human vastus lateralis muscle is maintained during fatiguing contractions. *Journal of Neurophysiology*, **90**, 2919–27.

Bangsbo, J., Krustrup, P., Gonzalez-Alonso, J. and Saltin, B. (2001). ATP production and efficiency of human skeletal muscle during intense exercise: effect of previous exercise. *American Journal of Physiology*, **280**, E956–64.

Bangsbo, J., Gibala, M.J., Krustrup, P., Gonzalez-Alonso, J. and Saltin, B. (2002). Enhanced pyruvate dehydrogenase activity does not affect muscle O_2 uptake at onset of intense exercise in humans. *American Journal of Physiology*, **282**, R273–80.

Barstow, T.J. and Molé, P. (1991). Linear and nonlinear characteristics of oxygen uptake kinetics during heavy exercise. *Journal of Applied Physiology*, **71**, 2099–106.

Bearden, S.E. and Moffatt, R.J. (2001). $\dot{V}O_2$ and heart rate kinetics in cycling: transitions from an elevated baseline. *Journal of Applied Physiology*, **90**, 2081–7.

Behnke, B.J., Kindig, C.A., Musch, T.I., Sexton, W.L. and Poole, D.C. (2002). Effects of prior contractions on muscle microvascular oxygen pressure at onset of subsequent contractions. *Journal of Physiology*, **539**, 927–34.

Bonhert, B., Ward, S.A. and Whipp, B.J. (1998). Effects of prior arm exercise on pulmonary gas exchange kinetics during high-intensity exercise in humans. *Experimental Physiology*, 83, 557–70.

Brooks, G.A., Hittleman, D.J., Faulknet, J.A. and Beyer, R.E. (1971). Temperature, skeletal muscle mitochondrial function, and oxygen debt. *American Journal of Physiology*, 220, 1053–59.

Buono, M.J. and Roby, F.B. (1982). Acid–base, metabolic, and ventilatory responses to repeated bouts of exercise. *Journal of Applied Physiology*, 53, 436–9.

Burnley, M., Jones, A.M., Carter, H. and Doust, J.H. (2000). Effects of prior heavy exercise on phase II pulmonary oxygen uptake kinetics during heavy exercise. *Journal of Applied Physiology*, 89, 1387–96.

Burnley, M., Doust, J.H., Carter, H. and Jones, A.M. (2001). Effects of prior exercise and recovery duration on oxygen uptake kinetics during heavy exercise in humans. *Experimental Physiology*, 86, 417–25.

Burnley, M., Doust, J.H., Ball, D. and Jones A.M. (2002a). Effects of prior heavy exercise on heavy exercise $\dot{V}O_2$ kinetics are related to changes in muscle activity. *Journal of Applied Physiology*, 93, 167–74.

Burnley, M., Doust, J.H. and Jones, A.M. (2002b). Effects of prior heavy exercise, prior sprint exercise and passive warming on oxygen uptake kinetics during heavy exercise in humans. *European Journal of Applied Physiology*, 87, 424–32.

Campbell-O'Sullivan, S.P., Constantin-Teosiu, D., Peirce, N. and Greenhaff, P.L. (2002). Low intensity exercise in humans accelerates mitochondrial ATP production and pulmonary oxygen kinetics during subsequent more intense exercise. *Journal of Physiology*, 538, 931–9.

Cardus, J., Marrades, R.M., Roca, J., Barbera, J.A., Diaz, O., Masclans, J.R., Rodriguez-Roisin, R. and Wagner, P.D. (1998). Effects of F(I)O$_2$ on leg $\dot{V}O_2$ during cycle ergometry in sedentary subjects. *Medicine and Science in Sports and Exercise*, 30, 697–703.

Carpentier, A., Duchateau, J. and Hainaut, K. (2001). Motor unit behaviour and contractile changes during fatigue in the human first interosseus. *Journal of Physiology*, 534, 903–12.

Cunningham, D.A., St Croix, C.M., Paterson, D.H., Ozyener, F. and Whipp, B.J. (2000). The off-transient pulmonary oxygen uptake ($\dot{V}O_2$) kinetics following attainment of a particular $\dot{V}O_2$ during heavy-intensity exercise in humans. *Experimental Physiology*, 85, 339–47.

De Bruyn-Prevost, P. (1980). The effects of various warming up intensities and durations upon some physiological variables during an exercise corresponding to the WC170. *European Journal of Applied Physiology*, 43, 93–100.

De Luca, C.J. (1985). Control properties of motor units. *Journal of Experimental Biology*, 115, 125–36.

Fukuba, Y., Hayashi, N., Koga, S. and Yoshida, T. (2002). $\dot{V}O_2$ kinetics in heavy exercise is not altered by prior exercise with a different muscle group. *Journal of Applied Physiology*, 92, 2467–74.

Fukuba, Y., Ohe, Y., Miura, A., Kitano, A., Endo, M., Sato, H., Miyachi, M., Koga, S. and Fukuda, O. (2004). Dissociation between the time courses of femoral artery blood flow and pulmonary $\dot{V}O_2$ during repeated bouts of heavy knee extension exercise in humans. *Experimental Physiology*, 89, 243–53.

Gaesser, G.A. and Poole, D.C. (1996). The slow component of oxygen uptake kinetics in humans. *Exercise and Sport Sciences Reviews*, 24, 35–70.

Gerbino, A., Ward, S.A and Whipp, B.J. (1996). Effects of prior exercise on pulmonary gas exchange kinetics during high-intensity exercise in humans. *Journal of Applied Physiology*, 80, 99–107.

Grassi, B. (2000). Skeletal muscle $\dot{V}O_2$ on-kinetics: set by O_2 delivery or by O_2 utilization? New insights into an old issue. *Medicine and Science in Sports and Exercise*, **32**, 108–116.

Grassi, B., Gladden, L.B., Stary, C.M. and Wagner, P.D. (1998). Peripheral O_2 diffusion does not affect $\dot{V}O_2$ -on kinetics in isolated in situ canine muscle. *Journal of Applied Physiology*, **85**, 1404–12.

Grassi, B., Hogan, M.C., Greenhaff, P.L., Hamann, J.J., Kelley, K.M., Aschenbach, W.G., Constantin-Teodosiu, D. and Gladden, L.B. (2002). Oxygen uptake on-kinetics in dog gastrocnemius in situ following activation of pyruvate dehydrogenase by dichloroacetate. *Journal of Physiology* **538**, 195–207.

Greenhaff, P.L. and Timmons, J.A. (1998). Interaction between aerobic and anaerobic metabolism during intense muscle contraction. *Exercise and Sports Sciences Reviews*, **26**, 1–30.

Greenhaff, P.L., Campbell-O'Sullivan, S.P., Constantin-Teosiu, D., Poucher, S.M., Roberts, P.A. and Timmons, J.A. (2002). An acetyl group deficit limits mitochondrial ATP production at the onset of exercise. *Biochemical Society Transactions*, **30**, 275–80.

Gutin, B, Stewart, K., Lewis, S. and Kruper, J. (1976). Oxygen consumption in the first stages of strenuous work as a function of prior exercise. *Journal of Sports Medicine*, **16**, 60–5.

Haddy, F.J. and Scott, J.B. (1968). Metabolically linked vasoactive chemicals in local regulation of blood flow. *Physiological Reviews*, **48**, 688–707.

Hansen, J., Sander, M. and Thomas, G.D. (2000). Metabolic modulation of sympathetic vasoconstriction in exercising skeletal muscle. *Acta Phyiologica Scandinavica*, **168**, 489–503.

Henneman, E. (1985). The size principle: a deterministic output emerges from a set of probabilistic connections. *Journal of Experimental Biology*, **115**, 105–12.

Hester, R.L. and Choi, J. (2002). Blood flow control during exercise: role for the venular endothelium? *Exercise and Sport Sciences Reviews*, **30**, 147–51.

Hogan, M.C. (2000). Fall in intracellular PO_2 at the onset of contractions in *Xenopus* single skeletal muscle fibers. *Journal of Applied Physiology*, **90**, 1871–6.

Howlett, R.A., Heigenhauser, J.F., Hultman, E., Hollide-Horvat, M.G. and Spriet, L.L. (1999). Effects of dichloroacetate infusion on human skeletal muscle metabolism at the onset of exercise. *American Journal of Physiology*, **277**, E18–25.

Hughson, R.L. and Tschakovsky, M.E. (1999). Cardiovascular dynamics at the onset of exercise. *Medicine and Science in Sports and Exercise*, **31**, 1005–10.

Hughson, R.L., Cochrane, J.E. and Butler, G.C. (1993). Faster O_2 uptake kinetics at onset of supine exercise with than without lower body negative pressure. *Journal of Applied Physiology*, **75**, 1962–7.

Hunter, S.K. and Enoka, R.M. (2003). Changes in muscle activation can prolong the endurance time of a submaximal isometric contraction in humans. *Journal of Applied Physiology*, **94**, 108–18.

Inbar, O. and Bar-Or, O. (1975). The effects of intermittent warm-up on 7–9 year-old boys. *European Journal of Applied Physiology*, **34**, 81–9.

Ingjer, F. and Stromme, S.B. (1979). Effects of active, passive or no warm-up on the physiological response to heavy exercise. *European Journal of Applied Physiology*, **40**, 273–82.

Jones, A.M., Carter, H., Pringle, J.S.M. and Campbell, I.T. (2002). Effect of creatine loading on oxygen uptake kinetics during submaximal exercise. *Journal of Applied Physiology*, **92**, 2571–7.

Jones, A.M., Wilkerson, D.P., Burnley, M. and Koppo, K. (2003). Prior heavy exercise enhances performance during subsequent perimaximal exercise. *Medicine and Science in Sports and Exercise*, **35**, 2085–92.

Koga, S., Shiojiri, T., Kondo, N. and Barstow, T.J. (1997). Effects of increased muscle temperature on oxygen uptake kinetics during exercise. *Journal of Applied Physiology*, **83**, 1333–8.

Koga, S., Shiojiri, T., Shibasaki, M., Kondo, N., Fukuba, Y. and Barstow, T.J. (1999). Kinetics of oxygen uptake during supine and upright exercise. *Journal of Applied Physiology*, **87**, 253–60.

Koppo, K. and Bouckaert, J. (2000). In humans the oxygen uptake slow component is reduced by prior exercise of high as well as low intensity. *European Journal of Applied Physiology*, **83**, 559–65.

Koppo, K. and Bouckaert, J. (2001). The effect of prior high-intensity cycling exercise on the $\dot{V}O_2$ kinetics during high-intensity cycling exercise is situated at the additional slow component. *International Journal of Sports Medicine*, **22**, 21–6.

Koppo, K. and Bouckaert, J. (2002). The decrease in the $\dot{V}O_2$ slow component induced by prior exercise does not affect the time to exhaustion. *International Journal of Sports Medicine*, **23**, 262–7.

Koppo, K., Jones, A.M., Vanden Bossche, L. and Bouckaert, J. (2002). Effect of prior exercise on $\dot{V}O_2$ slow component is not related to muscle temperature. *Medicine and Science in Sports and Exercise*, **34**, 1600–04.

Koppo, K., Jones, A.M. and Bouckaert, J. (2003). Effect of prior heavy arm and leg exercise on $\dot{V}O_2$ kinetics during heavy leg exercise. *European Journal of Applied Physiology*, **88**, 593–600.

Krustrup, P., Gonzalez-Alonso, J., Quistorff, B. and Bangsbo, J. (2001). Muscle heat production and anaerobic energy turnover during repeated intense dynamic exercise in humans. *Journal of Physiology*, **536**, 947–56.

Krustrup, P., Soderlund, K., Mohr, M. and Bangsbo, J. (2004). The slow component of oxygen uptake during intense, sub-maximal exercise in man is associated with additional fibre recruitment. *Pflugers Archives*, **447**, 855–66.

MacDonald, M., Pedersen, P.K. and Hughson, R.L. (1997). Acceleration of $\dot{V}O_2$ kinetics in heavy submaximal exercise by hyperoxia and prior high-intensity exercise. *Journal of Applied Physiology*, **83**, 1318–25.

Mahler, M. (1980). Kinetics and control of oxygen consumption in skeletal muscle. In P. Cerretelli and B.J. Wjipp (Eds) *Exercise Bioenergetics and Gas Exchange*. Elsevier/North-Holland Biomedical Press, Amsterdam, pp. 53–66.

Martin, B.J., Robinson, S., Wiegman, D.L. and Aulick, L.H. (1975). Effect of warm-up on metabolic responses to strenuous exercise. *Medicine and Science in Sports*, **7**, 146–9.

Meyer, R.A. and Foley, J.M. (1996). Cellular processes integrating metabolic response to exercise. In L.B. Rowell and J.T. Shepherd (Eds) *Handbook of Physiology Exercise Section 12: Regulation and Integration of Multiple Organ Systems*. American Physiological Society, Bethesda, pp. 841–69.

Mitchell, P. (1978). David Keilin's respiratory chain concept and its chemiosmotic consequences. In *Nobel Lectures Chemistry 1971–1980*, pp. 295–330 (available online at: www.nobel.se/chemistry/laureates/1978/mitchell-lecture.html).

Moritani, T. and Yoshitake, Y. (1998). The use of electromyography in applied physiology. *Journal of Electromyography and Kinesiology*, **8**, 363–81.

Moritani, T., Sherman, M., Shibata, M., Matsumoto, T. and Shinohara, M. (1992). Oxygen availability and motor unit activity in humans. *European Journal of Applied Physiology*, **64**, 552–6.

Patel, R., Rossiter, H.B. and Whipp, B.J. (2001). The effect of recovery time between repeated bouts of high-intensity exercise on the on-transient $\dot{V}O_2$ kinetics in humans. *Journal of Physiology*, 533P, 123–4P.

Paterson, D.H. and Whipp, B.J. (1991). Asymmetries of oxygen uptake transients at the on- and offset of heavy exercise in humans. *Journal of Physiology*, **443**, 575–86.

Perrey, S., Betik, A., Candau, R., Rouillon, J.D. and Hughson, R.L. (2001). Comparison of oxygen uptake kinetics during concentric and eccentric cycle exercise. *Journal of Applied Physiology*, **91**, 2135–42.

Perrey, S., Scott, J., Mourot, L. and Rouillon, J.-D. (2003). Cardiovascular and oxygen uptake kinetics during sequential heavy cycling exercises. *Canadian Journal of Applied Physiology*, **28**, 283–98.

Poole, D.C., Barstow, T.J., Gaesser, G.A., Willis, W.T. and Whipp, B.J. (1994). $\dot{V}O_2$ slow component: physiological and functional significance. *Medicine and Science in Sports and Exercise*, **26**, 1354–8.

Pringle, J.S.M., Doust, J.H., Carter, H., Tolfrey, K., Campbell, I.T. and Jones, A.M. (2003). Oxygen uptake kinetics during moderate, heavy and severe intensity 'submaximal' exercise in humans: the influence of muscle fibre type and capillarisation. *European Journal of Applied Physiology*, **89**, 289–300.

Rossiter, H.B., Howe, F.A., Ward, S.A., Kowalchuck, J.M., Doyle, V.L., Griffiths, J.R. and Whipp, B.J. (2001). Effects of prior exercise on oxygen uptake and phosphocreatine kinetics during high-intensity knee-extension exercise in humans. *Journal of Physiology*, **537**, 291–303.

Rossiter, H.B., Ward, S.A., Howe, F.A., Wood, D.M., Kowalchuck, J.M., Griffiths, J.R. and Whipp, B.J. (2003). Effects of dichloroacetate on $\dot{V}O_2$ and intramuscular ^{31}P metabolite kinetics during high-intensity exercise in humans. *Journal of Applied Physiology*, **95**, 1105–15.

Rowell, L.B. and O'leary, D.S. (1990). Reflex control of the circulation during exercise: chemoreflexes and mechanoreflexes. *Journal of Applied Physiology*, **69**, 407–18.

Saunders, M.J., Evans, E.M., Arngrimsson, S.A., Allison, J.D., Warren, G.L. and Cureton, K.J. (2000). Muscle activation and the slow component rise in oxygen uptake during cycling. *Medicine and Science in Sports and Exercise*, **32**, 2040–45.

Scheuermann, B., Hoelting, B.D., Noble, M.L. and Barstow, T.J. (2001). The slow component of O_2 uptake is not accompanied by changes in muscle EMG during repeated bouts of heavy exercise in humans. *Journal of Physiology*, **531**, 245–56.

Scheuermann, B., Bell, C., Paterson, D.H., Barstow, T.J. and Kowalchuck, J.M. (2002). Oxygen uptake kinetics for moderate exercise are speeded in older humans by prior heavy exercise. *Journal of Applied Physiology*, **92**, 609–16.

Shinohara, M. and Moritani, T. (1992). Increase in neuromuscular activity and oxygen uptake during heavy exercise. *Annals of Physiology and Anthropology*, **11**, 257–62.

Stringer, W., Wasserman, K., Casaburi, R., Porszasz, J., Maehara, K. and French, W. (1994). Lactic acidosis as a facilitator of oxyhemoglobin dissociation during exercise. *Journal of Applied Physiology*, **76**, 1462–7.

Timmons, J.A., Gustafsson, T., Sundberg, C.J., Jansson, E. and Greenhaff, P.L. (1998a). Muscle acetyl group availability is a major determinant of oxygen deficit in humans during submaximal exercise. *American Journal of Physiology*, **274**, E377–80.

Timmons, J.A., Gustafsson, T., Sundberg, C.J., Jansson, E., Hultman, E., Kaijser, L., Chwalbinska-Moneta, J., Constantin-Teodosiu, D., Macdonald, I.A. and Greenhaff, P.L. (1998b). Substrate availability limits human skeletal muscle oxidative ATP generation at the onset of ischemic exercise. *Journal of Clinical Investigation*, **101**, 79–85.

Tordi, N., Perrey, S., Harvey, A. and Hughson, R.L. (2003). Oxygen uptake kinetics during two bouts of heavy cycling separated by fatiguing sprint exercise in humans. *Journal of Applied Physiology*, **94**, 533–41.

Tschakovsky, M.E. and Hughson, R.L. (1999). Interaction of factors determining oxygen uptake at the onset of exercise. *Journal of Applied Physiology*, **86**, 1101–13.

Van Teeffelen, J.W.G.E. and Segal, S.S. (2000). Effect of motor unit recruitment on functional vasodilatation in hamster retractor muscle. *Journal of Physiology*, **524**, 267–78.

Ward, S.A., Skasick, A. and Whipp, B.J. (1994). Skeletal muscle oxygenation profiles and oxygen uptake kinetics during high-intensity exercise in humans. *Federation Proceedings*, **8**, A288.

Weltman, A., Stamford, B.A. and Fulco, C. (1979). Recovery from maximal effort exercise: lactate disappearence and subsequent performance. *Journal of Applied Physiology*, **47**, 677–82.

Whipp, B.J. (1994). The slow component of O_2 uptake kinetics during heavy exercise. *Medicine and Science in Sports and Exercise*, **26**, 1319–26.

Whipp, B.J. and Mahler, M. (1980). Dynamics of pulmonary gas exchange during exercise. In J.B. West (Ed.) *Pulmonary Gas Exchange*, Vol. II *Organism and Environment*. Academic Press, London, pp. 33–96.

Whipp, B.J. and Ward, S.A. (1990). Physiological determinants of pulmonary gas exchange kinetics during exercise. *Medicine and Science in Sports and Exercise*, **22**, 62–71.

Whipp, B.J. and Ward, S.A. (1992). Pulmonary gas exchange dynamics and tolerance to muscular exercise: effects of fitness and training. *Annals of Physiology and Anthropology*, **11**, 207–14.

Whipp, B.J. and Wasserman, K. (1972). Oxygen uptake kinetics for various intensities of constant load work. *Journal of Applied Physiology*, **33**, 351–6.

Whipp, B.J., Rossiter, H.B. and Ward S.A. (2002). Exertional oxygen uptake kinetics: a stamen of stamina? *Biochemical Society Transactions*, **30**, 237–47.

Williamson, J.W., Raven, P.B. and Whipp, B.J. (1996). Unaltered oxygen uptake kinetics at exercise onset with lower-body positive pressure in humans. *Experimental Physiology*, **81**, 695–705.

Willis, W.T. and Jackman, M.R. (1994). Mitochondrial function during heavy exercise. *Medicine and Science in Sports and Exercise*, **26**, 1347–54.

11 Influence of muscle fibre type and motor unit recruitment on $\dot{V}O_2$ kinetics

Andrew M. Jones, Jamie S.M. Pringle and Helen Carter

Introduction

Contraction of skeletal muscle produces the forces that enable movement to occur. When force requirement is low, only a relatively small volume of muscle needs to be recruited. However, as muscle force requirement increases, for example at higher work rates during cycle ergometer exercise, progressively more muscle mass has to be recruited. Human skeletal muscle comprises muscle cells (fibres) with distinct metabolic properties. There is generally thought to be an orderly hierarchy in fibre recruitment strategy with smaller low-threshold fibres being recruited first and larger high-threshold fibres being recruited as force requirement increases (Henneman *et al.*, 1965). Furthermore, during sustained exercise at the same constant work rate, there may be alterations in fibre recruitment as 'fresh' fibres replace 'fatigued' fibres (Vøllestad *et al.*, 1984; Vøllestad and Blom, 1985). There is also evidence that higher-order fibres make a proportionately greater contribution to force production at higher contraction frequencies (e.g. Beelen and Sargeant, 1993).

Given the well-known differences in energy metabolism and efficiency in the different muscle fibre types (see later), it has been suggested that alterations in muscle fibre recruitment might, at least in part, be responsible for the aetiology of the $\dot{V}O_2$ slow component phenomenon at work rates above the lactate threshold (LT) (Poole *et al.*, 1994; Whipp, 1994). This theory is indirectly supported by glycogen depletion studies that indicate that type II fibres are indeed active at heavy and severe work-rates (e.g. Gollnick *et al.*, 1974; Vøllestad *et al.*, 1984; Vøllestad and Blom, 1985; Ivy *et al.*, 1987; Beelen *et al.*, 1993). Differences in efficiency (in terms of differences in the ATP cost of force production and/or the O_2 cost of ATP resynthesis) or in the time constant for the increase in O_2 consumption following the onset of contractions in fibres of different 'types', might also impact upon the muscle (and pulmonary) $\dot{V}O_2$ response. However, while, in theory, differences and/or changes in fibre recruitment at higher work rates provide a strong explanation for the changes in $\dot{V}O_2$ kinetics at higher work rates, in practice this has been difficult to demonstrate conclusively.

Several approaches have been used to investigate the relationship between muscle fibre type and/or fibre recruitment and the parameters of the pulmonary

$\dot{V}O_2$ response to ramp and square-wave exercise. These include

(1) examination of differences in $\dot{V}O_2$ kinetics between individuals with different muscle fibre type distribution (Barstow et al., 1996, 2000; Mallory et al., 2002; Pedersen et al., 2002; Pringle et al., 2003a; Jones et al., 2004);

(2) assessment of the temporal relationship between the development of the $\dot{V}O_2$ slow component and changes in neuromuscular activation as assessed with electromyography (EMG) or magnetic resonance imaging (Lucia et al., 2000; Saunders et al., 2000; Borrani et al., 2001; Perrey et al., 2001; Scheuermann et al., 2001, 2002; Burnley et al., 2002; Pringle and Jones, 2002);

(3) assessment of the effect of manipulations of movement frequency/muscle contraction velocity (in an attempt to modify fibre recruitment patterns) on $\dot{V}O_2$ kinetics (Barstow et al., 1996; Pringle et al., 2003b; Jones et al., 2004);

(4) assessment of the effect of alterations in substrate availability (by the performance of exercise/dietary regimes designed to deplete specific muscle fibre pools of their glycogen content and so alter recruitment) on $\dot{V}O_2$ kinetics (Perrey et al., 2003; Bouckaert et al., 2004; Carter et al., 2004).

As might be anticipated, there are problems with each of these essentially indirect approaches. The establishment of relationships between muscle fibre type distribution, *per se*, and $\dot{V}O_2$ kinetics assumes that the muscle fibre type proportions determined from a small muscle biopsy from one muscle represents the muscle fibre type proportions across the entire muscle mass engaged during exercise and that the muscle fibres are recruited in these same proportions during exercise. While the former assumption may be reasonable, the latter is almost certainly not. Inherent noise in the measurement of both pulmonary $\dot{V}O_2$ (see Chapters 2 and 3) and EMG makes it difficult to establish relationships between the two variables. This is made even more difficult because muscle fibre recruitment will vary with work-rate, over time, across different muscles, with fatigue, and in different exercise modes. Although interventions such as the manipulation of muscle contraction frequency (by altering pedal rate) and the alteration of muscle glycogen availability should theoretically result in predictable alterations in muscle fibre recruitment, this is also difficult to confirm experimentally. It should also be cautioned that quantitative changes in muscle $\dot{V}O_2$ cannot be estimated precisely from whole-body $\dot{V}O_2$ in the transition from rest or unloaded cycling to exercise (see Chapter 6). It is possible, for example, that the $\dot{V}O_2$ associated with metabolic processes during the baseline period is altered upon the transition to exercise (Stainsby et al., 1980; Kautz and Neptune, 2002). For all these reasons, causality between changes in muscle fibre recruitment and changes in $\dot{V}O_2$ kinetics between low and higher work-rates have proven difficult to establish. Nevertheless, the approaches outlined above have provided substantial circumstantial evidence that muscle fibre recruitment impacts upon $\dot{V}O_2$ kinetics during exercise.[1]

Muscle fibre type, energetics and efficiency

There is great heterogeneity in skeletal muscle, both between muscles in the same species, and across different species. This heterogeneity is important in allowing the same muscles to be used for a variety of different activities from the maintenance of posture to the generation of maximal power. This is facilitated by the presence of numerous different fibre types possessing distinctly different functional features such as maximal shortening velocity, peak power and fatigue resistance (see Bottinelli and Reggiani (2000) and Sieck and Regnier (2001) for review).

Muscle fibre type has most frequently been classified histochemically by using acid and alkaline pre-incubation for the assessment of differences in myofibrillar ATPase activity (e.g. Brooke and Kaiser, 1970). With this approach, three main groups of muscle fibres, namely I, IIA and IIB were defined. The different functional and metabolic properties in these fibres also led to them being termed 'slow-twitch, oxidative' (type I), 'fast-twitch oxidative glycolytic' (type IIA), and 'fast-twitch glycolytic' (type IIB) to reflect the differences in contraction time and oxidative (and glycolytic) capacity. In general, mitochondrial density and capillary density is higher in type I muscle fibres than in type IIA muscle fibres, with type IIB fibres having lower values still. However, this histochemical classification of muscle fibre types is now regarded as being somewhat misleading (Staron, 1997). First, for example, while it is true that type I muscle fibres are generally more oxidative than type IIB, it is known that there is a wide range of metabolic enzyme activity within the same fibre type such that there can be significant overlap between muscle fibres of different 'types'. Second, it is now known that muscle fibres express several different specific myosin heavy chain (MHC) isoforms (which determine ATPase activity, maximum shortening velocity and rate of power output) and that there are numerous 'hybrid' fibres. There is therefore a continuum of contractile and metabolic properties across the 'different' types of muscle fibre. The electrophoretical identification of MHC isoform has also revealed that the fibre type previously classified as type IIB in human muscle does not contain MHC IIB but rather MHC IIX, and therefore the principal human muscle fibre 'types' have recently been reclassified as type I, type IIA, and type IIX (Bottinelli and Reggiani, 2000).

Human skeletal muscle fibres show a large variability in maximal shortening velocity and peak power. The force–velocity curves for the different types of muscle fibre demonstrate that type I muscle fibres develop peak power at a lower load and at a much lower velocity compared to type IIX fibres (with type IIA fibres being intermediate). As alluded to earlier, this is a useful design feature in that it ensures that muscle is capable of responding to a number of different tasks and challenges. Type I fibres are well suited to isometric and slow isotonic contractions due to their low tension cost, development of maximum power at low velocity and fatigue resistance. Type IIX muscle fibres are well suited to very fast and powerful contractions due to their high power and high efficiency at high velocities. Type IIA fibres are well suited to a wide range of movements at intermediate speeds due to their intermediate (in relation to type I and type IIX fibres) optimal velocity, power and tension cost. From the above, it is not surprising that 'postural' muscles have a higher percentage of type I (denoted as % type I hereafter) muscle fibres compared to, for example, muscles of the upper arm (Saltin and Gollnick, 1983), and that sprint and endurance athletes generally have lower and higher % type I fibres, respectively, in the locomotory muscles compared to the norm (Saltin and Gollnick, 1983).

The energy cost of isometric contractions (expressed as the amount of ATP split to develop a given amount of force) is considerably lower in type I than in type II and type IIX fibres (Steinen et al., 1996; Han et al., 2001, 2003). However, whether or not efficiency (calculated from the rate of energy liberated by ATP hydrolysis and the power produced) is different between type I and type II muscle fibres is unclear. When slow and fast muscles of small mammals have been compared, using different techniques, efficiency has generally, though not universally, been reported to be greater in slow muscles compared to fast muscles (cf. Gibbs and Gibson, 1972; Wendt and Gibbs, 1973; Crow and Kushmerick, 1982; Heglund and Cavagna, 1987; Barclay et al., 1993). The P/O ratio in mitochondria extracted from type I muscle fibres has been reported to be 18% higher than in mitochondria from type II fibres, which might reflect the use of different NADH shuttles (Willis and Jackman, 1994). In single fibres from the rat, Reggiani et al. (1997) reported that thermodynamic efficiency was higher in type I fibres than in type IIX fibres. In addition, it is known that the ATP utilisation for sarcoplasmic reticulum calcium pumping, which represents a significant fraction (30–55%) of the total cell ATPase activity, is appreciably greater in type IIB than type I muscle fibres (e.g. Szentesi et al., 2001). There is therefore some evidence, at least from animal muscle, that type II muscle fibres have both a higher ATP cost of force production and a higher O_2 cost of ATP turnover. This suggests that the recruitment of type II muscle fibres during high-intensity exercise could result in an additional O_2 cost of exercise, therefore potentially explaining the $\dot{V}O_2$ slow component. Unfortunately, however, very few studies have examined differences in efficiency between type I and type II fibres in human muscle.

In human fibres obtained from the vastus lateralis, He et al. (2000) reported that peak thermodynamic efficiency was not significantly different between type I and type IIA or type IIA/X fibres, although peak efficiency was obtained at a significantly lower relative load and speed of shortening in the type I fibres. However, it has recently been reported that the ATP cost of submaximal force development is lower in voluntary contractions (presumed to recruit only or predominantly type I muscle fibres) compared to contractions evoked by electrical stimulation (presumed to recruit both type I and type II fibres) (Ratkevicius et al., 1998). Overall, studies of both human and other muscle demonstrate that while differences in efficiency do exist between type I and type II fibres, these differences are not nearly as large as differences in maximal power or maximal speed of shortening. In whole human muscle, it is also clear that efficiency will depend greatly upon factors such as the exercise intensity and the rate of muscle contraction and corresponding changes in fibre recruitment. For example, at relatively slow movement speeds (e.g. at a pedal rate of ~60 rev · min⁻¹ during cycle exercise), the efficiency of recruited type I fibres would be close to optimal but the efficiency of any recruited type II fibres would be sub-optimal; the opposite situation would exist at higher movement speeds (e.g. at a pedal rate of ~120 rev · min⁻¹) (Sargeant, 1999).

In addition to possible effects on efficiency, it is also possible that the recruitment of type II muscle fibres might impact upon the time constant for the increase in muscle $\dot{V}O_2$ at the onset of exercise. For example, it has been reported that the time constant for the rise in $\dot{V}O_2$ in mouse soleus muscle (almost exclusively comprising type I and IIA fibres; ~36 s) is significantly faster than that in extensor digitorum lungus muscle (mainly type IIA and IIX fibres; ~138 s) (Crow and Kushmerick, 1982), presumably because of the greater oxidative enzyme activity in type I muscle fibres and/or the lower PCr concentration and faster PCr kinetics in type I compared to type II muscle fibres (Soderlund and Hultman, 1991). Assuming that similar differences in the rate at which $\dot{V}O_2$ increases at the onset of contractions exist in human muscle fibres, it is likely that if type II fibres comprised a large proportion of the total fibres recruited at the onset of heavy exercise, that this could result in a slowing of the primary $\dot{V}O_2$ response relative to an exercise domain in which only type I fibres were recruited. Alternatively, if type II fibres are 'progressively' recruited as heavy exercise proceeds, the slower kinetics in these fibres could be superimposed on the primary response and explain the 'slow' continued rise in $\dot{V}O_2$ with time. Therefore, while more studies of human muscle fibres are required, it appears that changes in muscle fibre recruitment patterns may provide a viable explanation for the $\dot{V}O_2$ slow component (see also Chapter 12).

Muscle fibre type and $\dot{V}O_2$ kinetics

The first study to directly investigate the relationship between muscle fibre type and $\dot{V}O_2$ kinetics was that of Barstow *et al.* (1996). In this study, nine subjects of heterogeneous fitness completed 8 min of heavy-intensity constant work-rate exercise (at 50% of the difference between the gas exchange threshold (GET) and $\dot{V}O_{2\,max}$; 50% Δ) and consented to a muscle biopsy of the vastus lateralis muscle for determination of muscle fibre type (i.e. % type I, IIA and IIX) by standard histochemistry. In support of the experimental hypothesis, the % type I muscle fibres was significantly correlated with the relative contribution made by the $\dot{V}O_2$ slow component to the end-exercise $\dot{V}O_2$ ($r = -0.83$ at a pedal rate of 60 rev · min⁻¹; $P < 0.01$). Although there was no difference in the gain ($\Delta\dot{V}O_2$ / ΔWR) of the $\dot{V}O_2$ response at the end of the 8 min of exercise, the greater slow component amplitude in subjects with a low % type I muscle fibres suggested that $\dot{V}O_2$ would have been higher in these subjects if exercise had been extended (Figure 11.1). These results are therefore consistent with reports that the % type I muscle fibres was associated with a reduced $\dot{V}O_2$ for the same work rate (i.e. improved efficiency) during cycling (Coyle *et al.*, 1992; Horowitz *et al.*, 1994), treadmill running (Bosco *et al.*, 1987) and leg extension exercise following

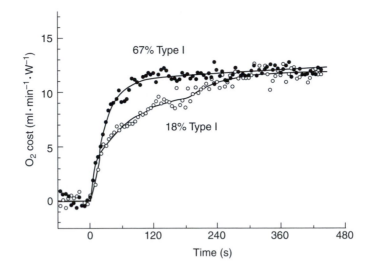

Figure 11.1 Representative $\dot{V}O_2$ responses to heavy exercise in subjects with a high % type I fibres and a low % type I fibres. Reproduced from Barstow *et al.* (1996) with permission.

pre-stretch (Aura and Komi, 1987). An unexpected observation in the study of Barstow *et al.* (1996) was that the % type I muscle fibres was also significantly correlated with the gain of the primary component $\dot{V}O_2$ response (G_p; $r = 0.78$ at 60 rev $\cdot$ min^{-1}; $P < 0.01$). Unfortunately, because of the positive relationship between aerobic fitness (as $\dot{V}O_{2\,max}$) and % type I muscle fibres, it was not possible for the authors to rule out the possibility that differences in fitness, *per se*, also influenced the results. However, the difference in the $\dot{V}O_2$ response to square-wave exercise in individuals with high vs low % type I fibres was striking (Figure 11.1).

Russell *et al.* (2002) examined the influence of % type I muscle fibres, citrate synthase (CS) activity and mitochondrial uncoupling proteins 2 and 3 (UCP2 and UCP3) mRNA levels on the relative magnitude of the $\dot{V}O_2$ slow component (calculated from the increase in $\dot{V}O_2$ after the first 3 min of heavy exercise) in groups of trained and untrained subjects. Similar to Barstow *et al.* (1996), these authors reported that both the % type I muscle fibres and markers of aerobic fitness were significantly negatively correlated with the relative magnitude of the slow component. Compared to the untrained subjects, the trained subjects had a lower relative magnitude of the slow component along with a lower expression of UCP2 and UCP3. Higher levels of UCP3 mRNA were associated with greater % type IIA muscle fibres and with a greater relative magnitude of the slow component. It has been shown that UCP3 expression is greatest in type IIX fibres, followed by type IIA, and then type I fibres, but is lower in all fibre types of trained subjects compared to untrained subjects (Hesselink *et al.*, 2001; Russell *et al.*, 2003). The precise function of UCP3 is uncertain but it has been suggested that it might uncouple the respiratory chain resulting in a reduction of aerobic ATP production. Further research is required to elucidate the possible role of UCP3 in altering muscle efficiency during heavy exercise.

Mallory *et al.* (2002) extended investigation of muscle fibre type on $\dot{V}O_2$ kinetics to the moderate exercise intensity domain. In this study, there was no significant correlation between % type I muscle fibres and the $\Delta\dot{V}O_2/\Delta WR$ slope established over four moderate-intensity work rates. Chilibeck *et al.* (1997) also reported that there was no significant relationship between % type I fibres and $\dot{V}O_2$ kinetics during moderate-intensity plantar flexion exercise either in young or old subjects. However, it was reported by Mallory *et al.* (2002) that $\dot{V}O_{2\,max}$ was weakly but significantly correlated with the $\Delta\dot{V}O_2/\Delta WR$ slope. In contrast, Pringle *et al.* (2003a) reported that % type I muscle fibres was significantly, albeit relatively weakly, correlated with G_p for moderate exercise ($r = 0.65$). Also, in contrast to Mallory *et al.* (2002), there was no significant relationship between $\dot{V}O_{2\,max}$ and G_p for moderate exercise. It is therefore unclear whether or not muscle fibre type or aerobic fitness is related to the $\Delta\dot{V}O_2/\Delta WR$ slope during moderate-intensity constant work-rate exercise. If a predominance of type I muscle fibres are recruited during moderate exercise, as might be reasoned, then no relationship between % type I muscle fibres and $\dot{V}O_2$ kinetics might be expected. However, it is equally difficult to explain why subjects of higher aerobic fitness might be relatively less efficient than less fit subjects during moderate exercise.

Pringle *et al.* (2003a) confirmed and extended the results of Barstow *et al.* (1996) by demonstrating that % type I fibres was significantly correlated with the relative amplitude of the $\dot{V}O_2$ slow component during both heavy ($r = -0.74$) and severe ($r = -0.64$) exercise in 14 subjects. Furthermore, % type I fibres was significantly correlated with G_p for both heavy and severe exercise (both $r = 0.57$). However, in contrast to Barstow *et al.* (1996), Pringle *et al.* (2003a) reported that % type I fibres was significantly negatively correlated with the time constant for the primary component $\dot{V}O_2$ response (τ_p) during heavy exercise ($r = -0.68$). This is consistent with the observation that the time constant for the rise in $\dot{V}O_2$ in predominantly type II mouse muscle is appreciably longer than that for predominantly type I muscle (Crow and Kushmerick, 1982). Interestingly, Pringle *et al.* (2003a) did not find a significant relationship between measures of muscle capillarity and τ_p, and suggested that the correlation between % type I muscle fibres and τ_p might be linked to the greater oxidative enzyme activity in type I compared to type II fibres.

Similar to Barstow *et al.* (1996), the data of Pringle *et al.* (2003a) clearly demonstrate that a subject's muscle fibre type has the potential to influence $\dot{V}O_2$ kinetics following the onset of exercise (Figure 11.2). However, given the inherent measurement error in both the dependent and independent variables, large sample sizes are preferable in studies designed to investigate the influence of muscle fibre type on $\dot{V}O_2$ kinetics. In Figure 11.3, we have combined the data from three studies (Barstow *et al.*, 1996; Pringle *et al.*, 2003a; Carter *et al.* (2004), making a total of 35 subjects) in order to more clearly define the relationship

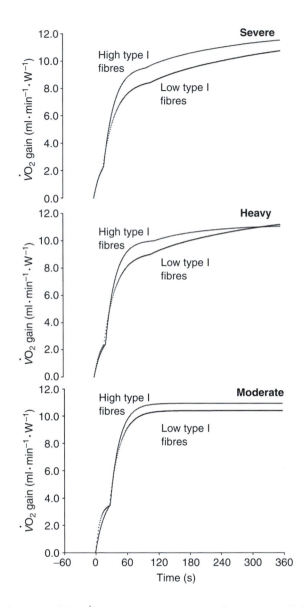

Figure 11.2 Schematic of the $\dot{V}O_2$ response to moderate (bottom panel), heavy (middle panel) and severe (top panel) exercise in subjects with a high and low % type I fibres. Reproduced from Pringle *et al.* (2003a) with permission.

between muscle fibre type and the amplitude of the $\dot{V}O_2$ slow component relative to the end-exercise $\dot{V}O_2$. The strength of this relationship is remarkable given the assumptions with this approach and the limitations to the methods outlined earlier.

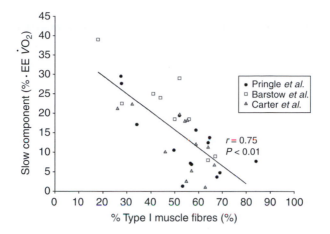

Figure 11.3 Relationship between the relative contribution made by the $\dot{V}O_2$ slow component to the end-exercise $\dot{V}O_2$ during 6 min of heavy-intensity cycle exercise and the % type I muscle fibres in the vastus lateralis. Data are from Barstow *et al.* (1996), Pringle *et al.* (2003a) and Carter *et al.* (2004).

The relationship between muscle fibre type and $\dot{V}O_2$ kinetics has also been assessed during ramp exercise (Barstow *et al.*, 2000; Lucia *et al.*, 2002; Pedersen *et al.*, 2002; Jones *et al.*, 2004), but the results are inconclusive. Barstow *et al.* (2000) reported that % type I muscle fibres was significantly correlated with the $\Delta\dot{V}O_2/\Delta WR$ slope for exercise both below and above the GET during ramp cycle exercise, but not with the mean response time of the response (a measure analogous to the sum of the initial time delay and the τ_p for constant work-rate exercise). The results of this study were therefore consistent with the results obtained by the same researchers for constant work-rate exercise (Barstow *et al.*, 1996). Pedersen *et al.* (2002), however, could not discern any relationship between muscle fibre type and indices of upward curvilinearity in the $\dot{V}O_2$ response for exercise above the GET. (NB The 'excess' $\dot{V}O_2$ observed above the GET during slow ramp exercise tests (e.g. Hansen *et al.*, 1988; Zoladz *et al.*, 1995) has been presumed to be of similar mechanistic origin to the $\dot{V}O_2$ slow component observed during constant work-rate exercise above the GET). Lucia *et al.* (2002) reported that % type IIX fibres was significantly correlated with the non-linear increase in $\dot{V}O_2$ above the GET, although it is possible that this relationship was skewed by 1–2 subjects with very high values for % type IIX fibres. Most recently, Jones *et al.* (2004) have reported that % type I fibres was significantly negatively correlated with the $\Delta\dot{V}O_2/\Delta WR$ slope for exercise above (but not below) the GET. In this study, subjects with a low % type I fibres had a significantly higher $\Delta\dot{V}O_2/\Delta WR$ slope for exercise above the GET compared to subjects with a high % type I fibres.

There is therefore no consensus on the influence of muscle fibre type on $\dot{V}O_2$ kinetics during ramp exercise. For exercise above the GET, the $\Delta\dot{V}O_2/\Delta WR$ slope has been reported to be not significantly correlated with % type I fibres (Pedersen *et al.*, 2002), and to be significantly correlated with % type I fibres (Barstow *et al.*, 2000), % type II fibres (Jones *et al.*, 2004), and % type IIX fibres (Lucia *et al.*, 2002). To add a further level of complication, Perez *et al.* (2003) have recently shown that the $\Delta \dot{V}O_2/\Delta WR$ slope for exercise above the GET was reduced from 9.8 to 8.6 ml $\cdot$ min^{-1} $\cdot$ W^{-1} on average following six weeks of electrical stimulation of the quadriceps which resulted in a significant increase in the % type II muscle fibres. The differences in the results are likely explained by a number of factors including variability in the measurement of the dependent and independent variables and differences in ramp test protocol (including ramp rate and time to exhaustion) and data analysis. The extent to which the $\Delta \dot{V}O_2 / \Delta WR$ slope changes for exercise above compared to below the GET may be an important factor in determining whether or not (and in which manner) muscle fibre type influences $\dot{V}O_2$ kinetics. In this respect, investigating the relationship between muscle fibre type and the ratio between the $\Delta \dot{V}O_2/\Delta WR$ slope for exercise above as compared to below the GET (Jones *et al.*, 2004) may be a useful approach.

Neuromuscular activation and $\dot{V}O_2$ kinetics

Progressive increases over time of the amplitude of the surface electromyogram (EMG) and the integrated electromyogram (iEMG) of the contracting muscles have been reported during sustained constant work rate, sub-maximal (typically <50% MVC) but fatiguing, isometric contractions, intermittent isometric contractions, and dynamic contractions (for review see De Luca, 1997). This increase in iEMG has also been reported for locomotory exercise such as cycling and running and the increases are generally greater at higher work rates (De Luca, 1997). In light of the evidence that the vast majority of the $\dot{V}O_2$ slow component originates from within the exercising limbs (Poole *et al.*, 1991), and given the strong theoretical arguments that type II fibre recruitment might, in some way, be related to the $\dot{V}O_2$ slow component (Poole *et al.*, 1994; Whipp, 1994; Barstow *et al.*, 1996; Gaesser and Poole, 1996; see earlier text), it is not surprising that a number of investigators have attempted to relate this progressive increase in iEMG with time to the $\dot{V}O_2$ slow component (Saunders *et al.*, 2000; Borrani *et al.*, 2001; Scheuermann *et al.*, 2001; Pringle and Jones, 2002).

It is not within the scope of this chapter to comprehensively examine all the factors that affect the EMG signal. However, where the muscle tension requirement presumably remains constant, for example during constant work-rate exercise, the common theory is that to compensate for a decrease in contractility of fatigued or impaired motor units (i.e. a slowed propagation of the neuromuscular action potential), the increase in iEMG represents (i) increased firing rate (rate-coding); and/or (ii) synchronisation of the activated fibres; and/or (iii) recruitment of previously inactive fibres. It is the latter mechanism that has received the most attention in the $\dot{V}O_2$ kinetics literature on the basis that the 'size principle' (e.g. Henneman, 1985) predicts that any additional motor units recruited will be of larger size and of higher threshold (i.e. type IIA and IIX fibres). This progressive and, it is assumed, hierarchical recruitment of additional motor units is believed to occur predominantly in muscles of mixed fibre type (i.e. a combination of both types I and II). Alternatively (or additionally), the increased rate-coding of the already recruited motor units is believed to occur in muscles which are predominantly composed of type I fibres and during large-muscle activity (De Luca, 1997). The relative importance of either process is believed to be dependent on the fibre type population and other factors such as the initial force requirement and speed of contraction, blood flow and the oxygen availability at the start of and during exercise, along with the initial state of fatigue and its subsequent rate of development (De Luca, 1997).

The higher EMG signal of type II motor units is due to their higher spike amplitude and, in muscles where the fast fibres are nearer the surface, their close proximity to the surface electrodes (De Luca, 1997). In certain conditions, the rate of increase in iEMG over time appears to be directly correlated with the % type II fibres of the active musculature and closely associated with the onset of fatigue. Thus, a concurrent slow rise in pulmonary $\dot{V}O_2$ and increases in iEMG from the exercising muscles during supra-threshold exercise has been interpreted as evidence that the serial (i.e. additional) recruitment of the supposedly less-efficient type II motor units is mechanistically linked to the development of the $\dot{V}O_2$ slow component (Shinohara and Moritani, 1992; Saunders *et al.*, 2000).

During incremental exercise, an increase in iEMG has often been associated with the commencement of an increase in blood lactate accumulation above baseline (i.e. the LT) and a disproportionate increase in $\dot{V}CO_2$ and $\dot{V}_E$ (relative to $\dot{V}O_2$; i.e. the GET), and it has been suggested that increased type II fibre recruitment underpins both the increase in lactate accumulation and the increase in EMG (e.g. Nagata *et al.*, 1981; Helal *et al.*, 1987; Mateika and Duffin, 1994; but see also Scheuermann *et al.*, 2002). During constant work-rate exercise, Shinohara and Moritani (1992) were the first researchers to present EMG evidence suggesting a link between an increase in neuromuscular activity with time and the $\dot{V}O_2$ slow component. They observed no change in either iEMG or $\dot{V}O_2$ with time during moderate exercise. However, during heavy exercise, an increase in iEMG of the quadriceps muscle was observed that was significantly correlated ($r = 0.53$) with the slow increase in pulmonary $\dot{V}O_2$ from 4 to 7 min. It should be noted, however, that the increase in $\dot{V}O_2$ beyond ~4 min of exercise in this early study is temporally inconsistent with evidence that the slow component either begins to emerge or at least becomes detectable at 2–3 min following the onset of exercise. Others have reported similar patterns of change in $\dot{V}O_2$ and root mean square (RMS) EMG activity during moderate and heavy cycling (e.g. Arnaud *et al.*, 1997; Jammes *et al.*, 1998). Fulco *et al.* (1995; 1996) reported a progressive increase in iEMG of the quadriceps muscle, concurrent with rising $\dot{V}O_2$ in subjects performing dynamic single-leg extension exercise at a work rate equivalent to 83% $\dot{V}O_{2\,max}$ (force of ~13% of the maximum voluntary contraction, MVC). In this research, subjects were also required to perform maximal voluntary contractions (MVCs) periodically throughout the protocol. The progressive decline in MVC was paralleled by a decline in iEMG elicited during the MVC and at exhaustion (to ~50% of their initial values). However, the iEMG measured at the end of the exhausting dynamic exercise equalled the iEMG value elicited by the MVC, indicating that the 'spare' capacity for force generation was attenuated. In similar experiments, Vøllestad and colleagues reported an increased $\dot{V}O_2$ (similar in nature and amplitude to the $\dot{V}O_2$ slow component phenomenon) during repeated isometric contractions at 30% MVC, and a gradual, concurrent decline in MVC (Vøllestad et al., 1990; Saugen and Vøllestad, 1996). During these experiments, a parallel increase in metabolic heat production was observed and the authors therefore attributed the increase in $\dot{V}O_2$ to a change in the energy cost of contraction.

More recently, Saunders et al. (2000) examined the contrast shifts (T_2, broadly indicative of muscle and/or muscle fibre recruitment/activation) in magnetic resonance images (MRI) and the EMG response in the vastus lateralis and rectus femoris to 15 min of moderate and heavy cycle exercise. During moderate exercise, there was no significant change between 3 and 15 min of exercise in either $\dot{V}O_2$ or in most (though not all) measures of muscle activation. However, during heavy exercise, a 285 ml·min^{-1} increase in $\dot{V}O_2$ was associated with significant increases in RMS EMG and mean power frequency (MPF) of the vastus lateralis (but not the rectus femoris) and in MRI T_2 measures of both muscles. The increase in $\dot{V}O_2$ with time was significantly correlated with the increase in T_2 but not with the increase in EMG. It should be noted here that although T_2 measures provide a broad index of muscle activation, it is presently not clear whether this reflects increased recruitment of fibres, *per se*, or increases in rate coding or metabolic changes in already recruited fibres. Interestingly, Saunders et al. (2000) found no correlation between changes in the T_2 measures and changes in the EMG measures.

Similar to Saunders et al. (2000), Borrani et al. (2001) reported an increase in the EMG mean power frequency (MPF) of the vastus lateralis and gastrocnemius muscles during a high-intensity treadmill run to exhaustion, with the increased MPF occurring simultaneously with the onset of the $\dot{V}O_2$ slow component. Interestingly, the MPF fell during the first two minutes of exercise (i.e. during the $\dot{V}O_2$ primary component phase). The explanation for this effect is not clear but it is possible that changes in MPF resulting from altered fibre type recruitment in this phase were masked. Unfortunately, Borrani et al. (2001) did not include a 'control' bout of moderate exercise in their study design and so were unable to categorically demonstrate that an increase in MPF only occurred during heavy exercise in which a $\dot{V}O_2$ slow component developed.

The results of Perrey et al. (2001) also provide some support for the theory that the $\dot{V}O_2$ slow component is associated with increased neuromuscular activity. In this study, the EMG and $\dot{V}O_2$ responses to moderate- and high-intensity concentric cycle exercise and high-intensity eccentric cycle exercise were measured. There was no change in MPF with time in any of the conditions. Furthermore, there was no change in iEMG with time for those conditions that did not elicit a $\dot{V}O_2$ slow component response (i.e. moderate concentric and high-intensity eccentric exercise) in any of the four muscles examined. However, there was a significant increase in iEMG in the rectus femoris and vastus medialis muscles (but not in the other muscles) during high-intensity concentric exercise where a $\dot{V}O_2$ slow component was observed. Burnley et al. (2002) have also shown an increase in iEMG (but no change in MPF) with time in the vastus lateralis, vastus medialis and gluteus maximus muscles during heavy exercise. In this study, the temporal profiles of iEMG and $\dot{V}O_2$ were altered in a corresponding fashion both before and after a bout of 'priming' exercise (see Chapter 10).

In contrast to these investigations, some investigators have not observed significant changes in EMG measurements even though a $\dot{V}O_2$ slow component was evident (Lucia et al., 2000; Scheuermann et al., 2001; Perrey et al., 2003; Tordi et al., 2003). Conversely, Takaishi et al., (1992, 1996) have reported an increase in iEMG *without* an increase in $\dot{V}O_2$ in some subjects. Lucia et al. (2000) reported that there was no change in either RMS-EMG or MPF during 20 min of cycling at ~80% $\dot{V}O_{2\ max}$ in professional cyclists. However, it is debatable whether or not this exercise intensity was sufficiently challenging to elicit appreciable alterations in the physiological responses in these subjects. Scheuermann et al. (2001) also reported no change in either iEMG or MPF during moderate exercise or during either the first or second bouts of heavy exercise. The iEMG was higher for heavy exercise compared to moderate exercise, but there was no difference in MPF. The results of Scheuermann et al. (2001) contrast with those of Burnley et al. (2002; see before). However, comparison is thwarted by differences in the way the data were normalised (to the initial value by Burnley et al., and to the end-exercise value by Scheuermann et al.). Using a similar model, Tordi et al. (2003) reported that there was no change in either iEMG or MPF with time in either the first or a subsequent bout of heavy exercise separated by fatiguing sprint exercise. Although iEMG was higher in the second bout in this study, substantial variability in the response precluded the attainment of statistical significance. In contrast, Perrey et al. (2003) reported that iEMG was generally lower in the latter part of a second bout of heavy exercise compared to the first bout (when these bouts were separated by 90 min moderate exercise). In this study, the MPF of the vastus medialis increased with time in both bouts, but there was no change in MPF in the other three muscles tested (vastus lateralis, biceps femoris, gluteus maximus).

In a recent study, we manipulated the amplitude of the $\dot{V}O_2$ slow component by having subjects run at the same relative intensity (separate bouts at 80% GET and 50% Δ) at treadmill gradients of 0% and 10% (Pringle et al., 2002), and simultaneously measured the iEMG in eight leg muscles (unpublished data). We hypothesized that increasing the $\dot{V}O_2$ slow component by increasing the treadmill gradient (and thus increasing the concentric/eccentric muscle contraction ratio; Minetti et al., 1994) during heavy exercise would be associated with a concurrent increase in neuromuscular activity. Concentric muscle action is associated with a lower mechanical work efficiency and greater fatigue (see Chapter 4). Uphill running resulted in a 40% larger $\dot{V}O_2$ slow component amplitude compared to running on the flat (397 vs 283 ml $\cdot$ min^{-1}; Pringle et al., 2002). Generally, there was a greater absolute iEMG at the heavy compared to the moderate running speeds. However, with the exception of the gluteus maximus and rectus femoris in heavy exercise, there was little change in iEMG with time in any of the individual muscles tested for either moderate or heavy exercise at either gradient (Figure 11.4). In those muscles where there was an increase in iEMG with time, there were only limited associations with the $\dot{V}O_2$ changes. When only the time period during

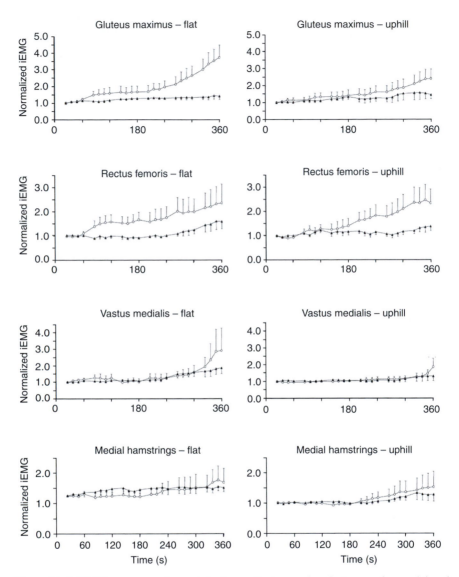

Figure 11.4 iEMG responses from eight lower limb muscles during moderate (closed symbols) and heavy (open symbols) intensity running on both a flat (0% grade) and inclined (10% grade) treadmill. Data are normalised to the value measured at 10 s into exercise. The $\dot{V}O_2$ slow component was significantly greater during heavy intensity running at 10% grade compared to 0% grade. Unpublished data from Pringle, Carter, Doust and Jones.

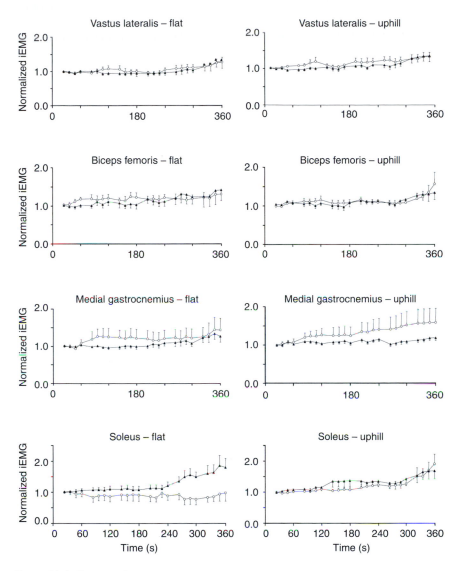

Figure 11.4 Continued.

which the $\dot{V}O_2$ slow component was developing was considered, there was no correlation between the relative amplitude of the slow component and the increases in the normalized iEMG at either gradient. Furthermore, for some muscles, the correlations were negative indicating that those subjects who had the greater changes in iEMG activity exhibited a lower $\dot{V}O_2$ slow component amplitude, and *vice versa*.

In another study (Pringle and Jones, 2002), we examined the relationship between the critical power, defined as the asymptote of the hyperbolic relationship between work-rate and time to fatigue (CP; Monod and Scherrer, 1965; Moritani *et al.*, 1981), the maximal lactate steady state (MLSS; i.e. highest work rate at which blood [lactate] increases by less than 1.0 mM between 10 and 30 min of constant work rate exercise; Beneke and von Duvillard, 1996), and the electromyographic fatigue threshold, defined as the highest work rate that can be maintained without an increase in iEMG over time (EMG$_{FT}$; Moritani *et al.*, 1993). If the $\dot{V}O_2$ slow component is associated with increased neuromuscular activity then, because $\dot{V}O_2$ increases inexorably with time for work rates exceeding CP/MLSS, these three 'thresholds' should be coincident. Indeed, Le Chevalier *et al.* (2000) reported that the work rates associated with a steady state in $\dot{V}O_2$, blood [La], and iEMG during local knee-extension exercise were significantly correlated and not significantly different (within 3%). However, during cycle exercise, we were unable to determine an EMG$_{FT}$ in the vastus lateralis in 4 out of 8 subjects. This was largely because iEMG often decreased over time at higher work rates. Indeed, it has been shown that during fatiguing moderate exercise (Fuglevand *et al.*, 1993), iEMG will increase with time as higher threshold units are recruited to maintain power output, whereas during near-maximal exercise, iEMG may decrease with time as motor units become de-recruited (Peters and Fuglevand, 1999). This feature of the iEMG response to fatiguing exercise, of course, adds greater complexity to interpretation of iEMG data in relation to the $\dot{V}O_2$ slow component. In the remaining 4 subjects in our study, there was no agreement between the work rates at the CP/MLSS and the EMG$_{FT}$. In the same study, we also examined the relationship between iEMG, $\dot{V}O_2$, and blood [lactate] during sustained exercise performed below, at, and above the pre-determined MLSS. Significant inter-individual variability meant that there were no significant changes in iEMG with time at any work rate. However, at the work rate below the MLSS, where neither $\dot{V}O_2$ nor blood [lactate] increased with time, iEMG actually tended to increase; on the other hand, at the work rate above the MLSS, where $\dot{V}O_2$ and blood [lactate] both increased significantly with time, iEMG tended to decrease.

It is clear from this discussion that there is no consensus concerning the relationship between neuromuscular activation and $\dot{V}O_2$ kinetics with some studies supporting such a relationship (Shinohara and Moritani, 1992; Saunders *et al.*, 2000; Borrani *et al.*, 2001; Perrey *et al.*, 2001; Burnley *et al.*, 2002) and others reporting no association between the two variables (Lucia *et al.*, 2000; Scheuermann *et al.*, 2001; Pringle and Jones, 2002; Perrey *et al.*, 2003; Tordi *et al.*, 2003). However, it is also clear from the above that measures of surface EMG which, in any case, are limited to detecting changes in activation of a limited amount of superficial muscle, may not be sufficiently sensitive to discriminate changes in neuromuscular activity (much less changes in fibre recruitment) and the measurement may be confounded by a variety of other factors. It is, therefore, perhaps not surprising that a strong relationship between EMG and pulmonary $\dot{V}O_2$ measurements (which are, in themselves, subject to variability and measurement error) are so rarely reported. It is interesting that all the studies that were unable to detect a significant alteration in iEMG with time either only assessed the response of the vastus lateralis muscle (Lucia *et al.*, 2000; Scheuermann *et al.*, 2001; Pringle and Jones, 2002) or the vastus lateralis was one of a few muscles examined (Perrey *et al.*, 2003; Tordi *et al.*, 2003). The study of a single muscle (perhaps especially the vastus lateralis), or a limited number of muscles, in previous studies may weaken the conclusions drawn regarding fibre recruitment and the origins of the $\dot{V}O_2$ slow component. In whole-body exercise, the muscle recruitment pattern is complex and the study of one muscle is unlikely to allow inferences to be made regarding activation patterns in other muscles. Also, ascribing the temporal changes in iEMG activity to fatigue processes assumes that the tension requirement of individual muscles remains constant. However, it is possible that fatigue-related changes in EMG activity of an agonist muscle could cause a change in EMG activity in a 'non-fatigued' antagonist muscle (or *vice versa*) (De Luca and Mambrito, 1987).

With regard to the MPF, some studies suggest that this increases with time during heavy exercise (Saunders *et al.*, 2000; Borrani *et al.*, 2001; Perrey *et al.*, 2003) while others suggest that it remains essentially constant (Lucia *et al.*, 2000; Perrey *et al.*, 2001; Scheuermann *et al.*, 2001; Burnley *et al.*, 2002; Tordi *et al.*, 2003). A shift to a higher frequency content in the power density spectrum (i.e. increased MPF) has been suggested to represent the recruitment of type II muscle fibres (Wretling *et al.*, 1987; Gerdle *et al.*, 1991). Saunders *et al.* (2000) and Borrani *et al.* (2001) therefore suggested that the increase in MPF they observed with time during heavy exercise was consistent with there having been a progressive recruitment of the type II fibre pool. Similarly, Scheuermann *et al.* (2001) proposed that the lack of change in MPF either over time during heavy exercise or between moderate and heavy work rates might mean that no additional type II fibres were recruited at higher work rates. The tendency for MPF to fall with time in the study of Burnley *et al.* (2002) might be interpreted to indicate that muscle fibres (perhaps particularly type II fibres) are becoming fatigued and/or de-recruited. However, interpretations of MPF data should be made with caution since it is known that MPF is increased by elevated muscle temperature (Bigland-Ritchie *et al.*, 1981), decreased by muscular fatigue (Ament *et al.*, 1993), and may be influenced by changes in the firing frequency of type I fibres as well as type II fibres.

In conclusion to this section, it is clear that pulmonary gas exchange responses and EMG activity are not, and should not be expected to be, related in any simple way. This is especially true when EMG is recorded from only one of a large number of muscles that are producing force and consuming O_2 during exercise. The complexity of the neuromuscular responses to fatigue indicate that it is impossible to use surface EMG to directly identify whether or not a specific muscle fibre type population has been recruited. On this basis we would suggest that the results of EMG studies should be interpreted carefully, with full acknowledgement of the limitations to the methods.

Interventions designed to modify fibre recruitment

Pedal rate

The force–velocity curves of type I and type II muscle fibres indicate that power and efficiency are optimised at higher velocities of contraction in type II than in type I muscle fibres (Sargeant, 1999). Consistent with this, it is notable that at high work rates (where type II fibres are likely to be recruited), subjects will tend to select higher pedal rates (compared to lower work rates) when given the choice (Marsh and Martin, 1993). Elite cyclists also select surprisingly high pedal rates (i.e. ~100 rev · min^{-1}) during competition. These high, freely chosen, pedal rates are higher than those that would result in the lowest gross $\dot{V}O_2$. It has been argued that this strategy is optimal because it minimizes the muscle tension per pedal thrust (MacIntosh *et al.*, 2000) and maximises the reserve power output generating capacity (Ferguson *et al.*, 2002). Figure 11.5 shows that the optimal velocity for muscle efficiency will vary according to the power output required along with the underlying muscle fibre type and recruitment strategy.

It is generally accepted that the proportional contribution of type II fibres to force production is enhanced at high compared to low pedal rates (Beelen and Sargeant, 1993; Beelen *et al.*, 1993; Marsh *et al.*, 2000; but see also Ahlquist *et al.*, 1992).

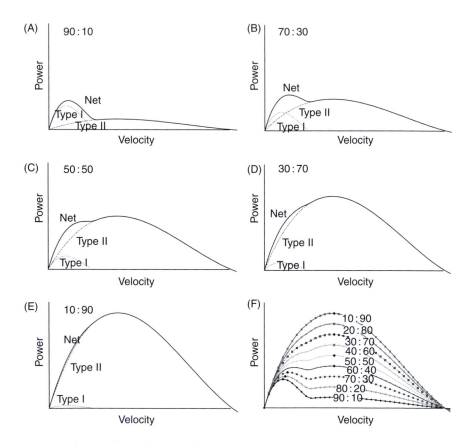

Figure 11.5 Hypothetical power–velocity profiles in subjects with different muscle fibre type distribution. The values in the top left corner of each panel refers to the relative proportions of type I to type II fibres. Notice how the velocity for peak power output (and also for optimal efficiency) shifts to the right as % type II fibres increases.

Therefore, the manipulation of pedal rate at the same relative exercise intensity is potentially useful in exploring the relationship between alterations in type II fibre recruitment and $\dot{V}O_2$ kinetics. Notwithstanding the potential complications arising from the different proportional recruitment of different muscles at higher pedal rates and of changes in efficiency of the principal fibre types at higher forces and contraction velocities, the results of such studies have proven insightful.

Barstow *et al.* (1996) examined the $\dot{V}O_2$ response to heavy-intensity constant work rate exercise at four different pedal rates (45, 60, 75, and 90 rev $\cdot$ min^{-1}) after adjusting the baseline and exercise work rates to account for differences in the O_2 cost of 'unloaded' pedalling across the pedal rates. There was no significant difference in the relative contribution of the $\dot{V}O_2$ slow component to the total increase in $\dot{V}O_2$ above baseline across the pedal rates (16–22 %). Although not specifically discussed in that paper, the G_p was significantly lower at 90 rev $\cdot$ min^{-1} (~9.4 ml $\cdot$ min^{-1} $\cdot$ W^{-1}) compared to the three lower pedal rates (~11.4–11.9 ml $\cdot$ min^{-1} $\cdot$ W^{-1}). Pringle *et al.* (2003b) employed a similar approach to Barstow *et al.* (1996) but extended the range of pedal rates used (35, 75 and 115 rev $\cdot$ min^{-1}) in order to amplify any differences in the effect of fibre recruitment on $\dot{V}O_2$ kinetics. At higher pedal rates, the G_p was significantly reduced whereas the absolute and relative amplitude of the slow component was significantly increased, such that the total end-exercise gain was not significantly different across pedal rates (Figure 11.6). Indirect evidence that type II fibre recruitment was indeed enhanced at the highest pedal rate came from the observation that the peak power output generated in a 6 s maximal cycle ergometer sprint performed within 10 s of the completion of the constant work rate bouts was

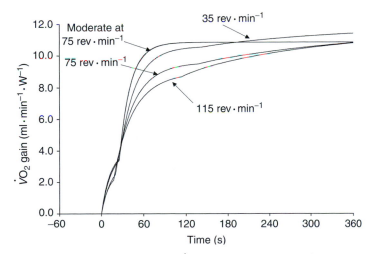

Figure 11.6 Schematic demonstrating the $\dot{V}O_2$ response to heavy cycle exercise at pedal rates of 35, 75 and 115 rev $\cdot$ min^{-1}. Notice the fall in the primary component gain, and the increase in the slow component gain, at higher pedal rates. The $\dot{V}O_2$ response to moderate exercise at 75 rev $\cdot$ min^{-1} is shown for comparison. Reproduced, with permission, from Pringle *et al.* (2003b).

significantly lower following heavy exercise at 115 compared to 35 rev·min^{-1}. Therefore, greater fatigue (presumably of the type II fibre population) was apparently associated with a greater amplitude of the $\dot{V}O_2$ slow component.

Consistent with the results of Pringle *et al.* (2003b), Jones *et al.* (2004) reported that the $\Delta\dot{V}O_2/\Delta WR$ slope for exercise below the GET (which should broadly reflect 'delta efficiency' (Mallory *et al.*, 2002) without contamination from non-linearities in the $\dot{V}O_2$ response for exercise > GET) was significantly steeper at 35 rev·min^{-1} compared to that at 75 and 115 rev·min^{-1}. However, there was no difference in the $\Delta\dot{V}O_2/\Delta WR$ slope across pedal rates for exercise above the GET. This latter result could be considered to be consistent with the results of Pringle *et al.* (2003b) for heavy constant work rate exercise in that the lower G_p was countered by a higher slow component gain at higher pedal rates with there being no difference in end-exercise gain across the pedal rates. The reduction in the $\Delta\dot{V}O_2/\Delta WR$ slope for exercise below the GET at higher pedal rates during ramp exercise is intriguing. However, a similar effect is evident in the data of Zoladz *et al.* (2000). Moreover, Scheuermann *et al.* (2002) reported that the $\Delta\dot{V}O_2/\Delta WR$ slope for exercise below the GET was reduced in very fast compared to slowly incremented ramp tests. Again, these data might be interpreted to suggest that type II fibre recruitment reduces $\dot{V}O_2$ at least early in the transition to a higher work rate, either as a result of a limitation in the potential to increase $\dot{V}O_2$ or because of slow adaptation of oxidative metabolism when compared to type I fibres.

Glycogen depletion/prior exercise

Another way in which muscle fibre recruitment during exercise might be modified is by using prior exercise and/or dietary regimes in order to fatigue specific muscle fibre populations. For example, depleting type I muscle fibres of their glycogen content (i.e. glycogen would be the principal substrate used during heavy exercise) might be hypothesised to result in increased recruitment of type II muscle fibres, and *vice versa*.

Bouckaert *et al.* (2004) recently examined the effect of glycogen depletion of the type I fibres on $\dot{V}O_2$ kinetics during constant work rate exercise at 85% $\dot{V}O_{2\,max}$. The glycogen depletion regimen used (a carbohydrate-free diet for 24 h and 2 h cycling at 60% $\dot{V}O_{2\,max}$) had been shown previously to result in almost complete glycogen depletion in type I muscle fibres (Gollnick *et al.*, 1974). Measurements of RER, and blood glucose, glycerol, lactate, ammonia, and free fatty acids all indicated that the glycogen depletion regimen had been successful. In the glycogen depleted condition, $\dot{V}O_2$ was ~100–150 ml·min^{-1} higher throughout exercise compared to the control condition, but there were no significant differences in the primary or slow component amplitudes or τ_p. Perrey *et al.* (2003) examined the effect of a 90 min bout of cycle exercise at ~60% $\dot{V}O_{2\,max}$ on $\dot{V}O_2$ kinetics and EMG during constant work rate exercise at ~90% $\dot{V}O_{2\,max}$. This study differed from that of Bouckaert *et al.* (2004) in that the glycogen depleting exercise bout was separated from the 90% $\dot{V}O_{2\,max}$ trial by just 30 min. Nevertheless, the results for $\dot{V}O_2$ kinetics were almost identical in these two studies. Specifically, Perrey *et al.* (2003) also reported that $\dot{V}O_2$ was higher at baseline (~100 ml · min^{-1}) and throughout exercise (140–200 ml · min^{-1}) when it was preceded by the 90 min moderate intensity exercise bout but there were no differences in the parameters of either the primary or slow components. Additionally, there were no differences in iEMG or MPF during exercise after, compared to before, the 90 min moderate exercise bout.

Perrey *et al.* (2003) suggested that the higher $\dot{V}O_2$ they observed throughout exercise following glycogen depletion might have been consequent to a greater recruitment of type II muscle fibres, elevated core and muscle temperature, or to a greater $\dot{V}O_2$ associated with the higher heart rate and minute ventilation. However, a similar elevation in exercise $\dot{V}O_2$ was noted by Bouckaert *et al.* (2004). despite the longer recovery period (~20 h) following the glycogen depleting exercise bout and the consequent equivalence of heart rate, minute ventilation, and presumably temperature between the control and experimental exercise bouts. Therefore, the higher exercise $\dot{V}O_2$ is most likely explained by a shift in substrate metabolism (the P/O ratio is lower for fat compared to carbohydrate metabolism). The data of Perrey *et al.* (2003) and Bouckaert *et al.* (2004) might be interpreted to indicate that alterations in muscle fibre recruitment caused by prior fatiguing exercise do not influence $\dot{V}O_2$ kinetics. However, to the extent that EMG data can be used to infer changes in motor unit recruitment, the data of Perrey *et al.* (2003) suggest that no changes in fibre recruitment occurred. Moreover, Bouckaert *et al.* (2004) argued that glycogen depletion of low-order muscle fibres might not be expected to alter fibre recruitment because these fibres could simply increase their use of free fatty acids as a metabolic substrate. In this respect, selective glycogen depletion of the type II muscle fibre population would be more likely to result in a change in fibre recruitment because type II fibres are not well suited to using fat as a metabolic substrate.

We recently addressed this latter possibility in a comprehensive study of the influence of glycogen depletion on $\dot{V}O_2$ kinetics (Carter *et al.*, 2004). In this study, 19 subjects performed repeated bouts of moderate and heavy exercise preceded by no prior exercise (control), 3 h of cycling at 30% $\dot{V}O_{2\,max}$ (to deplete type I muscle fibres), and 10 × 1 min bouts of high-intensity exercise at 120% $\dot{V}O_{2\,max}$ separated by 5 min recovery (to deplete type II fibres). Preliminary experiments in the same subject group with muscle biopsies had confirmed that these procedures successfully and selectively depleted the type I and type II fibre pools respectively. For example, the periodic acid Schiff (PAS) reaction for glycogen concentration demonstrated that 6%, 70% and 96% of type I, IIA and IIX fibres, respectively, were PAS dark (i.e. indicating the presence of muscle glycogen) following the low-intensity exercise protocol whereas 85%, 1% and 1% of type I, IIA and IIX fibres, respectively, were PAS dark following the high-intensity exercise protocol. Neither of the glycogen depletion regimens had any effect on $\dot{V}O_2$ kinetics during moderate exercise. Furthermore, consistent with Bouckaert *et al.* (2004), glycogen depletion of the type I fibres did not significantly affect $\dot{V}O_2$ kinetics during heavy exercise. However, glycogen depletion of the type II fibres resulted in a significant increase in the amplitude of the $\dot{V}O_2$ primary component along with a significantly later emergence and reduced amplitude of the $\dot{V}O_2$ slow component. Indirect confirmation that type II muscle fibres were glycogen depleted in this condition came from the finding that blood lactate accumulation was significantly reduced compared to the control condition. The increase in G_p and the reduced gain of the slow component in a condition where the recruitment of type II muscle fibres was presumably reduced (Figure 11.7) is consistent with the responses observed in subjects with a high proportion of type I muscle fibres (Barstow *et al.*, 1996; Pringle *et al.*, 2003a) and with the alteration in $\dot{V}O_2$ kinetics when muscle fibre recruitment is altered with extreme pedal rates (Pringle *et al.*, 2003b).

Interestingly, when heavy constant work rate exercise is performed within 6–12 min of a prior bout of high-intensity exercise, there is a significant increase in $\dot{V}O_2$ over the first 2–3 min of exercise and a significant reduction in the amplitude of the $\dot{V}O_2$ slow component (see Chapter 10 for detailed coverage of this topic). It is reasonable to suggest that prior sprint or heavy-intensity constant work rate exercise (which will elevate blood [lactate] to 5–10 mM) is likely to result in selective fatigue of the recruited type II fibres and that these might not have completely recovered their force-generating capacity before the onset of the subsequent heavy exercise bout. It is noteworthy, therefore, that the characteristic $\dot{V}O_2$ response (i.e. elevated G_p and reduced slow component gain) is identical to the $\dot{V}O_2$ response

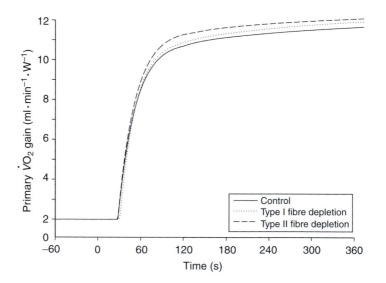

Figure 11.7 $\dot{V}O_2$ response to heavy exercise following glycogen depletion of the type I and type II fibre pools. The solid line represents the $\dot{V}O_2$ response in the control condition, the dotted line represents the $\dot{V}O_2$ response following a low-intensity exercise regime which resulted in substantial glycogen depletion of the type I fibre pool, and the dashed line represents the $\dot{V}O_2$ response following a high-intensity exercise regime which resulted in substantial glycogen depletion of the type II fibre pool. Note the increased primary component gain and reduced slow component gain with similar end-exercise gain following glycogen depletion of the type II fibres. Data from Carter *et al.* (2004).

observed following selective glycogen depletion of the type II fibre population (Carter *et al.*, 2004) and in subjects with a high proportion of type I fibres (Barstow *et al.*, 1996; Pringle *et al.*, 2003a), and opposite to the $\dot{V}O_2$ response observed when type II fibre recruitment is enhanced by performing cycle exercise at a high pedal rate (Pringle *et al.*, 2003b), (compare Figure 10.5A in Chapter 10 with Figures 11.2, 11.6 and 11.7 in this chapter). Consistent with this, there is evidence that the iEMG response changes in parallel with the $\dot{V}O_2$ response in two bouts of heavy exercise separated by a short recovery period (Burnley *et al.*, 2002). However, prior high-intensity exercise may also influence the $\dot{V}O_2$ kinetics during subsequent heavy exercise (when it is performed shortly afterwards) by a number of other mechanisms also (Jones *et al.*, 2003; see Chapter 10). One other situation in which an elevated G_p and a relatively small slow component response is observed is in exercising children (Williams *et al.*, 2001; see Chapter 13, Figure 13.2). However, for obvious ethical reasons, it is not presently known whether this response derives from there being a proportionately greater % type I fibres in the muscles of children.

Summary and conclusions

Although the data linking an increase in neuromuscular activity over time with the $\dot{V}O_2$ slow component is inconclusive, presumably due to the many technical and physiological complexities outlined in this chapter, there is nevertheless a raft of experimental evidence which suggests that muscle fibre type distribution and patterns of motor unit recruitment influence $\dot{V}O_2$ kinetics (Barstow *et al.*, 1996; Pringle *et al.*, 2003a,b; Carter *et al.*, 2004). Indeed, given the numerous factors which might conspire to confound the demonstration of a simple relationship between these variables, the consistency of the findings from the cross-sectional (i.e. % fibre type distribution) and 'manipulative' (i.e. pedal rate, glycogen depletion) studies is quite remarkable (see also note 1). Specifically, an increased activity/recruitment of type II muscle fibres is associated with a reduction in the G_p and an increase in the gain of the $\dot{V}O_2$ slow component. While a relationship between type II fibre activation and the $\dot{V}O_2$ slow component had been hypothesized (Poole *et al.*, 1994; Whipp, 1994), the consistent finding of a concurrently reduced G_p term had not been anticipated. It is clear, however, that any model designed to explain the complex $\dot{V}O_2$ kinetics observed during heavy exercise has to account for both these phenomena.

The finding that the % type I muscle fibres is significantly positively correlated with G_p during heavy and severe exercise (i.e. subjects with a greater proportion of type I fibres evidence a higher G_p) (Barstow *et al.*, 1996; Pringle *et al.*, 2003a) is worthy of comment. It is also necessary to note, however, that several studies have reported that G_p is lower for heavy/severe exercise compared to moderate exercise (Carter *et al.*, 2002; Jones *et al.*, 2002; Pringle *et al.*, 2003a,b; Scheuermann and Barstow, 2003). With the assumptions that subjects with a greater proportion of type I fibres recruit proportionately more type I fibres during heavy exercise of the same relative intensity (e.g. 50% Δ) compared to subjects with a low % type I fibres, and that type II fibres are recruited during heavy and severe exercise, these data suggest that the recruitment of type II fibres results in a fall in the G_p.

However, this is difficult to reconcile with *in vitro* data obtained in other species which appears to indicate a higher O_2 cost of contraction in type II compared to type I fibres (see earlier). However, in general, type II fibres have a lower oxidative capacity (reflected in a lower mitochondrial volume and capillary density), and a greater glycolytic capacity compared to type I fibres. It might therefore be reasonable to suggest that type II fibres have an inherently limited gain in comparison to type I fibres such that they might be obligated to meet some of the energy demand of contraction through O_2-independent pathways (Jones *et al.*, 2002; Pringle *et al.*, 2003b; Scheuermann and Barstow, 2003). The recent data of Behnke *et al.* (2003) showing a lower amplitude of both muscle blood flow and $\dot{V}O_2$ (derived from phosphorescence quenching measurements of microvascular PO_2) in peroneal compared to soleus muscle is potentially consistent with this view.

Another possibility for the reduced G_p in subjects with a low % type I fibres and for the falling G_p at higher work rates is that type II fibres have a large eventual gain but very slow kinetics. If a large proportion of the recruited type II fibres become active soon after the onset of exercise, this would tend to 'drag down' the G_p (because $\dot{V}O_2$ measured at the mouth will reflect the net O_2 consumption of all recruited fibres) but still result in a slow component (Koppo *et al.*, 2004; see Figure 15.3 in Chapter 15). It has been noted previously that changes in muscle fibre type and/or fibre activation with endurance training might at least partially explain the altered $\dot{V}O_2$ kinetics (e.g. faster kinetics, reduced $\dot{V}O_2$ slow component) evidenced in the trained state (Carter *et al.*, 2000). It is also of interest that interventions designed to increase muscle O_2 availability (e.g. prior exercise, hyperoxia) result in an increased G_p (e.g. MacDonald *et al.*, 1997; Burnley *et al.*, 2002) whereas some interventions designed to reduce muscle O_2 availability (e.g. supine exercise) have the opposite effect (Koga *et al.*, 1999). It is possible that the G_p is itself sensitive to O_2 availability or that muscle O_2 availability influences muscle fibre recruitment patterns which, in turn, influence the $\dot{V}O_2$ kinetics. The tendency for G_p to fall at higher work rates is discussed in more detail in Chapter 12.

Notwithstanding the difficulties in interpreting EMG data as highlighted earlier, there are several possible explanations for observed associations between changes in neuromuscular activity and the $\dot{V}O_2$ slow component. The mechanism responsible for the $\dot{V}O_2$ slow component has often been assumed to be the progressive and serial recruitment of type II fibres with time as heavy exercise proceeds and the initially recruited fibres become fatigued. Alternatively, it is possible that any increase in iEMG with time represents either an increased recruitment of both principal fibre types or an increased firing frequency of the initially activated fibres. It has been suggested that in the heavy and severe exercise intensity domains most of the available motor units, including the fatigue sensitive motor units, are recruited at or soon after the onset of exercise (cf. Sargeant, 1999). In response to the increasing deficit of contractile force in fatiguing fibres, an increase in iEMG might therefore represent rate-coding or synchronization of already recruited type I and IIA fibres which are fatigue resistant and have metabolic capacity to spare. On the other hand, the apparent constancy of the surface iEMG response seen in some studies could be interpreted differently. It may be that at very high forces the increases in iEMG due to rate coding or synchronization of fibres (i.e. type I and IIA) are masked somewhat by decreases in iEMG from other fibres that are mechanically failing (i.e. type IIX). However, in either scenario, fatigue in the type II (or type I) fibre pool as exercise continues might necessitate an increased activity (through increased activation, firing frequency or synchronization) of type I motor units.

The suggestion that type II fibres are recruited initially during heavy exercise and that these may drop out due to fatigue as exercise proceeds is consistent with reports of an increased or unchanged iEMG but no change in the mean power frequency during heavy exercise (Perrey *et al.*, 2001; Scheuermann *et al.*, 2001; Burnley *et al.*, 2002). Acceptance of this explanation, however, requires that the mechanistic basis for the $\dot{V}O_2$ slow component be re-considered. Specifically, in this scenario, the $\dot{V}O_2$ slow component need not necessarily nor wholly be explained by a progressive recruitment of type II fibres with inherently 'low efficiency'; rather, an alternative or complementary explanation is that the $\dot{V}O_2$ slow component arises due to the effects of fatigue on the initially recruited type II fibres.

In connection with this suggestion, it is instructive to consider the data of Pringle *et al.* (2003b). The reduced G_p observed at the highest pedal rate in this study and in a previous study (Barstow *et al.*, 1996) is consistent with the notion that type II fibres are operating closer to their optimal velocity of contraction for mechanical efficiency (Sargeant, 1999; He *et al.*, 2000; MacIntosh *et al.*, 2000). However, if type II fibre recruitment is enhanced at high pedal rates and the recruited type II fibres are operating at a velocity that is close to optimal for efficiency, then how might the greater amplitude of the $\dot{V}O_2$ slow component at the highest pedal rate in the study of Pringle *et al.* (2003b) be explained? One possibility is that the powerful but fatigue-sensitive type II fibres that are recruited during exercise at the highest pedal rate become fatigued as exercise progresses. The consequences of this might be increased fibre recruitment (of any 'remaining' type II fibres; i.e. the 'traditional' explanation for the evolution of the slow component) or increased rate coding of the already recruited and non-fatigued muscle fibres. In the latter case, type I fibres might be increasingly activated at a high contraction velocity that is sub-optimal in terms of their efficiency (He *et al.*, 2000) thus increasing $\dot{V}O_2$ with time. It is also possible that the fatigued fibres continue to require significant energy (as ATP) and to consume O_2 as they recover. Type II fibres have significantly greater calcium and sodium–potassium pump activity compared to type I fibres (Gibbs and Gibson, 1972; Szentesi *et al.*, 2001) such that the energy cost for the restoration of homeostasis in these fibres may be substantial although they may contribute only minimally, if at all, to force production.

This hypothesis (which does not exclude the 'traditional' explanation for the $\dot{V}O_2$ slow component that less efficient higher-order fibres are progressively recruited with time at high work rates) is attractive in that the continued phosphate turnover and O_2 consumption in recovering type II fibres is consistent with recent evidence that ATP turnover increases with time at high work rates with commensurate increases in $\dot{V}O_2$, that is that the $\dot{V}O_2$ slow component is associated with an increased phosphate turnover and need not be explained by altered P/O (Bangsbo *et al.*, 2001; Rossiter *et al.*, 2002; Krustrup *et al.*, 2003). Furthermore, it is perhaps unlikely that initially recruited type I fibres, which are by definition fatigue-resistant, would become fatigued and be replaced by type II fibres as heavy exercise progresses. Indeed, there is evidence that both type I and type II fibres are recruited at or close to the onset of heavy-intensity square-wave exercise (Vøllestad *et al.*, 1984; Vøllestad and Blom, 1985) and that type II fibres become fatigued first (Sargeant, 1999). The hypothesis that the $\dot{V}O_2$ slow component is related to the progressive 'de-recruitment' of fatigued type II fibres (Pringle *et al.*, 2003b), rather than or in addition to the progressive recruitment of type II fibres with time, is worthy of further study.

Glossary of terms

ATP	adenosine triphosphate
CP	critical power
CS	citrate synthase, mitochondrial enzyme
Δ	'delta', that is, difference or change in a value
% Δ	% difference (in $\dot{V}O_2$) between gas exchange threshold and $\dot{V}O_{2\,max}$
EMG	electromyogram
GET	gas exchange threshold
G_p	primary component 'gain' ($\Delta\dot{V}O_2/\Delta WR$)
LT	lactate threshold
MHC	myosin heavy chain
MLSS	maximal lactate steady state
MRI	magnetic resonance imaging
MPF	mean power frequency (of EMG signal)
MVC	maximum voluntary contraction
NADH	nicotinamide adenine dinucleotide reduced
O_2	oxygen
PCr	phosphocreatine
P-to-O ratio	ratio of ADP rephosphorylated to oxygen consumed
RER	respiratory exchange ratio
RMS	root mean square (EMG)
τ_p	time constant (time taken to reach 63% of the final amplitude) of the primary component $\dot{V}O_2$ response
UCP	uncoupling protein
$\dot{V}O_2$	oxygen uptake
$\dot{V}O_{2\,max}$	the maximum $\dot{V}O_2$ attained during for example an incremental exercise test to exhaustion
$\dot{V}CO_2$	carbon dioxide output
$\dot{V}_E$	pulmonary ventilation
WR	work rate

Note

1 While this chapter was in production, Peter Krustrup and colleagues at the University of Copenhagen published two papers which provide the first direct evidence that type II fibre recruitment is associated with the $\dot{V}O_2$ slow component (Krustrup *et al.*, 2004a,b). In the first of these studies, Krustrup *et al.* (2004b) measured PCr and glycogen concentrations in single muscle fibres of discrete types and reported that only type I fibres were recruited cycle exercise at 50% $\dot{V}O_{2\ max}$, where a steady state $\dot{V}O_2$ was attained after a few minutes. In contrast, during exercise at 80% $\dot{V}O_{2\ max}$, both type I and type II fibres were recruited from (close to) the onset of exercise, and additional fibres (of both types) were recruited with time in temporal association with the development of the $\dot{V}O_2$ slow component. However, the authors were unable to discriminate between (a) a shift in fibre recruitment pattern towards 'less-efficient' type II fibres and (b) an increased energy cost of recovery processes in previously active fibres, as the principal determinant of the $\dot{V}O_2$ slow component. In another study, Krustrup *et al.* (2004a) used a combination of low-intensity exercise and fasting to cause selective glycogen depletion of type I muscle fibres. This resulted in the recruitment of type II fibres and a significant elevation of pulmonary $\dot{V}O_2$ during moderate-intensity cycle exercise, compared to the control (glycogen replete) condition. Furthermore, there appeared to be a small continued increase in $\dot{V}O_2$ with time following glycogen depletion. The authors suggested that this represented the first demonstration of the $\dot{V}O_2$ slow component during moderate-intensity exercise where there is no blood lactate accumulation. It is unclear why the results of Krustrup *et al.* (2004b) differ from those obtained by other groups using similar procedures (Carter *et al.*, 2004). However, the elevated $\dot{V}O_2$ during moderate exercise suggests that the recruitment of higher order fibres reduces exercise efficiency, at least in the moderate domain (see also Brittain *et al.*, 2001). (Note, however, that the situation appears to be much more complicated during exercise $>$ LT; see main text for discussion.)

References

Ahlquist, L.E., Bassett, D.R., Sufit, R., Nagle, F.J. and Thomas, D.P. (1992). The effect of pedaling frequency on glycogen depletion rates in type I and type II quadriceps muscle fibers during submaximal cycling exercise. *European Journal of Applied Physiology*, **65**, 360–4.

Ament, W., Bonga, G.J.J., Hof, A.L. and Verkerke, G.J. (1993). EMG median power frequency in an exhausting muscle. *Journal of Electromyography and Kinesiology*, **3**, 214–20.

Arnaud, S., Zattara-Hartmann, M.C., Tomei, C. and Jammes, Y. (1997). Correlation between muscle metabolism and changes in M-wave and surface electromyogram: dynamic constant load leg exercise in untrained subjects. *Muscle and Nerve*, **20**, 1197–9.

Aura, O. and Komi, P. (1987). Effects of muscle fibre distribution on the mechanical efficiency of human locomotion. *International Journal of Sports Medicine*, **8**, 30–7.

Bangsbo, J., Krustrup, P., Gonzalez-Alonso, J. and Saltin, B. (2001). ATP production and efficiency of human skeletal muscle during intense exercise: effect of previous exercise. *American Journal of Physiology*, **280**, E956–64.

Barclay, C.J., Constable, J.K. and Gibbs, C.L. (1993). Energetics of fast- and slow-twitch muscles of the mouse. *Journal of Physiology*, **472**, 61–80.

Barstow, T.J., Jones, A.M., Nguyen, P. and Casaburi, R. (1996). Influence of muscle fibre type and pedal frequency on oxygen uptake kinetics of heavy exercise. *Journal of Applied Physiology*, **75**, 755–62.

Barstow, T.J., Jones, A.M., Nguyen, P. and Casaburi, R. (2000). Influence of muscle fibre type and fitness on the oxygen uptake/power output slope during incremental exercise in humans. *Experimental Physiology*, **85**, 109–16.

Beelen, A. and Sargeant, A.J. (1993). Effect of prior exercise at different pedalling frequencies on maximal power in humans. *European Journal of Applied Physiology*, **66**, 102–7.

Beelen, A., Sargeant, A.J., Lind, A., de Haan, A., Kernell, D. and van Mechelen, W. (1993). Effect of contraction velocity on the pattern of glycogen depletion in human muscle fibre types. In A. J. Sargeant and D. Kernell (Eds) *Neuromuscular Fatigue*. North Holland, Amsterdam, pp. 93–5.

Behnke, B.J., McDonough, P., Padilla, D.J., Musch, T.I. and Poole, D.C. (2003). Oxygen exchange profile in rat muscles of contrasting fibre types. *Journal of Physiology*, **549**, 597–605.

Beneke, R. and von Duvillard, S.P. (1996). Determination of maximal lactate steady state response in selected sports events. *Medicine and Science in Sports and Exercise*, **28**, 241–6.

Bigland-Ritchie, B., Donovan, E.F. and Roussos, C.S. (1981). Conduction velocity and EMG power spectrum changes in fatigue of sustained maximal efforts. *Journal of Applied Physiology*, **51**, 1300–5.

Borrani, F., Candau, R., Millet, G.Y., Perrey, S., Fuchslocher, J. and Rouillon, J.D. (2001). Is the $\dot{V}O_2$ slow component dependent on progressive recruitment of fast-twitch fibers in trained runners? *Journal of Applied Physiology*, **90**, 2212–20.

Bosco, C., Montanari, G., Ribacchi, R., Giovenali, P., Latteri, F., Iachelli, G., Faina, M., Colli, R., Dal Monte, A., La Rosa, M., Cortili, G. and Saibene, F. (1987). Relationship between the efficiency of muscular work during jumping and the energetics of running. *European Journal of Applied Physiology*, **56**, 138–43.

Bottinelli, R. and Reggiani, C. (2000). Human skeletal muscle fibres: molecular and functional diversity. *Progress in Biophysics and Molecular Biology*, **73**, 195–262.

Bouckaert, J., Jones, A.M. and Koppo, K. (2004). Effect of glycogen depletion on the oxygen uptake slow component in humans. *International Journal of Sports Medicine*, **25**(5), 351–6.

Brittain, C.J., Rossiter, H.B., Kowalchuk, J.M. and Whipp, B.J. (2001). Effect of prior metabolic rate on the kinetics of oxygen uptake during moderate-intensity exercise. *European Journal of Applied Physiology*, **86**, 125–34.

Brooke, M.H. and Kaiser, K.K. (1970). Muscle fiber types: how many and what kind? *Archives of Neurology*, **23**, 369–79.

Burnley, M., Doust, J.H., Ball, D. and Jones, A.M. (2002). Effects of prior heavy exercise on $\dot{V}O_2$ kinetics during heavy exercise are related to changes in muscle activity. *Journal of Applied Physiology*, **93**, 167–74.

Carter, H., Pringle, J.S.M., Jones, A.M. and Doust, J.H. (2002). Oxygen uptake kinetics during treadmill running across exercise intensity domains. *European Journal of Applied Physiology*, **86**, 347–54.

Carter, H., Jones, A.M., Barstow, T.J., Burnley, M., Williams, C. and Doust, J.H. (2000). Effect of endurance training on oxygen uptake kinetics during treadmill running. *Journal of Applied Physiology*, **89**, 1744–52.

Carter, H., Pringle, J.S.M., Boobis, L., Jones, A.M. and Doust, J.H. (2004). Muscle glycogen depletion alters oxygen uptake kinetics during heavy exercise. *Medicine and Science in Sports and Exercise*, **36**, 965–72.

Chilibeck, P.D., Paterson, D.H., Cunningham, D.A., Taylor, A.W. and Noble, E.G. (1997). Muscle capillarization O_2 diffusion distance, and $\dot{V}O_2$ kinetics in old and young individuals. *Journal of Applied Physiology*, **82**, 63–9.

Coyle, E.F., Sidossis, L.S., Horowitz, J.F. and Beltz, J.D. (1992). Cycling efficiency is related to the percentage of type I muscle fibres. *Medicine and Science in Sports and Exercise*, **24**, 782–8.

Crow, M.T. and Kushmerick, M.J. (1982). Chemical energetics of slow- and fast-twitch muscles of the mouse. *Journal of General Physiology*, **79**, 147–66.

De Luca, C.J. (1997). The use of surface electromyography in biomechanics. *Journal of Applied Biomechanics*, **13**, 135–63.

De Luca, C.J. and Mambrito, B. (1987). Voluntary control of motor units in human antagonist muscles: coactivation and reciprocal activation. *Journal of Neurophysiology*, **58**, 525–42.

Ferguson, R.A., Ball, D. and Sargeant, A.J. (2002). Effect of muscle temperature on rate of oxygen uptake during exercise in humans at different contraction frequencies. *Journal of Experimental Biology*, **205**, 981–7.

Fuglevand, A.J., Zackowski, K.M., Huey, K.A. and Enoka, R.M. (1993). Impairment of neuromuscular propagation during human fatiguing contractions at submaximal forces. *Journal of Physiology*, **460**, 549–72.

Fulco, C.S., Lewis, S.F., Frykman, P.N., Boushel, R., Smith, S., Harman, E.A., Cymerman, A. and Pandolf, K.B. (1995). Quantitation of progressive muscle fatigue during dynamic leg exercise in humans. *Journal of Applied Physiology*, **79**, 2154–62.

Fulco, C.S., Lewis, S.F., Frykman, P.N., Boushel, R., Smith, S., Harman, E.A., Cymerman, A. and Pandolf, K.B. (1996). Muscle fatigue and exhaustion during dynamic leg exercise in normoxia and hypobaric hypoxia. *Journal of Applied Physiology*, **81**, 1891–900.

Gaesser, G.A. and Poole, D.C. (1996). The slow component of oxygen uptake kinetics in humans. *Exercise and Sport Science Reviews*, **24**, 35–71.

Gerdle, B., Henriksson-Larsen, K., Lorentzon, R. and Wretling, M.L. (1991). Dependence of the mean power frequency of the electromyogram on muscle force and fibre type. *Acta Physiologica Scandinavica*, **142**, 457–65.

Gibbs, C.L. and Gibson, W.R. (1972). Energy production of rat soleus muscle. *American Journal of Physiology*, **223**, 864–71.

Gollnick, P.D., Piehl, K. and Saltin, B. (1974). Selective glycogen depletion pattern in human muscle fibres after exercise of varying intensity and at varying pedalling rates. *Journal of Physiology*, **241**, 45–57.

Han, Y.S., Proctor, D.N., Geiger, P.C. and Sieck, G.C. (2001). Reserve capacity for ATP consumption during isometric contraction in human skeletal muscle fibres. *Journal of Applied Physiology*, **90**, 657–64.

Han, Y.S., Geiger, P.C., Cody, M.J., Macken, R.L. and Sieck, G.C. (2003). ATP consumption rate per cross bridge depends on myosin heavy chain isoform. *Journal of Applied Physiology*, **94**, 2188–96.

Hansen, J.E., Casaburi, R., Cooper, D.M. and Wasserman, K. (1988). Oxygen uptake as related to work rate increment during cycle ergometer exercise. *European Journal of Applied Physiology*, **57**, 140–5.

He, Z.-H., Bottinelli, R., Pellegrino, M.A., Ferenczi, M.A. and Reggiani, C. (2000). ATP consumption and efficiency of human single muscle fibres with different myosin isoform composition. *Biophysical Journal*, **79**, 945–61.

Heglund, N.C. and Cavagna, G.A. (1987). Mechanical work, oxygen consumption, and efficiency in isolated frog and rat muscle. *American Journal of Physiology*, **253**, C22–9.

Helal, J.N., Guezennec, C.Y. and Goubel, F. (1987). The aerobic–anaerobic transition: re-examination of the threshold concept including an electromyographic approach. *European Journal of Applied Physiology*, **56**, 643–9.

Henneman, E. (1985). The size-principle: a deterministic output emerges from a set of probabilistic connections. *Journal of Experimental Biology*, **115**, 105–12.

Henneman, E., Somjen, G. and Carpenter, D.O. (1965). Excitability and inhibitability of motoneurons of different sizes. *Journal of Neurophysiology*, **28**, 599–620.

Hesselink, M.K., Keizer, H.A., Borghouts, L.B., Schaart, G., Kornips, C.F., Slieker, L.J., Sloop, K.W., Saris, W.H. and Schrauwen, P. (2001). Protein expression of UCP3 differs between human type 1, type 2a, and type 2b fibers. *FASEB Journal*, 15, 1071–3.

Horowitz, J.F., Sidossis, L.S. and Coyle, E.F. (1994). High efficiency of type I muscle fibers improves performance. *International Journal of Sports Medicine*, 15, 152–7.

Ivy, J.L., Chi, M.M.-Y., Hintz, C.S., Sherman, W.M., Hellendall, R.P. and Lowry, O.H. (1987). Progressive metabolite changes in individual human muscle fibers with increasing work rates. *American Journal of Physiology*, 252, C630–9.

Jammes, Y., Caquelard, F. and Badier, M. (1998). Correlation between surface electromyogram, oxygen uptake and blood lactate concentration during dynamic leg exercises. *Respiration Physiology*, 112, 167–74.

Jones, A.M., Carter, H., Pringle, J.S.M. and Campbell, I.T. (2002). Effect of creatine supplementation on oxygen uptake kinetics during submaximal cycle exercise. *Journal of Applied Physiology*, 92, 2571–7.

Jones, A.M., Koppo, K. and Burnley, M. (2003). Effects of prior exercise on metabolic and gas exchange responses to exercise. *Sports Medicine*, 33, 949–71.

Jones, A.M., Campbell, I.T. and Pringle, J.S.M. (2004). Influence of muscle fibre type and pedal rate on the $\dot{V}O_2$–work rate slope during ramp exercise. *European Journal of Applied Physiology*, 91(2–3), 238–45.

Kautz, S.A. and Neptune, R.R (2002). Biomechanical determinants of pedaling energetics: internal and external work are not independent. *Exercise and Sport Science Reviews*, 30(4), 159–65.

Koga, S., Shiojiri, T., Shibasaki, M., Kondo, N., Fukuba, Y. and Barstow, T.J. (1999). Kinetics of oxygen uptake during supine and upright heavy exercise. *Journal of Applied Physiology*, 87, 253–60.

Koppo, K., Bouckaert, J. and Jones A.M. (2004). Effect of training status and exercise intensity on phase II $\dot{V}O_2$ kinetics. *Medicine and Science in Sports and Exercise*, 36(2), 225–32.

Krustrup, P., Ferguson, R.A., Kjar, M. and Bangsbo, J. (2003). ATP and heat production in human skeletal muscle during dynamic exercise: higher efficiency of anaerobic than aerobic ATP resynthesis. *Journal of Physiology*, 549, 255–69.

Krustrup, P., Soderlund, K., Mohr, M. and Bangsbo, J. (2004a). Slow-twitch fiber glycogen depletion elevates moderate-exercise fast-twitch fiber activity and O_2 uptake. *Medicine and Science in Sports and Exercise*, 36, 973–82.

Krustrup, P., Soderlund, K., Mohr, M. and Bangsbo, J. (2004b). The slow component of oxygen uptake during intense, sub-maximal exercise in man is associated with additional fibre recruitment. *Pflugers Archives*, 447, 855–66.

Le Chevalier, J.M., Vandewalle, H., Thepaut-Mathieu, C., Stein, J.F. and Caplan, L. (2000). Local critical power is an index of local endurance. *European Journal of Applied Physiology*, 81, 120–7.

Lucia, A., Hoyos, J. and Chicharro, J.L. (2000). The slow component of $\dot{V}O_2$ in professional cyclists. *British Journal of Sports Medicine*, 34, 367–74.

Lucia, A., Rivero, J.-L.L., Perez, M., Serrano, A.L., Calbet, J.A.L., Santalla, A. and Chicharro, J.L. (2002). Determinants of $\dot{V}O_2$ kinetics at high power outputs during a ramp exercise protocol. *Medicine and Science in Sports and Exercise*, 34, 326–31.

Macdonald, M., Pedersen, P.K. and Hughson, R.L. (1997). Acceleration of $\dot{V}O_2$ kinetics in heavy submaximal exercise by hyperoxia and prior high-intensity exercise. *Journal of Applied Physiology*, 83, 1318–25.

MacIntosh, B.R., Neptune, R.R. and Horton, J.F. (2000). Cadence, power, and muscle activation in cycle ergometry. *Medicine and Science in Sports and Exercise*, 32, 1281–7.

Mallory, L.A., Scheuermann, B.W., Hoelting, B.D., Weiss, M.L., McAllister, R.M. and Barstow, T.J. (2002). Influence of peak $\dot{V}O_2$ and muscle fibre type on the efficiency of moderate exercise. *Medicine and Science in Sports and Exercise*, **34**, 1279–87.

Marsh, A.P. and Martin, P.E. (1993). The association between cycling experience and preferred and most economical cadences. *Medicine and Science in Sports and Exercise*, **25**, 1269–74.

Marsh, A.P., Martin, P.E. and Foley, K.O. (2000). Effect of cadence, cycling experience, and aerobic power on delta efficiency during cycling. *Medicine and Science in Sports and Exercise*, **32**, 1630–4.

Mateika, J.H. and Duffin, J. (1994). Coincidental changes in ventilation and electromyographic activity during consecutive incremental exercise tests. *European Journal of Applied Physiology*, **68**, 54–61.

Minetti, A.E., Ardigo, L.P. and Saibene, F. (1994). Mechanical determinants of the minimum energy cost of gradient running in humans. *Journal of Experimental Biology*, **195**, 211–25.

Monod, H. and Scherrer, J. (1965). The work capacity of a synergic muscle group. *Ergonomics*, **8**, 329–38.

Moritani, T., Nagata, A., deVries, H.A. and Muro, M. (1981). Critical power as a measure of physical work capacity and anaerobic threshold. *Ergonomics*, **24**, 339–50.

Moritani, T., Takaishi, T. and Matsumoto, T. (1993). Determination of maximal power output at neuromuscular fatigue threshold. *Medicine and Science in Sports and Exercise*, **74**, 1729–34.

Nagata, A., Muro, M., Moritani, T. and Yoshida, T. (1981). Anaerobic threshold determination by blood lactate and myoelectric signals. *Japanese Journal of Physiology*, **31**, 585–97.

Pedersen, P.K., Sorensen, J.B., Jensen, K., Johansen, L. and Levin, K. (2002). Muscle fibre type distribution and nonlinear $\dot{V}O_2$–power output relationship in cycling. *Medicine and Science in Sports and Exercise*, **34**, 655–61.

Perez, M., Lucia, A., Santalla, A. and Chicharro, J.L. (2003). Effects of electrical stimulation on $\dot{V}O_2$ kinetics and delta efficiency in healthy young men. *British Journal of Sports Medicine*, **37**, 140–3.

Perrey, S., Betik, A., Candau, R., Rouillon, J.D. and Hughson, R.L. (2001). Comparison of oxygen uptake kinetics during concentric and eccentric cycle exercise. *Journal of Applied Physiology*, **91**, 2135–42.

Perrey, S., Candau, R., Rouillon, J.D. and Hughson, R.L. (2003). The effect of prolonged submaximal exercise on gas exchange kinetics and ventilation during heavy exercise in humans. *European Journal of Applied Physiology*, **89**, 587–94.

Peters, E.J. and Fuglevand, A.J. (1999). Cessation of human motor unit discharge during sustained maximal voluntary contraction. *Neuroscience Letters*, **274**, 66–70.

Poole, D.C., Schaffartzik, W., Knight, D.R., Derion, T., Kennedy, B., Guy, H.J., Prediletto, R. and Wagner, P.D. (1991). Contribution of excising legs to the slow component of oxygen uptake kinetics in humans. *Journal of Applied Physiology*, **71**, 1245–60.

Poole, D.C., Barstow, T.J., Gaesser, G.A., Willis, W.T. and Whipp, B.J. (1994). $\dot{V}O_2$ slow component: physiological and functional significance. *Medicine and Science in Sports and Exercise*, **26**, 1354–8.

Pringle, J.S.M. and Jones, A.M. (2002). Maximal lactate steady state, critical power and EMG during cycling. *European Journal of Applied Physiology*, **88**, 214–26.

Pringle, J.S.M., Carter, H., Doust, J.H. and Jones, A.M. (2002). Oxygen uptake kinetics during horizontal and uphill treadmill running. *European Journal of Applied Physiology*, **88**, 163–9.

Pringle, J.S.M., Doust, J.H., Carter, H., Tolfrey, K., Campbell, I.T. and Jones, A.M. (2003a). Oxygen uptake kinetics during constant-load 'submaximal' exercise in humans: the influence of muscle fibre type and capillarisation. *European Journal of Applied Physiology*, **89**, 289–300.

Pringle, J.S.M., Doust, J.H., Carter, H., Tolfrey, K. and Jones, A.M. (2003b). Effect of pedal rate on primary and slow component oxygen uptake responses during heavy cycle exercise. *Journal of Applied Physiology*, **94**, 1501–7.

Ratkevicius, A., Mizuno, M., Povilonis, E. and Quistorff, B. (1998). Energy metabolism of the gastrocnemius and soleus muscles during isometric voluntary and electrically induced contractions in man. *Journal of Physiology*, **507**, 593–602.

Reggiani, C., Potma, E.J., Bottinelli, R., Canepari, M., Pellegrino, M.A. and Steinen, G.J.M. (1997). Chemo-mechanical energy transduction in relation to myosin isoform composition in skeletal muscle fibres of the rat. *Journal of Physiology*, **502**, 449–60.

Rossiter, H.B., Ward, S.A., Kowalchuk, J.M., Howe, F.A., Griffiths, J.R. and Whipp, B.J. (2002). Dynamic asymmetry of phosphocreatine concentration and O_2 uptake between the on- and off-transients of moderate- and high-intensity exercise in humans. *Journal of Physiology*, **541**, 991–1002.

Russell, A., Wadley, G., Snow, R., Giacobino, J.P., Muzzin, P., Garnham, A. and Cameron-Smith, D. (2002). Slow component of $\dot{V}O_2$ kinetics: the effect of training status, fibre type, UCP3 mRNA and citrate synthase activity. *International Journal of Obesity and Related Metabolic Disorders*, **26**, 157–64.

Russell, A.P., Wadley, G., Hesselink, M.K., Schaart, G., Lo, S., Leger, B., Garnham, A., Kornips, E., Cameron-Smith, D., Giacobino, J.P., Muzzin, P., Snow, R. and Schrauwen, P. (2003). UCP3 protein expression is lower in type I, IIa and IIx muscle fiber types of endurance-trained compared to untrained subjects. *Pflugers Archives*, **445**, 563–9.

Saltin, B. and Gollnick, P.D. (1983). Skeletal muscle adaptability: significance for metabolism and performance. In *Handbook of Physiology, Skeletal Muscle*. American Physiological Society, Bethesda USA, pp. 555–631.

Sargeant, A.J. (1999). Neuromuscular determinants of human performance. In B.J. Whipp, and A.J. Sargeant (Eds) *Physiological Determinants of Exercise Tolerance in Humans*. Portland Press, London, pp. 13–28.

Saugen, E. and Vøllestad, N.K. (1996). Metabolic heat production during fatigue from voluntary repetitive isometric contractions in humans. *Journal of Applied Physiology*, **81**, 1323–30.

Saunders, M.J., Evans, E.M., Arngrimsson, S.A., Allison, J.D., Warren, G.L. and Cureton, K.J. (2000). Muscle activation and the slow component rise in oxygen uptake during cycling. *Medicine and Science in Sports and Exercise*, **32**, 2040–5.

Scheuermann, B.W. and Barstow, T.J. (2003). O_2 uptake kinetics during exercise at peak O_2 uptake. *Journal of Applied Physiology*, **95**, 2014–22.

Scheuermann, B.W., Hoelting, B.D., Noble, M.L. and Barstow, T.J. (2001). The slow component of O_2 uptake is not accompanied by changes in muscle EMG during repeated bouts of heavy exercise in humans. *Journal of Physiology*, **531**, 245–56.

Scheuermann, B.W., McConnell, J.H.T. and Barstow, T.J. (2002). EMG and oxygen uptake responses during slow and fast ramp exercise in humans. *Experimental Physiology*, **87**, 91–100.

Shinohara, M. and Moritani, T. (1992). Increase in neuromuscular activity and oxygen uptake during heavy exercise. *Annals of Physiological Anthropology*, **11**, 257–62.

Sieck, G.C. and Regnier, M. (2001). Invited Review: plasticity and energetic demands of contraction in skeletal and cardiac muscle. *Journal of Applied Physiology*, **90**, 1158–64.

Soderlund, K. and Hultman, E. (1991). ATP and phosphocreatine changes in single human muscle fibers after intense electrical stimulation. *American Journal of Physiology*, **261**, E737–41.

Stainsby, W.N., Gladden, L.B., Barclay, J.K. and Wilson, B.A. (1980). Exercise efficiency: validity of baseline subtractions. *Journal of Applied Physiology*, **48**, 518–33.

Staron, R.S. (1997). Human skeletal muscle fiber types: delineation, development, and distribution. *Canadian Journal of Applied Physiology*, **22**, 307–27.

Stienen, G.J., Kiers, J.L., Bottinelli, R. and Reggiani, C. (1996). Myofibrillar ATPase activity in skinned human skeletal muscle fibres: fibre type and temperature dependence. *Journal of Physiology*, **493**, 299–307.

Szentesi, P., Zaremba, R., van Mechelen, W. and Stienen, G.J. (2001). ATP utilization for calcium uptake and force production in different types of human skeletal muscle fibres. *Journal of Physiology*, **531**, 393–403.

Takaishi, T., Ono, T. and Yasuda, Y. (1992). Relationship between muscle fatigue and oxygen uptake during cycle ergometer exercise with different ramp slope increments. *European Journal of Applied Physiology*, **65**, 335–9.

Takaishi, T., Yasuda, Y., Ono, T. and Moritani, T. (1996). Optimal pedaling rate estimated from neuromuscular fatigue for cyclists. *Medicine and Science in Sports and Exercise*, **28**, 1492–7.

Tordi, N., Perrey, S., Harvey, A. and Hughson, R.L. (2003). Oxygen uptake kinetics during two bouts of heavy cycling separated by fatiguing sprint exercise in humans. *Journal of Applied Physiology*, **94**, 533–41.

Vøllestad, N.K. and Blom, P.C.S. (1985). Effect of varying exercise intensity on glycogen depletion in human muscle fibres. *Acta Physiologica Scandinavica*, **125**, 395–405.

Vøllestad, N.K., Vaage, O. and Hermansen, L. (1984). Muscle glycogen depletion patterns in type I and subgroups of type II fibres during prolonged severe exercise in man. *Acta Physiologica Scandinavica*, **122**, 433–41.

Vøllestad, N.K., Wesche, J. and Sejersted, O.M. (1990). Gradual increase in leg oxygen uptake during repeated submaximal contractions in humans. *Journal of Applied Physiology*, **68**, 1150–6.

Wendt, I.R. and Gibbs, C.L. (1973). Energy production of rat extensor digitorum longus muscle. *American Journal of Physiology*, **224**, 1081–6.

Whipp, B.J. (1994). The slow component of O_2 uptake kinetics during heavy exercise. *Medicine and Science in Sports and Exercise*, **26**, 1319–26.

Willis, W.T. and Jackman, M.R. (1994). Mitochondrial function during heavy exercise. *Medicine and Science in Sports and Exercise*, **26**, 1347–54.

Williams, C.A., Carter, H., Jones, A.M. and Doust, J.H. (2001). Oxygen uptake kinetics during treadmill running in boys and men. *Journal of Applied Physiology*, **90**(5), 1700–6.

Wretling, M.L., Gerdle, B. and Henriksson-Larsen, K. (1987). EMG: a non-invasive method for determination of fibre type proportion. *Acta Physiologica Scandinavica*, **131**, 627–8.

Zoladz, J.A., Rademaker, A.C.H.J. and Sargeant, A.J. (1995). Non-linear relationship between O_2 uptake and power output at high intensities of exercise in humans. *Journal of Physiology*, **488**, 211–17.

Zoladz, J.A., Rademaker, A.C.H.J. and Sargeant, A.J. (2000). Human muscle power generating capability during cycling at different pedalling rates. *Experimental Physiology*, **85**, 117–24.

12 Towards an understanding of the mechanistic bases of $\dot{V}O_2$ kinetics

Summary of key points raised in Chapters 2–11

David C. Poole and Andrew M. Jones

Introduction

The foregoing chapters of this book have described the essential features of the $\dot{V}O_2$ response to exercise both at the level of the muscle and the lung (Chapters 1, 3 and 6); outlined the important theoretical and practical considerations in the measurement and analysis of $\dot{V}O_2$ kinetics (Chapters 2 and 3); highlighted similarities and differences in the response across species (Chapter 5) and in different exercise modalities in humans (Chapter 4); and debated the nature of the physiological mechanisms underpinning both the 'primary' and 'slow' components of the $\dot{V}O_2$ response to exercise of different intensities (Chapters 7–11). The latter section has included treaties on the possible influence of metabolic factors (Chapters 7 and 9), oxygen availability (Chapter 8) and muscle fibre type (Chapters 10 and 11) on $\dot{V}O_2$ kinetics. The purpose of the present chapter is to summarize much of the preceding discussion in an attempt to move towards a 'unifying' concept through which $\dot{V}O_2$ kinetics and their sensitivity to a variety of interventions can be better understood. To facilitate this process, Chapter 12 poses and attempts to answer six key questions:

1 How closely do pulmonary $\dot{V}O_2$ kinetics represent muscle $\dot{V}O_2$ kinetics?
2 Does muscle $\dot{V}O_2$ increase immediately at exercise onset?
3 Does O_2 delivery, metabolic inertia or something else, limit the speed of the $\dot{V}O_2$ kinetics?
4 Are the primary component $\dot{V}O_2$ kinetics slowed above the lactate threshold?
5 What is the mechanistic basis for the $\dot{V}O_2$ slow component?
6 How does 'priming exercise' influence $\dot{V}O_2$ kinetics?

How closely do pulmonary $\dot{V}O_2$ kinetics represent muscle $\dot{V}O_2$ kinetics?

Chapters 2 and 3 collectively demonstrate that, with certain reasonable assumptions and with careful attention paid to accuracy both in measurement and subsequent analysis, pulmonary $\dot{V}O_2$ kinetics can provide a close reflection of the kinetics of muscle O_2 consumption. Using a mathematical modelling approach, Barstow *et al.* (1990) demonstrated that the time constant (τ) describing the rise in pulmonary $\dot{V}O_2$ in phase II provided a very close approximation of the τ of the rise in muscle $\dot{V}O_2$ following the onset of exercise. It is important to remember, however, that pulmonary $\dot{V}O_2$ kinetics represent a conflation of the 'instantaneous' muscle $\dot{V}O_2$ kinetics, the kinetics of cardiac output and muscle blood flow, and the intervening venous volume and O_2 stores. In this respect, the computer simulations of Barstow *et al.* (1990) revealed that, for the same muscle $\dot{V}O_2$ kinetics, a slowing of cardiac output kinetics (as may occur in certain pathological conditions and with certain pharmacological interventions) may extend the duration of Phase I and cause an 'apparent' speeding of pulmonary $\dot{V}O_2$ kinetics in Phase II. Interestingly, however, this distortion did not influence the accuracy of the estimation of the intramuscular O_2 deficit from the pulmonary $\dot{V}O_2$ kinetics. In an important recent paper, Grassi *et al.* (1996) experimentally confirmed the model predictions of Barstow *et al.* (1990) by showing that Phase II pulmonary $\dot{V}O_2$ kinetics (half-time: ~25.5 s) provided a close reflection of muscle $\dot{V}O_2$ kinetics (half-time: ~27.9 s) in the transition from unloaded pedalling to moderate-intensity cycle exercise. It has also been demonstrated that >90% of the $\dot{V}O_2$ measured at the lung derives from $\dot{V}O_2$ at the level of the working muscles during cycle ergometry (Poole *et al.*, 1992) and that ~86% of the $\dot{V}O_2$ slow component measured at the lung derives from a continued increase in muscle $\dot{V}O_2$ with time (Poole *et al.*, 1991).

The papers of Barstow *et al.* (1990) and Grassi *et al.* (1996) collectively show that careful measurements of pulmonary $\dot{V}O_2$ kinetics can provide an accurate estimate (to *within* $\pm 10\%$) of the τ for muscle $\dot{V}O_2$ following the onset of exercise (reviewed in Chapter 6). However, as eloquently described by Koga (Chapter 2) and Whipp and Rossiter (Chapter 3), there are a number of potential 'pitfalls' in the measurement and analysis of pulmonary $\dot{V}O_2$ kinetics that should be avoided if such an approach is to have maximal utility. The first of these pitfalls is the inherent breath-to-breath 'noise' in measurements of pulmonary $\dot{V}O_2$. This can, however, be minimized by increasing the amplitude of the $\dot{V}O_2$ response above baseline (achieved, for example, by recruiting larger subjects of high fitness and/or by selecting an exercise modality which requires a large muscle mass) and/or by averaging together the responses to an appropriate number of identical transitions. Careful data editing and averaging procedures and the application of appropriate 'alveolar correction' algorithms can also reduce breath-to-breath variability in pulmonary $\dot{V}O_2$ data. A second important point in the analysis of $\dot{V}O_2$ kinetics is to attempt to 'isolate' the region of interest in the response. For example, where the τ of the Phase II response is of principal experimental interest, it is important that phase I is appropriately accounted for to prevent 'contamination' of the estimate. Strategies for achieving this goal are outlined in Chapters 2 and 3. It should also be noted that more complex models should only be preferred over simple models where there is a sound theoretical rationale for their use. While more complex models will generally improve the goodness of fit, this may reduce the confidence in each of the model parameters including that/those of primary experimental interest.

Although direct measures of $\dot{V}O_2$ across a working muscle are theoretically the 'ideal' in elucidating the limiting factors for aerobic respiration in the exercising human, this approach is highly invasive and technically complex. Analysis of pulmonary $\dot{V}O_2$ kinetics, while introducing further technical constraints (see before), obviates some of these problems and is applicable in a wide variety of experimental and clinical conditions. Furthermore, it is our contention that measurement of pulmonary $\dot{V}O_2$ kinetics is at least as accurate in inferring muscle $\dot{V}O_2$ kinetics as is repeated muscle biopsy sampling in which the difference between (an assumed) energy demand and the energy equivalent represented, for example, by changes in [PCr] and [lactate] are used to estimate the contribution of oxidative phosphorylation to the energy turnover. Factors such as the time taken from excision to freezing of the biopsy sample will influence the concentration of substrates and metabolites in the sample, as will differences in the efflux of metabolites (e.g. lactate) from muscle to blood. The contribution of muscles to force production varies between exercise activities, across exercise intensities, and over time, and there are marked spatial and temporal variations in metabolic rate even within small regions of the same muscle during exercise (Richardson et al., 2001). For this reason, we believe that conclusions concerning the control of muscle $\dot{V}O_2$ kinetics and the O_2 deficit that are based solely upon changes in muscle metabolites (e.g. Greenhaff et al., 2002) should be viewed with some caution. It should be pointed out here that the use of magnetic resonance spectroscopy (e.g. Rossiter et al., 1999) allows a non-invasive measurement or estimation of intramuscular [ATP], [ADP], [Pi], [PCr] and pH dynamics and circumvents a number of the problems alluded to here. Unfortunately, however, the type of exercise that can be performed and the volume of muscle that can be interrogated with ^{31}P-MRS methods are presently restricted.

Does muscle $\dot{V}O_2$ increase immediately at exercise onset?

The first measurements of $\dot{V}O_2$ kinetics across the exercising human leg demonstrated the presence of a pronounced delay (6–20 s) in the increase of $\dot{V}O_2$ for both moderate (Grassi et al., 1996) and severe (Bangsbo et al., 2000) intensity cycle exercise. Such a delay in $\dot{V}O_2$ increase has also been observed across the electrically stimulated dog gastrocnemius–plantaris complex (Grassi et al., 1998a,b). It is also pertinent that muscle microvascular (Behnke et al., 2001, 2002c) and intramyocyte (Hogan, 2001) O_2 pressures do not fall immediately at the onset of contractions. However, without knowing whether or not O_2 delivery is increasing in those particular experiments, it is not possible to state whether or not this corresponds to a delayed increase in $\dot{V}O_2$. The interpretation of the delay in $\dot{V}O_2$ increase at exercise onset seen across human and dog muscles is that blood flow (and thus O_2 delivery, $\dot{Q}O_2$) increases more rapidly than $\dot{V}O_2$ (Shoemaker and Hughson, 1999; Sheriff and Hakeman, 2001; Kindig et al., 2002b) such that muscle venous effluent O_2 content rises as the fractional extraction of O_2 falls

(Grassi *et al.*, 1996; Bangsbo *et al.*, 2000). Whereas these findings suggest that $\dot{Q}O_2$ is not limiting $\dot{V}O_2$ kinetics at exercise onset, they present a quandary with respect to our understanding of metabolic control.

Specifically, most models of metabolic control incorporate either [PCr] or some phosphate-linked mechanism that serves to drive increased mitochondrial function, for example (1) Changes in $[ADP]_{free}$ (and/or Pi) in accordance with Michaelis–Menten enzyme kinetics (Chance and Williams, 1955). (2) Thermodynamic control through the phosphorylation potential ([ATP]/[ADP]/[Pi]) (Balaban, 1990). (3) Changes in Gibbs free energy of cytosolic ATP hydrolysis (Meyer and Foley, 1996). Thus, the finding of a reduced [PCr] within the first few muscle contractions (Binzoni *et al.*, 1992; Yoshida and Watari, 1993; Rossiter *et al.*, 1999, 2001) conflicts directly with the presence of a delayed increase in muscle $\dot{V}O_2$ of the order demonstrated by Grassi and colleagues or Bangsbo *et al.* When measuring $\dot{V}O_2$ either across the exercising limb (Grassi *et al.*, 1996; Bangsbo *et al.*, 2000) or muscle complex (Grassi *et al.*, 1998 a,b), the possibility must be acknowledged that there will be a transit delay between the site of O_2 exchange (i.e. the capillary) and the effluent venous blood, the duration of which will be dictated by the relationship between the vascular volume and blood flow. To calculate the size of this transit delay, Grassi and colleagues estimated the size of the vascular volume relative to the measured blood flow and could only account for a modest portion of the delay. Bangsbo *et al.* attempted to measure directly the actual transit time and likewise could not account for all of the delay in muscle $\dot{V}O_2$ increase at exercise onset.

One obvious approach to this problem is to measure $\dot{V}O_2$ at the site of utilization or exchange within the microcirculation. As detailed in Chapter 6, Behnke and colleagues (2002a, see Chapter 6, Figure 6.9) have combined direct measurement of capillary red blood cell flux (Kindig *et al.*, 2002b) with phosphorescence quenching determination of microvascular O_2 pressures within the spinotrapezius muscle at the onset of electrically induced contractions. In contrast to the delay found in human and canine muscle at exercise onset, $\dot{V}O_2$ began increasing simultaneously with the first contraction cycles. Indeed, the latest experiments performed in canine muscle (Grassi *et al.*, 2002) and also single muscle fibres of the frog (Kindig *et al.*, 2003, Figure 12.1) confirm this essentially immediate increase in $\dot{V}O_2$. In conclusion therefore, whilst there appears to be a delay in muscle $\dot{V}O_2$ increase at the onset of contractions in human and some canine studies, measurements of an immediate $\dot{V}O_2$ increase made at the site of O_2 exchange concur with currently accepted models of metabolic control.

Does O_2 delivery, metabolic inertia or something else, limit the speed of the $\dot{V}O_2$ kinetics?

This argument is analogous to 'feed forward' (O_2 delivery) vs 'feedback' (metabolic inertia) control of $\dot{V}O_2$. As presented by Hughson (Chapter 8) and Grassi (Chapter 9), there is substantial evidence that can be marshalled in support of either the O_2 delivery or metabolic inertia hypothesis for limiting the speed of the $\dot{V}O_2$ kinetics. For example, the 'O_2 delivery' proponents point out

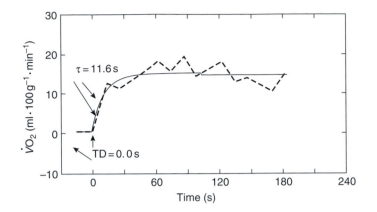

Figure 12.1 Within single muscle fibres, $\dot{V}O_2$ increases in the first contraction cycle (redrawn from Kindig *et al.*, 2003). This has also been demonstrated recently at the capillary level in rat muscle (Behnke *et al.*, 2002a) and across the canine gastrocnemius–plantaris complex (Grassi *et al.*, 2002).

that acute conditions associated with a reduced muscle O_2 delivery such as inspired hypoxia (Engelen *et al.*, 1996), β-blockade (Hughson and Smyth, 1983), supine exercise (Hughson *et al.*, 1993), and arm exercise with the arm above heart level (Hughson *et al.*, 1996), as well as chronic disease conditions, that is diabetes (Regensteiner *et al.*, 1998) and heart failure (Hepple *et al.*, 1999), all slow $\dot{V}O_2$ kinetics. In addition, conditions that are expected to enhance muscle O_2 delivery, for example priming exercise (Gerbino *et al.*, 1996; Macdonald *et al.*, 1997; Burnley *et al.*, 2000) and inspired hyperoxia (MacDonald *et al.*, 1997) do speed the overall $\dot{V}O_2$ kinetics but usually only in the heavy and severe (above the lactate/ventilatory thresholds) exercise domains. This effect is manifested as a faster MRT which usually occurs via a reduced $\dot{V}O_2$ slow component rather than any change in the primary component time constant. The counter position to some of these observations is that muscle O_2 delivery *per se* has not always been measured in these investigations. With respect to priming exercise, Krustrup *et al.* (2001) have shown that muscle blood flow is elevated at the beginning of the second bout of exercise. However, such an increase is not requisite for increasing blood–muscle O_2 exchange (Behnke *et al.*, 2002c). Moreover, it is well known that lowering the arterial PO_2 causes a compensatory vasodilation whereas raising the arterial PO_2 induces vasoconstriction. Both responses act to normalize muscle O_2 delivery albeit at very different inflowing capillary PO_2 values. This, in itself, may be crucial because according to Fick's Law of diffusion, a reduced O_2 pressure head in the microcirculation will limit blood–muscle O_2 transfer. A further consideration is that the different disease conditions are accompanied by profound structural and functional perturbations within the exercising muscles that confound interpretation of the relationship between O_2 delivery and $\dot{V}O_2$ kinetics (rev. Xu *et al.*, 1998; Kindig *et al.*, 1998, 1999; Behnke *et al.*, 2002b; Richardson *et al.*, 2003).

In contrast to this, the 'metabolic inertia' proponents consider that the rate of oxidative phosphorylation across the on-transient is determined by the concentrations of cellular metabolic controllers and/or mitochondrial enzyme activation (rev. Chance and Williams, 1955; Mahler, 1985; Balaban, 1990; Hochachka and Matheson, 1992; Meyer and Foley, 1996; Timmons *et al.*, 1998b; Tschakovsky and Hughson, 1999; Walsh *et al.*, 2001). Key evidence comes from a range of different models and includes the following:

1   Lack of a reduction and sometimes even an increase in muscle microvascular (Behnke *et al.*, 2001) and effluent venous PO_2 (Grassi *et al.*, 1996; Bangsbo *et al.*, 2000) for the initial 6–20 s of muscle contractions suggesting that O_2 delivery is equal to or in excess of demand (or at least utilization). Moreover, in healthy muscle beyond this initial period, there is no subsequent decrease of microvascular or effluent venous PO_2 below that found in the steady-state. The latter would be the expected consequence of muscle $\dot{V}O_2$ being limited by O_2 delivery and is in fact evident in diseased muscle (diabetes, Behnke *et al.* (2002b); heart failure, Diederich *et al.* (2002)) and in hypotensive states (Ross *et al.*, 2003).

2   Heart rate, cardiac output and muscle blood flow dynamics are almost always faster than $\dot{V}O_2$ kinetics (rev. Delp, 1999; Tschakovsky and Hughson, 1999). If the blood flow and O_2 delivery is distributed effectively to the active muscle fibres (which may not always be the case given the spatial disparity in motor and microvascular units (Richardson *et al.*, 2001)), it is difficult to appreciate how a slower process can be temporally limited by a faster one. One caveat here is that it is not technically feasible to measure the distribution of that blood flow relative to the metabolic needs of the active muscle fibres. It is also pertinent that Yoshida and colleagues (1995) have dissociated cardiac output and pulmonary $\dot{V}O_2$ dynamics using a one-leg exercise paradigm and Fukuba *et al.* (2004) found that priming knee extension exercise speeded pulmonary $\dot{V}O_2$ kinetics in the absence of altered leg blood flow kinetics.

3   Experimental perturbations demonstrated to improve muscle O_2 delivery such as local vasodilation (Grassi *et al.*, 1998a) and right-shifting the O_2 dissociation curve to elevate microvascular PO_2 (Grassi *et al.*, 1998b) do not speed $\dot{V}O_2$ kinetics for moderate exercise and only slightly speed $\dot{V}O_2$ kinetics for heavy/severe exercise in pump-perfused, electrically stimulated dog muscles.

4   Phase II $\dot{V}O_2$ kinetics are exponential and match closely those of muscle [PCr] (Mahler, 1985; Rossiter *et al.*, 1999, 2001; see Chapter 7). It is difficult to conceive of such a response if $\dot{V}O_2$ is controlled by a muscle O_2 delivery profile that follows a markedly biphasic increase at exercise onset (e.g. Kindig *et al.*, 2002b).

5   Decreasing mitochondrial enzyme inertia by the following: (A) Improving the activation of pyruvate dehydrogenase using dichloroacetate speeds the fall in intracellular PO_2 (Howlett and Hogan, 2003) and reduces the decrease in [PCr] (Timmons *et al.*, 1998a,b), which is the expected consequence of faster $\dot{V}O_2$ kinetics. However, direct measurements of $\dot{V}O_2$ kinetics have not

supported this observation (e.g. Bangsbo *et al.*, 2002; Grassi *et al.*, 2002; Rossiter *et al.*, 2003; Jones *et al.*, 2004). (B) Nitric oxide (NO) synthase inhibition which reduces/removes the inhibitory effect of NO on the electron transport chain and elsewhere, speeds $\dot{V}O_2$ kinetics during moderate and heavy exercise in horses (Kindig *et al.*, 2001, 2002a) and humans (Jones *et al.*, 2003, 2004). This effect is present despite a possible reduction in cardiac output (Kindig *et al.*, 2000) and muscle blood flow (Hirai *et al.*, 1994) resulting from removal of NO-mediated muscle vasodilation and in agreement with point number 1, suggests that muscle O_2 availability is not limited across the transition (see Chapter 8).

Towards a unifying concept

In part, the controversy between the 'O$_2$ delivery' and 'metabolic inertia' camps has been fostered by the range and complexity of models studied from the intact upright human down to the isolated single muscle fibre or isolated mitochondria. The O_2 delivery proponents have argued that shortcomings of animal preparations that usually include the necessity for anaesthesia and electrical stimulation abrogates study of the true physiological response. At the same time, it is true that experimental constraints and technical limitations have precluded measurements of muscle O_2 delivery and its microvascular temporal and spatial distribution in human muscle. It is also evident that there exists a plethora of different models and modalities as well as four different exercise intensity domains across which the balance of factors limiting $\dot{V}O_2$ kinetics may change. In addition, the elegant modelling of Hughson and colleagues (2001) suggests that the ability to resolve substantial non-linearities in metabolic control even from well-behaved data is extremely poor.

The original work of David F. Wilson at the University of Pennsylvania has demonstrated *in vitro* that mitochondrial regulation can be profoundly sensitive to altered PO_2 values even at levels above those which compromise $\dot{V}O_2$ (Wilson *et al.*, 1977, 1983, 1984). More recently, Michael C. Hogan and Peter Arthur and colleagues at the University of California, San Diego showed the interdependence of the phosphorylation potential ($[ATP]/[ADP] * [Pi]$) and PO_2 in the contracting dog gastrocnemius–plantaris muscle complex (Arthur *et al.*, 1992; Hogan *et al.*, 1992, 1996). Specifically, as PO_2 was lowered, a greater perturbation of the phosphorylation potential was required to achieve a given $\dot{V}O_2$ (see Figure 12.2 for a mechanistic explanation of this effect). This is consistent with the notion that the oxidative phosphorylation reaction is a function of the cumulative drive of the phosphorylation potential (see Chapter 7), the PO_2, the redox potential and $[H^+]$:

$$6ADP + 6Pi + O_2 + 2(NADH + H^+) \rightarrow 6ATP + 2NAD + 2H_2O$$

Irrespective of whether PCr functions simply as an energy store or alternatively constitutes an essential signal to accelerate oxidative phosphorylation, its dependence on PO_2 implies that an altered intracellular PO_2 has the potential to impact upon $\dot{V}O_2$ kinetics. Indeed, the NMR studies of Haseler *et al.* (1998) suggest that PCr kinetics are slowed in hypoxia. However, this will only occur at

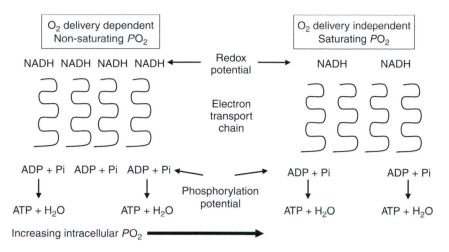

Figure 12.2 Schematization of the effect of intracellular PO_2 on the redox and phosphorylation potentials and flux rate through the electron transport chain. Note that
when intracellular PO_2 reaches saturating levels, the number of NADH and
ADP + Pi necessary to meet the required ATP production rate is reduced.
When this threshold is reached, $\dot{V}O_2$ kinetics become independent of intracellular PO_2 and thus O_2 delivery (see Figure 12.3). This figure was developed
in part from Hughson *et al.* (2001). One very recent finding that apparently
flies in the face of this concept is the inability of Marcinek *et al.* (2003) to
detect complimentary alterations in PO_2 and the phosphorylation state of the
cell. However, the observations by Marcinek *et al.* were restricted to the non-
contracting mouse muscle under ischaemic and hypermetabolic conditions.

non-saturating PO_2 levels. At present, the minimum PO_2 that constitutes a saturating level in human muscle during exercise and the interdependence of this
value on metabolic rate or the physicochemical environment present in contracting muscle are not known. Notwithstanding these uncertainties, Figures 12.2
and 12.3 attempt to explain the apparently disparate experimental findings
from the 'O₂ delivery' and 'metabolic inertia' camps along a continuum of muscle O_2 deliveries that transcends O_2 delivery dependent and independent zones
based upon their effect on intracellular PO_2. Table 12.1 separates different exercise conditions/circumstances between O_2 delivery dependent and independent
conditions based upon the presiding experimental evidence.

Overarching problems with current models of metabolic control

The dependence of $\dot{V}O_2$ kinetics and the metabolic status of the myocyte upon
intracellular PO_2 is an attractive hypothesis that explains observed behaviour
in vitro (Wilson *et al.*, 1977) and in intact animal (Arthur *et al.*, 1992; Hogan
et al., 1992, 1996) and human (Richardson *et al.*, 1995; Haseler *et al.*, 1998)

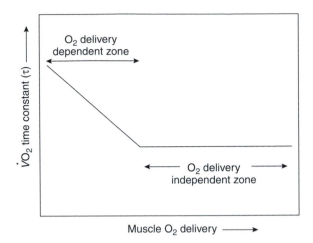

Figure 12.3 Schematic that explains the dependence of $\dot{V}O_2$ kinetics on muscle O_2
delivery in some, but not all, circumstances. See text for details and Table
12.1 for specific conditions lying in the O_2 delivery dependent and independent zones. This concept was developed, in part, through discussions with
Drs S. Koga and T.J. Barstow.

Table 12.1 List of exercise models and conditions residing in the O_2 delivery dependent
and independent zones (see Figure 12.3)

O_2 delivery dependent	Ambiguous	O_2 delivery independent
Dog gastroc.–plantaris complex >60% $\dot{V}O_{2\,max}$ Supine cycling exercise Arm exercised above heart β-blockade Exercise with blood flow impeded Diabetes Chronic heart failure Systemic hypotension	Upright cycling in heavy/ severe domains	Upright cycling in moderate domain Horse exercising in moderate and heavy domains Rat muscles stimulated in moderate domain Dog gastroc.–plantaris complex <60% $\dot{V}O_{2\,max}$

contracting muscle as noted above. However, the control of ATP turnover rates
may not be dependent upon the concentration of pathway intermediates such as
the adenylates, phosphagen, Pi, etc. which exhibit relatively modest alterations
in the face of metabolic rate increases up to two (human muscle, Richardson
et al., 1993) or even three (locust flight muscle, Hochachka, 1994) orders of magnitude. Indeed, these observations have inspired the notion that pivotal control
elements in the ATP utilization and ATP yielding pathways have to be located
externally to the pathways themselves. Moreover, given that ATP levels change

very little during transition to elevated metabolic rates, there must be parallel and simultaneous control of ATP demand and ATP supply (Hochachka, 1994). Thus, some activating signal must arrive essentially instantaneously at all parts of the cell and influence the majority of proteins in each step of the ATP demand and supply pathways. It is difficult to envisage a second messenger system such as Ca^{2+} operating with the required speed and efficacy for this to occur.

Peter W. Hochachka and Gerald W. Pollack have independently considered that a crucial element absent from all current models of the control of muscle function and ATP turnover is the specific nature of myocyte cytosol. Specifically, they have considered the possibility that cytosol may resemble a gel rather than a sol. Cytoplasm is over ten times more viscous than water and microviscosities in different cell regions may vary with contractions and metabolic activity (Dix and Verkman, 1990). Microviscosities within the mitochondria are even higher and also change with mitochondrial activity – being highest during state 3 respiration (i.e. ADP saturating conditions). The cytosol resembles a highly organized poly-meric matrix with cross-linked polymers containing structured water that excludes solutes and may exhibit large electrical potentials. Such organized gels are expected to exhibit 'schizophrenic' behaviour. For instance, akin to water changing from a solid to a liquid, gels undergo phase transitions that can be prop-agated by water depolarizations and polymer condensation. Phase transitions constitute a massively potent trigger such that, within protein-like gels a ratio of one phosphate molecule to three hundred kinase molecules can induce a complete transition. Thus, gels potentially possess the kind of amplification mechanisms necessary for increasing metabolic rate several orders of magnitude. X-ray diffrac-tion of muscle reveals a tight structural regularity at the single nanometer scale which is necessary for such a homogeneous phase transition trigger. Pollack (2001) has considered that such phase transitions may explain muscle contraction more accurately than the sliding filament theory. If they do occur, they may also be central to metabolic control at the onset of those contractions.

Although highly speculative, it is possible that upon contraction, myocytes experience a phase transition within the cytoplasm and mitochondrial matrices, that is partial gel to partial sol that is transmitted instantaneously throughout the myocyte. The question then arises, could such a phase transition be affected by intracellular PO_2, possibly through Ca^{2+}? If so, it would explain both the O_2 reg-ulation of ATPases and ATP synthesis and provide a mechanistic explanation for the up- or down-regulation of ATP turnover rate in the absence of substantial changes in ATP utilization/production pathway intermediates (Hochachka, 1994). Resolution of these issues is essential if we are to fully understand the dynamics of metabolic control within muscle.

Are the primary component $\dot{V}O_2$ kinetics slowed above the lactate threshold?

One of the long-standing debates in the field concerns whether or not the time constant of the primary component (τ_p) is slower for work rates above the LT compared to those below the LT. A slowing of the primary component $\dot{V}O_2$ kinetics in the heavy exercise domain (where, by definition, blood [lactate] will be elevated appreciably above baseline values) has been interpreted to indicate that O_2 availability may be (increasingly) limiting the $\dot{V}O_2$ kinetics (Hughson et al., 2001). The literature is equivocal on this issue with some studies finding no difference between the τ_p for heavy compared to moderate exercise (e.g. Barstow and Mole, 1991; Ozyener et al., 2001; Scheuermann and Barstow, 2003) and others reporting a significant lengthening of τ_p at higher work rates (e.g. Paterson and Whipp, 1991; Jones et al., 2002; Koppo et al., 2004). However, as pointed out by Hughson and his colleagues (e.g. Perrey et al., 2001; see Chapter 8), large inter-individual variability in the value of the primary component τ along with small sample sizes may have conspired to result in non-significant differences in τ_p between moderate and heavy exercise even when the mean difference in the values appears to be substantial.

As a first step towards reconciling differences of opinion on this issue, Table 12.2 provides a summary of the results of those studies that have measured τ_p during

Table 12.2 Effect of exercise intensity (moderate vs heavy/severe) on the time constant of the Phase II $\dot{V}O_2$ kinetics

Authors	Moderate τ_p(s)	Heavy τ_p(s)	Exercise mode	Subject no.
Barstow and Mole, 1991	16.1	23.4	Cycling	4
Paterson and Whipp, 1991	31.3	40.2	Cycling	6
Engelen et al., 1996	19.1	28.1	Cycling	5
Koga et al., 1997	28.1	31.2	Cycling	7
Koga et al., 1999	21.2	26.9	Cycling	9
Koga et al., 2001	18.4	27.8	Cycling	6
Carter et al., 2000a	18.0	22.4	Cycling	7
Scheuermann et al., 2001	20.4	28.2	Cycling	7
Scheuermann and Barstow, 2003	24.7	24.7	Cycling	8
Perrey et al., 2003	20.9	20.6	Cycling	10
Burnley et al., 2000	15.6	23.9	Cycling	10
Jones et al., 2002	17.3	27.1	Cycling	7
Perrey et al., 2001	20.6	24.0	Cycling	6
Ozyener et al., 2001	33	32	Cycling	6
Pringle et al., 2003a	19.5	22.6	Cycling	14
Koppo et al., 2004	11.7	15.2	Cycling	7 trained
Koppo et al., 2004	21.5	23.5	Cycling	8 untrained
Pringle et al., 2002	16.7	19.1	Running, flat	9
Carter et al., 2002	12.7	19.1	Running	9
Carter et al., 2000a	15.0	20.1	Running	7
Carter et al., 2000b	16.3	19.4	Running	23 (pre-training)
Williams et al., 2001	14.7	19.0	Running	8
Rossiter et al., 2002b	35	39	Prone leg extension	9
Koga et al., 2001	16.8	26.8	One-legged cycling	6
Koga et al., 1999	27.7	24.5	Supine cycling	9
Mean	20.8	25.5	Cycling only	127
Mean	20.2	24.4	All exercise	207

both moderate and heavy/severe exercise. It should be noted that a comparison of τ_p between moderate and heavy/severe exercise was not always the sole purpose of these studies. Furthermore, the studies differ in a number of ways including the number of subjects studied, the number of repeat transitions performed, and the approach used to model the data. In addition, the work rates used (as a %LT or GET for moderate exercise, and as the %Δ for >GET/LT exercise) differed somewhat, although we were careful to ensure that the comparisons are only between work rates that are clearly moderate and clearly heavy or severe. We have also limited our analysis to young, ostensibly healthy, populations. Finally, it was not possible to perform a meta-analysis on these data because most of the studies report only the mean (and not individual) data. Nevertheless, it is clear from Table 12.2 that there is a strong trend for τ_p to become longer (i.e. for the primary component $\dot{V}O_2$ kinetics to become slower) for heavy/severe exercise compared to moderate exercise. For conventional cycle ergometry, Table 12.2 shows that τ_p increases by 23% (from 20.8 s for moderate exercise to 25.5 s for heavy/severe exercise; $n=127$). When the results of studies using other exercise modalities (e.g. running, leg extension, supine and one-legged cycling) are combined with those of upright cycle exercise, τ_p increases by 21% (from 20.2 s for moderate exercise to 24.4 s for heavy/severe exercise; $n=207$). Furthermore, the τ_p was longer for heavy/severe exercise compared to moderate exercise in 21 of the 25 studies examined.

This analysis clearly indicates that τ_p is slower for heavy/severe exercise compared to moderate exercise. It is possible that this difference was not detected in some studies due to low statistical power (i.e. too much noise in the data or too few subjects). It is also possible, however, that there is inherent variability in the response of individual subjects that is of physiological origin. For example, in a recent study in which we examined the $\dot{V}O_2$ responses to a wide range of work rates (moderate, heavy, severe and extreme), we found that τ_p was essentially unchanged in 5 subjects but became substantially greater (by ~100%) at higher work rates in the other 2 subjects studied (Figure 12.4). The reason for this differential slowing of τ_p in some subjects but not others is presently unclear but could potentially involve a limitation in bulk O_2 delivery and/or regional mismatch between metabolic rate and O_2 availability. However, evidence against this position was reviewed earlier (see 'Does O_2 delivery, metabolic inertia or something else, limit the speed of the $\dot{V}O_2$ kinetics?').

The law of superposition (Fujihara *et al.*, 1973) states that, in a linear first-order system, the key response parameters to a higher work rate (i.e. the gain and the time constant) can be predicted from the response to a lower work rate. The fact that τ_p becomes longer at higher work rates therefore indicates that the primary component $\dot{V}O_2$ kinetics are not under linear first-order control throughout the continuum of ostensibly submaximal exercise. The view is generally held, however, that the asymptotic gain of the primary component (G_p) response is essentially constant over a wide range of exercise intensities (from moderate to extreme) (e.g. Whipp and Mahler, 1980). However, there are recent data that challenge this view. Jones *et al.* (2002) first demonstrated

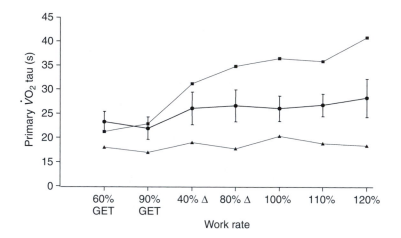

Figure 12.4 The influence of exercise intensity on the time constant of the fundamental component of $\dot{V}O_2$ (τ_p). The filled circles with the solid line represents the group mean ($\pm$ SEM) response. There was no significant difference in τ_p across the range of exercise intensities studied. The lower line (filled triangles) denotes the response of a representative participant from a subgroup of the five participants in whom τ_p was essentially unchanged from 60% GET (25.2 $\pm$ 2.3 s) to 120% $\dot{V}O_{2\,max}$ (23.9 $\pm$ 4.2 s). The higher line (closed squares) denotes the response from one of two participants in whom there was an appreciable lengthening of τ_p at higher work rates (from 18.2 $\pm$ 1.5 s at 60% GET to 38.6 $\pm$ 1.2 s at 120% $\dot{V}O_{2\,max}$). See text for further discussion. Data from Wilkerson *et al.*, 2004.

that G_p fell significantly from moderate (80% GET; 10.8 ml $\cdot$ min^{-1} $\cdot$ W^{-1}) to heavy (50%Δ; 9.9 ml $\cdot$ min^{-1} $\cdot$ W^{-1}) exercise. Pringle *et al.* (2003a,b) also reported that G_p fell progressively from 80% GET (10.6 ml $\cdot$ min^{-1} $\cdot$ W^{-1}) to 50% Δ (9.6 ml $\cdot$ min^{-1} $\cdot$ W^{-1}) and 70% Δ (9.1 ml $\cdot$ min^{-1} $\cdot$ W^{-1}) and that the G_p for heavy exercise fell further at higher pedal rates. Scheuermann and Barstow (2003) have also reported recently that the G_p is significantly lower during severe-intensity exercise compared to moderate-intensity exercise. A trend for the G_p to become reduced at higher work rates is also evident in several earlier studies in both cycling (Barstow *et al.*, 1993; Carter *et al.*, 2000a; Ozyener *et al.*, 2001) and running (Carter *et al.*, 2002). It also appears that the projected asymptote of the primary component response falls substantially and progressively for exercise within the extreme domain (Scheuermann and Barstow, 2003; Wilkerson *et al.*, 2004; Figure 12.5).

The cause of the reduced G_p at higher work rates is presently unclear. However, changes in muscle efficiency resulting from an increase in carbohydrate oxidation at higher work rates can only explain a small portion of the effect (Mallory *et al.*, 2002). One possibility is that the G_p is itself sensitive to O_2 availability. Evidence in support of this includes the reduction in G_p during supine compared to upright heavy cycle exercise (Koga *et al.*, 1999) and the

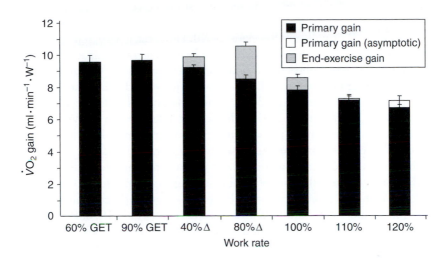

Figure 12.5 The influence of exercise intensity on the gain of the fundamental component of $\dot{V}O_2$ (black bars) and the total (i.e. end-exercise) gain (i.e. including
the contribution of the $\dot{V}O_2$ slow component to the end-exercise $\dot{V}O_2$). The
asymptote of the fundamental gain is also shown at 110% and 120% $\dot{V}O_2$ peak.
Data from Wilkerson *et al.*, 2004.

increase in G_p with inspiratory hyperoxia during heavy exercise (MacDonald *et al.*,
1997). Another possibility is that the metabolic acidosis during heavy/severe
exercise alters respiratory control in some fashion. For example, Conley *et al.*
(2001) have suggested that the fall in pH resulting from high rates of glycolysis
inhibits the rise in [ADP] by altering the creatine kinase reaction equilibrium
(i.e. [ADP] = [ATP][Cr]/([PCr][H$^+$]K$_{eq}$)) and therefore limits the extent to
which $\dot{V}O_2$ can rise. More recently, Jubrias *et al.* (2003) have measured a reduction
in estimated oxidative flux during exercise which elicits a metabolic acidosis,
suggesting a direct inhibition of mitochondrial respiration with acidosis
(pH < 6.88). Finally, it is feasible that alterations in the population of muscle
fibres recruited might account for both the lower G_p and the longer τ_p that is
observed at higher work rates. As schematized by Koppo *et al.* (2004), the metabolic properties of the type II muscle fibres would be expected to make a greater
proportional contribution to the pulmonary $\dot{V}O_2$ signal when their recruitment
is enhanced, for example at higher work rates (see Chapter 15, Figure 15.3). The
τ for the increase in $\dot{V}O_2$ has been reported to be appreciably slower in muscles
comprising predominantly type II fibres (e.g. extensor digitorum longus; 138 s)
compared to muscles comprising predominantly type I fibres (e.g. soleus; 36 s),
(Crow and Kushmerick, 1982). If a similar differentiation exists between muscle
fibres of low and high oxidative capacity in the same muscle during human exercise, then the recruitment of type II fibres at higher work rates might cause a net
slowing of pulmonary $\dot{V}O_2$ kinetics measured at the mouth. *In vitro* studies suggest

that type II fibres have a higher phosphate cost for a given force production and a higher oxygen cost for the same phosphate turnover compared to type I fibres (for review, see Bottinelli and Reggiani, 2000). However, *in vivo*, it might be considered that the low oxidative capacity and high 'anaerobic' capacity of type II fibres relative to type I fibres might limit the extent to which $\dot{V}O_2$ can rise and/or obligate a greater proportion of the ATP cost of force production through anaerobic mechanisms (Jones *et al.*, 2002; Scheuermann and Barstow, 2003). The recent data of Behnke *et al.* (2003) indicate that differences in the $\dot{V}O_2$ response at exercise onset between the principal muscle fibre types might be at least partially related to differences in perfusion and microvascular O_2 exchange.

That muscle fibre recruitment is at least partially responsible for the fall in G_p (and possibly the lengthening of τ_p also) at higher work rates is supported by evidence that muscle fibre type distribution is significantly correlated with G_p during moderate, heavy and severe exercise (Barstow *et al.*, 1996; Pringle *et al.*, 2003a). Furthermore, a number of interventions that alter muscle fibre recruitment during heavy/severe exercise have consistent and predictable effects on G_p. For example (1) the performance of prior heavy exercise increases both the G_p and the integrated electromyogram during subsequent heavy exercise (Burnley *et al.*, 2002); (2) glycogen depletion of the type II fibre pool results in an increased G_p during heavy exercise (Carter *et al.*, 2004); and (3) at the same relative work rate during heavy exercise, a higher pedal rate is associated with a reduced G_p (Pringle *et al.*, 2003b) (see Chapter 11 for further discussion). The gain of the primary component of $\dot{V}O_2$ appears to be inversely related to the gain of the slow component of $\dot{V}O_2$ (Burnley *et al.*, 2002; Pringle *et al.*, 2003a,b; Carter *et al.*, 2004) and therefore exposition of the factors influencing the G_p will also shed light on the mechanisms responsible for the $\dot{V}O_2$ slow component. It is interesting to note, however, that if it is accepted that type II fibres have an inherently low gain (Barstow *et al.*, 1996; Jones *et al.*, 2002; Pringle *et al.*, 2003a; Scheuermann and Barstow, 2003), then the common explanation for the slow component (i.e. the 'progressive' recruitment of *low-efficiency* type II fibres with time at higher work rates) may need to be reconsidered (Pringle *et al.*, 2003b; see later).

What is the mechanistic basis for the $\dot{V}O_2$ slow component?

Despite the substantial magnitude of the $\dot{V}O_2$ slow component (up to $1\,l\cdot min^{-1}$ or more) and its temporal association with the maximal $\dot{V}O_2$ (i.e. for exercise in the severe domain, the $\dot{V}O_2$ slow component drives $\dot{V}O_2$ to $\dot{V}O_{2\,max}$) and the fatigue process(es), key exercise physiology textbooks have been reluctant to acknowledge the very existence of the $\dot{V}O_2$ slow component (e.g. Astrand and Rodahl, 1986; Fox *et al.*, 1988; DeVries and Housh, 1994; McArdle *et al.*, 1996). In part, this attitude is understandable because the slow component challenges some of the fundamental concepts in exercise physiology including the notion of the 'steady-state $\dot{V}O_2$,' O_2 deficit, work efficiency and the control of muscle energetics. However, resolution of the mechanistic bases of this phenomenon is crucial to our understanding of muscle function and dysfunction and in the past two decades or so considerable efforts have been made in this regard.

Indirect experimental approaches

A plethora of putative mediators of the $\dot{V}O_2$ slow component has been proposed (Figure 12.6). In the 1970s and 1980s, the most popular experimental approaches to try and link cause and effect with respect to these mediators was to either (1) derive an O_2 cost for a given process (e.g. temperature or respiratory muscle O_2 cost of ventilation) and calculate how much of the $\dot{V}O_2$ slow component could be attributed to this process (Hagberg *et al.*, 1978), or (2) correlate the temporal profile of change of each mediator with that of the $\dot{V}O_2$ slow component during heavy or severe exercise (Roston *et al.*, 1987; Poole *et al.*, 1988; Casaburi *et al.*, 1987). These approaches were necessarily indirect and fraught with assumptions. For example, Hagberg and colleagues (1978) used previously published values for the O_2 cost of breathing and elevated core temperature to estimate the contribution of these two processes to the $\dot{V}O_2$ slow component during heavy exercise. By so doing, they could account for more than 100% of the $\dot{V}O_2$ slow component! As demonstrated by McKerrow and Otis

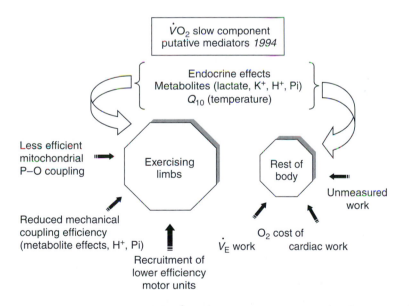

Figure 12.6 Putative mediators of the $\dot{V}O_2$ slow component as considered in 1994. The relative sizes of the octagons indicates the greater contribution of the exercising limbs to the $\dot{V}O_2$ slow component. Please note that less efficient mitochondrial P–O coupling and reduced mechanical coupling efficiency can occur within already recruited fibres and therefore does not necessitate increasing fibre recruitment.

(1956) and very elegantly by Aaron and colleagues (1992), there is a substantial inter-individual variation in the O_2 cost of breathing. Unless it is measured in a given subject over the precise range of ventilations in question using the appropriate ventilatory pattern present during exercise, errors can arise (rev. Aaron et al., 1992; Gaesser and Poole, 1996). Similarly when assuming an O_2 cost of exercise-induced elevations of temperature (i.e. the so-called Q_{10} effect) it is important to measure the temperature change within the tissues that generate the metabolic response, that is contracting muscles, rather than body core temperature as measured by Hagberg et al. (1978). Temperature changes within the exercising muscle can be much greater than those of core temperature and also follow a different temporal profile (Saltin et al., 1968). Subsequent investigations have demonstrated that it is possible to dissociate the profiles of changing ventilation and muscle temperature from the $\dot{V}O_2$ slow component (Poole et al., 1991; Gaesser and Poole, 1996) and that increased muscle temperature does not elevate pulmonary $\dot{V}O_2$ during exercise (Koga et al., 1997).

In many investigations (e.g. Whipp and Wasserman, 1986; Roston et al., 1987; Poole et al., 1988), the temporal profile of change in blood lactate concentration has correlated significantly with that of the $\dot{V}O_2$ slow component. The strength of that correlation has typically been better than that for other potential mediators such as catecholamines, ventilation or temperature (Poole et al., 1988). Moreover, Casaburi et al., (1987) reported an excellent correlation between the decrease in the $\dot{V}O_2$ slow component and the fall in blood lactate concentration induced by an exercise training regimen. As with ventilation and temperature discussed earlier, there is a solid theoretical and empirical basis for considering elevated blood lactate as a candidate for driving at least a portion of the $\dot{V}O_2$ slow component. Sodium L-(+)-lactate infusion elevates $\dot{V}O_2$ at rest and during exercise in humans (Ryan et al., 1979). The mechanism for this effect may involve stimulation of gluco/glyconeogenesis particularly within the exercising skeletal muscle which contains the enzymes essential for this process (Talmadge et al., 1989; rev. Gaesser and Poole, 1996). Alternatively, there may have been an alkalinizing effect of the lactate infused that resulted in stimulation of metabolism in a manner unlike that present during heavy exercise (Karetsky and Cain, 1969). The case for blood lactate as the major causative factor in the $\dot{V}O_2$ slow component is weakened by a few reported instances where blood lactate is elevated and rising progressively whilst $\dot{V}O_2$ is in a steady state (e.g. Scheen et al., 1981). Moreover, during treadmill running, there may be a significant slow component in the presence of blood lactate concentrations close to resting values (Steed et al., 1994). Finally, infusion of norepinephrine during exercise may elevate blood lactate significantly without increasing exercise $\dot{V}O_2$ (Gaesser et al., 1994).

That the predominant portion of the $\dot{V}O_2$ slow component occurs within the exercising limbs/muscles focused attention on the possibility that some aspect of fibre type specific recruitment or energetics may be involved in this process. However, before we examine that complex issue, there are several other important and, to a certain extent, definitive studies that allow us to disregard some more of the putative mediators given in Figure 12.6.

Lactate. L-(+)-lactate infusions sufficient to raise lactate concentration by ~10 mM in the arterial blood and ~9 mM in the contracting muscle failed to elevate $\dot{V}O_2$ in the dog gastrocnemius (Poole *et al.*, 1994). However, the lactate infusion was associated with a reproducible fall in muscle tension (Hogan *et al.*, 1995). Because pH can alter $\dot{V}O_2$ (Karetsky and Cain, 1969), an important facet of these experiments was that arterial pH was not altered by the lactate infusion.

Catecholamines. Gaesser and colleagues (1994) infused sufficient epinephrine into subjects exercising at a $\dot{V}O_2$ of $3\,L \cdot min^{-1}$ to raise the venous epinephrine concentrations by four- to fivefold which is consistent with subjects performing supramaximal exercise. There was absolutely no difference in pulmonary $\dot{V}O_2$ from the control exercise bout which is in agreement with the lack of effect of β-blockade on the $\dot{V}O_2$ response to heavy exercise (Davis *et al.*, 1994).

Muscle temperature. Using hot water-perfused pants, Koga and colleagues (1997) increased muscle temperature from 35.4°C to 38.9°C at the beginning and from 38.8°C to 40.3°C at the end of heavy exercise. They found that this elevation of temperature which was as large or larger than that expected during the development of the $\dot{V}O_2$ slow component, did not increase exercising $\dot{V}O_2$. Indeed, if anything the $\dot{V}O_2$ slow component was reduced compared with the control condition. Thus, these three series of experiments provide strong evidence that none of these potential mediators (lactate, epinephrine, muscle temperature) are likely, in and of themselves, to generate the $\dot{V}O_2$ slow component.

In science, it is axiomatic that correlations do not establish cause and effect. During heavy/severe-intensity exercise all putative mediators may be changing simultaneously and it is not always possible to measure a given mediator at its site of action or predict exactly what that action might be. In the early 1990s, it became apparent that a more direct experiment approach to resolving the mechanistic bases for the $\dot{V}O_2$ slow component was necessary.

Direct experimental approaches

To discriminate between candidate mechanisms that may participate in the $\dot{V}O_2$ slow component, Poole and colleagues (1991) simultaneously measured pulmonary and leg $\dot{V}O_2$ during cycle ergometry. Processes such as ventilatory muscle and cardiac work, increased body temperature, accessory muscle work (e.g. pulling on the handlebars of the ergometer) and metabolic effects (e.g. lactate, catecholamines, potassium) acting outside the active legs would contribute to the pulmonary $\dot{V}O_2$ but not to the leg $\dot{V}O_2$. Thus, by subtraction, the $\dot{V}O_2$ slow component arising from the exercising muscles and that from the rest of the body could be determined. These experiments demonstrated that for a pulmonary $\dot{V}O_2$ slow component of ~$700\,ml \cdot min^{-1}$, 86% on average emanated from processes occurring within the exercising limbs (Figure 12.6). Elegant NMR studies have recently confirmed these findings by demonstrating that intramuscular PCr concentrations fall in synchrony with the rising pulmonary $\dot{V}O_2$ slow component (Rossiter *et al.*, 2001, 2002a).

Obviously, location of over four-fifths of the pulmonary $\dot{V}O_2$ slow component within the exercising muscles severely constrains the potential participation of energetic demands from respiratory, cardiac or accessory muscles to a relatively minor portion of the overall $\dot{V}O_2$ slow component. The same is true for any additional metabolic stimulatory effects of hormonal, metabolite or temperature changes acting outside the exercising muscles. One caveat here is that although the respiratory muscles are relatively minor contributors to the $\dot{V}O_2$ slow component in healthy individuals (Poole *et al.*, 1991; Engelen *et al.*, 1996), this may not be so for patients afflicted with diseases such as emphysema or fibrosis or those who experience elevated flow resistance consequent to a narrowing or blockage of the large airways resulting from other pathological conditions. Addition of inspiratory resistance significantly increases the amplitude of the $\dot{V}O_2$ slow component (Carra *et al.*, 2003). This latter study suggested that the respiratory muscles themselves, as well as contributing to the overall increase in pulmonary $\dot{V}O_2$, may also elicit a slow component of their own under these circumstances.

Muscle fibre energetics

By process of elimination, as detailed in the preceding section, many scientists have settled on the notion that some aspect of fibre type recruitment patterns or energetic processes occurring within discrete fibre populations underlie the $\dot{V}O_2$ slow component (Figure 12.6). Despite intense interest and many published papers, an unequivocal linkage between fibre type effects and the $\dot{V}O_2$ slow component has remained elusive. In many respects this has resulted from the lack of temporal and spatial resolution of the electromyographical and NMR imaging and spectroscopy techniques available to the human exercise physiologist. Before reviewing the most recent experimental evidence for the involvement of muscle fibre recruitment patterns in the aetiology of the $\dot{V}O_2$ slow component, a brief review of the principal energetic differences between type I (slow twitch) and type II (fast twitch) fibres is useful.

In vitro *fibre type energetic differences*

The energetic cost of force production is fibre type specific and many investigations using muscles from a range of animal preparations have demonstrated that the energetic cost of tension production is higher for type II than type I muscles. For example, in the rat extensor digitorum longus muscle (EDL, predominantly type II fibres), a given isometric tension development increased initial heat production several-fold more than found in the type I soleus muscle (Gibbs and Gibson, 1972; Wendt and Gibbs, 1973). Similarly, Crow and Kushmerick (1982) found that the high-energy phosphate splitting during contraction of the mouse EDL was three-fold that of the soleus. Interestingly, this difference was reduced to ~50% for tetani >12 s in duration. This greater chemical energy requirement of type II fibres may result from either a different chemical-to-mechanical coupling efficiency or alternatively from faster actomyosin turnover. In addition, calcium pump activity is five- to ten-fold faster in type II versus type I fibres (Gibbs and Gibson, 1972; Wendt and Gibbs, 1973) and the greater α-glycerophosphate shuttle activity (which is FAD rather than NAD-linked) reduces the P:O ratio ~18% in type II fibres (Willis and Jackman, 1994).

Few investigators have addressed this issue in human muscle fibres *in vitro*. In a series of extremely elegant experiments, He and colleagues (2000) demonstrated that there was a four-fold higher ATP hydrolysis rate and maximal power in single human vastus lateralis type II vs type I fibres performing shortening (isotonic) contractions. However, the peak thermodynamic efficiencies were not significantly different between fibre types (type I, 0.21; type II, 0.27). These studies also demonstrated that type II fibres achieved their peak efficiency at greater shortening velocities and higher relative loads than type I fibres. Thus, depending on the fibre shortening velocity, which will be determined in large part by the pedal frequency during cycle exercise, the $\dot{V}O_2$ cost of force production from type II compared with type I fibres may not be excessive.

In vivo *fibre type energetic differences*

The conflicting results cited in the previous section emphasize the importance of examining muscle fibre energetics during isotonic rather than isometric conditions in order to apply the results to dynamic exercise in humans. Coyle and colleagues (1992) found that cycling efficiency at 80 rev·min^{-1} correlated significantly with the proportion of type I fibres in the vastus lateralis which was attributed to the close proximity of this pedal rate to that yielding the peak efficiency of type I fibres (for type II fibres this pedal rate is typically above 100 rpm, Sargeant, 1999). Although some authors have argued against the necessity for recruitment of a substantial population of type II fibres during cycling at submaximal $\dot{V}O_2$ values (Scheuermann *et al.*, 2001), there is credible evidence that virtually all Type II muscle fibres in the vastus lateralis are recruited at these intensities (Vollestad and Blom, 1985; Ivy *et al.*, 1987). This is consistent with the correlation between % type II muscle fibres in the musculature recruited and the relative amplitude of the $\dot{V}O_2$ slow component (Barstow *et al.*, 1996; Pringle *et al.*, 2003a).

Thus, type II fibres contribute proportionally more to the power output at higher pedal rates, that is 100–135 rev·min^{-1} (Beelen and Sargeant, 1993; He *et al.*, 2000) and these pedal rates also engender greater $\dot{V}O_2$ slow components compared to frequencies of 35–75 rev·min^{-1} (Gaesser and Brooks, 1975; Pringle *et al.*, 2003b). At first glance, it seems counterintuitive that type II fibres operating at shortening speeds closer to those that yield their optimum velocity with respect to mechanical efficiency (Sargeant, 1999) should generate a larger $\dot{V}O_2$ slow component. However, this greater slow component occurs concomitant with a reduced primary gain of the $\dot{V}O_2$ response such that the end exercise (i.e. 6 min) $\dot{V}O_2$ is not greater at 115 rev·min^{-1} than either 35 or 75 rev·min^{-1} (Pringle *et al.*, 2003b). The reason for the influence of pedal rate on the primary gain is addressed in the section entitled 'Are the primary fast $\dot{V}O_2$ kinetics slowed above the lactate threshold?'

Relationship between muscle (fibre) recruitment patterns and $\dot{V}O_2$ slow component

In the last decade or so, many investigations have attempted to establish the profile of muscle (integrated EMG, iEMG; and magnetic resonance imaging, MRI) and muscle fibre (analysis of the mean power frequency, MPF) recruitment patterns and their temporal association with the $\dot{V}O_2$ slow component. Increased MPF has been interpreted as a reflection of type II fibre recruitment (Wretling *et al.*, 1987; Borrani *et al.*, 2001). Alternatively, it is possible that MPF may increase consequent to an increased firing frequency of type I motor units or a rise in muscle temperature. Overall, the results have provided conflicting evidence as to whether the $\dot{V}O_2$ slow component by necessity arises from the recruitment of previously quiescent fibres and whether such fibres, if recruited, have to be type II fibres. The reasons for the differing findings relate, perhaps, to the inherent noise within the EMG signal, the variety of muscles evaluated, the size and temporal profile of the associated $\dot{V}O_2$ slow component and possibly inter-subject variability (e.g. degree of training, inherent fibre type distribution).

In 1992, Shinohara and Moritani demonstrated a weak, though significant, relationship between iEMG increases and the amplitude of the $\dot{V}O_2$ slow component. However, the iEMG increases became apparent only after ~240 s of exercise which is somewhat later than the onset of the $\dot{V}O_2$ slow component in most studies (i.e. 120–180 s, Casaburi *et al.*, 1987; Roston *et al.*, 1987; Barstow and Mole, 1991; Paterson and Whipp, 1991; Barstow *et al.*, 1993; Koga *et al.*, 1999). Since then, there has been more compelling evidence: (1) Within two major muscles (vastus lateralis, gastrocnemius lateralis) recruited in heavy-intensity cycling, the start of the MPF increase corresponds with that of the $\dot{V}O_2$ slow component (Borrani *et al.*, 2001). (2) Following priming exercise that increases the primary $\dot{V}O_2$ response and reduces the $\dot{V}O_2$ slow component, there is ~19% increase in gluteus maximus, vastus lateralis and vastus medialis iEMG in the first two minutes of the subsequent bout (Burnley *et al.*, 2002). In addition, the iEMG during minutes 3–6 of the subsequent bout was reduced in concert with the reduced $\dot{V}O_2$ slow component. MPF was unchanged. These data were interpreted to mean that additional fibre recruitment (type I and type II) at the onset of the second bout effectively spread the work rate over more myofibrils such that the metabolic disturbance of each was reduced. Moritani *et al.* (1992) have demonstrated that the motor unit recruitment strategy can be altered by metabolic disturbances within the exercising muscle and that this is detectable by surface EMG. (3) Using MRI, Saunders and colleagues (2000) found progressive increases in vastus lateralis, rectus femoris and whole leg T2 (indicative of muscle recruitment) that correlated with the $\dot{V}O_2$ slow component during heavy-intensity exercise. Both iEMG and MPF of the vastus lateralis (the only muscle so evaluated) also increased progressively. (4) Most recently, Krustrup *et al.* (a) selectively trained quadriceps type II fibres and demonstrated a reduced muscle $\dot{V}O_2$ slow component during heavy intensity knee extensor exercise (30W, see figure 4A of Krustrup *et al.* (2004a) and (b) created a $\dot{V}O_2$ slow component at a sub-LT work rate by using type I fibre glycogen depletion to de-recruit type I fibres and force greater type II fibre recruitment (Krustrup *et al.*, 2004b).

In contrast to these, other investigations have failed to find evidence that increased muscle fibre recruitment is associated with the slow component. Each of the following studies utilized some permutation of the repeated exercise paradigm employed by Burnley *et al.* (2002) discussed earlier. Scheuermann and colleagues (2001) assessed the profiles of iEMG and $\dot{V}O_2$ of the vastus lateralis muscle during repeated bouts of heavy/severe exercise. iEMG and MPF remained constant and at the same level throughout the second exercise bout despite the smaller $\dot{V}O_2$ slow component. Tordi *et al.* (2003) found similar results in the vastus lateralis, rectus femoris, vastus medialis and gastrocnemius medialis muscles during heavy/severe exercise that followed 30 s bouts of sprint exercise. Finally, Perrey *et al.* (2003) utilized a prolonged (90 min at 60% $\dot{V}O_2$ peak) exercise bout to lower the subsequent $\dot{V}O_2$ slow component by ~25% during heavy exercise. Again, this effect occurred in the absence of detectable changes in iEMG and MPF. The ensemble of data presented in these four latter studies is consistent with the notion that the $\dot{V}O_2$ slow component is coupled to a progressive increase in ATP requirements of the already recruited motor units rather than to changes in the recruitment pattern of type I vs type II muscle fibres. It should be mentioned, however, that there was enormous variability evident in the EMG signals in the second exercise bout that may have precluded identification of altered muscle recruitment (see figure 3 of Tordi *et al.*, 2003).

In summary to this section, the $\dot{V}O_2$ slow component arises predominantly from within the exercising limbs and therefore, presumably, the contracting muscles. However, there is not incontrovertible evidence that this $\dot{V}O_2$ slow component is dependent solely upon the recruitment of additional type II muscle fibres. Specifically, iEMG, MPF and also MRI indices of muscle activation have been shown to increase with $\dot{V}O_2$ (Saunders *et al.*, 2000; Borrani *et al.*, 2001; Burnley *et al.*, 2002) and selective training of type II muscle fibres reduces the slow component of muscle $\dot{V}O_2$ (Krustrup *et al.* 2004a) whereas selectively increasing type II fibre recruitment can create a slow component at work rates $<$ LT (Krustrup *et al.*, 2004b). However, notwithstanding the concerns expressed relative to the fidelity of the EMG signal, the $\dot{V}O_2$ slow component has been manipulated independently from iEMG and MPF in other investigations (Scheuermann *et al.*, 2001; Perrey *et al.*, 2003; Tordi *et al.*, 2003).

Is it possible that the $\dot{V}O_2$ cost of force production increases during heavy/severe-intensity exercise irrespective of whether additional type II fibres are recruited or not? The falling PCr profile observed during the $\dot{V}O_2$ slow component suggests that there is a high phosphate cost of force generation rather than a high O_2 cost of phosphate production (Rossiter *et al.*, 2001, 2002a). This is consistent with the unchanged O_2 cost of ATP resynthesis (i.e. P:O ratio) found in mitochondria isolated from the vastus lateralis of humans performing repeated bouts of fatiguing exercise (work-rate corresponding to 130% of that required to elicit $\dot{V}O_{2\,max}$) (Tonkonogi *et al.*, 1999). Energetically speaking, one of the most expensive processes during muscle contraction is Ca^{2+} handling by the sarcoplasmic reticulum

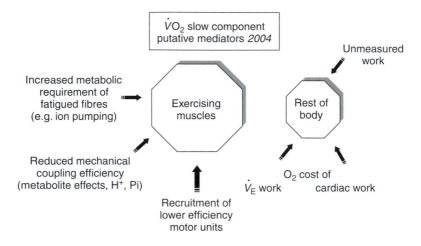

Figure 12.7 The current array of potential mediators of the slow $\dot{V}O_2$ component is somewhat less cluttered than in 1994. See text for details of those experiments that have removed potential candidate mediators.

which may account for up to 50% of the total ATP requirement (Bergstrom and Hultman, 1988). Accumulation of metabolites or ions (hydrogen ions, inorganic phosphate [particularly the diprotonated form], magnesium, potassium) in fatiguing muscle does affect sarcoplasmic reticulum Ca^{2+} dynamics, troponin sensitivity to Ca^{2+} and the contraction force of the cross-bridge attachments (rev. Allen *et al.*, 1992). Consequently, there is the potential for alterations in the intracellular milieu, if they result in the need for either elevated cytosolic $[Ca^{2+}]$ or Ca^{2+} turnover rates, to raise the O_2 cost of generating a given power output. This scenario may explain the tight coupling between the reduction in intramuscular pH and the $[PCr]$ and $\dot{V}O_2$ slow components reported by Rossiter *et al.* (2002b).

Given these facts, one can envisage several possible scenarios within the contracting muscle during heavy exercise as a consequence of the accumulation of metabolites. The most likely of these are as follows: (1) Those fibres experiencing a pronounced metabolite accumulation increase their ATP turnover to sustain power output (consistent with Scheuermann *et al.*, 2001; Perrey *et al.*, 2003; Tordi *et al.*, 2003). (2) Alternatively, some of these fibres may fatigue thereby necessitating either the recruitment of additional motor units (most likely type II but possibly type I) or greater power output from other already recruited muscle fibres (Pringle *et al.*, 2003b). The O_2 cost of ion pumping and related activities within the fatigued fibres (either type I or II) might be substantial even in the absence of force output from these fibres (consistent with Saunders *et al.*, 2000; Borrani *et al.*, 2001; Burnley *et al.*, 2002). Figure 12.7 summarizes the current and much abbreviated (cf. Figure 12.6) list of potential mediators of the $\dot{V}O_2$ slow component. Unequivocal discrimination between these remaining candidate mechanisms within the exercising muscle beckons rigorous scientific attention.

How does 'priming exercise' influence $\dot{V}O_2$ kinetics?

Since the seminal work of Gerbino *et al.* (1996), a large number of studies have utilized the 'prior exercise' model to examine the influence of increased O_2 availability on $\dot{V}O_2$ kinetics during heavy and severe exercise (see Chapter 10 for review). For upright cycle exercise in young healthy subjects, all of the studies conducted to date (with one exception; Tordi *et al.*, 2003) have reported that the performance of prior heavy exercise has no significant influence on τ_p during subsequent heavy exercise (e.g. Burnley *et al.*, 2000; Koppo and Bouckaert, 2001; Scheuermann *et al.*, 2001). On the other hand, in situations in which O_2 availability may be compromised in the control condition (e.g. in the senescent individual and in exercise modes where the working muscle is level with or above the heart), prior heavy exercise has been found to result in a reduction of τ_p (e.g. MacDonald *et al.*, 2001; Rossiter *et al.*, 2001; Scheuermann *et al.*, 2002). These differences between studies are consistent with the model presented in Figure 12.3.

One general similarity between all the 'priming' studies is that prior heavy exercise results in a reduction in the amplitude of the $\dot{V}O_2$ slow component (note that for upright cycle exercise, this effect may be secondary to an increased amplitude of the $\dot{V}O_2$ primary component; e.g. Burnley *et al.*, 2002). The cause of this effect remains somewhat obscure. However, the effect of prior exercise on muscle temperature has been ruled out (Koppo *et al.*, 2002). Given the known relationship between muscle fibre type composition and the gains of the primary and slow components (Barstow *et al.*, 1996; Pringle *et al.*, 2003a), and the sensitivity of these gain terms to interventions designed to alter fibre recruitment such as muscle glycogen depletion and pedal rate (Pringle *et al.*, 2003b; Carter *et al.*, 2004), the most likely cause of the altered $\dot{V}O_2$ kinetics following priming exercise may be an alteration in muscle fibre recruitment (Burnley *et al.*, 2002) which may or may not be related to altered O_2 availability.

Conclusions

Before we progress to Part IV, which deals with the plasticity of $\dot{V}O_2$ kinetics and metabolic control within the context of human maturation and ageing, disease and exercise training, it is instructive to briefly summarize some of the major points from Parts I–III. These parts have reinforced the notion that pulmonary $\dot{V}O_2$ measurements – though not without their problems of data collection, analysis and interpretation – can provide valuable insights into metabolic control processes within exercising muscle. More direct or invasive techniques such as muscle biopsy, NMRS or catheterization procedures have their own inherent limitations and are simply not available to many laboratories for ethical or technical reasons.

Although temporally displaced, the primary component of pulmonary $\dot{V}O_2$ kinetics can provide a faithful representation of muscle $\dot{V}O_2$ – which begins to increase within the first contraction cycle. For upright moderate-intensity exercise with large muscle groups the speed of those kinetics can be accelerated by reducing mitochondrial inertia but not by increasing O_2 delivery. Thus, intracellular PO_2

may be considered to be at some 'saturating' level with respect to $\dot{V}O_2$ kinetics. For heavy and severe exercise, the weight of evidence suggests that the primary $\dot{V}O_2$ kinetics are slowed and the primary gain is reduced. A $\dot{V}O_2$ slow component is also manifested at these work-rates which is responsible for increasing the total gain at these exercise intensities. That augmented O_2 delivery can speed the overall $\dot{V}O_2$ kinetics, increase the gain of the primary $\dot{V}O_2$ component and reduce the $\dot{V}O_2$ slow component suggests that intracellular PO_2 may be non-saturating in these exercise intensity domains. Thus, for heavy/severe exercise $\dot{V}O_2$ kinetics reflect a complex interaction between intracellular PO_2 and mitochondrial inertia. Metabolic regulation within specific fibre populations and the recruitment and derecruitment among and within specific fibre type populations are likely to play a crucial role in these processes. However, despite concerted efforts and the implementation of elegant experimental designs, our understanding in this regard is hamstrung by the lack of spatial resolution and the inability to unequivocally identify specific fibre populations within voluntarily contracting muscle(s).

As emphasized throughout this text, slower $\dot{V}O_2$ kinetics obligate an increased O_2 deficit and greater perturbation of the intracellular milieu that is accompanied by reduced exercise tolerance. The $\dot{V}O_2$ slow component represents an 'excess' $\dot{V}O_2$ that may drive $\dot{V}O_2$ to $\dot{V}O_{2\,max}$ (severe exercise) or mandate an accelerated glycogenolysis (heavy exercise) both of which accelerate the fatigue process(es). Recent elegant glycogen depletion and one-legged training studies provide some of the strongest support yet for the integral involvement of type II fibre recruitment in the aetiology of the $\dot{V}O_2$ slow component (Krustrup et al., 2004 a,b). Whereas Part III has presented a range of acute experimental manipulations designed to investigate the determinants of $\dot{V}O_2$ kinetics, Part IV focuses on chronic adaptations that impact the human condition. Emphasis is placed upon integration of the principles and information developed in the previous parts as a basis for understanding the structural and functional bases for impaired (Chapters 13 and 14) or improved (Chapter 15) $\dot{V}O_2$ kinetics and exercise tolerance. This topic is particularly germane to the (unfortunately) burgeoning populations of patients whose mobility and therefore quality of life is restricted by pathological limitations in the ability to load, transport and utilize O_2. For such individuals, a greater understanding of $\dot{V}O_2$ kinetics and the therapeutic ability to speed those kinetics and/or reduce the magnitude of the $\dot{V}O_2$ slow component may substantially improve their quality of life.

Glossary of terms

ADP	adenosine diphosphate (ADP_{free}, the metabolically important fraction of intracellular ADP)
ATP	adenosine triphosphate
Ca^{2+}	calcium ion
Cr	creatine
$\Delta \dot{V}O_2/\Delta$ work rate	slope of the $\dot{V}O_2$-to-work-rate relationship, usually considered synonymous with gain (G)

%Δ	% of the difference between the GET (or LT) and $\dot{V}O_{2\,max}$
EDL	extensor digitorum longus muscle
FAD	flavine adenine dinucleotide
GET	gas exchange threshold
G_i	gain of the primary component increase in $\dot{V}O_2$, that is increase in $\dot{V}O_2$ per unit increase in external work rate
Half-time	time required to reach 50% of total $\dot{V}O_2$ increase
iEMG	integrated electromyogram
K_{eq}	equilibrium constant
LT	lactate threshold
MPF	mean power frequency of the EMG
MRI	magnetic resonance imaging
MRS	magnetic resonance spectroscopy
MRT	mean response time (time delay + time constant, τ or tau, denotes time to 63% of final response)
NADH	reduced form of nicotinamide adenine nucleotide
NAD	nicotinamide adenine nucleotide
NMR	nuclear magnetic resonance
NO	nitric oxide
PCr	phosphocreatine
Pi	inorganic phosphate
Phase I	initial increase in $\dot{V}O_2$ following exercise onset caused by elevated pulmonary blood flow (also called the cardiodynamic phase)
Phase II	(same as primary component) the exponential increase in $\dot{V}O_2$ that is initiated when venous blood from the exercising muscles arrives at the lungs. Corresponds closely with muscle $\dot{V}O_2$ dynamics under normal circumstances
Phase II τ	time constant of Phase II $\dot{V}O_2$ response
Pi	inorganic phosphate
P:O ratio	ATP yield per atom of oxygen
PO_2	partial pressure of O_2
τ or tau,	time constant, denotes time to 63% of final response from onset of exponential
τ_p	time constant of Phase II or primary component
$\dot{V}O_2$	oxygen uptake
$\dot{V}O_{2\,max}$	maximal oxygen uptake (achieved under conditions of large muscle mass exercise unless otherwise specified, and considered synonymous with $\dot{V}O_2$ peak)
$\dot{V}O_2$ slow component	a slowly developing $\dot{V}O_2$ response initiated beyond ~2 min of heavy and severe exercise. Also termed 'excess' $\dot{V}O_2$ (see Chapter 1)
VT	ventilatory threshold
[ ]	denotes concentration

References

Aaron, E.A., Johnson, B.D., Seow, C.K. and Dempsey, J.A. (1992). Oxygen cost of exercise hyperpnea: measurement. *Journal of Applied Physiology*, **72**, 1810–17.

Allen, D.G., Westerblad, H., Lee, J.A. and Lannergren, J. (1992). Role of excitation–contraction coupling in muscle fatigue. *Sports Medicine*, **13**, 116–26.

Arthur, P.G., Hogan, M.C., Bebout, D.E., Wagner, P.D. and Hochachka, P.W. (1992). Modeling the effects of hypoxia on ATP turnover in exercising muscle. *Journal of Applied Physiology*, **73**, 737–42.

Astrand, P.-O. and Rodahl, K. (1986) Textbook *of Work Physiology: Physiological Basis of Exercise*. McGraw-Hill, New York, pp. 299–303.

Balaban, R.S. (1990). Regulation of oxidative phosphorylation in the mammalian cell. *American Journal of Physiology*, **258**, C377–89.

Bangsbo, J., Krustrup, P., Gonzalez-Alonso, J., Boushel, R. and Saltin, B. (2000). Muscle oxygen kinetics at onset of intense dynamic exercise in humans. *American Journal of Physiology*, **279**, R899–906.

Bangsbo, J., Gibala, M.J., Krustrup, P., Gonzalez-Alonso, J. and Saltin, B. (2002). Enhanced pyruvate dehydrogenase activity does not affect muscle O_2 uptake at onset of intense exercise in humans. *American Journal of Physiology*, **282**, R273–80.

Barstow, T.J. and Mole, P.A. (1991). Linear and nonlinear characteristics of oxygen uptake kinetics during heavy exercise. *Journal of Applied Physiology*, **71**, 2099–106.

Barstow, T.J., Lamarra, N. and Whipp, B.J. (1990). Modulation of muscle and pulmonary O_2 uptakes by circulatory dynamics during exercise. *Journal of Applied Physiology*, **68**, 979–89.

Barstow, T.J., Casaburi, R. and Wasserman, K. (1993). O_2 uptake kinetics and the O_2 deficit as related to exercise intensity and blood lactate. *Journal of Applied Physiology*, **75**, 755–62.

Barstow, T.J., Jones, A.M., Nguyen, P.H. and Casaburi, R. (1996). Influence of muscle fiber type and pedal frequency on oxygen uptake kinetics of heavy exercise. *Journal of Applied Physiology*, **81**, 1642–50.

Beelen, A. and Sargeant, A.J. (1993). Effect of prior exercise at different pedalling frequencies on maximal power in humans. *European Journal of Applied Physiology*, **66**, 102–7.

Behnke, B.J., Kindig, C.A., Musch, T.I., Koga, S. and Poole, D.C. (2001). Dynamics of microvascular oxygen pressure across the rest–exercise transition in rat skeletal muscle. *Respiration Physiology and Neurobiology*, **126**, 53–63.

Behnke, B.J., Barstow, T.J., Kindig, C.A., McDonough, P., Musch, T.I. and Poole, D.C. (2002a). Dynamics of oxygen uptake following exercise onset in rat skeletal muscle. *Respiration Physiology and Neurobiology*, **133**, 229–39.

Behnke, B.J., Kindig, C.A., McDonough, P., Poole, D.C. and Sexton, W.L. (2002b). Dynamics of microvascular oxygen pressure during rest–contraction transition in skeletal muscle of diabetic rats. *American Journal of Physiology*, **283**, H926–32.

Behnke, B.J., Kindig, C.A., Musch, T.I., Sexton, W.L. and Poole, D.C. (2002c). Effects of prior contractions on muscle microvascular oxygen pressure at onset of subsequent contractions. *Journal of Physiology*, **539**, 927–34.

Behnke, B.J., McDonough, P., Padilla, D.J., Musch, T.I. and Poole, D.C. (2003). Oxygen exchange profile in rat muscles of contrasting fibre types. *Journal of Physiology*, **549**, 597–605.

Bergstrom, M. and Hultman, E. (1988). Energy cost and fatigue during intermittent electrical stimulation of human skeletal muscle. *Journal of Applied Physiology*, **65**, 1500–5.

Binzoni, T., Ferretti, G., Schenker, K. and Cerretelli, P. (1992). Phosphocreatine hydrolysis by 31P-NMR at the onset of constant-load exercise in humans. *Journal of Applied Physiology*, **73**, 1644–9.

Borrani, F., Candau, R., Millet, G.Y., Perrey, S., Fuchslocher, J. and Rouillon, J.D. (2001). Is the $\dot{V}O_2$ slow component dependent on progressive recruitment of fast-twitch fibers in trained runners. *Journal of Applied Physiology*, **90**, 2212–20.

Bottinelli, R. and Reggiani, C. (2000). Human skeletal muscle fibres: molecular and functional diversity. *Progress in Biophysics and Molecular Biology*, **73**, 195–262.

Burnley, M., Jones, A.M., Carter, H. and Doust, J.H. (2000). Effects of prior heavy exercise on phase II pulmonary oxygen uptake kinetics during heavy exercise. *Journal of Applied Physiology*, **89**, 1387–96.

Burnley, M., Doust, J.H., Ball, D. and Jones, A.M. (2002). Effects of prior heavy exercise on $\dot{V}O_2$ kinetics during heavy exercise are related to changes in muscle activity. *Journal of Applied Physiology*, **93**, 167–74.

Carra, J., Candau, R., Keslacy, S., Giolbas, F., Borrani, F., Millet, G.P., Varray, A. and Ramonatxo, M. (2003). Addition of inspiratory resistance increases the amplitude of the slow component of O_2 uptake kinetics. *Journal of Applied Physiology*, **94**, 2448–55.

Carter, H., Jones, A.M., Barstow, T.J., Burnley, M., Williams, C.A. and Doust, J.H. (2000a). Oxygen uptake kinetics in treadmill running and cycle ergometry: a comparison. *Journal of Applied Physiology*, **89**, 899–907.

Carter, H., Jones, A.M., Barstow, T.J., Burnley, M., Williams, C.A. and Doust, J.H. (2000b). Effect of endurance training on oxygen uptake kinetics during treadmill running. *Journal of Applied Physiology*, **89**, 1744–52.

Carter, H., Pringle, J.S., Jones, A.M. and Doust, J.H. (2002). Oxygen uptake kinetics during treadmill running across exercise intensity domains. *European Journal of Applied Physiology*, **86**, 347–54.

Carter, H., Pringle, J.S., Boobis, L., Jones, A.M. and Doust, J.H. (2004). Muscle glycogen depletion alters pulmonary oxygen uptake kinetics during heavy constant-load cycle exercise. *Medicine and Science in Sports and Exercise*, **36**(6), 965–72.

Casaburi, R., Storer, T.W., Ben-Dov, I. and Wasserman K. (1987). Effect of endurance training on possible determinants of $\dot{V}O_2$ during heavy exercise. *Journal of applied physiology*, **62**, 199–207.

Chance, B. and Williams, G.R. (1955). Respiratory enzymes in oxidative phosphorylation. I. Kinetics of oxygen utilization. *Journal of Biological Chemistry*, **217**, 383–93.

Conley, K.E., Kemper, W.F. and Crowther, G.J. (2001). Limits to sustainable muscle performance: interaction between glycolysis and oxidative phosphorylation. *Journal of Experimental Biology*, **204**, 3189–94.

Coyle, E.F., Sidossis, L.S., Horowitz, J.F. and Beltz, J.D. (1992). Cycling efficiency is related to the percentage of type I muscle fibers. *Medicine and Science in Sports and Exercise*, **24**, 782–8.

Crow, M.T. and Kushmerick, M.J. (1982). Chemical energetics of slow- and fast-twitch muscles of the mouse. *Journal of General Physiology*, **79**, 147–66.

Davis, S.E., Womack, C.J., Gutgesell, M., Barrett, E., Weltman, A. and Gaesser, G.A. (1994). Effects of β-blockade on slow component of $\dot{V}O_2$ during moderate and heavy exercise. *Medicine and Science in Sports and Exercise*, **26**, S208.

Delp, M.D. (1999). Control of skeletal muscle perfusion at the onset of dynamic exercise. *Medicine and Science in Sports and Exercise*, **31**, 1011–18.

De Vries, H.A. and Housh, T.J. (1994). *Physiology of Exercise: For Physical Education, Athletics, and Exercise Science*. Brown & Benchmark, Madison, WI, pp. 216–22.

Diederich, E.R., Behnke, B.J., McDonough, P., Kindig, C.A., Barstow, T.J., Poole, D.C. and Musch, T.I. (2002). Dynamics of microvascular oxygen partial pressure in contracting skeletal muscle of rats with chronic heart failure. *Cardiovascular Research*, **56**, 479–86.

Dix, J.A. and Verkman, A.S. (1990). Mapping of fluorescence anisotropy in living cells by ratio imaging. Application to cytoplasmic viscosity. *Biophysical Journal*, **57**, 231–40.

Engelen, M., Porszasz, J., Riley, M., Wasserman, K., Maehara, K. and Barstow, T.J. (1996). Effects of hypoxic hypoxia on O_2 uptake and heart rate kinetics during heavy exercise. *Journal of Applied Physiology*, **81**, 2500–8.

Fox, E.L., Bowers, R.W. and Foss, M.L. (1988). *The Physiological Basis of Physical Education and Athletics* (4th edition) W.B. Saunders, Philadelphia, pp. 32–3.

Fujihara, Y., Hildebrandt, J.R. and Hildebrandt, J. (1973). Cardiorespiratory transients in exercising man. I. Tests of superposition. *Journal of Applied Physiology*, **35**, 58–67.

Gaesser, G.A. and Brooks, G.A. (1975). Muscular efficiency during steady-rate exercise: effects of speed and work rate. *Journal of Applied Physiology*, **38**, 1132–9.

Gaesser, G.A. and Poole, D.C. (1996). The slow component of oxygen uptake kinetics in humans. In J.O. Holloszy (Ed.) *Exercise and Sports Science Reviews*, Vol. 25. Williams and Wilkins, Philadelphia, pp. 35–70.

Gaesser, G.A., Ward, S.A., Baum, V.C. and Whipp, B.J. (1994). Effects of infused epinephrine on slow phase of O_2 uptake kinetics during heavy exercise in humans. *Journal of Applied Physiology*, **77**, 2413–19.

Gerbino, A., Ward, S.A. and Whipp, B.J. (1996). Effects of prior exercise on pulmonary gas-exchange kinetics during high-intensity exercise in humans. *Journal of Applied Physiology*, **80**, 99–107.

Gibbs, C.L. and Gibson, W.R. (1972). Energy production of rat soleus muscle. *American Journal of Physiology*, **223**, 864–71.

Grassi, B., Poole, D.C., Richardson, R.S., Knight, D.R., Erickson, B.K. and Wagner, P.D. (1996). Muscle O_2 uptake kinetics in humans: implications for metabolic control. *Journal of Applied Physiology*, 80, 988–98.

Grassi, B., Gladden, L.B., Samaja, M., Stary, C.M. and Hogan, M.C. (1998a). Faster adjustment of O_2 delivery does not affect $\dot{V}O_2$ on-kinetics in isolated in situ canine muscle. *Journal of Applied Physiology*, **85**, 1394–403.

Grassi, B., Gladden, L.B., Stary, C.M., Wagner, P.D. and Hogan, M.C. (1998b). Peripheral O_2 diffusion does not affect $\dot{V}O_2$ on-kinetics in isolated in situ canine muscle. *Journal of Applied Physiology*, **85**, 1404–12.

Grassi, B., Hogan, M.C., Greenhaff, P.L., Hamann, J.J., Kelley, K.M., Aschenbach, W.G., Constantin-Teodosiu, D. and Gladden, L.B. (2002). Oxygen uptake on-kinetics in dog gastrocnemius in situ following activation of pyruvate dehydrogenase by dichloroacetate. *Journal of Physiology*, **538**, 195–207.

Greenhaff, P.L., Campbell-O'Sullivan, S.P., Constantin-Teodosiu, D., Poucher, S.M., Roberts, P.A. and Timmons, J.A. (2002). An acetyl group deficit limits mitochondrial ATP production at the onset of exercise. *Biochemical Society Transactions*, **30**, 75–80.

Hagberg, J.M., Mullin, J.P. and Nagle, F.J. (1978). Oxygen consumption during constant-load exercise. *Journal of Applied Physiology*, **45**, 381–4.

Haseler, L.J., Richardson, R.S., Videen, J.S. and Hogan, M.C. (1998). Phosphocreatine hydrolysis during submaximal exercise: the effect of F_1O_2. *Journal of Applied Physiology*, **85**, 1457–63.

He, Z.H., Bottinelli, R., Pellegrino, M.A., Ferenczi, M.A. and Reggiani, C. (2000). ATP consumption and efficiency of human single muscle fibers with different myosin isoform composition. *Biophysical Journal*, **79**, 945–61.

Hepple, R.T., Liu, P.P., Plyley, M.J. and Goodman, J.M. (1999). Oxygen uptake kinetics during exercise in chronic heart failure: influence of peripheral vascular reserve. *Clinical Science*, **97**, 569–77.

Hirai, T., Visneski, M.D., Kearns, K.J., Zelis, R. and Musch, T.I. (1994). Effects of NO synthase inhibition on the muscular blood flow response to treadmill exercise in rats. *Journal of Applied Physiology*, **77**, 1288–93.

Hochachka, P.W. (1994). *Muscles as Metabolic Machines*. CRC Press, Ann Arbor, pp. 95–118.

Hochachka, P.W. and Matheson, G.O. (1992). Regulating ATP turnover rates over broad dynamic work ranges in skeletal muscles. *Journal of Applied Physiology*, **73**, 1697–703.

Hogan, M.C. (2001). Fall in intracellular PO_2 at the onset of contractions in Xenopus single skeletal muscle fibers. *Journal of Applied Physiology*, **90**, 1871–6.

Hogan, M.C., Arthur, P.G., Bebout, D.E., Hochachka, P.W. and Wagner, P.D. (1992). Role of O_2 in regulating tissue respiration in dog muscle working in situ. *Journal of Applied Physiology*, **73**, 728–36.

Hogan, M.C., Gladden, L.B., Kurdak, S.S. and Poole, D.C. (1995). Increased [lactate] in working dog muscle reduces tension development independent of pH. *Medicine and Science in Sports and Exercise*, **27**, 371–7.

Hogan, M.C., Kurdak, S.S. and Arthur, P.G. (1996). Effect of gradual reduction in O_2 delivery on intracellular homeostasis in contracting skeletal muscle. *Journal of Applied Physiology*, **80**, 1313–21.

Howlett, R.A. and Hogan, M.C. (2003). Dichloroacetate accelerates the fall in intracellular PO_2 at onset of contractions in Xenopus single muscle fibers. *American Journal of Physiology*, **284**, R481–5.

Hughson, R.L. and Smyth, G.A. (1983). Slower adaptation of $\dot{V}O_2$ to steady-state of submaximal exercise with beta-blockade. *European Journal of Applied Physiology*, **52**, 107–10.

Hughson, R.L., Cochrane, J.E. and Butler, G.C. (1993). Faster O_2 uptake kinetics at onset of supine exercise with than without lower body negative pressure. *Journal of Applied Physiology*, ,**75**, 1962–7.

Hughson, R.L., Shoemaker, J.K., Tschakovsky, M.E. and Kowalchuk, J.M. (1996). Dependence of muscle $\dot{V}O_2$ on blood flow dynamics at onset of forearm exercise. *Journal of Applied Physiology*, **81**, 1619–26.

Hughson, R.L., Tschakovsky, M.E. and Houston, M.E. (2001). Regulation of oxygen consumption at the onset of exercise. *Exercise and Sport Science Reviews*, **29**, 129–33.

Ivy, J.L., Chi, M.M., Hintz, C.S., Sherman, W.M., Hellendall, R.P. and Lowry, O.H. (1987). Progressive metabolite changes in individual human muscle fibers with increasing work-rates. *American Journal of Physiology*, **252**, C630–9.

Jones, A.M., Carter, H., Pringle, J.S. and Campbell, I.T. (2002). Effect of creatine supplementation on oxygen uptake kinetics during submaximal cycle exercise. *Journal of Applied Physiology*, **92**, 2571–7.

Jones, A.M., Wilkerson, D.P., Koppo, K., Wilmshurst, S. and Campbell, I.T. (2003). Inhibition of nitric oxide synthase by L-NAME speeds phase II pulmonary $\dot{V}O_2$ kinetics in the transition to moderate intensity exercise in man. *Journal of Physiology*, **552**, 265–72.

Jones, A.M., Koppo, K., Wilkerson, D.P., Wilmshurst, S. and Campbell, I.T. (2004). Influence of L-NAME on pulmonary O_2 uptake kinetics during heavy-intensity cycle exercise. *Journal of Applied Physiology*, **96**, 1033–8.

Jubrias, S.A., Crowther, G.J., Shankland, E.G., Gronka, R.K. and Conley, K.E. (2003). Acidosis inhibits oxidative phosphorylation in contracting skeletal muscle in vivo. *Journal of Physiology*, **533**, 589–99.

Karetzky, M.S. and Cain, S.M. (1969). Oxygen uptake stimulation following Na-L-lactate infusion in anesthetized dogs. *American Journal of Physiology*, **216**, 1486–90.

Kindig, C.A., Sexton, W.L., Fedde, M.R. and Poole, D.C. (1998). Skeletal muscle micro-circulatory structure and hemodynamics in diabetes. *Respiration Physiology and Neurobiology*, **111**, 163–75.

Kindig, C.A., Musch, T.I., Basaraba, R.J. and Poole, D.C. (1999). Impaired capillary hemodynamics in skeletal muscle of rats in chronic heart failure. *Journal of Applied Physiology*, **87**, 652–60.

Kindig, C.A., Gallatin, L.L., Erickson, H.H., Fedde, M.R. and Poole, D.C. (2000). Cardiorespiratory impact of the nitric oxide synthase inhibitor L-NAME in the exercising horse. *Respiration Physiology and Neurobiology*, **120**, 151–66.

Kindig, C.A., McDonough, P., Erickson, H.H. and Poole, D.C. (2001). Effect of L-NAME on oxygen uptake kinetics during heavy-intensity exercise in the horse. *Journal of Applied Physiology*, **91**, 891–6.

Kindig, C.A., McDonough, P., Erickson, H.H. and Poole, D.C. (2002a). Nitric oxide synthase inhibition speeds oxygen uptake kinetics in horses during moderate domain running. *Respiration Physiology and Neurobiology*, **132**, 169–78.

Kindig, C.A., Richardson, T.E. and Poole, D.C. (2002b). Skeletal muscle capillary hemodynamics from rest to contractions: implications for oxygen transfer. *Journal of Applied Physiology*, **92**, 2513–20.

Kindig, C.A., Kelley, K.M., Howlett, R.A., Stary, C.M. and Hogan, M.C. (2003). Assessment of O_2 uptake dynamics in isolated single skeletal myocytes. *Journal of Applied Physiology*, **94**, 353–7.

Koga, S., Shiojiri, T., Kondo, N. and Barstow, T.J. (1997). Effect of increased muscle temperature on oxygen uptake kinetics during exercise. *Journal of Applied Physiology*, **83**, 1333–8.

Koga, S., Shiojiri, T., Shibasaki, M., Kondo, N., Fukuba, Y. and Barstow, T.J. (1999). Kinetics of oxygen uptake during supine and upright heavy exercise. *Journal of Applied Physiology*, **87**, 253–60.

Koga, S., Barstow, T.J., Shiojiri, T., Takaishi, T., Fukuba, Y., Kondo, N., Shibasaki, M. and Poole, D.C. (2001). Effect of muscle mass on $\dot{V}O_2$ kinetics at the onset of work. *Journal of Applied Physiology*, **90**, 461–8.

Koppo, K. and Bouckaert, J. (2001). The effect of prior high-intensity cycling exercise on the $\dot{V}O_2$ kinetics during high-intensity cycling exercise is situated at the additional slow component. *International Journal of Sports Medicine*, **22**, 21–6.

Koppo, K., Jones, A.M., Vanden Bossche, L. and Bouckaert, J. (2002). Effect of prior exercise on $\dot{V}O_2$ slow component is not related to muscle temperature. *Medicine and Science in Sports and Exercise*, 34, 1600–4.

Koppo, K., Bouckaert, J. and Jones, A.M. (2004). Effect of training status and exercise intensity on the on-transient $\dot{V}O_2$ kinetics. *Medicine and Science in Sports and Exercise* **36**(2), 225–32.

Krustrup, P., Gonzalez-Alonso, J., Quistorff, B. and Bangsbo, J. (2001). Muscle heat production and anaerobic energy turnover during repeated intense dynamic exercise in humans. *Journal of Physiology*, **536**, 947–56.

Krustrup, P., Hellsten, Y. and Bangsbo, J. (2004a). Intense interval training enhances human skeletal muscle oxygen uptake in the initial phase of dynamic exercise at high but not at low intensities. *Journal of Physiology*, **559**, 335–45.

Krustrup, P., Soderlund, K., Mohr, M. and Bangsbo, J. (2004b). Slow-twitch fiber glycogen depletion elevates moderate-exercise fast-twitch fiber activity and O_2 uptake. *Medicine and Science in Sports and Exercise*, **36**, 973–82.

McArdle, W.D., Katch, F.I. and Katch, V.L. (1996). *Exercise Physiology: Energy, Nutrition, and Human Performance* (4th edition) Lea and Febiger, Philadelphia, 1991, pp. 127–34.

MacDonald, M.J., Pedersen, P.K. and Hughson, R.L. (1997). Acceleration of $\dot{V}O_2$ kinetics in heavy submaximal exercise by hyperoxia and prior high-intensity exercise. *Journal of Applied Physiology*, **83**, 1318–25.

MacDonald, M.J., Naylor, H.L.,Tachakovsky, M.E. and Hughson, R.L. (2001). Peripheral circulatory factors limit rate of increase in muscle O(2) uptake at onset of heavy exercise. *Journal of Applied Physiology*, **90**(1), 83–9.

McKerrow, C.B. and Otis, A.B. (1956). Oxygen cost of hyperventilation. *Journal of Applied Physiology*, **9**, 375–9.

Mahler, M. (1985). First-order kinetics of muscle oxygen consumption, and an equivalent proportionality between QO_2 and phosphorylcreatine level. Implications for the control of respiration. *Journal of General Physiology*, **86**, 135–65.

Mallory, L.A., Scheuermann, B.W., Hoelting, B.D., Weiss, M.L., McAllister, R.M. and Barstow, T.J. (2002). Influence of peak $\dot{V}O_2$ and muscle fiber type on the efficiency of moderate exercise. *Medicine and Science in Sports and Exercise*, **34**, 1279–87.

Marcinek, D.J., Ciesielski, W.A., Conley, K.E. and Schenkman, K.A. (2003). Oxygen regulation and limitation to cellular respiration in mouse skeletal muscle *in vivo*. *American Journal of Physiology*, **285**, H1900–8.

Meyer, R.A. and Foley, J.M. (1996). Cellular processes integrating the metabolic response to exercise. In: *Handbook of Physiology. Exercise: Regulation and Integration of Multiple Systems*. Am. Physiol. Soc., Bethesda, MD, Section, 12, Ch. 18, pp. 841–69.

Moritani, T., Sherman, W.M., Shibata, M., Matsumoto, T. and Shinohara, M. (1992). Oxygen availability and motor unit activity in humans. *European Journal of Applied Physiology*, **64**, 552–6.

Ozyener, F., Rossiter, H.B., Ward, S.A. and Whipp, B.J. (2001). Influence of exercise intensity on the on- and off-transient kinetics of pulmonary oxygen uptake in humans. *Journal of Physiology*, **533**, 891–902.

Paterson, D.H. and Whipp, B.J. (1991). Asymmetries of oxygen uptake transients at the on- and offset of heavy exercise in humans. *Journal of Physiology*, **443**, 575–86.

Perrey, S., Betik, A., Candau, R., Rouillon, J.D. and Hughson, R.L. (2001). Comparison of oxygen uptake kinetics during concentric and eccentric cycle exercise. *Journal of Applied Physiology*, **91**, 2135–42.

Perrey, S., Candau, R., Rouillon, J.D. and Hughson, R.L. (2003). The effect of prolonged submaximal exercise on gas exchange kinetics and ventilation during heavy exercise in humans. *European Journal of Applied Physiology*, **89**, 587–94.

Pollack, G.W. (2001). *Cells, Gels and the Engines of Life*. Ebner & Sons, Seattle, 2001.

Poole, D.C., Ward, S.A., Gardner, G.W. and Whipp, B.J. (1988). Metabolic and respiratory profile of the upper limit for prolonged exercise in man. *Ergonomics*, **31**, 1265–79.

Poole, D.C., Schaffartzik, W., Knight, D.R., Derion, T., Kennedy, B., Guy, H.J., Prediletto, R. and Wagner, P.D. (1991). Contribution of excising legs to the slow component of oxygen uptake kinetics in humans. *Journal of Applied Physiology*, **71**, 1245–60.

Poole, D.C., Gaesser, G.A., Hogan, M.C., Knight, D.R. and Wagner, P.D. (1992). Pulmonary and leg $\dot{V}O_2$ during submaximal exercise: implications for muscular efficiency. *Journal of Applied Physiology*, **72**, 805–10.

Poole, D.C., Gladden, L.B., Kurdak, S. and Hogan, M.C. (1994). L-(+)-lactate infusion into working dog gastrocnemius: no evidence lactate per se mediates $\dot{V}O_2$ slow component. *Journal of Applied Physiology*, **76**, 787–92.

Pringle, J.S., Doust, J.H., Carter, H., Tolfrey, K., Campbell, I.T. and Jones, A.M. (2003a). Oxygen uptake kinetics during moderate, heavy and severe intensity 'submaximal' exercise in humans: the influence of muscle fibre type and capillarisation. *European Journal of Applied Physiology*, **89**, 289–300.

Pringle, J.S.M., Doust, J.H., Carter, H., Tolfrey, K. and Jones, A.M. (2003b). Effect of pedal rate on primary and slow-component oxygen uptake responses during heavy-cycle exercise. *Journal of Applied Physiology*, **94**, 1501–7.

Regensteiner, J.G., Bauer, T.A., Reusch, J.E., Brandenburg, S.L., Sippel, J.M., Vogelsong, A.M., Smith, S., Wolfel, E.E., Eckel, R.H. and Hiatt, W.R. (1998). Abnormal oxygen uptake kinetic responses in women with type II diabetes mellitus. *Journal of Applied Physiology*, **85**, 310–17.

Richardson, R.S., Poole, D.C., Knight, D.R., Kurdak, S.S., Hogan, M.C., Grassi, B., Johnson. E.C., Kendrick, K.F., Erickson, B.K. and Wagner, P.D. (1993). High muscle blood flow in man: is maximal O_2 extraction compromised? *Journal of Applied Physiology*, **75**, 1911–16.

Richardson, R.S., Knight, D.R., Poole, D.C., Kurdak, S.S., Hogan, M.C., Grassi, B. and Wagner, P.D. (1995). Determinants of maximal exercise $\dot{V}O_2$ during single leg knee-extensor exercise in humans. *American Journal of Physiology*, **268**, H1453–61.

Richardson, R.S., Haseler, L.J., Nygren, A.T., Bluml, S. and Frank, L.R. (2001). Local perfusion and metabolic demand during exercise: a noninvasive MRI method of assessment. *Journal of Applied Physiology*, **91**, 1845–53.

Richardson, T.E., Kindig, C.A., Musch, T.I. and Poole, D.C. (2003). Effects of chronic heart failure on skeletal muscle capillary hemodynamics at rest and during contractions. *Journal of Applied Physiology*, **95**, 1055–62.

Ross, K.D., Abbo, L.A., Behnke, B.J., Padilla, D.J., Musch, T.I. and Poole, D.C. (2003). Hypovolemic hypotension alters the dynamic balance between O_2 delivery and utilization in contracting skeletal muscle. *Medicine and Science in Sports and Exercise*, **35**, S309.

Rossiter, H.B., Ward, S.A., Doyle, V.L., Howe, F.A., Griffiths, J.R. and Whipp, B.J. (1999). Inferences from pulmonary O_2 uptake with respect to intramuscular [phosphocreatine] kinetics during moderate exercise in humans. *Journal of Physiology*, **518**, 921–32.

Rossiter, H.B., Ward, S.A., Kowalchuk, J.M., Howe, F.A., Griffiths, J.R. and Whipp, B.J. (2001). Effects of prior exercise on oxygen uptake and phosphocreatine kinetics during high-intensity knee-extension exercise in humans. *Journal of Physiology*, **537**, 291–303.

Rossiter, H.B., Ward, S.A., Howe, F.A., Kowalchuk, J.M., Griffiths, J.R. and Whipp, B.J. (2002a). Dynamics of intramuscular 31P-MRS P_i peak splitting and the slow components of PCr and O_2 uptake during exercise. *Journal of Applied Physiology*, **93**, 2059–69.

Rossiter, H.B., Ward, S.A., Kowalchuk, J.M., Howe, F.A., Griffiths, J.R. and Whipp, B.J. (2002b). Dynamic asymmetry of phosphocreatine concentration and O_2 uptake between the on- and off-transients of moderate- and high-intensity exercise in humans. *Journal of Physiology*, **541**, 991–1002.

Rossiter, H.B., Ward, S.A., Howe, F.A., Wood, D.M., Kowalchuk, J.M., Griffiths, J.R and Whipp, B.J. (2003). Effects of dichloroacetate on $\dot{V}O_2$ and intramuscular ^{31}p metabolite kinetics during high-intensity exercise in humans. *Journal of Applied Physiology*, **95**, 1105–15.

Roston, W.L., Whipp, B.J., Davis, J.A., Cunningham, D.A., Effros, R.M. and Wasserman, K. (1987). Oxygen uptake kinetics and lactate concentration during exercise in humans. *American Review of Respiratory Disease*, **135**, 1080–4.

Ryan, W.J., Sutton, J.R., Toews, C.J. and Jones, N.L. (1979). Metabolism of infused L(+)-lactate during exercise. *Clinical Science*, **56**, 139–46.

Saltin, B., Gagge, A.P. and Stolwijk, J.A. (1968). Muscle temperature during submaximal exercise in man. *Journal of Applied Physiology*, **25**, 679–88.

Sargeant, A.J. (1999). Neuromuscular determinants of human performance. In B.J. Whipp and A.J. Sargeant (Eds) *Physiological Determinants of Exercise Tolerance in Humans*. The Physiological Society, Portland Press, London, pp. 13–28.

Saunders, M.J., Evans, E.M., Arngrimsson, S.A., Allison, J.D., Warren, G.L. and Cureton, K.J. (2000). Muscle activation and the slow component rise in oxygen uptake during cycling. *Medicine and Science in Sports and Exercise*, **32**, 2040–5.

Scheen, A., Juchmes, J. and Cession-Fossion, A. (1981). Critical analysis of the 'anaerobic threshold' during exercise at constant workloads. *European Journal of Applied Physiology*, **46**, 367–77.

Scheuermann, B.W. and Barstow, T.J. (2003). O_2 uptake kinetics during exercise at peak O_2 uptake. *Journal of Applied Physiology*, **95**, 2014–22.

Scheuermann, B.W., Hoelting, B.D., Noble, M.L. and Barstow, T.J. (2001). The slow component of O_2 uptake is not accompanied by changes in muscle EMG during repeated bouts of heavy exercise in humans. *Journal of Physiology*, **531**, 245–56.

Scheuermann, B.W., Bell., C., Paterson, D.H., Barstow, T.J. and Kowalchuk, J.M. (2002). Oxygen uptake kinetics for moderate exercise are speeded in older humans by prior heavy exercise. *Journal of Applied Physiology*, **92**(2), 609–16.

Sheriff, D.D. and Hakeman, A.L. (2001). Role of speed vs grade in relation to muscle pump function at locomotion onset. *Journal of Applied Physiology*, **91**, 269–76.

Shinohara, M. and Moritani, T. (1992). Increase in neuromuscular activity and oxygen uptake during heavy exercise. *Annals of Physiological Anthropology*, **11**, 257–62.

Shoemaker, J.K. and Hughson, R.L. (1999). Adaptation of blood flow during the rest to work transition in humans. *Medicine and Science in Sports and Exercise*, **31**, 1019–26.

Steed, J., Gaesser, G.A. and Weltman, A. (1994). Rating of perceived exertion and blood lactate concentration during submaximal running. *Medicine and Science in Sports and Exercise*, **26**, 797–803.

Talmadge, R.J., Scheide, J.I. and Silverman, H. (1989). Glycogen synthesis from lactate in a chronically active muscle. *Journal of Applied Physiology*, **66**, 2231–8.

Tschakovsky, M.E. and Hughson, R.L. (1999). Interaction of factors determining oxygen uptake at the onset of exercise. *Journal of Applied Physiology*, **86**, 1101–13.

Tonkonogi, M., Walsh, B., Tiivel, T., Saks, V. and Sahlin, K. (1999). Mitochondrial function in human skeletal muscle is not impaired by high intensity exercise. *Pflugers Archives*, **437**, 562–8.

Timmons, J.A., Gustafsson, T., Sundberg, C.J., Jansson, E. and Greenhaff, P.L. (1998a). Muscle acetyl group availability is a major determinant of oxygen deficit in humans during submaximal exercise. *American Journal of Physiology*, **274**, E377–80.

Timmons, J.A., Gustafsson, T., Sundberg, C.J., Jansson, E., Hultman, E., Kaijser, L., Chwalbinska-Moneta, J., Constantin-Teodosiu, D., Macdonald, I.A. and Greenhaff, P.L. (1998b). Substrate availability limits human skeletal muscle oxidative ATP regeneration at the onset of ischemic exercise. *Journal of Clinical Investigations*, **101**, 79–85.

Tordi, N., Perrey, S., Harvey, A. and Hughson, R.L. (2003). Oxygen uptake kinetics during two bouts of heavy cycling separated by fatiguing sprint exercise in humans. *Journal of Applied Physiology*, **94**, 533–41.

Vøllestad, N.K. and Blom, P.C. (1985). Effect of varying exercise intensity on glycogen depletion in human muscle fibres. *Acta Physiologica Scandinavica*, **125**, 395–405.

Walsh, B., Tonkonogi, M., Soderlund, K., Hultman, E., Saks, V. and Sahlin, K. (2001). The role of phosphorylcreatine and creatine in the regulation of mitochondrial respiration in human skeletal muscle. *Journal of Physiology*, **537**, 971–8.

Wendt, I.R. and Gibbs, C.L. (1973). Energy production of rat extensor digitorum longus muscle. *American Journal of Physiology*, **224**, 1081–6.

Whipp, B.J. and Mahler, M. (1980). Dynamics of pulmonary gas exchange during exercise. In J.B. West, (Ed.) *Pulmonary Gas Exchange* (Vol. II) *Organism and Environment*, Academic Press, London, pp. 33–96.

Whipp, B.J. and Wasserman, K. (1986). Effect of anaerobiosis on the kinetics of O_2 uptake during exercise. *Federation Proceedings*, **45**, 2942–7.

Wilkerson, D.P., Koppo, K., Barstow, T.J. and Jones, A.M. (2004). Effect of work rate on the functional 'gain' of Phase II pulmonary O_2 uptake response to exercise. *Respiration Physiology and Neurobiology*, in press.

Willis, W.T. and Jackman, M.R. (1994). Mitochondrial function during heavy exercise. *Medicine and Science in Sports and Exercise*, **26**, 1347–53.

Wilson, D.F., Erecinska, M., Drown, C. and Silver, I.A. (1977). Effect of oxygen tension on cellular energetics. *American Journal of Physiology*, **233**, C135–40.

Wilson, D.F., Erecinska, M. and Silver, I.A. (1983). Metabolic effects of lowering oxygen tension *in vivo*. *Advances in Experimental Medicine and Biology*, **159**, 293–301.

Wilson, D.F., Erecinska, M., Nuutinen, E.M. and Silver, I.A. (1984). Dependence of cellular metabolism and local oxygen delivery on oxygen tension. *Advances in Experimental Medicine and Biology*, **180**, 629–34.

Wretling, M.L., Gerdle, B. and Henriksson-Larsen, K. (1987). EMG: a non-invasive method for determination of fibre type proportion. *Acta Physiologica Scandinavica*, **131**, 627–8.

Xu, L., Poole, D.C. and Musch, T.I. (1998). Effect of heart failure on muscle capillary geometry: implications for O_2 exchange. *Medicine and Science in Sports and Exercise*, **30**, 1230–7.

Yoshida, T. and Watari, H. (1993). ^{31}P-nuclear magnetic resonance spectroscopy study of the time course of energy metabolism during exercise and recovery. *European Journal of Applied Physiology*, **66**, 494–9.

Yoshida, T., Kamiya, J. and Hishimoto, K. (1995). Are oxygen uptake kinetics at the onset of exercise speeded up by local metabolic status in active muscles? *European Journal of Applied Physiology*, **70**, 482–6.

Part IV

Practical applications to the study of $\dot{V}O_2$ kinetics

13 $\dot{V}O_2$ kinetics

Effects of maturation and ageing

Thomas J. Barstow and Barry W. Scheuermann

Introduction

Within the lifespan of an individual there are several discrete stages that include periods of rapid growth, adolescence and maturation followed by adult life leading to senescence and eventually, death. During growth and maturation the different organs and physiological systems develop and increase their capacities, for example, to perform physical work. Later in adult life with approaching senescence these same organs and systems experience a reduced integrity and capacity and the tolerance for physical work is reduced. In this text, it has been stressed that several organ systems – cardiopulmonary, vascular and muscular – must operate in a highly coordinated fashion to effectively conduct O_2 from the inspired air to its site of utilization within the mitochondria. The effect of advancing age in reducing $\dot{V}O_{2\,max}$, has been well described (Docherty, 1990; Folkow and Svanborg, 1993; Lakatta, 1999; Conley *et al.*, 2000a; McGuire *et al.*, 2001), however, apart from contrived laboratory tests and a select few athletic events, humans rarely exercise at $\dot{V}O_{2\,max}$, and this is even more true for children and aged individuals.

By comparison with the infrequent excursions to $\dot{V}O_{2\,max}$, the vast majority of children and adults undergo many dozens of metabolic transitions each day (see Figure 13.1). Other chapters (e.g. Chapter 1) have stressed the importance of achieving rapid $\dot{V}O_2$ kinetics across those transitions in order to preserve the integrity of the intramyocyte milieu and the capacity for sustained physical activity. Whereas there is some ambiguity as to whether it is cardiovascular O_2 delivery to, or metabolic inertia within, the contracting myocytes that ultimately determines the speed of those $\dot{V}O_2$ kinetics (see Chapters 8–12), it is certain that dysfunction or discoordination at any step in the O_2 pathway can impair O_2 transduction and thus $\dot{V}O_2$ kinetics. Consequently, during growth there is likely to be an altered balance of cardiopulmonary, vascular and muscle capacities compared with the adult. By the same token, these systems will degrade at different rates with approaching senescence. Thus, both growth and senescence represent states in which $\dot{V}O_2$ kinetics are likely to be very different from those in the young adult and it is the purpose of this chapter to describe those differences and to seek out clues as to their mechanistic bases. We are all ageing and with the average life expectancy approaching 80 years, this is a particularly important and relevant topic. Indeed, preservation of

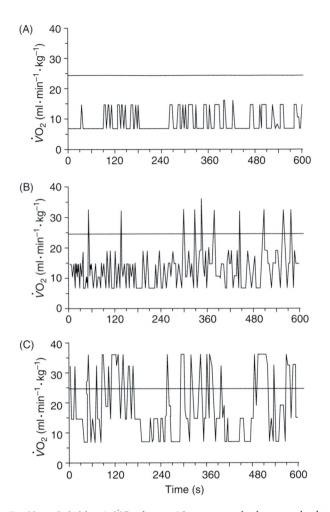

Figure 13.1 Profiles of children's $\dot{V}O_2$ during 10 min periods showing the highly transi-
tory nature of spontaneous, natural activity in free-ranging children aged
6–10 years. The solid horizontal line represents the lactate threshold (LT)
estimated from gas exchange. (A) Profile of a girl's $\dot{V}O_2$ during a representative 10 min period of relatively low activity. (B) Profile of a girl's $\dot{V}O_2$ during
a representative 10 min period of moderate activity (5% of observations are
above LT). (C) Profile of a boy's $\dot{V}O_2$ during a 10 min period of relatively
intense activity (26.5% of observations are above LT). Redrawn from Bailey
et al. (1995).

our quality of life into old age may be intrinsically dependent on sustaining some
minimal speed of $\dot{V}O_2$ kinetics. To this end, the potential for exercise training to
either speed $\dot{V}O_2$ kinetics and thereby constrain (or prevent) the effects of ageing
in senescent populations will be addressed in brief (see Chapter 15 for a comprehensive treatment of this topic). Because of their nature, it is often impractical to

perform longitudinal studies on humans, therefore much of the information presented in this chapter is drawn from cross-sectional comparisons of different age
groups and studies in animals that have a more limited lifespan such as the rat.

$\dot{V}O_2$ kinetics in children

Resolution of $\dot{V}O_2$ kinetics in children, and whether or not the responses to
moderate, heavy and severe exercise differ from those found in adults, has proved
challenging. In children, as the maximal work capacity is less than that for their
young adult counterparts, the scope of the metabolic transitions to exercise possible
within each domain is necessarily reduced. Coupled with a generally more erratic
breathing pattern, that is greater breath-to-breath variability in tidal volume and
timing of breaths, the low signal-to-noise ratio reduces confidence in resolving
parameters of the $\dot{V}O_2$ response, in particular τ for the primary component (Phase II).
To a certain extent, problems related to low signal-to-noise behaviour may be constrained by averaging multiple transitions (Lamarra et al., 1987; see Chapter 2).
However, this remains a significant problem when interpreting the literature in the
field. Moreover, in kinetics studies of children, the issue is compounded by a lack of
rigorous adherence to a specific work-rate domain, small subject populations, limited or sub-optimal numbers of repeated transitions and a confusingly eclectic array
of analytic models. Notwithstanding these concerns, the literature supports a pattern for faster primary component τ (moderate- and heavy/severe-intensity domain
exercise) and a higher gain (reduced work efficiency) in pre-pubertal children. This
topic has been comprehensively reviewed by Fawkner and Armstrong (2003).

Moderate exercise

Phase I

As discussed in Chapter 1, Phase I or the cardiodynamic component of the $\dot{V}O_2$
kinetics is driven by the almost immediate increase of cardiac output and therefore
pulmonary blood flow following exercise onset. In children, the increase of cardiac
output as a function of exercising $\dot{V}O_2$ is lower than that found in adults consequent
to a reduced stroke volume which mandates a greater peripheral O_2 extraction
(Cooper et al., 1985). One logical hypothesis, therefore, would be that Phase I might
be smaller in children than adults. However, the data have not provided unequivocal support for this notion. Specifically, Cooper et al. (1985) found no difference in
the magnitude of Phase I between a group of 7–10 year-old children and their
15–18 year-old counterparts. On the other hand, Springer et al. (1991) reported that
although mass-specific Phase I $\dot{V}O_2$ was not different between groups of 6–10- and
18–33-year-olds, it did represent a greater percentage of the steady-state $\dot{V}O_2$
response in adults. It is also pertinent that, at very light exercise intensities, Phase I
$\dot{V}O_2$ may actually overshoot the steady-state. Given the challenges presented by
trying to resolve $\dot{V}O_2$ kinetics in children, discriminating the length of Phase I is
particularly difficult. However, Hebestreit et al. (1998) noted that, unlike in adults,
the duration of Phase I does not appear to decrease with increased work rates.

Phase II

At first glance, there appears to be no consensus in the literature regarding whether or not $\dot{V}O_2$ kinetics at the onset of moderate exercise (i.e. below LT or the gas exchange threshold, GET) are faster in pre-pubertal children vs adults. Specifically, in comparison with subjects aged from 15 to 40 years, the primary component (Phase II) τ was not different in 6–12 year-old children following the onset of cycling (Cooper *et al.*, 1985; Springer *et al.*, 1991; Zanconato *et al.*, 1991; Hebestreit *et al.*, 1998) or treadmill running (Williams *et al.*, 2001). In contrast, other studies have reported faster time constants in children vs adults (Figure 13.2,

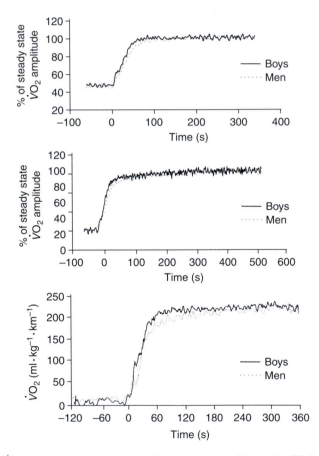

Figure 13.2 $\dot{V}O_2$ response at the onset of moderate (upper) and heavy (middle) cycle ergometer and heavy treadmill (lower) exercise in boys (11–12 years) and men (>18 years). Upper and middle panels demonstrate significantly faster $\dot{V}O_2$ kinetics in boys than men for cycle ergometry. Data have been time-aligned and averaged to show group mean responses. Upper panel is drawn from data of Fawkner *et al.* (2002), middle panel is from S.G. Fawkner, personal communication. Lower panel demonstrates faster $\dot{V}O_2$ kinetics in a representative boy vs man from Williams *et al.* (2001) with permission.

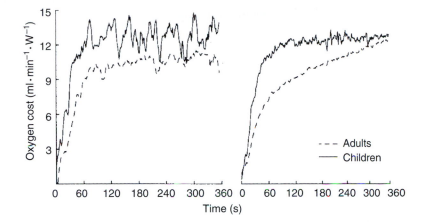

Figure 13.3 Group mean O_2 cost of lowest (left panel, 80% LT) and highest (right panel, 75% Δ) intensity exercise in children and adults. For both low- and high-intensity exercise, average O_2 cost was significantly higher in children. Note difference in response time between the two groups at high-intensity exercise. Adults achieve the children's value only toward the end of exercise. During the last minute of exercise, O_2 cost in adults was significantly higher at 75% Δ than at 80% LT exercise. From Armon *et al.* (1991) with permission.

upper panel and Figure 13.3, left panel; Macek and Vavra, 1980; Armon *et al.*, 1991; Fawkner *et al.* 2002). In their review, Fawkner and Armstrong (2003) have criticized many of these studies on the basis of their lack of adequate exercise transitions, modelling procedures and/or limitations within their subject populations. In an extremely well-designed investigation, Fawkner *et al.*, (2002) evaluated the on-kinetics in 11–12 year-old boys and girls and 19–26 year-old adults to exercise at 80% of their ventilation thresholds (VT). Up to 10 transitions were analysed for each subject using the criteria defined by Lamarra *et al.* (1987) after which, any subjects in whom the confidence interval exceeded 5 s were removed from the study. This criterion left the data from 13 men, 12 women, 12 boys and 11 girls in the final analysis. The data after the end of Phase I (i.e. beyond 15 s) were modelled using an exponential term that followed a delay by means of least-squares non-linear regression. These procedures are vastly superior to those utilized in some of the previous studies where sometimes only a single transition was analysed with an exponential term constrained to pass through the origin. In this investigation, Fawkner *et al.* (2002) demonstrated that the Phase II response was significantly faster in the boys than the men (τ, 19 s vs 28 s, Figure 13.2, upper panel) and the girls compared with the women (τ, 21 s vs 26 s).

With respect to the possibility of a sexual dimorphism in $\dot{V}O_2$ kinetics, Fawkner *et al.* (2002) reported no difference in the Phase II τ between boys and girls. This lack of a difference was surprising in these particular children because the boys had a higher $\dot{V}O_{2\,max}$ than the girls and the speed of the $\dot{V}O_2$ kinetics is generally positively related to $\dot{V}O_{2\,max}$ (see Chapters 5 and 15 and also Obert *et al.*, 2000). In addition, Cooper and colleagues (1985) did find that this relationship between $\dot{V}O_{2\,max}$ and Phase II τ was present in their mixed population of boys and girls but was not significant for the boys alone. This particular issue warrants further investigation.

O_2 cost of exercise

To avoid interpretational problems arising from inappropriate normalization procedures (rev. Welsman and Armstrong, 2000), differences in the O_2 cost of work in children are most clearly addressed using cycle ergometry. The O_2 cost per unit of work, that is, ml $\dot{V}O_2 \cdot min^{-1} \cdot W^{-1}$ (also termed 'gain') is substantially elevated for children performing cycle ergometry (Figure 13.3, left panel) (Armon *et al.*, 1991; Zanconato *et al.*, 1991). Thus, Armon *et al.* (1991) observed that $\Delta\dot{V}O_2/\Delta$ work rate was 11.9 ± 1.1 ml $O_2 \cdot min^{-1} \cdot W^{-1}$ in children vs 9.3 ± 1.8 ml $O_2 \cdot min^{-1} \cdot W^{-1}$ in adults exercising at 80% VT. Similarly, Springer *et al.* (1991) found an almost 50% higher O_2 cost of performing work in children than adults. In contrast, another study found a smaller and non-significant difference between boys and men (10.9 ± 2.2 ml $O_2 \cdot min^{-1} \cdot W^{-1}$ vs 9.7 ± 0.9 ml $O_2 \cdot min^{-1} \cdot W^{-1}$) (Hebestreit *et al.*, 1998).

Consonant with the cycle ergometer studies presented here, during walking or running exercise, children have a higher O_2 cost than adults (Cooper *et al.*, 1985; Springer *et al.*, 1991; Williams *et al.*, 2001). For example, in the study of Williams *et al.* (2001), the O_2 cost per kg per km was 239 ± 8 ml for children vs 168 ± 3 ml for adults. The conclusion that children are somehow less efficient that their adult counterparts has been challenged on the basis that the body mass ratio was incorrectly normalized (rev. Welsman and Armstrong, 2000). Irrespective of normalization procedures *per se*, there is solid, though not unopposed, data that cycling efficiency is lower and the O_2 cost of locomotion higher in children than adults. The biochemical and physiological mechanisms for this effect remain to be resolved. However, it is pertinent that muscle metabolic capacity, in particular the balance of oxidative and glycolytic enzymatic activities may change during maturation with children exhibiting lower glycolytic and higher oxidative enzyme activities than their adult counterparts (see 'Putative mechanistic bases…' section). Within the adult population, individuals with a greater proportion of Type I fibres (and fewer highly glycolytic Type II fibres) evince a larger primary component gain during moderate-, heavy and severe-intensity exercise than those with proportionally more Type II fibres (Barstow *et al.*, 1996; Pringle *et al.*, 2003, see Chapter 11). The ethics of muscle fibre type determination by biopsy in healthy children is questionable. Nonetheless, it remains an interesting question whether the energetic differences found in children compared with adults (greater $\dot{V}O_2$ gain and faster $\dot{V}O_2$ kinetics) can be explained by either muscle fibre type composition or metabolic capacity.

Exercise above the gas exchange (GET) or ventilatory threshold (VT)

As delineated in Chapter 1, the GET (considered synonymous with the lactate threshold, LT, and approximated by VT) demarcates the moderate and heavy exercise intensity domains whereas the critical power (CP) separates the heavy and severe domains. Whereas both the heavy and severe domains are characterized by elevated blood [lactate] and a slowly developing component of $\dot{V}O_2$, their metabolic profiles and mechanisms of fatigue differ significantly. For instance, during heavy exercise blood [lactate] becomes elevated for the entire exercise bout but both blood [lactate] and $\dot{V}O_2$ do stabilize if exercise is sufficiently prolonged. Fatigue may not occur for an hour or more and is characterized by extremely low muscle glycogen contents. In marked contrast, within the severe domain, blood [lactate] rises inexorably to the point of fatigue, $\dot{V}O_{2\,max}$ is achieved and both intramuscular [PCr] and pH fall to extremely low levels. Given these profoundly different metabolic profiles, it is important to equate exercise tests in both adults and children with respect to their heavy or severe-intensity domains. Unfortunately, this can prove problematic, in part, because of the compression of the GET-to-$\dot{V}O_{2\,max}$ region. It is evident that, without formal identification of CP, an arbitrary work rate, set as a % $\dot{V}O_{2\,max}$ or ΔGET-to-$\dot{V}O_{2\,max}$ (e.g. Δ40% or Δ50%), will likely result in some children and adults exercising in the heavy whilst others exercise in the severe domain. This eventuality confounds interpretation of the $\dot{V}O_2$ kinetics and impairs identification of any differences present between children and adults. Consequently, in the next section, the heavy and severe exercise intensity domains had to be combined for those studies in which there is ambiguity with respect to the work-rate domain. In contrast, the following section entitled 'Severe exercise' presents those studies where the exercise intensity is clearly above CP. CP has recently been measured in children where the average values obtained, that is, 73–79% $\dot{V}O_{2\,max}$ (Fawkner and Armstrong, 2002) are not systematically different from those found in adults (Poole *et al.*, 1988). In future studies, rigorous adherence to either heavy or severe-intensity exercise would be valuable.

Heavy/severe exercise

At the onset of heavy exercise $\dot{V}O_2$ kinetics are faster for children than adults and their $\dot{V}O_2$ reaches a greater percentage of their end-exercise $\dot{V}O_2$ during Phase II. Moreover, the $\dot{V}O_2$ slow component is either quantitatively less pronounced than in adults or absent altogether. For example, Armon *et al.* (1991) evaluated six children (6–12 years) and seven adults (27–40 years) performing cycle ergometer exercise within the heavy and/or severe domain (Δ25%, Δ50% and Δ75%). The half-time of the $\dot{V}O_2$ response to the highest work-rate was 20 s for the children and 45 s for the adults (Figure 13.3, right panel). Moreover, when the slow component was modelled as a linear response, the mean slope was far lower in the children (0.24 vs 0.97 ml $O_2 \cdot kg^{-1} \cdot min^{-1}$). This very small mean slow component arose, in part, because no slowly developing $\dot{V}O_2$ was evident in many of the children's tests. In fact, for the Δ75% condition, a slow component was only detected in 25% of the tests. In Figure 13.3, it is striking that the gain of the primary component and overall response for children is the same for moderate (13.1 $\pm$ 1.3) and heavy/severe (12.7 $\pm$ 1.5 ml $O_2 \cdot min^{-1} \cdot W^{-1}$)

exercise (Δ75%). This was certainly not true for the adults where after 6 min of exercise in the heavy/severe domain the $\dot{V}O_2$ gain was significantly higher than that seen for moderate exercise (heavy/severe, 12.4 ± 1.4, moderate, 10.9 ± 2.2 ml $O_2 \cdot min^1 \cdot W^{-1}$) (compare left and right panels in Figure 13.3).

These differences noted for children and adults performing cycle ergometer exercise in the heavy/severe domain appear to be common features of the response, being also found for treadmill exercise. For instance, Williams and colleagues (2001) demonstrated that the Phase II τ was over 20% faster in boys (aged 11–12 years) than men (aged 21–36 years). Moreover the $\dot{V}O_2$ slow component comprised only 0.9% of the overall response in the children compared with 8.3% in the adults. This greater $\dot{V}O_2$ slow component was accompanied by an approximately six-fold higher blood [lactate] increase in the adults. A reduced blood [lactate] increase in children performing heavy/severe exercise is described throughout the literature and several authors have attributed it to either a reduced glycolytic (or 'anaerobic') enzyme capacity in children than adults (Eriksson, 1972; Haralambie, 1982) or to the faster $\dot{V}O_2$ kinetics that reduce the requirement for substrate level phosphorylation (e.g. Zanconato et al., 1991).

As for moderate-intensity exercise, the gain of the primary component $\dot{V}O_2$ response is greater for boys than men performing heavy exercise of a similar relative intensity (cycling, Armon et al., 1991; Hebestreit et al., 1998; treadmill running, Williams et al., 2001). Indeed, Figure 13.3 (right panel) demonstrates that both the child and the adult project towards the same gain of the $\dot{V}O_2$ response at 360 s. However, the profile of $\dot{V}O_2$ change is markedly different with the $\dot{V}O_2$ slow component comprising a significant portion of the end-exercise $\dot{V}O_2$ only in the adult (cycling, Armon et al., 1991; treadmill running, Williams et al., 2001). It is quite possible that the mechanisms underlying the reduction in the primary component gain in adults are involved in, if not wholly responsible for, the generation of the slow component in adults (Chapters 1, 12; see also Fawkner and Armstrong, 2004). Poole and colleagues (1991) determined that over 80% of the $\dot{V}O_2$ slow component arises from within the exercising muscles and, as detailed in Chapters 11 and 12, some aspect of either fibre type recruitment patterns (e.g. less efficient Type II fibres) and/or fatigue processes within select fibre populations is thought to underlie this phenomenon. Consequently, it is plausible that either a reduced recruitment of the Type II fibre population or an altered metabolic profile (less glycolytic activity and lower lactate and hydrogen ion accumulation) that reduces fatigue within certain fibre types, may decrease or abolish the $\dot{V}O_2$ slow component during heavy exercise in children.

Severe exercise

Even for adults, resolution of $\dot{V}O_2$ kinetics during severe-intensity exercise is problematic when the achievable $\dot{V}O_2$ (i.e $\dot{V}O_{2\,max}$) is below the estimated requirement for the work-rate. Not only is the process of estimating that $\dot{V}O_2$ requirement contentious but different models (logarithmic vs exponential) yield very different kinetics parameters (Hughson et al., 2000). Notwithstanding these concerns, several studies have suggested that $\dot{V}O_2$ kinetics are faster for children than adults for exercise that almost certainly falls within the severe-intensity domain, whereas others have not. For example, during supramaximal cycling the half-time of the $\dot{V}O_2$ response (mono-exponential fit) was significantly shorter in pre-pubescent boys vs men (Sady, 1981). This latter study has been criticized on the basis of their data collection methods (every 15 s), modelling the fit with a single exponential constrained to start simultaneously with exercise onset and permitting the subjects to decrease their power output during the test (rev. Fawkner and Armstrong, 2003). Two additional studies that assessed $\dot{V}O_2$ at 30 s intervals (Douglas bag collection) demonstrated that boys (aged 10–11 years) exercising at 100% $\dot{V}O_{2\,max}$ reached over 55% of their $\dot{V}O_{2\,max}$ within 30 s of exercise onset compared with 35% in men (Robinson, 1938; Macek and Vavra, 1980). In contrast, Zanconato *et al.* (1991) and Hebestreit *et al.* (1998) utilized breath-by-breath technology and determined that, for exercise at 100% and either 125% or 130% $\dot{V}O_{2\,max}$, the half-time of the response was not different between children and adults. With one of these latter investigations, it was determined that the O_2 cost per unit of work was higher in the children (Zanconato *et al.*, 1991). This highlights the issue mentioned above that for modelling $\dot{V}O_2$ kinetics parameters, it is absolutely critical to have a precise estimate of the O_2 requirement for the exercise. This is problematic for adults and even more so for children given that the O_2 cost may be different than for adults.

In contrast to the absent or reduced $\dot{V}O_2$ slow component found in children vs adults performing heavy-intensity exercise, Obert *et al.* (2000) found a similar relative contribution of the $\dot{V}O_2$ slow component in both populations during exercise that was estimated to require 90% $\dot{V}O_{2\,max}$ which, according to Fawkner and Armstrong's (2002) data should be well within the severe-intensity domain for most children. Following on from the fibre type recruitment or fatigue hypothesis advanced for heavy exercise, it may be that in children it requires a far higher relative metabolic stress to either recruit and/or fatigue those fibres that generate the $\dot{V}O_2$ slow component. Hence the $\dot{V}O_2$ slow component is present for exercise in the severe but not the heavy-intensity domain.

Putative mechanistic bases for different $\dot{V}O_2$ kinetics in children vs adults

The previous sections present substantial evidence that children exhibit faster $\dot{V}O_2$ kinetics for moderate, heavy and possibly severe-intensity exercise than adults. Moreover, the gain of the primary component (Phase II) is increased and at least during heavy-intensity exercise, the $\dot{V}O_2$ slow component is either absent or significantly reduced. These differences between children and adults are qualitatively similar to comparisons between groups of adults with distinct fibre type populations. Specifically, the children's responses show commonality with the adults who have a greater Type I fibre type profile than their counterparts with proportionally more Type II fibres (Barstow *et al.*, 1996; Pringle *et al.*, 2003; see Chapter 11). Is it possible that children have either a greater Type I fibre population or a higher oxidative:glycolytic enzymatic ratio that may help explain these findings?

The paediatric literature is replete with evidence supporting the notion that maturation affects exercise energetics such that the balance between aerobic and so-called 'anaerobic' metabolism is shifted towards aerobic in pre-pubescent children. Specifically, children exhibit lower peak blood [lactate], higher arterial blood pH and a reduced 'anaerobic' power (Eriksson *et al.*, 1971, 1973, 1974; Macek and Vavra, 1971; Inbar and Bar-Or, 1986; Paterson *et al.*, 1986; Saavedra *et al.*, 1991; Falk and Bar-Or, 1993). Whereas, the percentage fibre type composition is not thought to evidence substantial changes from childhood to adulthood (rev. Baldwin, 1984), some of the few studies of muscle enzymatic profiles in children reveal either an enhanced oxidative enzyme potential (13–15 year-old vs 22–42 year-old females, lipoamide dehydrogenase (+40%), NADP-isocitrate dehydrogenase (+44%), fumarase (+24.5%), total malate dehydrogenase (+42.2%) and NADH-dehydrogenase (+39%); Haralambie, 1982) or a reduced glycolytic enzyme potential (11–13-year olds vs adults, decreased phosphofructokinase, PFK, Eriksson *et al.*, 1973). Also, in rats there is a ~17-fold increase in total PFK activity that occurs over the first two months of age (equivalent to birth–puberty in humans) accompanied by an increase in the muscle-type PFK subunit at the expense of the cardiac-type subunit (Dunaway *et al.*, 1986; rev. Zanconato *et al.*, 1993). This isozyme subunit profile has a greater affinity for fructose-6-phosphate and reduced inhibition by ATP, both of which would be expected to enhance glycolytic activity under exercising conditions in adults.

Because of the difficulty and questionable ethics of obtaining muscle samples from healthy children for analysis of fibre type and/or histochemical determination of enzymatic profiles, non-invasive magnetic resonance spectroscopy (MRS) has become a valuable tool for investigation of muscle energetics in children. One of the first MRS studies which compared pre-pubertal children (aged 7–10 years, 8 boys, 2 girls) to 20–42-year olds (5 males, 3 females) during progressive calf muscle exercise to volitional fatigue found a reduced increase in gastrocnemius Pi/PCr and decrease of pH in the children (Zanconato *et al.*, 1993). The authors concluded that these children therefore relied less on 'anaerobic' metabolism than their adult counterparts. However, a more recent MRS study (Petersen *et al.*, 1999) considered the possibility that in the relatively small calves of children, MRS may tend to sample the deeper lying slow twitch soleus as well as the gastrocnemius muscle and that this may have biased the findings of Zanconato *et al.* (1993). Moreover, the progressive nature of the test may have preferentially fatigued the children before they could achieve Pi/PCr and pH levels equivalent to the adults. Thus Petersen and colleagues (1999) evaluated a pre- and a post-pubertal group of female swimmers during plantar flexion exercise at light (40% maximal work capacity) and supramaximal (140%) intensities. Whilst no significant difference was found for either the gastrocnemius Pi/PCr ratio or pH, there was an interaction effect between Pi/PCr ratio and pubertal status with a strong tendency for a lower Pi/PCr ratio in the pre-pubertal girls. Indeed, their results were so variable within groups that a 66% difference could

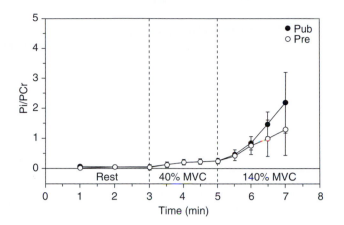

Figure 13.4 Ratio between inorganic phosphate (Pi) and phosphocreatine (PCr) at rest and during submaximal and supramaximal (140%) exercise in pre-pubescent ($n = 9$) and pubescent ($n = 9$) girls. Notice the high variability in the maximal response at 7 min that confounds statistical interpretation of the ~66% difference in Pi/PCr ratio between pre- and post-pubescent girls. From Petersen *et al.* (1999) with permission.

not be detected statistically (Figure 13.4) and therefore the possibility remains that there are energetic differences in children that support an enhanced oxidative function and reduced reliance on substrate level phosphorylation (lower increase in Pi/PCr and decrease in PCr). This supposition is consistent with the faster $\dot{V}O_2$ kinetics that occur despite the presence of a reduced cardiac output and presumably lower muscle blood flows (O_2 delivery) to exercising skeletal muscle.

$\dot{V}O_2$ kinetics with ageing (senescence) in adults

As discussed earlier for children, resolution of the effects of ageing *per se* on $\dot{V}O_2$ kinetics in adult populations presents multiple challenges for the investigator. These include recruitment of a suitably aged population that is free from chronic cardiorespiratory disease or medications that may affect the exercising response, compression of the work-rate domains such that the size of the metabolic transient is reduced, widely disparate exercise/activity histories and cardiorespiratory fitness levels, frequent presence of high breath-to-breath variability, and often a reduced willingness to tolerate intense exercise. In addition, institutional human subject protection committees are sometimes extremely conservative in the type and intensity of exercise that the older subject is allowed to perform. Accordingly, the literature is lacking in a detailed analysis of the Phase I $\dot{V}O_2$ kinetics (magnitude and duration) and also the response to severe exercise. However, some excellent studies have been published which demonstrate that $\dot{V}O_2$ kinetics are profoundly slowed in aged individuals. This effect is probably secondary to decreased activity and fitness levels and other structural and functional alterations that may alter the balance between O_2 delivery and O_2 utilization within the working muscles from that found in young healthy adults (Chapters 1, 8, 9 and 12).

The cardiovascular and muscular systems within the senescent individual experience structural and functional adaptations that may impair muscle O_2 delivery, the matching of that O_2 delivery to $\dot{V}O_2$ requirements, and mitochondrial oxidative function. Accordingly, the majority of studies in senescent individuals demonstrate a decreased ability to elevate cardiac output during exercise (Docherty, 1990; Folkow and Svanborg, 1993; Lakatta, 1999) such that muscle blood flow is impaired in both humans (Jorfeldt and Wahren, 1971; Wahren *et al.*, 1974) and rats (Irion *et al.*, 1987). There is also recent evidence in the rat that there may be a preferential redistribution of blood flow away from the highly oxidative Type I and IIA fibres towards the low oxidative, highly glycolytic Type IIX/B fibres (Musch *et al.*, 2004). In addition, capillary density, capillary-to-fibre ratio and mitochondrial volume density and oxidative function all decline with age (Coggan *et al.*, 1993; Conley *et al.*, 2000a,b). In these studies it was not possible to distinguish the effects of ageing *per se* from the effects of decreased activity (detraining effect). In one superbly designed 30-year longitudinal investigation in five humans, McGuire and colleagues (2001) made the discovery that the well-known decrease in maximal heart rate (~1 beat per year) was not accompanied by a reduction in maximum cardiac output. Rather, an increased stroke volume compensated for the reduced heart rate and thus the decreased $\dot{V}O_{2\,max}$, observed in these individuals, arose from an impaired muscle O_2 extraction. Ageing is associated with muscle microcirculatory changes such as capillary rarefaction (Russell *et al.*, 2003) and a redistribution of muscle blood flow amongst and within different organs and muscles (Musch *et al.*, 2004) that may contribute to an impaired O_2 diffusing capacity and the decreased O_2 extraction documented by McGuire *et al.* (2001).

Moderate exercise

Given that most, if not all, steps in the O_2 transport and utilization pathway are downregulated in aged individuals, it is not surprising that these people also evidence a profound slowing of their $\dot{V}O_2$ kinetics during moderate-intensity exercise performed with a large muscle mass (Figure 13.5; Paterson *et al.*, 1989; Cunningham *et al.*, 1993; Babcock *et al.*, 1994b; Chilibeck *et al.*, 1996a,b; Bell *et al.*, 1999; Scheuermann *et al.*, 2002). For example, in 59–78-year olds the primary component $\dot{V}O_2$ time constant averages 50–70s (e.g. Babcock *et al.*, 1994b; Scheuermann *et al.*, 2002) which is about twice that found in the young healthy population (Figure 13.5, upper panel). One key feature of these slowed $\dot{V}O_2$ kinetics with ageing is their dependence on the mode of exercise and thus the size and degree of 'training' of the active muscles. For example, $\dot{V}O_2$ kinetics for plantar flexion, which recruits muscles used for walking, are significantly faster than those for cycling which was an activity to which these particular subjects were unaccustomed (Chilibeck *et al.*, 1996b). Indeed, nuclear magnetic resonance determination of PCr kinetics (considered functionally indicative of mitochondrial $\dot{V}O_2$ kinetics) has

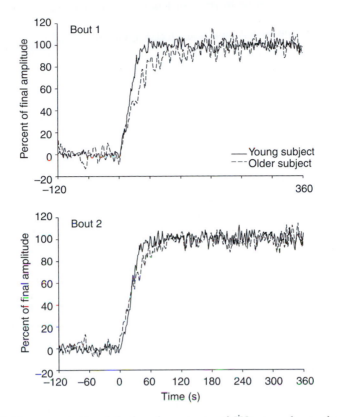

Figure 13.5 Upper panel: Breath-by-breath response of $\dot{V}O_2$ to a bout of moderate-intensity (80% VT) exercise for a representative young male (22 years old) and an older (67 years old) subject (Bout 1). Zero $\dot{V}O_2$ corresponds to unloaded cycling and 100 denotes end-exercise $\dot{V}O_2$. The line of best fit is given for each response. *Lower panel:* Bout 2 is the same moderate-intensity exercise but following a bout of heavy exercise. Notice that the $\dot{V}O_2$ kinetics are much faster for the older subject after heavy (or priming) exercise but not for the younger subject. Redrawn from the data of Scheuermann *et al.* (2002).

revealed that small muscle groups which are engaged in daily activities such as walking, retain PCr (and $\dot{V}O_2$) kinetics that are not different from their younger counterparts (Chilibeck *et al.*, 1998; Kent-Braun and Ng, 2000). However, declining activity levels resulting from either a sedentary lifestyle or illness-enforced inactivity will prejudice these muscles to the structural and functional impairments akin to detraining. This detraining effect will slow their PCr (and $\dot{V}O_2$) kinetics (McCully *et al.*, 1991, 1993). Given these effects of detraining, it is not surprising that older individuals respond to training with improved cardiovascular and muscle function that conspire to speed $\dot{V}O_2$ kinetics (cross-sectional studies, DeVries *et al.*, 1982; Chilibeck *et al.*, 1996a; longitudinal studies, Bell *et al.*, 1999). In fact, the proportional improvement in the speed of the primary component of the $\dot{V}O_2$ kinetics with training may be greater in the aged vs their younger counterparts (Babcock *et al.*, 1994b; Fukuoka *et al.*, 2002). One particularly interesting finding from these studies is that the speed of the $\dot{V}O_2$ kinetics is more tightly related to fitness than chronological age (Babcock *et al.*, 1994a; Chilibeck *et al.*, 1996a). Indeed, for three groups of subjects aged 37, 51, and 71 years, the correlation between the mean values for $\dot{V}O_{2\,max}$ and the primary component $\dot{V}O_2$ kinetics was 0.999 (Babcock *et al.*, 1994a). The response of the elderly to exercise training is dealt with in more detail in Chapter 15.

In Chapter 12, an attempt is made to explain the effect of experimentally or pathologically induced decreases (or increases) in muscle O_2 delivery or arterial O_2 content on $\dot{V}O_2$ kinetics (Figure 12.1 and 12.3). Accordingly, if the individual performing upright cycle ergometry in the moderate-intensity domain is subjected to lower body positive pressure (reduction in muscle O_2 delivery, Williamson *et al.*, 1996) or inspired hyperoxia (increased arterial O_2 content and muscle microvascular PO_2, MacDonald *et al.*, 1997), $\dot{V}O_2$ kinetics remain unaltered because they reside in the 'O_2 saturated' region of the response. In contrast, at the left-hand side of that figure (non-O_2 saturated) the $\dot{V}O_2$ kinetics are sensitive to either increased or decreased O_2 delivery. It is possible that ageing changes the location of the individual on Figure 12.3. Scheuermann *et al.* (2002) demonstrated that a bout of heavy priming exercise speeded $\dot{V}O_2$ kinetics at the onset of subsequent moderate-intensity exercise in the older but not the younger subjects (Figure 13.5, lower panel) and that this effect was greater in the least-fit older individuals (Figure 13.6). This was the first demonstration in healthy humans that an acute experimental intervention speeded the $\dot{V}O_2$ kinetics for moderate-intensity exercise (Kindig and colleagues in 2002 and Jones and colleagues in 2003 have subsequently demonstrated that inhibition of nitric oxide synthase can speed $\dot{V}O_2$ kinetics in the horse and human, respectively during moderate exercise). Because heart rate was elevated prior to initiating the second exercise bout, the authors proposed that $\dot{V}O_2$ kinetics in these older individuals (in contrast to their younger counterparts) may be O_2 delivery limited. In addition, Babcock *et al.* (1994a) demonstrated a significant correlation between the speeding of the $\dot{V}O_2$ kinetics and those of heart rate again raising the possibility that improved O_2 delivery may, in part, be responsible for the faster $\dot{V}O_2$ kinetics after training in this population. Unfortunately, in those studies it was not possible to discriminate with any certainty whether improved O_2 delivery or alternatively a more rapid activation of mitochondrial function was responsible for the faster kinetics in the old subjects. In contrast, Bell and colleagues (2001) employed a 9-week, one-leg training programme in older individuals which revealed that the training-induced faster $\dot{V}O_2$ kinetics were associated with increased muscle oxidative enzymes rather than an elevated femoral arterial blood flow (measured as velocity by Doppler ultrasound). Indeed, as for young individuals (see Chapters 9 and 12), the blood velocity (equated to blood flow) response following exercise onset was far faster than that of $\dot{V}O_2$. These findings suggest strongly that the effects of ageing on the $\dot{V}O_2$ kinetics following the onset

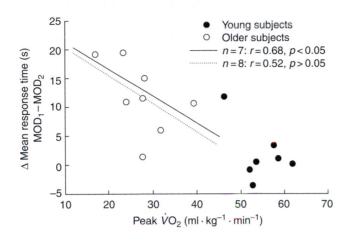

Figure 13.6 Change in mean response time (MRT) between two bouts of moderate-intensity exercise (MOD$_1$ and MOD$_2$) when MOD$_2$ is preceded by a bout of heavy exercise in younger and older subjects. Younger 22–29 years; older 59–71 years. The dashed line denotes the linear regression for all eight older subjects. When the subject who elicited the smallest change in MRT from MOD$_1$ to MOD$_2$ was excluded, the regression denoted by the solid line was obtained that demonstrates an inverse relationship between the MRT of the $\dot{V}O_2$ kinetics and fitness (peak or maximum $\dot{V}O_2$) in these seven older subjects. From Scheuermann *et al.* (2002) with permission.

of moderate-intensity exercise are modulated by altered structural (mitochondrial, microvascular) and/or functional alterations within the exercising musculatures. This conclusion is supported by the observation that, as in younger individuals, breathing hyperoxic gas mixtures does not speed the $\dot{V}O_2$ kinetics following the onset of moderate-intensity exercise in the elderly (Bell *et al.*, 1999).

Heavy exercise

In ageing or pathological conditions where the capacity of the cardiopulmonary, vascular and muscular systems is reduced, the presence of slowed $\dot{V}O_2$ kinetics and the 'excess' O_2 cost associated with the $\dot{V}O_2$ slow component may be of greater importance in limiting exercise tolerance than for their younger or healthier counterparts. As detailed in Chapter 12, it remains ambiguous if the primary component of the $\dot{V}O_2$ kinetics is slowed at work-rates above, compared to those below, the lactate threshold (although the compelling weight of evidence suggests that it is slowed). This issue has also not been completely resolved in the aged population.

With respect to the $\dot{V}O_2$ slow component and the potential role of the Type II muscle fibre type pool in evoking this response (Poole *et al.*, 1994, see Chapters 11 and 12), Bell *et al.* (1998) speculated that the preferential loss of (presumably) less efficient Type II motor units in aged individuals would be associated with a reduced $\dot{V}O_2$ slow component. As for young adults, exercise at 50% of the difference between the gas exchange threshold (GET) and $\dot{V}O_{2\,max}$ (determined during incremental/ramp cycle ergometry) elicited a significant $\dot{V}O_2$ slow component in older individuals. Whereas the magnitude of this slow component was inversely related to age, it correlated positively with the absolute work-rate performed. Moreover, when the O_2 cost of exercise was expressed as $\Delta \dot{V}O_2/\Delta$ work rate, there was no difference between age groups. One potential problem that emerges when trying to equate relative work rates between young and aged populations is that the frame of reference may be shifted. For example, the GET may be as high as 70% $\dot{V}O_{2\,max}$ in old vs ~50% for young individuals (Bell *et al.*, 1998). A plausible interpretation of this behaviour is that the relative level of fitness may be greater in the aged than reflected by their $\dot{V}O_{2\,max}$ *per se*. As alluded to in the introduction, one effect of this higher relative GET is that it compresses the range of heavy and severe-intensity exercise domains into a small range of absolute work rates that may challenge the limits of experimental design in old individuals (Neder *et al.*, 2000). What is certain is that the potential benefits of exercise training to promote structural and functional alterations that speed $\dot{V}O_2$ kinetics, reduce the $\dot{V}O_2$ slow component and improve exercise tolerance in the aged, is enormous (see Chapter 15).

Conclusions

As the individual progresses from childhood to adulthood, there may be a slowing of the primary component of the $\dot{V}O_2$ kinetics and a reduced gain, that is, $\Delta \dot{V}O_2/\Delta$ work-rate, in response to moderate exercise which occurs despite an elevated cardiac output-to-$\dot{V}O_2$ ratio (and therefore mean capillary O_2 pressure) in adults compared with children. In contrast, children evidence little or no $\dot{V}O_2$ slow component behaviour for heavy exercise but a slow component is discernible during severe-intensity exercise. Whereas there is a distinct paucity of relevant investigations in children, it is possible that the reduced oxidative and elevated glycolytic enzyme activities present in adulthood contribute to these responses. At the other end of the age spectrum, the primary component of the $\dot{V}O_2$ response is slowed during moderate-intensity exercise in aged/senescent individuals (this issue has not been resolved for heavy exercise). Exercise training profoundly speeds these kinetics and the strong correlation between fitness or $\dot{V}O_{2\,max}$ and $\dot{V}O_2$ kinetics irrespective of age suggests that the age-induced slowing of the $\dot{V}O_2$ kinetics is due primarily to a detraining effect that disproportionately compromises muscle oxidative capacity (and microvascular structure) rather than cardiovascular O_2 delivery kinetics. Whereas the magnitude of the $\dot{V}O_2$ slow component decreases in the aged, this occurs in proportion to the reduced work rate and it therefore is not necessary to invoke alterations in muscle fibre recruitment or energetic alterations within those muscle fibres to explain this phenomenon. The available evidence indicates that regular activity or exercise with either small or large muscle groups preserves metabolic integrity (PCr and $\dot{V}O_2$ kinetics) for subsequent exercise involving those muscles.

Glossary of terms

ADP	adenosine diphosphate (ADP$_{free}$, the metabolically important fraction of intracellular ADP)
ATP	adenosine triphosphate
CP	critical power. Asymptote of the hyperbolic power–time relationship, demarcates heavy and severe exercise intensity domains
Cr	creatine
$\Delta\dot{V}O_2/\Delta$ work rate	slope of the $\dot{V}O_2$ to-work rate relationship
GET	gas exchange threshold. Considered synonymous with the lactate threshold, LT. Sometimes estimated from the ventilatory threshold, VT
HR	heart rate
LT	lactate threshold
MRS	magnetic resonance spectroscopy
MRT	mean response time (time delay + time constant, τ or tau, denotes time to 63% of final response)
NADH	reduced form of nicotinamide adenine nucleotide
NADP	nicotinamide adenine nucleotide phosphate
PCr	phosphocreatine
%Δ	denotes the % of the work rate or speed difference between GET/VT and $\dot{V}O_{2\,max}$ as established during an incremental or ramp exercise test
PFK	phosphofructokinase
Phase I	initial increase in $\dot{V}O_2$ following exercise onset caused by elevated pulmonary blood flow (also called the cardiodynamic phase)
Phase II	(same as primary component) the exponential increase in $\dot{V}O_2$ that is initiated when venous blood from the exercising muscles arrives at the lungs. Corresponds closely with muscle $\dot{V}O_2$ dynamics under normal circumstances
Phase II τ	time constant of Phase II or primary component
Pi	inorganic phosphate
PO$_2$	partial pressure of O_2
Senescence	to grow old or age
τ or tau	denotes time to 63% of final response in the exponential function
$\dot{V}O_2$	oxygen uptake
$\dot{V}O_{2\,max}$	maximal oxygen uptake (achieved under conditions of large muscle mass exercise unless otherwise specified, and considered synonymous with $\dot{V}O_{2\,peak}$)
$\dot{V}O_2$ slow component	a slowly developing $\dot{V}O_2$ response initiated beyond ~2 min of heavy and severe exercise. Also termed 'excess' $\dot{V}O_2$ (see Chapter 1)
VT	ventilatory threshold

References

Armon, Y., Cooper, D.M., Flores, R., Zanconato, S. and Barstow, T.J. (1991). Oxygen uptake dynamics during high-intensity exercise in children and adults. *Journal of Applied Physiology*, **70**, 841–48.

Babcock, M.A., Paterson, D.H. and Cunningham, D.A. (1994a). Effects of aerobic endurance training on gas exchange kinetics of older men. *Medicine and Science in Sports and Exercise*, **26**, 447–52.

Babcock, M.A., Paterson, D.H., Cunningham, D.A. and Dickinson, J.R. (1994b). Exercise on-transient gas exchange kinetics are slowed as a function of age. *Medicine and Science in Sports and Exercise*, **26**, 440–6.

Bailey, R.C., Olson, J., Pepper, S.L., Porszasz, J., Barstow, T.J. and Cooper, D.M. (1995). The level and tempo of children's physical activities: an observational study. *Medicine and Science in Sports and Exercise*, **27**, 1033–41.

Baldwin, K.M. (1984). Muscle development: neonatal to adult. *Exercise and Sports Science Reviews*, **12**, 1–19.

Barstow, T.J., Jones, A.M., Nguyen, P.H. and Casaburi, R. (1996). Influence of muscle fiber type and pedal frequency on oxygen uptake kinetics of heavy exercise. *Journal of Applied Physiology*, **81**, 1642–50.

Bell, C., Paterson, D.H., Babcock, M.A. and Cunningham, D.A. (1998). Characteristics of the $\dot{V}O_2$ slow component during heavy exercise in humans aged 30 to 80 years. *Advances in Experimental Medicine and Biology*, **450**, 219–22.

Bell, C., Paterson, D.H., Kowalchuk, J.M. and Cunningham, D.A. (1999). Oxygen uptake kinetics of older humans are slowed with age but are unaffected by hyperoxia. *Experimental Physiology*, **84**, 747–59.

Bell, C., Paterson, D.H., Kowalchuk, J.M., Moy, A.P., Thorp, D.B., Noble, E.G., Taylor, A.W. and Cunningham, D.A. (2001). Determinants of oxygen uptake kinetics in older humans following single-limb endurance exercise training. *Experimental Physiology*, **86**, 659–65.

Chilibeck, P.D., Paterson, D.H., Petrella, R.J. and Cunningham, D.A. (1996a). The influence of age and cardiorespiratory fitness on kinetics of oxygen uptake. *Canadian Journal of Applied Physiology*, **21**, 185–96.

Chilibeck, P.D., Paterson, D.H., Smith, W.D. and Cunningham, D.A. (1996b). Cardiorespiratory kinetics during exercise of different muscle groups and mass in old and young. *Journal of Applied Physiology*, **81**, 1388–94.

Chilibeck, P.D., Paterson, D.H., McCreary, C.R., Marsh, G.D., Cunningham, D.A. and Thompson, R.T. (1998). The effects of age on kinetics of oxygen uptake and phosphocreatine in humans during exercise. *Experimental Physiology*, **83**, 107–17.

Coggan, A.R., Wailgum, T.D., Swanson, S.C., Earle, M.S., Farris, J.W., Mendenhall, L.A. and Robitaille, P.M. (1993). Muscle metabolism during exercise in young and old untrained and endurance-trained men. *Journal of Applied Physiology*, **75**, 2125–33.

Conley, K.E., Esselman, P.C., Jubrias, S.A., Cress, M.E., Inglin, B., Mogadam, C. and Schoene, R.B. (2000a). Ageing, muscle properties and maximal O_2 uptake rate in humans. *Journal of Physiology (London)*, **526**, 211–17.

Conley, K.E., Jubrias, S.A. and Esselman, P.C. (2000b). Oxidative capacity and ageing in human muscle. *Journal of Physiology (London)*, **526**, 203–10.

Cooper, D.M., Berry, C., Lamarra, N. and Wasserman, K. (1985). Kinetics of oxygen uptake and heart rate at onset of exercise in children. *Journal of Applied Physiology*, **59**, 211–17.

Cunningham, D.A., Himann, J.E., Paterson, D.H. and Dickinson, J.R. (1993). Gas exchange dynamics with sinusoidal work in young and elderly women. *Respiration Physiology*, **91**, 43–56.

DeVries, H.A., Wiswell, R.A., Romero, G., Moritani, T. and Bulbulian, R. (1982). Comparison of oxygen kinetics in young and old subjects. *European Journal of Applied Physiology and Occupational Physiology*, **49**, 277–86.

Docherty, J.R. (1990). Cardiovascular responses in aging: a review. *Pharmacological Reviews*, **42**, 103–25.

Dunaway, G.A., Kasten, T.P., Nickols, G.A. and Chesky, J.A. (1986). Regulation of skeletal muscle 6-phosphofructo-1-kinase during aging and development. *Mechanisms of Ageing and Development*, **36**, 13–23.

Eriksson, B.O. (1972). Physical training, oxygen supply and muscle metabolism in 11–13-year old boys. *Acta Physiologica Scandinavica Supplement*, **384**, 1–48.

Eriksson, B.O., Karlsson, J. and Saltin, B. (1971). Muscle metabolites during exercise in pubertal boys. *Acta Paediatric Scandinavica Supplement*, **217**, 154–7.

Eriksson, B.O., Gollnick, P.D. and Saltin, B. (1973). Muscle metabolism and enzyme activities after training in boys 11–13 years old. *Acta Physiologica Scandinavica*, **87**, 485–97.

Eriksson, B.O., Gollnick, P.D. and Saltin, B. (1974). The effect of physical training on muscle enzyme activities and fiber composition in 11-year-old boys. *Acta Paediatrics Belgium Supplement*, **28**, 245–52.

Falk, B. and Bar-Or, O. (1993). Longitudinal changes in peak aerobic and anaerobic mechanical power of circumpubertal boys. *Pediatric Exercise Science*, **5**, 318–31.

Fawkner, S.G. and Armstrong, N. (2002). Assessment of critical power with children. *Pediatric Exercise Science*, **14**, 259–68.

Fawkner, S.G. and Armstrong, N. (2003). Oxygen uptake kinetic response to exercise in children. *Sports Medicine*, **33**, 651–69.

Fawkner, S.G. and Armstrong, N. (2004). Longitudinal changes in the kinetic response to heavy-intensity exercise in children. *Journal of Applied Physiology*, **97**, 460–66.

Fawkner, S.G., Armstrong, N., Potter, C.R. and Welsman, J.R. (2002). Oxygen uptake kinetics in children and adults after the onset of moderate-intensity exercise. *Journal of Sports Science*, **20**, 319–26.

Folkow, B. and Svanborg, A. (1993). Physiology of cardiovascular aging. *Physiological Reviews*, **73**, 725–64.

Fukuoka, Y., Grassi, B., Conti, M., Guiducci, D., Sutti, M., Marconi, C. and Cerretelli, P. (2002). Early effects of exercise training on on- and off- kinetics in 50-year-old subjects. *Pfleugers Archives*, **443**, 690–7.

Haralambie, G. (1982). Enzyme activities in skeletal muscle of 13–15 years old adolescents. *Bulletin of the European Physiopatholological Respiratory Society*, **18**, 65–74.

Hebestreit, H., Kriemler, S., Hughson, R.L. and Bar-Or, O. (1998). Kinetics of oxygen uptake at the onset of exercise in boys and men. *Journal of Applied Physiology*, **85**, 1833–41.

Hughson, R.L., O'Leary, D.D., Betik, A.C. and Hebestreit, H. (2000). Kinetics of oxygen uptake at the onset of exercise near or above peak oxygen uptake. *Journal of Applied Physiology*, **88**, 1812–19.

Inbar, O. and Bar-Or, O. (1986). Anaerobic characteristics in male children and adolescents. *Medicine and Science in Sports and Exercise*, **18**, 264–9.

Irion, G.L., Vasthare, U.S. and Tuma RF (1987). Age related changes in skeletal muscle blood flow in the rat. *Journal of Gerontology*, **42**, 660–5.

Jones, A.M., Wilkerson, D.P., Koppo, K., Wilmshurst, S. and Campbell, I.T. (2003). Inhibition of nitric oxide synthase by L-NAME speeds phase II pulmonary $\dot{V}O_2$ kinetics in the transition to moderate-intensity exercise in man. *Journal of Physiology (London)*, **552**, 265–72.

Jorfeldt, L. and Wahren, J. (1971). Leg blood flow during exercise in man. *Clinical Science (Colc)*, **41**, 459–73.

Kent-Braun, J.A. and Ng, A.V. (2000). Skeletal muscle oxidative capacity in young and older women and men. *Journal of Applied Physiology*, **89**, 1072–8.

Kindig, C.A., McDonough, P., Erickson, H.H. and Poole, D.C. (2002). Nitric oxide synthase inhibition speeds oxygen uptake kinetics in horses during moderate domain running. *Respiration Physiology and Neurobiology*, **132**, 169–78.

Lakatta, E.G. (1999). Cardiovascular aging research: the next horizons. *Journal of the American Geriatrics Society*, **47**, 613–25.

Lamarra, N., Whipp, B.J., Ward, S.A. and Wasserman, K. (1987). Effect of interbreath fluctuations on characterizing exercise gas exchange kinetics. *Journal of Applied Physiology*, **62**, 2003–12.

McCully, K.K., Forciea, M.A., Hack, L.M., Donlon, E., Wheatley, R.W., Oatis, C.A., Goldberg, T. and Chance, B. (1991). Muscle metabolism in older subjects using 31P magnetic resonance spectroscopy. *Canadian Journal of Physiological Pharmacology*, **69**, 576–80.

McCully, K.K., Fielding, R.A., Evans, W.J., Leigh, J.S.J. and Posner, J.D. (1993). Relationships between *in vivo* and *in vitro* measurements of metabolism in young and old human calf muscles. *Journal of Applied Physiology*, **75**, 813–19.

Macdonald, M., Pedersen, P.K. and Hughson, R.L. (1997). Acceleration of $\dot{V}O_2$ kinetics in heavy submaximal exercise by hyperoxia and prior high-intensity exercise. *Journal of Applied Physiology*, **83**, 1318–25.

Macek, M. and Vavra, J. (1971). Cardiopulmonary and metabolic changes during exercise in children 6–14 years old. *Journal of Applied Physiology*, **30**, 200–4.

Macek, M. and Vavra, J. (1980). The adjustment of oxygen uptake at the onset of exercise: a comparison between prepubertal boys and young adults. *International Journal of Sports Medicine*, **1**, 75–7 (Abstract).

McGuire, D.K., Levine, B.D., Williamson, J.W., Snell, P.G., Blomqvist, C.G., Saltin, B. and Mitchell, J.H. (2001). A 30-year follow-up of the Dallas Bedrest and Training Study: II. Effect of age on cardiovascular adaptation to exercise training. *Circulation*, **104**, 1358–66.

Musch, T.I., Eklund, K.E., Hageman, K.S. and Poole, D.C. (2004). Effects of age on the blood flow distribution amongst muscles of different fibre types. *Journal of Applied Physiology*, **96**, 81–8.

Neder, J.A., Jones, P.W., Nery, L.E. and Whipp, B.J. (2000). The effect of age on the power/duration relationship and the intensity-domain limits in sedentary men. *European Journal of Applied Physiology*, **82**, 326–32.

Obert, P., Cleuziou, C., Candau, R., Courteix, D., Lecoq, A.M. and Guenon, P. (2000). The slow component of O_2 uptake kinetics during high-intensity exercise in trained and untrained prepubertal children. *International Journal of Sports Medicine*, **21**, 31–6.

Paterson, D.H., Cunningham, D.A. and Bumstead, L.A. (1986). Recovery O_2 and blood lactic acid: longitudinal analysis in boys aged 11 to 15 years. *European Journal of Applied and Occupational Physiology*, **55**, 93–9.

Paterson, D.H., Cunningham, D.A. and Babcock, M.A. (1989). Oxygen kinetics in the elderly. In G.D. Swanson, F.S. Grodins and R.L. Hughson (Eds) *Respiratory Control: A Modelling Perspective*, Plenum Press, New York, pp. 171–8.

Petersen, S.R., Gaul, C.A., Stanton, M.M. and Hanstock, C.C. (1999). Skeletal muscle metabolism during short-term, high-intensity exercise in prepubertal and pubertal girls. *Journal of Applied Physiology*, **87**, 2151–6.

Poole, D.C., Ward, S.A., Gardner, G.W. and Whipp, B.J. (1988). Metabolic and respiratory profile of the upper limit for prolonged exercise in man. *Ergonomics*, **31**, 1265–79.

Poole, D.C., Schaffartzik, W., Knight, D.R., Derion, T., Kennedy, B., Guy, H.J., Prediletto, R. and Wagner P.D. (1991). Contribution of excising legs to the slow component of oxygen uptake kinetics in humans. *Journal of Applied Physiology*, **71**, 1245–60.

Poole, D.C., Barstow, T.J., Gaesser, G.A., Willis, W.T. and Whipp, B.J. (1994). $\dot{V}O_2$ slow component: physiological and functional significance. *Medicine and Science in Sports and Exercise*, **26**, 1354–8.

Pringle, J.S., Doust, J.H., Carter, H., Tolfrey, K., Campbell, I.T. and Jones, A.M. (2003). Oxygen uptake kinetics during moderate, heavy and severe intensity 'submaximal' exercise in humans: the influence of muscle fibre type and capillarisation. *European Journal of Applied Physiology*, **89**, 289–300.

Robinson, S. (1938). Experimental studies of physical fitness in relation to age. *Int Z Angew Physiol*, **10**, 251–323.

Russell, J.A., Kindig, C.A., Behnke, B.J., Poole, D.C. and Musch, T.I. (2003). Effects of aging on capillary geometry and hemodynamics in rat spinotrapezius muscle. *American Journal of Physiology Heart Circulatory Physiology*, **285**, H251–8.

Saavedra, C., Lagasse, P., Bouchard, C. and Simoneau, J.A. (1991). Maximal anaerobic performance of the knee extensor muscles during growth. *Medicine and Science in Sports and Exercise*, **23**, 1083–9.

Sady, S.P. (1981). Transient oxygen uptake and heart rate responses at the onset of relative endurance exercise in prepubertal boys and young adults. *International Journal of Sports Medicine*, **2**, 240–4.

Scheuermann, B.W., Bell, C., Paterson, D.H., Barstow, T.J. and Kowalchuk, J.M. (2002). Oxygen uptake kinetics for moderate exercise are speeded in older humans by prior heavy exercise. *Journal of Applied Physiology*, **92**, 609–16.

Springer, C., Barstow, T.J., Wasserman, K. and Cooper, D.M. (1991). Oxygen uptake and heart rate responses during hypoxic exercise in children and adults. *Medicine and Science in Sports and Exercise*, **23**, 71–9.

Wahren, J., Saltin, B., Jorfeldt, L. and Pernow, B. (1974). Influence of age on the local circulatory adaptation to leg exercise. *Scandinavian Journal of Clinical Laboratory Investigation*, **33**, 79–86.

Welsman, J.R. and Armstrong, N. (2000). Statistical techniques for interpreting body size-related exercise performance during growth. *Pediatric Exercise Science*, **12**, 112–27.

Williams, C.A., Carter, H., Jones, A.M. and Doust, J.H. (2001). Oxygen uptake kinetics during treadmill running in boys and men. *Journal of Applied Physiology*, **90**, 1700–6.

Williamson, J.W., Raven, P.B. and Whipp, B.J. (1996). Unaltered oxygen uptake kinetics at exercise onset with lower-body positive pressure in humans. *Experimental Physiology*, **81**, 695–705.

Zanconato, S., Cooper, D.M. and Armon, Y. (1991). Oxygen cost and oxygen uptake dynamics and recovery with 1 min of exercise in children and adults. *Journal of Applied Physiology*, **71**, 993–8.

Zanconato, S., Buchthal, S., Barstow, T.J. and Cooper, D.M. (1993). 31P-magnetic resonance spectroscopy of leg muscle metabolism during exercise in children and adults. *Journal of Applied Physiology*, **74**, 2214–8.

14 $\dot{V}O_2$ kinetics in different disease states

David C. Poole, Casey A. Kindig and Brad J. Behnke

Introduction

Oxygen uptake ($\dot{V}O_2$) measured via respired gas analysis ultimately reflects O_2 utilization by the mitochondria within the cells of the body. This is true despite the interposition of gas stores for example within the lungs, muscles and venous blood in addition to circulatory transit delays from the exercising muscles to the lungs. At the onset of contractions, the working skeletal muscles are the predominant users of the increased $\dot{V}O_2$ and as shown in Chapter 6, muscle $\dot{V}O_2$ begins to increase without discernible delay (Behnke *et al.*, 2002a). Despite $\dot{V}O_{2\,max}$ being lowered, the absolute $\dot{V}O_2$ necessary to perform a given amount of constant-load submaximal work may not be affected by the disease processes and thus the steady-state $\dot{V}O_2$ *per se* provides no information about the underlying pathology (Wasserman *et al.*, 1994). However, the superb coordination among the respiratory, cardiovascular and muscle systems required for the rapid $\dot{V}O_2$ kinetics observed in healthy individuals is very sensitive to dysfunction at multiple steps in the O_2 transport pathway (Figure 14.1). Thus, evaluation of $\dot{V}O_2$ kinetics can provide a powerful method for detecting problems within the oxygen transport/utilization systems. This chapter will present the broad alterations in $\dot{V}O_2$ kinetics manifested in disease conditions that perturb those key systems responsible for delivering O_2 to and within the exercising muscles and will address briefly changes in skeletal muscle oxidative enzymes that may contribute to those alterations (Dernevik *et al.*, 1988; Drexler *et al.*, 1992; Mattson and Poole, 1998; Casaburi, 2000; Diederich *et al.*, 2002). Recent mechanistic insights that link the slowed pulmonary $\dot{V}O_2$ kinetics to impaired microvascular exchange profiles within the contracting muscles will be presented.

Almost all diseases that impact one or more of the respiratory, cardiovascular and muscle systems slow $\dot{V}O_2$ kinetics. As early as 1927 the pioneering work of Meakins and Long demonstrated that patients in circulatory failure evidence extremely sluggish $\dot{V}O_2$ kinetics (Figure 14.2). As detailed earlier (Chapter 1), the consequence of this is that for any given increase in metabolic rate, the patient will incur a larger O_2 deficit and thus a greater perturbation of intracellular phosphates (e.g. ↓PCr, ↑Cr, ↑ADP$_{free}$, ↑inorganic phosphate) which in turn leads to accelerated glycolytic activity and glycogen utilization (↑lactate formation, ↑hydrogen ions). Irrespective of the presence of angina, dyspnea or

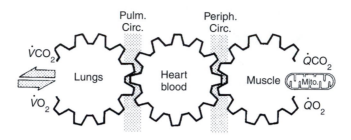

Figure 14.1 Schematic demonstrating that the passage of O_2 from the atmosphere to the muscle mitochondria depends on the coordinated function of the pulmonary, cardiovascular and muscle systems. Redrawn from Wasserman *et al.*, 1994.

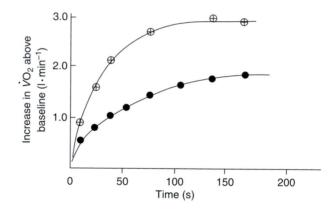

Figure 14.2 Grotesquely slowed $\dot{V}O_2$ response to running in place at 184 steps per minute in a patient with chronic heart disease (endocarditis with mitral stenosis and insufficiency, lower curve) compared to a normal healthy control (upper curve). Both individuals are of approximately the same body weight. Redrawn from Meakins and Long, 1927.

muscular discomfort, utilization of limited glycogen reserves within specific fibre population will contribute to premature fatigue in the affected individual.

Part III of this book has discussed the evidence for the competing notions that $\dot{V}O_2$ kinetics in healthy individuals are limited either by muscle O_2 delivery (Chapter 8) or alternatively by an inertia of mitochondrial respiration (Chapter 9). Whilst there can be no doubt that muscle mitochondrial function and therefore oxidative capacity are impacted by pulmonary disease (e.g. emphysema, COPD, Casaburi *et al.*, 1991; Mattson and Poole, 1998; Casaburi, 2000; Maltais *et al.*, 2000) and also myocardial pathologies (e.g. chronic heart failure, Dernevik *et al.*, 1988; Drexler *et al.*, 1992; Diederich *et al.*, 2002) it is certain that muscle O_2 delivery presents a major problem to these individuals. Figure 14.3 illustrates that $\dot{V}O_2$ kinetics for these patients may clearly be determined by O_2 delivery if that

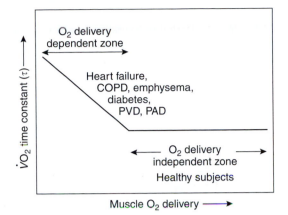

Figure 14.3 Schematic illustration of the relationship between muscle O_2 delivery and $\dot{V}O_2$ time constant (tau or τ) at the onset of moderate-intensity exercise. Notice that in patients with heart failure, COPD (chronic obstructive pulmonary disease), emphysema, diabetes and PVD or PAD (peripheral vascular or arterial occlusive disease), the compromised O_2 delivery has placed them in the O_2 delivery dependent zone where their $\dot{V}O_2$ kinetics are extremely sensitive to further alterations in O_2 delivery. See text associated with Figures 12.2 and 12.3 on pp. 300–301 for full explanation of the basis for this relationship.

individual resides in the 'O_2 delivery dependent zone' on the left-hand side of the relationship. In this zone, increases in the capacity to deliver O_2 to the working muscles speed $\dot{V}O_2$ kinetics whilst decreasing muscle O_2 delivery slows $\dot{V}O_2$ kinetics. There is experimental evidence that COPD patients (Palange *et al.*, 1995) and some (Cerretelli *et al.*, 1988) but not all chronic heart failure (CHF) patients (Grassi *et al.*, 1997) may evidence faster $\dot{V}O_2$ kinetics at the onset of moderate-intensity exercise when either arterial O_2 content or cardiac output is elevated. On the other hand, in healthy individuals who reside on the right-hand side of Figure 14.3 in the 'O_2 delivery independent zone' neither increasing the inspired O_2 fraction (MacDonald *et al.*, 1997) nor conditions that cause a modest reduction in muscle blood flow (lower body positive pressure (Williamson *et al.*, 1996) or nitric oxide inhibition (Kindig *et al.*, 2001, 2002a)) slow the $\dot{V}O_2$ kinetics.

Evaluating the $\dot{V}O_2$ kinetics literature in disease populations

There are several major concerns that emerge when trying to interpret the effects of chronic diseases on $\dot{V}O_2$ kinetics:

Lack of standardization of exercise intensity domains

When a CHF patient, for example, performs a task such as walking, climbing stairs or cycling, it seems intuitive that he or she is more concerned with the absolute work rate (e.g. how long it takes to cover a given vertical or horizontal distance) than whether the work constitutes 25% or 50% or 75% $\dot{V}O_{2\,max}$. However, because the maximal exercise tolerance (and $\dot{V}O_{2\,max}$) is reduced, evaluation of a given patient at the same absolute work rate as their healthy counterpart invariably means that the patient will be exercising at a greater percentage of their $\dot{V}O_{2\,max}$. This raises the possibility that the patient will be exercising in the heavy or severe domain whilst their healthy counterparts will be performing moderate-intensity exercise. Thus, for the patient, the primary $\dot{V}O_2$ kinetics may be slower (see Chapter 12 for a discussion of this issue) and a $\dot{V}O_2$ slow component will be present. It is crucial to realize that these effects can arise from the different exercise intensity domains and inasmuch they may be independent of the disease process *per se*. Whereas appropriate modelling of the $\dot{V}O_2$ response will remove the slow component effect, any slowing of the primary $\dot{V}O_2$ kinetics that is the result of exercising in the heavy vs moderate domain may obscure the true comparison between the disease response and the healthy response.

Differences in absolute work rate between healthy and patient populations

From the above, it is evident that accurate evaluation of the effects of disease on $\dot{V}O_2$ kinetics is dependent on both patients and healthy matched controls exercising in the same intensity domain. However, in extreme cases CHF can reduce work capacity and $\dot{V}O_{2\,max}$ by as much as 80% or 90%. Accordingly, if the work rate is set at a certain percentage of $\dot{V}O_{2\,max}$ in both healthy and CHF individuals so that the work is performed within the moderate-intensity domain, for example, the absolute work rate will be much lower for the patient. Figure 14.4 (upper panel) illustrates the effect of different work rates on the mean response time (MRT i.e. time to 63% of the final response) in healthy individuals (Sietsema et al., 1989). It is clear that, at a given fitness level (described here as $\dot{V}O_{2\,max}$) MRT increases as a function of increasing work rate. This results from two effects that are not removed by the modelling procedures undertaken in the investigation of Sietsema and colleagues. Specifically, within the domain of moderate-intensity exercise, the size of the immediate increase in $\dot{V}O_2$ within Phase I is relatively invariant with work rate (Figure 14.4, lower panel). Thus, for very light work rates, Phase I may comprise almost the entire $\dot{V}O_2$ response which is consequently very fast. Indeed, there are examples during very light exercise where the MRT approaches zero because Phase I either constitutes the entire $\dot{V}O_2$ response or $\dot{V}O_2$ may even overshoot the steady-state value. Higher work rates within the moderate domain will elicit progressively greater Phase II responses which are somewhat slower than the Phase I response and thus will tend to slow the overall response (i.e. MRT, Sietsema et al., 1989). Thus, it may not be appropriate to compare patient and healthy populations at the same relative but different absolute work rates *unless the Phase I response is removed* from the analysis (e.g. by disregarding the first 20s of data). It is unfortunate that there are many examples in the literature where this Phase I effect (and often the

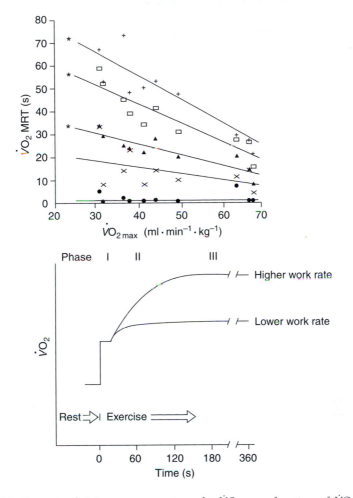

Figure 14.4 Upper panel: Mean response times for $\dot{V}O_2$ as a function of $\dot{V}O_{2\,max}$ for ten healthy subjects. Regression lines are drawn for each work rate (different symbols and regression lines refer to 0, 25, 50, 100, 150 W). * denotes work rates for which there was a significant correlation between $\dot{V}O_{2\,max}$ and mean response time. (From Sietsema *et al.*, 1989 with permission.) *Lower panel:* Schematic demonstrating how the Phase I response assumes a proportionally smaller role in the overall $\dot{V}O_2$ response as work rate increases. Redrawn from Sietsema *et al.*, 1986.

presence of a slow component) have contributed to the slowed MRT reported. In almost all instances, when comparisons are made at the same work rate which is constrained rigorously to be within the moderate domain (e.g. Sietsema *et al.*, 1994; Hepple *et al.*, 1999), the patient's $\dot{V}O_2$ kinetics are significantly slower than those of their healthy counterparts.

Are Phase I and Phase II responses truly independent of one another?

The sluggish cardiovascular response at exercise onset in CHF patients results in a prolonged Phase I. In agreement with the elegant modelling studies of Barstow and colleagues (1990), it is intuitively reasonable that the expression of Phase II at the mouth may be altered by prolongation of Phase I. As we shall see later, these considerations are further complicated in certain patient populations in which there may be independent effects of their pathology on Phase I and Phase II kinetics (Mettauer et al., 2000).

Diseases that impair the ventilatory response to exercise

O_2 delivery may be impacted by pulmonary diseases in two broad fashions: (1) Ventilation and gas exchange in the lung may be impaired and cause a low arterial O_2 content (termed hypoxemia). Conditions that may result in arterial hypoxemia include emphysema, COPD, chronic bronchitis, chronic airflow obstruction, bronchial asthma, fibrotic lung disease, alkalosing spondylitis, and respiratory muscle and motor nerve disorders. Although at a given submaximal $\dot{V}O_2$ minute ventilation may be elevated in some of these patients, they have difficulty in achieving the effective alveolar ventilation necessary for eliminating exercise-induced CO_2 (Wagner et al., 1977; Nery et al., 1982; Casaburi et al., 1991; Wasserman et al., 1994). Elevated arterial and alveolar CO_2 reduce alveolar PO_2 and further impair O_2 loading via the Bohr effect (rightward shift of the O_2 dissociation curve). Other conditions such as pulmonary oedema or alveolar proteinosis thicken the blood–gas barrier and impair O_2 diffusion which also results in arterial hypoxemia. (2) Pathological alterations within the pulmonary vasculature may reduce pulmonary blood flow and thus cardiac output (pulmonary emboli, idiopathic pulmonary hypertension). In addition, if right atrial pressures rise sufficiently in patients with a patent foramen ovale, right-to-left shunting will develop and cardiac output as well as arterial oxygenation may fall (Wasserman et al., 1994).

Unlike primary cardiac myopathies, diseases such as emphysema or COPD that reduce the ventilatory response to exercise often do not exhibit a reduced cardiovascular response to exercise and therefore the Phase I $\dot{V}O_2$ response is preserved (Nery et al., 1982). However, as demonstrated in Figure 14.5, Phase II is markedly slower and the O_2 deficit is enlarged at a given absolute work rate in COPD patients compared with their age- and gender-matched healthy counterparts. These patients are characterized by elevated ventilation-to-perfusion ($\dot{V}_A/\dot{Q}$) mismatch, increased dead space ventilation ($\dot{V}_D$) and a reduced alveolar surface area for gas exchange.

Pulmonary vascular diseases including idiopathic pulmonary vascular occlusion and pulmonary emboli decrease perfusion to regions of the lung. This creates alveolar dead space (elevates the dead space to total ventilation ratio, $\dot{V}_D/\dot{V}_T$) and elevates perfusion to alveoli with a patent vasculature. Consequently, red blood cell

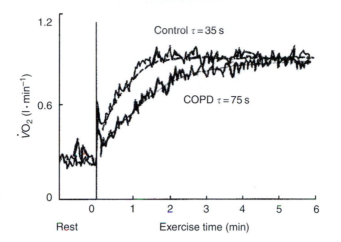

Figure 14.5 Effect of chronic obstructive pulmonary disease on $\dot{V}O_2$ response at exercise onset. Drawn from data of Nery *et al.*, 1982.

transit time in the patent pulmonary capillaries is reduced for any given cardiac output. Both effects exacerbate arterial hypoxemia and the situation becomes progressively worse with increasing work rates as is evident from the increasing alveolar to arterial O_2 pressure gradient (i.e. the so-called A-aPO_2). As mentioned earlier, arterial hypoxemia also arises from the development of right-to-left shunting consequent to the opening of the foramen ovale within the interatrial septum. The foramen ovale is believed to be potentially patent in one-fifth of the population which raises the possibility that, given the correct conditions, deoxygenated venous blood may pass from the right to the left atrium and thereby lower the arterial oxygenation (Wasserman *et al.*, 1994). Increased pulmonary vascular resistance during exercise will elevate right atrial pressure and when this exceeds left atrial pressure the foramen ovale is opened and venous blood bypasses the lungs and is shunted into the left atrium. Because this occurs close to the plateau of the O_2 dissociation curve, relatively small amounts of venous admixture will lower the arterial PO_2 substantially. The work of Engelen *et al.* (1996) among others have demonstrated that arterial hypoxemia induced by lowering the inspired fraction of O_2 to 12% or 15% for example, slows Phase II $\dot{V}O_2$ kinetics.

Although arterial hypoxemia constitutes one primary response to lung insult, it is now becoming evident that in certain diseases, emphysema for example, there is a reduction in locomotory muscle oxidative capacity over and above that resulting from disease enforced inactivity, that is, the detraining effect (Mattson and Poole, 1998; Casaburi, 2000; Maltais *et al.*, 2000). In addition, there may be augmented levels of metabolic stress (reactive oxygen species) within the muscles that may impair mitochondrial function (Mattson *et al.*, 2002). Thus, the slowed Phase II response may be induced by the arterial hypoxemia and this effect may be exacerbated by functional deficits within the exercising muscles.

Diseases that impair the cardiovascular response to exercise

Cardiac dysfunction

The cardinal function of the cardiovascular system is to transport oxygenated blood to the periphery and metabolically produced CO_2 from the periphery to the lungs for elimination. There are four principal classes of cardiac dysfunction: cardiomyopathic, coronary artery occlusive, valvular insufficiency and congenital defects. At exercise onset in healthy individuals, cardiac output increases almost instantaneously due to increased venous return, cardiac inotropy and elevated heart rate (HR) which drives the rapid Phase I $\dot{V}O_2$ response (sometimes termed the cardiodynamic phase) seen during the first ~15 s of exercise (Wasserman *et al.*, 1994). Cardiac myopathies such as cyanotic congenital heart disease (in addition to the pulmonary vascular diseases discussed earlier) prevent or constrain this elevation of cardiac output and thus pulmonary blood flow and consequently Phase I increases in $\dot{V}O_2$ are abolished or attenuated (Figure 14.6, Sietsema *et al.*, 1986). Reductions in stroke volume characteristic of many cardiac defects limit the O_2 pulse and result in an accentuated HR response at a given submaximal $\dot{V}O_2$. Exceptions to this include sinoatrial node defects and patients taking β-adrenergic blockers in whom the chronotropic (HR) response to exercise is blunted (Wasserman *et al.*, 1994).

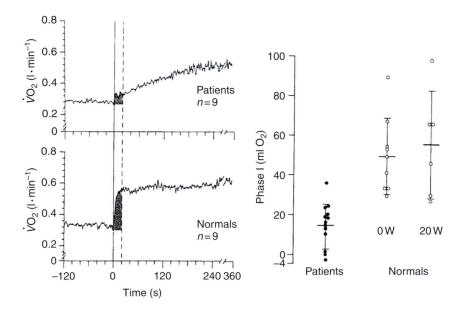

Figure 14.6 *Left panel*: Average $\dot{V}O_2$ response at the onset of unloaded cycling (~0 W) in patients with cyanotic congenital heart disease compared with normal healthy controls. Shaded area indicates Phase I. *Right panel*: Total size of the Phase I $\dot{V}O_2$ response in ml O_2 for patients and controls. Redrawn from Sietsema *et al.*, 1986.

In all these conditions, cardiac output is low but the $\dot{V}O_2$ for the exercise task is usually normal or in some instances, elevated (Zelis *et al.*, 1981). Elevated sympathetic activity and circulating vasoconstrictors (norepinephrine, angiotensin II) combined with a reduced endothelial nitric oxide response to exercise and impaired muscle pump effectiveness reduce the ability to increase blood flow to working skeletal muscles (Figure 14.7, rev. in Diederich *et al.*, 2002 and Richardson *et al.*, 2003). In this figure, it is evident that while the capillary haematocrit response at the onset of contractions is unchanged in heart failure, the elevated capillary red blood cell flux found in healthy muscle is greatly attenuated in muscle from heart failure animals. Consequently, fractional O_2 extraction within the exercising muscles must increase and this is expressed as a widening

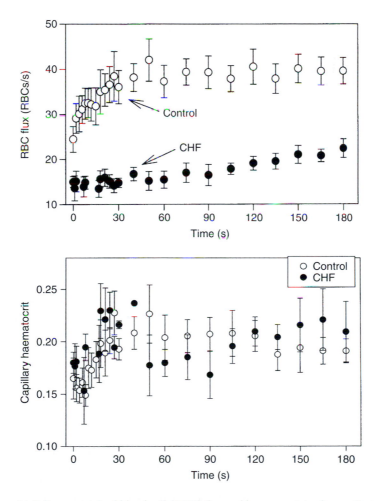

Figure 14.7 Response of red blood cell (RBC) flux and haematocrit in the capillaries of rat spinotrapezius muscle at the onset of 1 Hz contractions. Data from Kindig *et al.* (2002b) and Richardson *et al.* (2003), with permission.

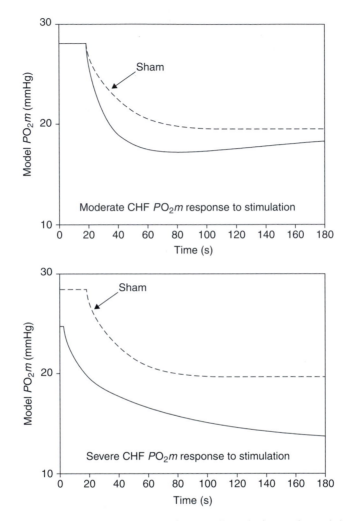

Figure 14.8 Effects of moderate (upper) and severe (lower) chronic heart failure (CHF)
on the partial pressure of O_2 (PO_2m) in the microvasculature of the rat
spinotrapezius muscle at the onset of 1 Hz contractions. Redrawn from
Diederich *et al.*, 2002.

of the arterial-to-venous O_2 difference (a-vO_2diff.) (see also Katz *et al.*, 2000).
Irrespective of whether there are associated changes in arterial O_2 content (e.g.
as in congestive heart failure and/or right-to-left shunting) this forces microvascular $\dot{Q}O_2$ to fall which lowers the pressure head for blood–myocyte O_2 diffusion
(PO_2m; Figure 14.8) thereby slowing muscle $\dot{V}O_2$ kinetics at exercise onset and
potentially reducing intramyocyte PO_2. This response is expressed as a precipitous
fall in microvascular PO_2 (PO_2m; i.e. the pressure of O_2 within the capillary bed and
adjacent small arterioles and venules) that undershoots the steady-state response

in moderate heart failure and in severe heart failure progresses slowly to extraordinarily low values (Figure 14.8, Diederich *et al.*, 2002). These lowered microvascular PO_2 values will exacerbate the degree of intracellular perturbation, accelerate glycolysis and lead to an elevated intracellular acidosis. Indeed, it has long been appreciated that heart disease patients evidence a lactic acidosis at very low work rates (Wasserman *et al.*, 1994).

As alluded to earlier, one of the problems that has arisen in the interpretation of the slowed $\dot{V}O_2$ kinetics response in CHF patients is whether there is an indication of a muscle impairment (Phase II) in addition to the reduction of Phase I (cardiodynamic response). It has been suggested that, following a prolonged (>30 s) Phase I, the absence of any slowing in Phase II is evidence that muscle function is preserved (Mettauer *et al.*, 2000). Contrary to this notion, it is likely that a sluggish muscle blood flow response combined with unimpaired muscle O_2 exchange will result in an accelerated Phase II response at the mouth (Barstow *et al.*, 1990) which is not seen. This becomes a crucial consideration in cardiac patients where statements are made about muscle function *per se* from the Phase II response. It can be argued that after a prolonged Phase I, the appearance of a quantitatively normal (healthy) Phase II is evidence of a muscle impairment (Mettauer *et al.*, 2000) because with healthy muscle it should actually be faster. Indeed, there is solid evidence that CHF and other forms of heart disease can induce a primary down-regulation of oxidative enzyme activity within skeletal muscle, impair capillary haemodynamics, microvascular PO_2 (PO_2m) and also blood–tissue O_2 exchange (Dernevik *et al.*, 1988; Drexler *et al.*, 1992; Delp *et al.*, 1997; Diederich *et al.*, 2002; Richardson *et al.*, 2003).

Diseases that impair blood flow to the periphery

Peripheral arterial disease (PAD)

PAD typically occludes lower extremity peripheral blood flow either unilaterally or bilaterally. This results in a reduced muscle blood flow response to exercise and often causes exercise-induced claudication (pain). As well as a reduced exercise capacity and $\dot{V}O_{2\,max}$, these patients exhibit a substantial slowing of their $\dot{V}O_2$ kinetics (Bauer *et al.*, 1999). Specifically, Bauer and colleagues have demonstrated that Phase II $\dot{V}O_2$ kinetics in PAD patients were about half the speed found in age-matched controls irrespective of their smoking history (Figure 14.9).One particularly interesting facet of these patients is that there is often an increased oxidative enzyme capacity within the active limb muscles of these patients which is due most likely to the prolonged state of muscle hypoxia present (Elander *et al.*, 1985; Lundgren *et al.*, 1989).

Diabetes

Diabetes elicits profound structural and functional changes within cardiac and skeletal muscle. Specifically, a reduced cardiac output and decreased muscle citrate

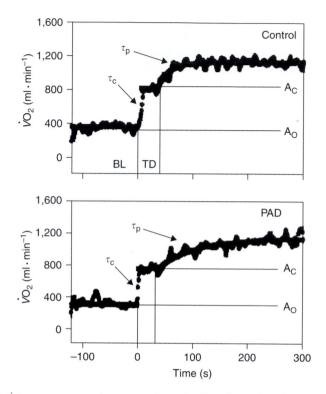

Figure 14.9 $\dot{V}O_2$ response at the onset of treadmill walking (2 mph, 4% grade) for a healthy control subject (upper) and a patient with bilateral peripheral arterial disease (PAD). (From Bauer *et al.* (1999) with permission.) τ_c is the time constant of the cardiodynamic component (Phase I), τ_p is the time constant of the primary component (Phase II). A_o is baseline, A_1 is amplitude of cardiodynamic component.

synthase activity conspire to reduce $\dot{V}O_{2\,max}$ and lower the $\dot{V}O_2$ to work rate slope during incremental exercise (Roy *et al.*, 1989; Regensteiner *et al.*, 1998; Simoneau and Kelley, 1997). Hence, it is not surprising that $\dot{V}O_2$ kinetics are severely slowed in diabetic patients (Figure 14.10, Regensteiner *et al.*, 1998). There is recent evidence that Type I diabetes induces capillary loss or involution in skeletal muscle and a reduction in capillary luminal diameter (Sexton *et al.*, 1994; Kindig *et al.*, 1998). In addition, 30–40% of those capillaries remaining do not support flowing red cells (Figure 14.11, Kindig *et al.*, 1998). Thus, diabetic pathology impairs arterial vasodilation, decreases the deformability of red cells and reduces the structural and functional capacities of the capillary bed. These structural and functional alterations accelerate the rate of decrease of PO_2m in diabetic muscle at the onset of contractions such that PO_2m values across the transition undershoot the steady-state values (Figure 14.12, Behnke *et al.*, 2002b). This will reduce the blood–muscle O_2 driving pressure and impair mitochondrial O_2 delivery.

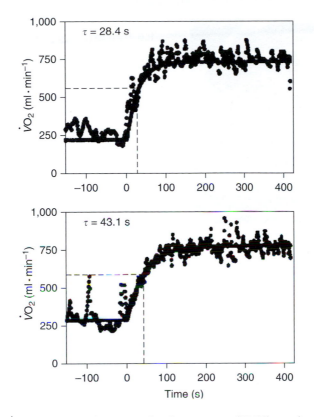

Figure 14.10 $\dot{V}O_2$ response at the onset of cycling exercise (30 W) in a healthy control
subject (upper) and a type II diabetic patient (lower). These data were fit by
a single exponential model and hence the τ (tau) denotes the mean
response time. From Regensteiner *et al.* (1998) with permission.

Effects of reduced muscle perfusive and diffusive conductance on muscle $\dot{V}O_2$ kinetics

Muscle O_2 delivery can be considered to be the net result of the perfusive
conductance ($\dot{Q}O_2$, number of red blood cells delivered per unit time each with
a finite quantity of accessible O_2) and diffusive conductance (DO_2, approximated
by the number of red cells adjacent to a muscle fibre volume at a given
time). Diseases such as CHF and Type I diabetes may reduce muscle blood flow
(perfusive conductance) as well as the number of red cell perfused capillaries
and thus the number of red cells per unit fibre volume (diffusive conductance,
Figure 14.13, upper panel). The reduced muscle $\dot{Q}O_2$ relative to $\dot{V}O_2$ means that
microvascular PO_2 falls faster and to a lower value than normal especially at the
onset of muscle contractions (Figure 14.8 and 14.12). Hence, the fractional O_2
extraction is elevated and femoral venous O_2 content falls below that found in

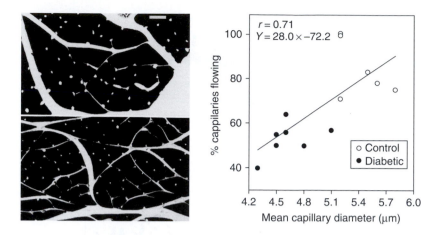

Figure 14.11 Left panel: Photomicrographs of perfusion-fixed plantaris muscle from control (upper) and streptozotocin-induced diabetic (lower) rats. Bar = 50 μm. Note extreme fibre atrophy and also smaller capillary luminal diameter in diabetic plantaris. (From Sexton *et al.* (1994) with permission.) *Right panel*: Within spinotrapezius muscle of Type I diabetic rats, the percentage of flowing capillaries decreases with the reduction in capillary luminal diameter. From Kindig *et al.* (1998) with permission.

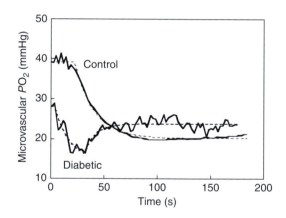

Figure 14.12 Effect of streptozotocin-induced diabetes on the partial pressure of O_2 in the microvasculature (PO_2m) of the rat spinotrapezius muscle at the onset of 1 Hz contractions. Notice the lowered PO_2m across the transition in diabetes. Data from Behnke *et al.*, 2002b.

healthy individuals (Katz *et al.*, 2000). In the past, this has been taken as evidence that microcirculatory O_2 exchange was functioning normally. However, it is evident from Figure 14.13 (upper panel) that very low microvascular PO_2 values can coexist with an impaired diffusing capacity (Kindig *et al.*, 1999; Diederich *et al.*,

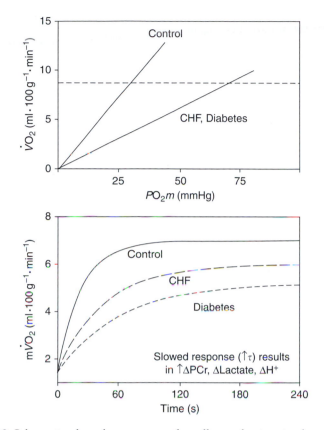

Figure 14.13 Schematic that demonstrates the effects of microcirculatory disorders associated with chronic heart failure (CHF) and Type 1 diabetes. *Upper panel:* illustrates the reduced O_2 diffusing capacity (given by the slope of the $\dot{V}O_2$-to-PO_2 relationship) that arises, in part, from the substantial loss of red blood cell perfused capillaries in skeletal muscle from CHF and Type I diabetic animals. *Lower panel:* demonstrates how the reduced perfusive (capillary red blood cell flux) and diffusive conductances conspire to slow $\dot{V}O_2$ kinetics across the rest–exercise transition. Note that the slowed $\dot{V}O_2$ kinetics for both disease conditions will elevate the muscle O_2 deficit and it is this effect that augments the breakdown of phosphocreatine, PCr, and accumulation of metabolites such as lactate and hydrogen ions.

2002; Richardson *et al.*, 2003). This effectively lowers the pressure head for diffusion of O_2 from the capillary to the myocyte. Consequently, net movement of O_2 is compromised, muscle $\dot{V}O_2$ kinetics are slowed and there will be a greater fall in intracellular PO_2 (Richardson *et al.*, 2003) and PCr and increased elevation of ADP_{free}, inorganic phosphate and Cr (Wilson *et al.*, 1977; Elander *et al.*, 1985; Haseler *et al.*, 1998, 1999). It is these slowed muscle $\dot{V}O_2$ kinetics that ultimately limit the pulmonary $\dot{V}O_2$ response. This effect will be seen subsequent to any initial slowing of the pulmonary $\dot{V}O_2$ response (Phase I) that results from an impaired venous return.

Conclusions

Any disease conditions that impair muscle O_2 delivery have the potential to reduce the speed of the $\dot{V}O_2$ kinetics (Figure 14.3). It is apparent that diseases which lower arterial O_2 content and decrease muscle O_2 delivery and thus microvascular PO_2 slow $\dot{V}O_2$ kinetics at the onset of exercise. In addition to pulmonary and cardiac dysfunction, there may also be profound structural and functional changes in the periphery that reduce local muscle blood flow and decrease capillary red blood cell flow and microvascular PO_2. Many of these pathologic changes are also associated with a down-regulation of mitochondrial oxidative capacity which will act to further slow O_2 utilization and $\dot{V}O_2$ kinetics. Indeed, if as Chapter 9 argues, the speed of the $\dot{V}O_2$ kinetics are determined locally by the mitochondrial enzymes then it is probable that the $\dot{V}O_2$ kinetics are more sensitive to reductions in those enzymes than subtle changes in O_2 delivery. This conclusion is certainly borne out by investigations in the human and the horse where reduction of nitric oxide via L-NAME *speeds* $\dot{V}O_2$ kinetics despite *reductions* in cardiac output and presumably muscle blood flow. It is likely that this is the result of L-NAME induced removal of nitric oxide inhibition of cytochrome oxidase and/or other steps in the electron transport chain (Kindig *et al.*, 2001,2002a). PAD patients are unusual in that chronic muscle ischaemic hypoxia actually increases mitochodrial enzyme activity (Elander *et al.*, 1985; Lundgren *et al.*, 1989) and in so doing may constrain the full effect of the reduced O_2 delivery. There is a compelling rationale for employing physical activity or training as a means to improve muscle oxidative function, restore $\dot{V}O_2$ kinetics towards control values and reduce the O_2 deficit and degree of intracellular perturbation incurred at exercise onset in patients suffering from diseases that impair pulmonary, cardiac or muscle function (Casaburi *et al.*, 1987; Poole *et al.*, 1994; Poole, 1997; Chapter 15). In addition to decreasing the O_2 deficit, exercise training has been demonstrated to reduce the $\dot{V}O_2$ cost of exercise performed in the heavy and sometimes the severe-intensity domain (Casaburi *et al.*, 1987; rev. Poole, 1997). Specifically, for a given absolute work rate that constituted heavy or severe-intensity exercise pre-training, after training this same work rate may reside within the moderate or lower extremes of the heavy-intensity domain. In either instance the $\dot{V}O_2$ will be reduced by the abolition or decrease of the $\dot{V}O_2$ slow component (rev. Gaesser and Poole, 1996, see Chapter 15).

Glossary of terms

A-aPO$_2$	alveolar-to-arterial O_2 partial pressure gradient
ADP	adenosine diphosphate (ADP$_{free}$, the metabolically important fraction of intracellular ADP)
ATP	adenosine triphosphate
a-vO$_2$diff.	arterial-to-venous O_2 difference
CHF	chronic heart failure
COPD	chronic obstructive pulmonary disease

Cr	creatine
HR	heart rate
L-NAME	L-nitro arginine methyl ester (inhibits nitric oxide synthase)
MRT	mean response time (time delay + time constant, τ or tau, denotes time to 63% of final response)
PAD	peripheral arterial disease
PO_2m	microvascular PO_2
PVD	peripheral vascular occlusive disease
$\dot{V}O_2$	partial pressure of O_2
$\dot{Q}O_2$	perfusive O_2 conductance (i.e. blood flow, $\dot{Q}$ × arterial O_2 content)
DO_2	diffusive O_2 conductance
τ or tau	denotes time to 63% of final response in the exponential function, τ_c cardiodynamic, τ_p primary
$\dot{V}_A/\dot{Q}$	alveolar ventilation to perfusion ratio
$\dot{V}_D$	dead space or wasted ventilation
$\dot{V}_D/\dot{V}_T$	dead space to tidal ventilation ratio (a measurement of the efficiency of ventilation)
$\dot{V}O_2$	oxygen uptake
$\dot{V}O_{2\,max}$	maximal oxygen uptake (achieved under conditions of large muscle mass exercise unless otherwise specified and considered synonymous with $\dot{V}O_{2\,peak}$)
Phase I	initial increase in $\dot{V}O_2$ at exercise onset caused by elevated pulmonary blood flow (also called the cardiodynamic phase)
Phase II	the exponential increase in $\dot{V}O_2$ that is initiated when venous blood from the exercising muscles arrives at the lungs. Corresponds closely with muscle $\dot{V}O_2$ dynamics.

References

Barstow, T.J., Lamarra, N. and Whipp, B.J. (1990). Modulation of muscle and pulmonary O_2 uptakes by circulatory dynamics during exercise. *Journal of Applied Physiology*, **68**, 979–89.

Bauer, T.A., Regensteiner, J.G., Brass, E.P. and Hiatt, W.R. (1999). Oxygen uptake kinetics during exercise are slowed in patients with peripheral arterial disease. *Journal of Applied Physiology*, **87**, 809–16.

Behnke, B.J., Barstow, T.J., Kindig, C.A., McDonough, P., Musch, T.I. and Poole, D.C. (2002a). Dynamics of oxygen uptake following exercise onset in rat skeletal muscle. *Respiration Physiology and Neurobiology*, **133**, 229–39.

Behnke, B.J., Kindig, C.A., McDonough, P., Poole, D.C. and Sexton, W.L. (2002b). Dynamics of microvascular oxygen pressure during rest–conraction transition in skeletal muscle of diabetic rats. *American Journal of Physiology*, **283**, H926–32.

Casaburi, R. (2000). Skeletal muscle function in COPD. *Chest*, **117**, 267S–71S.

Casaburi, R., Storer, T.W., Ben-Dov, I. and Wasserman, K. (1987). Effect of endurance training on possible determinants of $\dot{V}O_2$ during heavy exercise. *Journal of Applied Physiology*, **62**, 199–207.

Casaburi, R., Patessio, A., Ioli, F., Zanaboni, S., Donner, C.F. and Wasserman, K. (1991). Reductions in exercise lactic acidosis and ventilation as a result of exercise training in patients with obstructive lung disease. *American Review of Respiratory Disease*, **143**, 9–18.

Cerretelli, P., Grassi, B., Colombini, A., Caru, B. and Marconi, C. (1988). Gas exchange and metabolic transients in heart transplant recipients. *Respiration Physiology*, **74**, 355–71.

Delp, M.D., Duan, C., Mattson, J.P. and Musch, T.I. (1997). Changes in skeletal muscle biochemistry and histology relative to fiber type in rats with heart failure. *Journal of Applied Physiology*, **83**, 1291–9.

Dernevik, L., Bylund-Fellenius, A.C., Ekroth, R., Holm, J., Idstrom, J.P. and Schersten, T. (1988). Enzymatic activities in heart and skeletal muscle of children with cyanotic and noncyanotic congenital heart disease. *Thoracic and Cardiovascular Surgery*, **36**, 310–12.

Diederich, E.R., Behnke, B.J., McDonough, P., Kindig, C.A., Barstow, T.J., Poole, D.C. and Musch, T.I. (2002). Dynamics of microvascular oxygen partial pressure in contracting skeletal muscle of rats with chronic heart failure. *Cardiovascular Research*, **56**, 479–86.

Drexler, H., Riede, U., Munzel, T., Konig, H., Funke, E. and Just, H. (1992). Alterations of skeletal muscle in chronic heart failure. *Circulation*, **185**, 1751–9.

Elander, A., Idstrom, J.P., Schersten, T. and Bylund-Fellenius, A.C. (1985). Metabolic adaptation to reduced muscle blood flow. I. Enzyme and metabolite alterations. *American Journal of Physiology*, **249**, E63–9.

Engelen, M., Porszasz, J., Riley, M., Wasserman, K., Maehara, K. and Barstow, T.J. (1996). Effects of hypoxic hypoxia on O_2 uptake and heart rate kinetics during heavy exercise. *Journal of Applied Physiology*, **81**, 2500–8.

Gaesser, G.A. and Poole, D.C. (1996). The slow component of oxygen uptake kinetics in humans. In J.O. Holloszy (Ed.) *Exercise and Sports Science Reviews*, Vol. 25. Williams and Wilkins, pp. 35–70.

Grassi, B., Marconi, C., Meyer, M., Rieu, M. and Cerretelli, P. (1997). Gas exchange and cardiovascular kinetics with different exercise protocols in heart transplant recipients. *Journal of Applied Physiology*, **82**, 1952–62.

Haseler, L.J., Richardson, R.S., Videen, J.S. and Hogan, M.C. (1998). Phosphocreatine hydrolysis during submaximal exercise: the effect of FIO2. *Journal of Applied Physiology*, **85**, 1457–63.

Haseler, L.J., Hogan, M.C. and Richardson, R.S. (1999). Skeletal muscle phosphocreatine recovery in exercise-trained humans is dependent on O_2 availability. *Journal of Applied Physiology*, 86, 2013–18.

Hepple, R.T., Liu, P.P., Plyley, M.J. and Goodman, J.M. (1999). Oxygen uptake kinetics during exercise in chronic heart failure: influence of peripheral vascular reserve. *Clinical Science*, **97**, 569–77.

Katz, S.D., Maskin, C., Jondeau, G., Cocke, T., Berkowitz, R. and LeJemtel, T. (2000). Near-maximal fractional oxygen extraction by active skeletal muscle in patients with chronic heart failure. *Journal of Applied Physiology*, **88**, 2138–42.

Kindig, C.A., Sexton, W.L., Fedde, M.R. and Poole, D.C. (1998). Skeletal muscle microcirculatory structure and hemodynamics in diabetes. *Respiration Physiology and Neurobiology*, **111**, 163–75.

Kindig, C.A., Musch, T.I., Basaraba, R.J. and Poole, D.C. (1999). Impaired capillary hemodynamics in skeletal muscle of rats in chronic heart failure. *Journal of Applied Physiology*, **87**, 652–60.

Kindig, C.A., McDonough, P., Erickson, H.H. and Poole, D.C. (2001). Effect of L-NAME on oxygen uptake kinetics during heavy-intensity exercise in the horse. *Journal of Applied Physiology*, **91**, 891–6.

Kindig, C.A., McDonough, P., Erickson, H.H. and Poole, D.C. (2002a). Nitric oxide synthase inhibition speeds oxygen uptake kinetics in horses during moderate domain running. *Respiration Physiology and Neurobiology*, **132**, 169–78.

Kindig, C.A., Richardson, T.E. and Poole, D.C. (2002b). Skeletal muscle capillary hemodynamics from rest to contractions: implications for oxygen transfer. *Journal of Applied Physiology*, **92**, 513–20.

Lundgren, F., Dahllof, A.G., Schersten, T. and Bylund-Fellenius, A.C. (1989). Muscle enzyme adaptation in patients with peripheral arterial insufficiency: spontaneous adaptation, effect of different treatments and consequences on walking performance. *Clinical Science*, **77**, 485–93.

Macdonald, M., Pedersen, P.K. and Hughson, R.L. (1997). Acceleration of $\dot{V}O_2$ kinetics in heavy submaximal exercise by hyperoxia and prior high-intensity exercise. *Journal of Applied Physiology*, **83**, 1318–25.

Maltais, F., LeBlanc, P., Jobin, J. and Casaburi, R. (2000). Peripheral muscle dysfunction in chronic obstructive pulmonary disease. *Clinical Chest Medicine*, **21**, 665–77.

Mattson, J.P. and Poole, D.C. (1998). Pulmonary emphysema decreases hamster skeletal muscle oxidative enzyme capacity. *Journal of Applied Physiology*, **85**, 210–14.

Mattson, J.P., Sun, J., Murray, D.M. and Poole, D.C. (2002). Lipid peroxidation in the skeletal muscle of hamsters with emphysema. *Pathophysiology*, **8**, 215–21.

Meakins, J. and Long, C.N.H. (1927). Oxygen consumption, oxygen debt and lactic acid in circulatory failure. *Journal of Clinical Investigations*, **4**, 273–93.

Mettauer, B., Zhao, Q.M., Epailly, E., Charloux, A., Lampert, E., Heitz-Naegelen, B., Piquard, F., di Prampero, P.E. and Lonsdorfer, J. (2000). $\dot{V}O_2$ kinetics reveal a central limitation at the onset of subthreshold exercise in heart transplant recipients. *Journal of Applied Physiology*, **88**, 1228–38.

Nery, L.E., Wasserman, K., Andrews, D.J., Huntsman, D.J., Hansen, J.E. and Whipp, B.J. (1982). Ventilatory and gas exchange kinetics during exercise in chronic obstructive pulmonary disease. *Journal of Applied Physiology*, **53**, 1594–602.

Palange, P., Galassetti, P., Mannix, E.T., Farber, M.O., Manfredi, F., Serra, P. and Carlone, S. (1995). Oxygen effect on O_2 deficit and $\dot{V}O_2$ kinetics during exercise in obstructive pulmonary disease. *Journal of Applied Physiology*, **78**, 2228–34.

Poole, D.C. (1997). Influence of exercise training on skeletal muscle oxygen delivery and utilization. In R.G. Crystal, J.B. West, E.R. Weibel, P.J. Barnes (Eds) *The Lung: Scientific Foundations*, Raven Press, New York, pp. 1957–67.

Poole, D.C., Barstow, T.J., Gaesser, G.A., Willis, W.T. and Whipp, B.J. (1994). $\dot{V}O_2$ slow component: physiological and functional significance. *Medicine and Science in Sports and Exercise*, **26**, 1354–8.

Regensteiner, J.G., Bauer, T.A., Reusch, J.E., Brandenburg, S.L., Sippel, J.M., Vogelsong, A.M., Smith, S., Wolfel, E.E., Eckel, R.H. and Hiatt, W.R. (1998). Abnormal oxygen uptake kinetic responses in women with type II diabetes mellitus. *Journal of Applied Physiology*, **85**, 310–17.

Richardson, T.E., Kindig, C.A., Musch, T.I. and Poole, D.C. (2003). Effects of chronic heart failure on skeletal muscle capillary hemodynamics at rest and during contractions. *Journal of Applied Physiology*, **95**, 1055–62.

Roy, T.M., Peterson, H.R., Snider, H.L., Cyrus, J., Broadstone, V.L., Fell, R.D., Rothchild, A.H., Samols, E. and Pfeifer, M.A. (1989). Autonomic influence on cardiovascular performance in diabetic subjects. *American Journal of Medicine*, **87**, 382–8.

Sexton, W.L., Poole, D.C. and Mathieu-Costello, O. (1994). Microcirculatory structure–function relationships in skeletal muscle of diabetic rats. *American Journal of Physiology*, **266**, H1502–11.

Sietsema, K.E., Cooper, D.M., Perloff, J.K., Rosove, M.H., Child, J.S., Canobbio, M.M., Whipp, B.J. and Wasserman, K. (1986). Dynamics of oxygen uptake during exercise in adults with cyanotic congenital heart disease. *Circulation*, **73**, 1137–44.

Sietsema, K.E., Daly, J.A. and Wasserman, K. (1989). Early dynamics of O_2 uptake and heart rate as affected by exercise work rate. *Journal of Applied Physiology*, **67**, 2535–41.

Sietsema, K.E., Ben-Dov, I., Zhang, Y.Y., Sullivan, C. and Wasserman, K. (1994). Dynamics of oxygen uptake for submaximal exercise and recovery in patients with chronic heart failure. *Chest*, **105**, 1693–700.

Simoneau, J.A. and Kelley, D.E. (1997). Altered glycolytic and oxidative capacities of skeletal muscle contribute to insulin resistance in NIDDM. *Journal of Applied Physiology*, **83**, 166–71.

Wagner, P.D., Dantzker, D.R., Dueck, R., Clausen, J.L. and West, J.B. (1977). Ventilation–perfusion inequality in chronic obstructive pulmonary disease. *Journal of Clinical Investigations*, **59**, 203–16.

Wasserman, K., Hansen, J.E., Sue, D.S., Whipp B.J., and Casaburi, R. (1994). *Principles of Exercise Testing and Interpretation*. Lea & Febiger, London.

Williamson, J.W., Raven, P.B. and Whipp, B.J. (1996). Unaltered oxygen uptake kinetics at exercise onset with lower-body positive pressure in humans. *Experimental Physiology*, **81**, 695–705.

Wilson, D.F., Erecinska, M., Drown, C. and Silver, I.A. (1977). Effect of oxygen tension on cellular energetics. *American Journal of Physiology*, **233**, C135–40.

Zelis, R., Flaim, S.F., Liedtke, A.J. and Nellis, S.H. (1981). Cardiocirculatory dynamics in the normal and failing heart. *Annual Review of Physiology*, **43**, 455–76.

15 Effect of training on $\dot{V}O_2$ kinetics and performance

Andrew M. Jones and Katrien Koppo

Introduction

The rapidity with which the rate of adenosine triphosphate (ATP) supply through oxidative phosphorylation can adjust to meet the total ATP turnover rate in the transition to a higher metabolic rate is an important determinant of exercise tolerance (Chapter 1). 'Sluggish' $\dot{V}O_2$ on-kinetics is associated with a greater depletion of intra-muscular high-energy phosphates and a greater accumulation of lactate and hydrogen ions. This is illustrated in Figure 15.1 which shows the magnitude of the 'oxygen deficit' when the mean response time (MRT) for $\dot{V}O_2$ is both relatively fast (15 s) and relatively slow (45 s). The development of the $\dot{V}O_2$ 'slow component' during exercise performed above the lactate threshold (LT), which causes $\dot{V}O_2$ to rise above the predicted steady-state requirement, also appears to be associated with the fatigue process (Chapter 1). Interventions that facilitate either a speeding of the $\dot{V}O_2$ response towards the expected steady state or a reduction in the magnitude of the $\dot{V}O_2$ slow component should therefore result in improved exercise tolerance. The most potent intervention, in this regard, is endurance exercise training.

The purpose of this chapter is to review the effect of endurance training on $\dot{V}O_2$ kinetics in a variety of populations. The influence of training status on $\dot{V}O_2$ kinetics has been examined using two approaches: cross-sectional (in which the $\dot{V}O_2$ kinetic responses of well-trained individuals are compared with the responses of sedentary or less well-trained individuals); and longitudinal (in which $\dot{V}O_2$ kinetics are measured before and after a training intervention). Cross-sectional studies are useful in that they allow comparison to be made between 'extreme' groups (i.e. elite endurance athletes vs sedentary subjects). However, with this design, it is not possible to attribute differences in the response characteristics to differences in training performed, *per se*, since other factors (including genetics) may also be influential. In longitudinal studies, in which subjects perform a training programme for a few weeks, such extreme training responses are very unlikely to be elicited. On the other hand, longitudinal studies are important in exploring the cause–effect relationship between training and physiological adaptation.

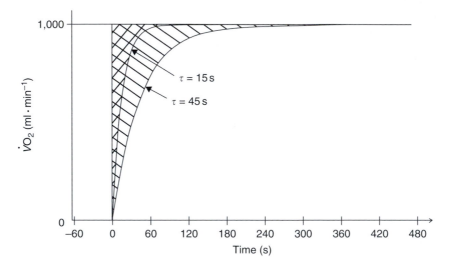

Figure 15.1 Schematic model of the oxygen uptake response following the onset of moderate-intensity exercise. The shaded areas correspond to the oxygen deficit incurred when the MRT of the $\dot{V}O_2$ on-response is 15 s and 45 s. Note the markedly longer time before a steady state is reached when the on-kinetics are slower. With an MRT of 15 s and an amplitude of $1 \, l \cdot min^{-1}$, the O_2 deficit is 0.25 l (i.e. $15/60 \times 1$). With an MRT of 45 s and an amplitude of $1 \, l \cdot min^{-1}$, the O_2 deficit is 0.75 l (i.e. $45/60 \times 1$).

Cross-sectional studies

One of the first cross-sectional studies that compared the $\dot{V}O_2$ responses of two groups of subjects with differing $\dot{V}O_{2 \, max}$ was that of Weltman and Katch (1976). In this study, 8 men with a high $\dot{V}O_{2 \, max}$ ($4.85 \pm 0.38 \, l \cdot min^{-1}$) and 8 men with a lower $\dot{V}O_{2 \, max}$ ($3.92 \pm 0.36 \, l \cdot min^{-1}$) performed a constant-load exercise bout below the gas exchange threshold (GET; i.e. 120 W). Although $\dot{V}O_2$ was not measured continuously, the results indicated that the group with the highest $\dot{V}O_{2 \, max}$ had a more rapid adjustment of $\dot{V}O_2$ toward the steady state. It was not clear, however, whether the differences in $\dot{V}O_2$ kinetics were related to differences in $\dot{V}O_{2 \, max}$ or to differences in training. Cerretelli *et al.* (1979) also showed that the half-time for the increase in $\dot{V}O_2$ during supine arm-cranking at the same absolute work rate of 125 W was significantly faster in kayakers compared to sedentary subjects (82 vs 47 s on average) and that the faster kinetics were associated with a reduced increase in blood lactate accumulation (~4 vs ~ 9 mM in the kayakers and sedentary subjects, respectively). Powers *et al.* (1985) compared the $\dot{V}O_2$ kinetics in highly trained athletes with similar training routines but who differed in $\dot{V}O_{2 \, max}$. They observed that for a constant-load test at 50% $\dot{V}O_{2 \, max}$, $\dot{V}O_2$ adjusted more rapidly towards the steady state in those subjects having a higher $\dot{V}O_{2 \, max}$. These data therefore indicate that $\dot{V}O_{2 \, max}$ is positively related to $\dot{V}O_2$ on-kinetics in athletes performing similar training programmes.

Zhang *et al.* (1991) conducted a more extensive study in which the effect of fitness on the $\dot{V}O_2$ kinetics was determined for different work rates. The subjects performed a 12 min incremental step test (4 × 3 min) where the work rates were chosen to be 25%, 50%, 75% and 100% of the subject's maximum work capacity. The $\dot{V}O_2$ kinetics became progressively slower at higher work-rate steps for all subjects. Furthermore, for each intensity, the $\dot{V}O_2$ kinetics were faster in the fitter subjects. Barstow *et al.* (1996a) however, reported that during constant-load exercise at 50%Δ (Δ = the difference between the GET and the $\dot{V}O_{2\,max}$), the time constant of the primary component $\dot{V}O_2$ response (τ_p) was not significantly correlated either with the $\dot{V}O_{2\,max}$ or the % type I fibres in the vastus lateralis. However, the gain of the $\dot{V}O_2$ primary component (G_p) was positively correlated with both the $\dot{V}O_{2\,max}$ and the % type I fibres, whereas the relative contribution of the $\dot{V}O_2$ slow component was negatively correlated with those parameters. In a later study, Barstow *et al.* (2000) reported that during incremental exercise, a higher $\dot{V}O_{2\,max}$ and a greater % type I fibres were correlated with a greater $\Delta\dot{V}O_2/\Delta WR$ (WR = work rate) both below and above the GET. The influence of muscle fibre type distribution and motor unit recruitment patterns on $\dot{V}O_2$ kinetics is addressed in Chapter 11.

In a recent study, Russell *et al.* (2002) compared the magnitude of the relative $\dot{V}O_2$ slow component to the muscle fibre type composition and citrate synthase activity in both highly trained endurance cyclists and recreationally active subjects. The subjects performed one constant-load test at 50%Δ for a duration of 6–10 min. As expected, the trained subjects had a greater % type I fibres and a higher citrate synthase activity. The relative magnitude of the slow component was lower in the trained subjects. When the trained and the recreationally active group were combined, the relative magnitude of the slow component was positively correlated with the % type IIa fibres ($r = 0.60$; $P < 0.01$), and negatively correlated with the % type I fibres ($r = -0.57$; $P = 0.003$). This led the authors to conclude that, since citrate synthase activity and $\dot{V}O_{2\,max}$ are indicators of aerobic fitness, the slow component is inversely correlated with aerobic fitness.

Because most of the cross-sectional studies compared the on-transient $\dot{V}O_2$ kinetics during constant-load exercise between trained and untrained subjects for one exercise intensity only, the interaction between training status and exercise intensity remained to be determined. Koppo *et al.* (2004) recently hypothesized that training status might influence whether or not the τ_p is slowed for exercise above compared to below the GET (see Chapter 12 for further discussion on this issue). Based on the work of Carter *et al.* (2000), which showed that τ_p did not differ significantly above and below the GET in a group of 23 subjects of heterogeneous fitness, but was significantly slower for supra-threshold exercise in the 6 subjects with the lowest $\dot{V}O_{2\,max}$ values, Koppo *et al.* (2004) reasoned that trained subjects would have an invariant time constant and untrained subjects would show a lengthening of τ_p for exercise above, compared with below the GET. In this study, seven trained competitive cyclists and eight untrained

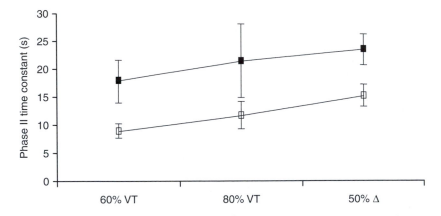

Figure 15.2 Influence of training status and work rate on the Phase II time constant τ_p. Open squares represent the values for highly trained cyclists; closed squares represent the values for untrained subjects. Note the trend for the kinetics to become slower at higher work rates in both groups, and the substantially faster kinetics in the trained subjects. Reproduced from Koppo *et al.* (2004) with permission.

subjects completed square-wave transitions to work rates requiring 60% and 80% of the GET and to 50%Δ. The results indicated that τ_p was significantly smaller in the trained compared to the untrained subjects and that, in contrast to the hypothesis, τ_p became progressively greater at higher work rates both in the trained and untrained subjects (Figure 15.2). Because τ_p was also slowed within the moderate-intensity domain, where O_2 availability is presumed not to be limiting, the authors suggested that this slowing may be linked to factors such as the recruitment of higher threshold motor units. Consistent with the results of Barstow *et al.* (1996a; 2000), Koppo *et al.* (2004) also observed a significantly greater G_p in the trained subjects. However, in contrast to the study of Russell *et al.* (2002), the relative contribution of the slow component was similar in the trained and untrained subjects. However, in the study of Koppo *et al.* (2004), the slow component emerged earlier and had faster kinetics in the trained compared to the untrained subjects. This indicates that, had the exercise been extended beyond 8 min, the relative contribution of the slow component would have been larger in the untrained subjects.

Koppo *et al.* (2004) attempted to explain the differences in $\dot{V}O_2$ response between trained and untrained subjects with a hypothetical model (Figure 15.3). They reasoned that for moderate exercise, in which type I muscle fibres are predominantly recruited, the greater mitochondrial density and oxidative enzyme activity in the muscles of trained subjects would lead to a faster $\dot{V}O_2$ response. Furthermore, for heavy exercise, in which both type I and type II fibres are likely to be recruited, the faster $\dot{V}O_2$ response of the trained subjects may have been related to the fact that trained subjects will have recruited relatively fewer type II fibres which are believed to have slower on-kinetics than type I fibres (Crow and Kushmerick, 1982) compared to the untrained subjects. Moreover,

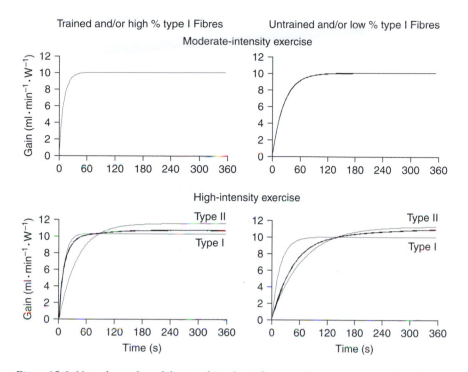

Figure 15.3 Hypothetical model to explain the influence of training status and work rate on $\dot{V}O_2$ kinetics. Subjects of higher training status are likely to recruit fewer type II fibres (with relatively slow on-kinetics) at any given relative work rate and to have greater mitochondrial density in all muscle fibres compared to untrained subjects. Reproduced from Koppo *et al.* (2004) with permission.

since it is likely that both principal fibre types have faster on-kinetics in the trained subjects compared to the untrained subjects, this might have resulted in the earlier onset and faster kinetics of the $\dot{V}O_2$ slow component in the trained subjects compared to the untrained subjects. However, it should be cautioned that alternative hypotheses also exist concerning the influence of muscle fibre type on $\dot{V}O_2$ kinetics (see Chapters 11 and 12).

Relatively few studies have reported values for the $\dot{V}O_2$ kinetic parameters for highly trained subjects ($\dot{V}O_{2\,max} > 65$ ml·kg^{-1}·min^{-1}) performing constant work-rate exercise. However, some examples can be found in the recent literature. In the study of Borrani *et al.* (2001), 13 regional-level competitive runners performed a running test at 95% $\dot{V}O_{2\,max}$ until exhaustion. The τ_p was 17.2 ± 5.8 s. In the study of Cleuziou *et al.* (2003) on-transient $\dot{V}O_2$ kinetics to cycling at 80% of the GET and to 50%Δ were determined for 10 well-trained male cyclists. The τ_p was similar for both transitions and averaged ~21 s. These values are shorter than the τ_p observed in healthy, young, non-specifically trained subjects (typically ~ 25–30 s). However, in the World record holder for

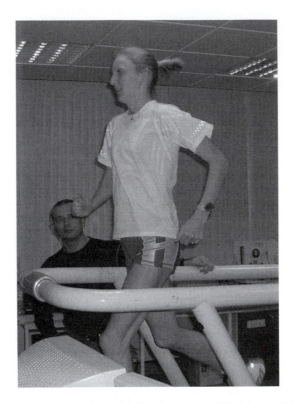

Figure 15.4 Photograph of Paula Radcliffe, the current World record holder for the women's marathon. Paula is pictured here warming up before undergoing a physiological evaluation with one of the chapter authors (AMJ).

the women' marathon, the τ_p is 8–10 s in the transition from standing rest to moderate-intensity treadmill running (Jones, unpublished observations; Figures 15.4 and 15.5). Also, τ_p values as fast as 9 s have been reported in highly trained cyclists (Barstow and Molé, 1991; Koppo *et al.*, 2004; Figure 15.5). Similarly fast $\dot{V}O_2$ kinetics have been reported in the Thoroughbred racehorse (Langsetmo *et al.*, 1997; see Chapter 5).

Longitudinal studies

It is clear from the previous section that enhanced physical 'fitness' leads to significant alterations in pulmonary $\dot{V}O_2$ kinetics, including a speeding of the kinetics of the primary component and a reduction in the amplitude of the slow component (at least at the same 'relative' exercise intensity). Relative to the 'control' condition (i.e. healthy sedentary young person), it is known that ageing and a variety of disease states result in changes to the kinetics that are associated

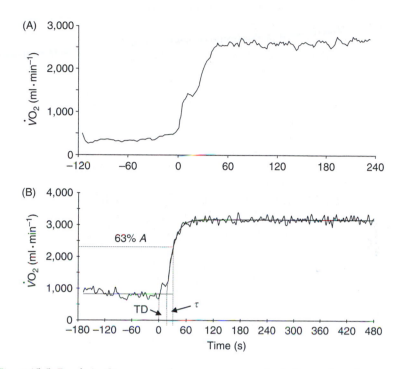

Figure 15.5 Panel A: Oxygen uptake response to a single bout of moderate-intensity treadmill running (at 16 km · h⁻¹) in the current World record holder for the women's marathon. Note the very fast on-kinetics which lead to the attainment of steady state within ~50 s. Panel B: Oxygen uptake response to moderate-intensity exercise (at 240 W) in a Belgian junior cycle champion. Data are the averaged response to six identical transitions. The model fit is superimposed.

with a reduced exercise tolerance (see Chapters 13 and 14), while physical training improves the kinetic profile such that exercise tolerance should be improved. As outlined earlier, faster $\dot{V}O_2$ kinetics at the same work rate will reduce the magnitude of the oxygen deficit, thereby sparing the fall in intra-muscular [PCr] and attenuating the production of lactic acid. There is therefore tighter metabolic control, that is the same $\dot{V}O_2$ is attained with less perturbation of the phosphorylation and redox potentials. At heavy and severe exercise intensities, a reduced slow component for the same work rate will extend time to fatigue because it will lower the metabolic cost of the exercise.

Endurance-type exercise training is known to result in significant improvements in the LT/GET (Davis *et al.*, 1979; Denis *et al.*, 1982), critical power (CP; Poole *et al.*, 1990), and $\dot{V}O_{2\,max}$ (Hickson *et al.*, 1981) (see Jones and Carter, 2000 for review). These parameters of aerobic fitness demarcate the boundaries between the various exercise intensity domains within which the metabolic and pulmonary gas exchange responses to exercise are predictable (see Chapter 1). It is therefore important to point out that the effects of training on $\dot{V}O_2$ kinetics will depend in part on whether the frame of reference is the same absolute work-rate or the same relative work rate. For example, an absolute work rate that was originally 'heavy' (i.e. above the LT) might become 'moderate' (i.e. below the LT) following a period of endurance training if the work rate at the LT increases appreciably. Similarly, a work rate that was originally 'severe' (i.e. above the CP) might become 'heavy' (i.e. below the CP) if, with training, the CP exceeds the original work rate. In these situations, if $\dot{V}O_2$ kinetics were measured at the same absolute work rate pre- vs post-training, a reduced end-exercise $\dot{V}O_2$, an attenuated slow component and faster $\dot{V}O_2$ kinetics (at least when expressed as the MRT over the entire response) would be anticipated. If, however, the $\dot{V}O_2$ kinetics were measured at the same relative work rate (e.g. 90% LT, or some percentage of the difference between LT and $\dot{V}O_{2\,max}$) as calculated from the pre- and post-training values of LT and $\dot{V}O_{2\,max}$, then relatively little change in the $\dot{V}O_2$ kinetics would be expected because these would essentially be 'normalized' in relation to the changes in the boundaries of the exercise intensity domains. It is of interest, however, that exercise at the same relative intensity post-training could result in larger amplitudes of the fundamental and slow components of the $\dot{V}O_2$ kinetics because this same relative intensity occurs at a higher absolute work rate. In this regard, it is notable that highly trained subjects often have larger slow component amplitudes (expressed in absolute values of $ml \cdot min^{-1}$) compared to untrained subjects exercising at the same relative intensity as a result of the much higher absolute work rate and hence $\dot{V}O_2$ requirement for the trained subjects. It is useful in this situation to functionally normalize the $\dot{V}O_2$ slow component term by expressing it as the percentage contribution it makes to the end-exercise $\dot{V}O_2$ (e.g. Carter *et al.*, 2000; Koppo *et al.*, 2002, 2004).

The parameters of aerobic function: efficiency, LT, $\dot{V}O_{2\,max}$, and $\dot{V}O_2$ kinetics (Whipp *et al.*, 1982), along with CP (Poole *et al.*, 1990), are sensitive to a number of features of the training programme that is undertaken. Factors that will influence the extent of the physiological response to training include: the initial training status of the subject; the total duration of the training programme; and the volume of the training per unit time (comprising the frequency, duration and intensity of all training sessions completed in a certain time frame which is typically one week; Wenger and Bell, 1986). Training studies are notoriously difficult to conduct, especially when the training sessions themselves are supervised by the experimenters and/or frequent or time-consuming measurements of the physiological responses to training are made. It is easier to detect physiological changes evoked by any training programme in subjects who are initially untrained; however, it is more difficult both to recruit and to retain such subjects. For all these reasons, the longitudinal studies conducted to date which have investigated the effects of training on $\dot{V}O_2$ kinetics have involved relatively short 'generic' endurance training programmes and young relatively fit students as subjects (although there is a growing literature base on the effects of training on $\dot{V}O_2$ kinetics and functional capacity in clinical populations).

Healthy populations

One of the earliest studies to investigate the influence of exercise training on $\dot{V}O_2$ kinetics was conducted by Hickson *et al.* (1978). In this study, 7 men performed 10 weeks of training (involving 3 × 40 min sessions of exhaustive running and 3 × 40 min sessions of exhaustive cycling per week). Before training, $\dot{V}O_2$ kinetics were assessed at 40%, 50%, 60% and 70% of the pre-training $\dot{V}O_{2\ max}$; after training, the subjects were tested at the same absolute and relative work rates. The $\dot{V}O_2$ kinetics were characterized as the time required for the attainment of 50%, 75% and 90% of the total increase in $\dot{V}O_2$ from the onset of exercise to the value recorded at 5 min. The training programme generally resulted in significantly faster $\dot{V}O_2$ kinetics, particularly at the higher absolute work rates. Interestingly, $\dot{V}O_2$ kinetics were also generally faster at the same relative work-rate post-training (Figure 15.6). The same research group extended these observations in a follow-up study (Hagberg *et al.*, 1980) in which 8 subjects performed a high-intensity training programme for 9 weeks. Using the same modelling approach, this study confirmed that training resulted in an overall speeding of the $\dot{V}O_2$ on and off response both when comparing the same absolute work rate and the same relative work rate (50% and 70% $\dot{V}O_{2\ max}$). At the same absolute work rate, the magnitudes of both the O_2 deficit and the O_2 debt were significantly reduced following training, consistent with evidence that there was a smaller decrement in muscle high-energy phosphates (Hultman *et al.*, 1967) and a reduction in the accumulation of muscle lactate (Karlsson *et al.*, 1972) following training. Although the authors did not specifically partition the fast and slow components, they rather insightfully noted that 'training accelerates the fast component, resulting in a smaller contribution of the slow component to the total increase in $\dot{V}O_2$'. Cerretelli *et al.* (1979) studied the separate effects of running and swimming training on the half-time for the increase in $\dot{V}O_2$ and showed that a speeding of the $\dot{V}O_2$ kinetics was highly specific to the muscle group

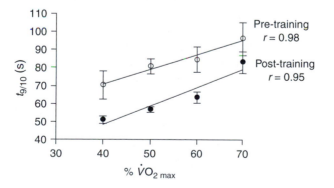

Figure 15.6 Relationship between speed of $\dot{V}O_2$ on-response (represented by the time taken to reach 90% of the steady-state value) and exercise intensity (as % $\dot{V}O_{2\ max}$) before (open symbols) and after (closed symbols) a period of endurance training. Redrawn from Hickson *et al.* (1978).

trained. A few years later, Convertino *et al.* (1984) reported that 7 days of continuous head-down bed rest resulted in a significant increase in the O_2 deficit (consistent with slowed $\dot{V}O_2$ kinetics) during upright, but not supine, cycle exercise. These early studies were important in providing general descriptions of the changes in the $\dot{V}O_2$ response to exercise and recovery elicited by physical training and by deconditioning. However, as pointed out elsewhere (e.g. Chapter 10), parameters derived from a single curve fitted from the onset to the end of exercise can mask whether any net 'speeding' derives from a more rapid primary component response or from a reduction in the amplitude of the $\dot{V}O_2$ slow component.

Phillips *et al.* (1995) assessed the time course for the adaptation of $\dot{V}O_2$ at a work rate requiring 60% of the pre-training $\dot{V}O_{2\,max}$ in 7 untrained young men before and after 4, 9 and 30 days of training. The training programme in this study involved 2 h of cycling per day on a stationary ergometer at 60% of pre-training $\dot{V}O_{2\,max}$ for 5 out of every 6 days. The results indicated a dissociation between changes in $\dot{V}O_2$ kinetics and changes in muscle metabolic potential with training. Specifically, both the $\dot{V}O_2$ on- and off-kinetics became significantly faster after only 4 days of training, and before there was a measurable increase in either muscle citrate synthase activity or $\dot{V}O_{2\,max}$. The τ_p in the on-transient was reduced from 37.2 s (pre-training) to 28.8 s (after 4 days training) and then further to 15.8 s (after 30 days training). As would be anticipated, the faster $\dot{V}O_2$ kinetics were associated with a reduced fall of muscle [PCr] and a reduced increase in blood [lactate]. This study demonstrated that the effect of endurance training on the speeding of τ_p may be extremely rapid. However, the cause of this speeding is not clear: while the authors proposed that this might be related to faster muscle blood flow kinetics or increased capillary-to-fibre ratio, it was not possible to rule out the influence of changes in the activity of other unmeasured oxidative enzymes on the $\dot{V}O_2$ kinetics. In another study from the same group, Shoemaker *et al.* (1996) reported that muscle blood flow kinetics were faster during knee-extension exercise following 10 days of endurance cycle training similar to that of Phillips *et al.* (1995). However, although this study demonstrates that muscle blood flow kinetics also adapt quickly following the onset of an endurance training programme, this does not prove that the faster blood flow kinetics caused the faster $\dot{V}O_2$ kinetics observed early following the onset of training by Phillips *et al.* (1995). Indeed, it is commonly observed that muscle blood flow kinetics are faster than $\dot{V}O_2$ kinetics even in the 'control' condition (Shoemaker *et al.*, 1994; MacDonald *et al.*, 1998; Bell *et al.*, 2001) suggesting that muscle blood flow does not limit $\dot{V}O_2$ kinetics at least at moderate intensities of exercise.

Noting that the majority of previous studies examining the effect of training on $\dot{V}O_2$ kinetics had utilized untrained subjects, Norris and Petersen (1998) studied the effect of 8 weeks of training on $\dot{V}O_2$ kinetics during moderate-intensity exercise in previously trained (but clearly not highly trained) cyclists ($\dot{V}O_{2\,max} \sim 57$ ml·kg^{-1}·min^{-1}). The training programme involved 5 training sessions at the work rate associated with the pre-training GET per week with the duration of each session increasing from 40 to 55 min as the programme continued.

The training programme resulted in significant improvements in $\dot{V}O_{2\,max}$, GET and 40 km time trial performance. The τ_p was significantly reduced from pre-training values (29.2 s on average) after both 4 (~ 24.4 s) and 8 weeks (~ 21.9 s) of training and this appeared to be dissociated from the response of $\dot{V}O_{2\,max}$ which did not improve between 4 to 8 weeks of training.

In a very recent study, Krustrup *et al.* (2004) reported that 7 weeks of single-leg high-intensity interval training resulted in an enchanced muscle $\dot{V}O_2$ response, compared to the untrained control leg, at 30W and 50W, though not at 10W, during knee extension exercise. The authors attributed this effect to a selective training effect on type II muscle fibres with this reducing the recruitment of type II fibres at the higher work rates. However, there were also improvements in muscle blood flow, capillarisation, and mitochondrial enzyme activity that might also have impacted on the enhanced $\dot{V}O_2$ response following training.

Demarle *et al.* (2001) investigated whether the increased time to exhaustion at high sub-maximal running speeds observed following endurance training was linked to a reduction in the oxygen deficit and/or to a reduction in the amplitude of the $\dot{V}O_2$ slow component. In their study, 6 trained runners ($\dot{V}O_{2\,max}$ ~ 61 ml $\cdot$ kg^{-1} $\cdot$ min^{-1}) underwent an 8-week training programme in which their training was supplemented with additional severe interval training sessions. They showed a significantly reduced τ_p (pre: 25.9 ± 1.2 s vs post: 14.2 ± 1.2 s) and a significantly reduced O_2 deficit, but no significant change in the amplitude of the slow component, following training. The reduction in the magnitude of the O_2 deficit was significantly correlated with the increase in the time to exhaustion at a high sub-maximal running speed observed after training ($r = -0.91$), although the strength of this relationship may have been influenced by the extreme response of a single subject. In a similar study, Billat *et al.* (2002) examined the effect of 4 weeks of severe interval training (two sessions per week) on some aspects of $\dot{V}O_2$ kinetics in 7 untrained young males. The subjects in this study performed an incremental treadmill test and exercise bouts at 90% and 95% of the running speed at the pre-training $\dot{V}O_{2\,max}$ both before and after training. Training resulted in a significant increase in the time to exhaustion (~ 40%) at both running speeds. Furthermore, training resulted in a significant reduction of τ_p at both speeds in the on-transient (from ~29 to ~22 s at 90% $\dot{V}O_{2\,max}$, and from ~28 to ~20 s at 95% $\dot{V}O_{2\,max}$), and the off-transient (from ~ 62 to ~ 44 s at 90% $\dot{V}O_{2\,max}$ and from ~63 to ~51 s at 95% $\dot{V}O_{2\,max}$).

Casaburi *et al.* (1987) examined the effect of endurance training on the magnitude of the $\dot{V}O_2$ slow component (defined as the increase in $\dot{V}O_2$ from 3 min to the end of exercise) and on a number of the variables that had been hypothesized to influence it, that is lactate accumulation; increased body temperature; increased ventilation; increased catecholamine concentration. These authors recruited 10 previously untrained university students (6 female; age ~ 23 years) and had them complete an 8-week programme of endurance exercise training (comprising 5 ×45 min sessions per week of supervised cycle ergometry). For the first 4 weeks of the programme, the subjects exercised at an intensity equivalent to 50% of the difference between the pre-training GET and $\dot{V}O_{2\,max}$ and for the next 4 weeks they trained at 70% of the difference between the pre-training

GET and $\dot{V}O_{2\,max}$. Before the training period, the subjects completed a ramp test and four square-wave tests (at 90% GET, and 25%, 50% and 75% of the difference between GET and $\dot{V}O_{2\,max}$). Following the training period, the subjects completed another ramp test and the four square-wave tests at the same absolute work-rate as before training.

The training programme in the Casaburi *et al.* (1987) study resulted in significant improvements in GET (+38%) and $\dot{V}O_{2\,max}$ (+15%). Furthermore, training resulted in significant reductions in the magnitude of the slow component at the three highest constant work rates. However, training was also associated with reductions in each of the variables that had been hypothesized to influence the slow component; that is, training resulted in significant reductions in blood lactate accumulation, rectal temperature, epinephrine and norepinephrine concentrations and minute ventilation. However, the time course of the increase in rectal temperature during exercise was not consistent with the time course for the development of the $\dot{V}O_2$ slow component. Furthermore, the changes in both rectal temperature and catecholamine concentrations across the training intervention were not significantly correlated with the changes in the magnitude of the slow component. In contrast, the change in the end-exercise blood [lactate] and the change in minute ventilation from 3 min to the end of exercise from pre- to post-training were both significantly correlated with the reduction in the slow component ($r = 0.64$ and $r = 0.51$, respectively). Casaburi *et al.* (1987) speculated that the cause of the association between blood lactate accumulation and the $\dot{V}O_2$ slow component might have been related to the O_2 cost associated with gluconeogenesis of some of the lactate (which, at least theoretically, is substantial; Whipp, 1994). It was suggested, therefore, that training caused a significant reduction in the rate of lactate catabolism for the same absolute work rate and/or substantially changed the fate of lactate from gluconeogenesis to oxidation. The authors acknowledged, however, that although the $\dot{V}O_2$ slow component appeared to be linked to lactate, another factor that was simultaneously linked to lactate accumulation and an increased O_2 cost of exercise might also be responsible for the results obtained; the influence of this causative agent would be attenuated for the same work rate after training (see Chapter 12 for a discussion of the mechanistic basis of the $\dot{V}O_2$ slow component).

Womack *et al.* (1995) pointed out that Casaburi *et al.* (1987) only assessed changes in the $\dot{V}O_2$ slow component and some of its putative mediators before and after 8 weeks of training such that important similarities or differences in the time course of adaptation of these factors to training could have been missed. Therefore, in their study, Womack *et al.* (1995) set out to better discriminate the time course of the reduction of the $\dot{V}O_2$ slow component during an endurance training programme and to assess this reduction in relation to changes in blood [lactate], minute ventilation and plasma [catecholamines]. Seven untrained young men underwent a 6-week programme of endurance training involving 5 days of cycle ergometer training per week. In each week, the training included a bout of exercise for 20 min at 60% of the pre-training Δ (the experimental test), two continuous exercise bouts for 40 min requiring ~68% of the pre-training $\dot{V}O_{2\,max}$, and two interval training sessions involving 6×5 min exercise bouts at ~77% of the pre-training $\dot{V}O_{2\,max}$

separated by 2 min recovery periods. Before and after the period of training, the subjects performed an incremental exercise test, and before and once per week during the training programme they performed a 20 min square-wave exercise bout at 60%Δ as calculated from the pre-training LT and $\dot{V}O_{2\,max}$ values. Subjects were therefore tested at the same absolute work-rate over the 6-week period with the magnitude of the $\dot{V}O_2$ slow component defined as the increase in $\dot{V}O_2$ from 3 min to the end of exercise. In addition, at the end of the training programme, the subjects were infused with epinephrine in order to examine the extent to which the reduction in the slow component with training could be attributed to the reduction in circulating catecholamines.

The results of the study of Womack *et al.* (1995) were, in large part, similar to those of Casaburi *et al.* (1987). The magnitude of the slow component was significantly reduced after 2 weeks of training and this was associated with significant reductions in blood [lactate], minute ventilation and plasma [norepinephrine] (see figure 3 in Womack *et al.*, 1995). The reduction in plasma [epinephrine] was significant after just one week however. The reduction in the $\dot{V}O_2$ slow component was not significantly correlated with the reductions in blood [lactate], minute ventilation or plasma [norepinephrine] in the first two weeks of training. Furthermore, infusion of epinephrine in the additional post-training exercise bout did not influence the magnitude of the $\dot{V}O_2$ slow component despite causing significant increases in plasma [epinephrine], minute ventilation and blood [lactate]. This latter result was consistent with a previous study in which epinephrine infusion did not influence the $\dot{V}O_2$ slow component (Gaesser *et al.*, 1994). Womack *et al.* (1995) suggested that the fact that the ~2.4 mM increase in blood [lactate] resulting from the epinephrine infusion did not influence $\dot{V}O_2$ was strong evidence against there being a causal relationship between lactate accumulation and the $\dot{V}O_2$ slow component (Casaburi *et al.*, 1987; Stringer *et al.*, 1994). Furthermore, it was calculated using the equations of Aaron *et al.* (1992) that the reduction in $\dot{V}_E$ with training could account for only ~18% of the reduction in the $\dot{V}O_2$ slow component. Because none of the variables they measured were able to adequately explain the cause of the reduction in the slow component with training, Womack *et al.* (1995) suggested that changes in motor unit recruitment patterns (i.e. a reduced recruitment of 'less efficient' type II fibres) with training might help to explain both the reduction in the slow component with training and the relationship between the slow component and blood [lactate].

Using a different mode of exercise (treadmill running), Carter *et al.* (2000) recruited 23 recreationally active young subjects (14 men) to a 6-week endurance running training programme incorporating both continuous and interval running sessions. Before and after the training programme, the subjects completed an incremental treadmill test for the determination of LT and $\dot{V}O_{2\,max}$ and repeat square-wave transitions to running speeds requiring 80% LT and 50%Δ (calculated from the pre-training values of LT and $\dot{V}O_{2\,max}$) for the determination of $\dot{V}O_2$ kinetics. In addition, 10 of the subjects completed transitions to 80% LT and 50%Δ as calculated from the post-training values of LT and $\dot{V}O_{2\,max}$. The training programme resulted in significant improvements in $\dot{V}O_{2\,max}$ and LT. Training had no effect on $\dot{V}O_2$ kinetics during moderate-intensity exercise. For heavy-intensity exercise, training had no effect on the G_p or τ_p (pre: 19.4 ± 1.2 s vs post: 18.8 ± 4.9 s). However, it was stressed by the authors that their subjects had a higher level of fitness on recruitment to the study ($\dot{V}O_{2\,max}$ ~ 55 ml · kg^{-1} · min^{-1}) such that the τ_p was already quite fast. Interestingly, however, when the 6 subjects with the lowest $\dot{V}O_{2\,max}$ values on recruitment to the study (~40 ml · kg^{-1} · min^{-1}) were analysed separately, the τ_p was significantly speeded by the training programme (pre: 31.5 ± 1.0 s vs post: 19.5 ± 1.5 s). This highlights the important interactive influences of initial training status and training programme on changes to the $\dot{V}O_2$ kinetics.

In the Carter *et al.* (2000) study, the amplitude of the $\dot{V}O_2$ slow component was significantly reduced with training (by ~100 ml · min^{-1}) and this resulted in a significant reduction in end-exercise $\dot{V}O_2$ (Figure 15.7). Training resulted in significant reductions in Δ blood [lactate] and $\Delta\dot{V}_E$ (when the latter was assessed over the same time frame as the $\dot{V}O_2$ slow component), but only the changes in $\Delta\dot{V}_E$ and the slow component amplitude with training were significantly correlated. However, in agreement with Womack *et al.* (1995), it was calculated that the reduction in $\Delta\dot{V}_E$ with training could account for only a relatively small proportion of the reduction in the slow component with training (~9–14%). In the subgroup of 10 subjects who were tested at 50%Δ when this was recalculated from the post-training LT and $\dot{V}O_{2\,max}$ values, the primary component amplitude was significantly higher (as would be expected for the higher running speed). The small but non-significant reduction in the amplitude of the slow component in these subjects resulted in a small reduction in the overall MRT (pre: 57.6 ± 2.6 s vs post: 53.4 ± 1.2 s; P<0.05). The authors argued that a similar (or slightly smaller slow component amplitude) for a higher running speed post-training was consistent with an enhanced exercise tolerance. Carter *et al.* (2000)

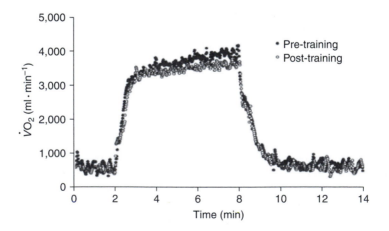

Figure 15.7 Effect of 6 weeks of endurance running training on $\dot{V}O_2$ kinetics during treadmill running. Note the slightly faster τ_p and the marked reduction in the amplitude of the $\dot{V}O_2$ slow component following training. Reproduced from Carter *et al.* (2000) with permission.

speculated that enhanced muscle mitochondrial density and/or capillarization (Anderson and Henriksson, 1977; Holloszy and Coyle, 1984) with training might result in the recruitment of fewer type II fibres post-training. The available data therefore indicate that the amplitude of the $\dot{V}O_2$ slow component may be reduced significantly after only 1–2 weeks of training (Womack et al., 1995), and that significant reductions in the slow component are also possible in subjects who are reasonably fit at the start of training and in whom 'traditional' markers of aerobic fitness such as $\dot{V}O_{2\,max}$ and LT do not therefore increase substantially (Carter et al., 2000).

To test the hypothesis that the lower $\dot{V}O_2$ slow component following endurance exercise training was the result of changes in motor unit recruitment, Saunders et al. (2003) assessed $\dot{V}O_2$ kinetics and muscle activation (by contrast shifts in MR images) during both moderate and heavy exercise before and after a 4-week endurance training programme in a group of untrained young subjects. The training programme involved 5 sessions per week of mixed continuous and interval-type training on a cycle ergometer. Before and after the training programme, the subjects completed an incremental cycle test and two 15-min constant-load exercise bouts, one below and one above the pre-training LT. The amplitude of the $\dot{V}O_2$ slow component was determined as the difference between the $\dot{V}O_2$ at 3 and at 15 min of exercise. Training had no effect on the $\dot{V}O_2$ or muscle transverse reaction times (T_2) during moderate-intensity exercise, but there were significant reductions in end-exercise $\dot{V}O_2$ and T_2 of the vastus lateralis during heavy-intensity exercise. The authors argued that these data provided evidence that the slow component is linked to changes in muscle activation (Saunders et al., 2000) and that the reduction in the slow component with training resulted from a reduced muscle activation. However, this conclusion is somewhat unconvincing because the reductions in the slow component (mean end-exercise $\dot{V}O_2$ pre: $2625\ ml \cdot min^{-1}$ vs post: $2567\ ml \cdot min^{-1}$) and T_2 of the vastus lateralis (mean pre: 35.6 ms vs mean post: 34.5 ms) evoked by the training were so small as to be within experimental error; furthermore, training did not result in significant changes in either T_2 of the whole muscle or of the rectus femoris.

Older populations

The τ_p response to moderate-intensity exercise tends to be longer in older sedentary subjects compared to young sedentary subjects (Babcock et al., 1994a; Chilibeck et al., 1996; Bell et al., 1999) although it is unclear whether this difference results from physiological changes resulting from the ageing process or from reductions in physical activity with increasing age (see Chapter 13). To examine this, Babcock et al. (1994b) trained 8 sedentary older men (aged 65–78 years) on a cycle ergometer three times per week for 40 min per session (at 20–50% of the pre-training Δ value) for 24 weeks. This training programme resulted in ~20% improvements in $\dot{V}O_{2\,max}$ and GET, as well as a marked speeding of τ_p at 80% GET (mean τ pre: 62.2 s vs mean τ post: 31.9 s). The faster $\dot{V}O_2$ kinetics and the greater $\dot{V}O_{2\,max}$ with training were not significantly correlated. The 49% speeding of $\dot{V}O_2$ kinetics in these older subjects is considerably greater than that reported in studies in which younger subjects were studied. Indeed, the τ_p at the end of training in the older subjects (~ 32 s) approached the values normally observed in healthy young subjects. A similarly impressive speeding of τ_p has recently been reported in middle-aged subjects (~ 51 years) during a 90-day programme of combined endurance and resistance training by Fukuoka *et al.* (2002). In this study, a significant reduction in τ_p was observed after just 15 days of training (pre-mean: 46.9 s; post-mean 34.4 s), after which there was a levelling-off in the rate of improvement. This study demonstrated a dissociation between improvements in $\dot{V}O_2$ kinetics and 'traditional' measures of aerobic fitness such as $\dot{V}O_{2\,max}$ (perhaps indicating different rates of adaptation of central and peripheral components of O_2 transport and utilization), and also demonstrates that improvements in $\dot{V}O_2$ kinetics with training can occur extremely rapidly both in young and older subjects. In this regard, it is of interest that the time course for the adaptation of several of the tricarboxylic acid cycle and electron transport chain enzymes with training is much faster than that of $\dot{V}O_{2\,max}$ (Gollnick and Saltin, 1982). Interestingly, it appears that changes in $\dot{V}O_2$ kinetics with ageing depend, in part, upon the mode of exercise used to assess the $\dot{V}O_2$ response. For example, Chilibeck *et al.* (1996) reported that slowing of the primary $\dot{V}O_2$ kinetics with advancing age was much more pronounced in activities to which subjects were unaccustomed (e.g. cycling) compared to activities to which they were accustomed (e.g. walking) or which used similar muscles (e.g. plantarflexion exercise).

The putative physiological mechanism(s) responsible for the speeding of the moderate exercise $\dot{V}O_2$ kinetics with training in older subjects are presumably the same as those for younger subjects. Mitochondrial density has been shown to be increased with training in older individuals (Coggan *et al.*, 1992; Meredith *et al.*, 1989). However, in the study of Babcock *et al.* (1994a) it was of interest that there was a correlation between the speeding of the $\dot{V}O_2$ kinetics and the speeding of the heart rate kinetics with training, suggesting that enhanced blood flow to muscle might be at least partly responsible for the 'normalized' $\dot{V}O_2$ kinetics in such subjects. Compromised vascular conductance and peripheral O_2 diffusion in older subjects (Wahren *et al.*, 1974; Dinenno *et al.*, 1999) might be at least partially reversed by training (Makrides *et al.*, 1990) possibly as a result of changes in capillarization (Coggan *et al.*, 1992; Hepple, 1997). Certainly, the dissociation between changes in $\dot{V}O_2$ kinetics and $\dot{V}O_{2\,max}$ (Babcock *et al.*, 1994a) with training in the elderly indicate that physiological adaptations resulting in faster $\dot{V}O_2$ kinetics might occur in the periphery. Scheuermann *et al.* (2002) recently reported that prior 'priming' exercise could reduce τ_p during subsequent moderate-intensity exercise, although the mechanism responsible for this effect is unclear. While the performance of 'warm-up' exercise enhances muscle blood flow during subsequent exercise, it may also influence intra-muscular enzyme activity and motor unit recruitment patterns (see Chapters 10 and 13).

In an attempt to examine the effect of left ventricular function on $\dot{V}O_2$ kinetics in older men, Harris *et al.* (2003) manipulated plasma volume using both exercise training and diuresis. Five days of exercise training altered peak cardiac early flow velocity but did not alter $\dot{V}O_2$ kinetics suggesting that left ventricular function does not limit $\dot{V}O_2$ kinetics in these conditions. However, in older men with impaired diastolic function, both the same training programme and calcium channel blockade (with verapamil) resulted in significant improvements in $\dot{V}O_{2\,max}$ and the time constant for the primary $\dot{V}O_2$ response in the transition to moderate-intensity exercise. The effects of exercise training and verapamil on $\dot{V}O_2$ kinetics were similar (from ~62 s (control) to ~48 s (with verapamil) and ~44 s (with training)), and the effects were not additive. Neither intervention improved heart rate kinetics, but both interventions resulted in greater estimated stroke volume. These data therefore demonstrate that improving left ventricular end-diastolic filling in individuals with impaired Frank–Starling function results in faster $\dot{V}O_2$ kinetics during moderate-intensity exercise. Chilibeck et al. (1996) reported that τ_p was significantly longer for cycle exercise than for plantar flexor exercise in older subjects (~67 years) and that this difference was associated with differences in heart rate kinetics. Furthermore, the τ_p for plantar flexor exercise was similar to that measured in a group of young subjects. These data appear to indicate that the primary $\dot{V}O_2$ kinetics may be limited by muscle O_2 delivery in older subjects since in small muscle group exercise (such as plantar flexor exercise), cardiovascular function is unlikely to be challenged and muscle perfusion should be in excess of metabolic demand.

In an elegant study designed to identify the primary mechanism (enhanced O_2 delivery or enhanced mitochondrial function) for the faster $\dot{V}O_2$ kinetics with training in older subjects, Bell et al. (2001) had 5 men (aged 77 ± 7 years) perform single-leg endurance training (4 × 40 min sessions per week at ~80% of $\dot{V}O_{2\,max}$) for 9 weeks. Before and after training, muscle biopsies were taken from both legs for the determination of citrate synthase activity (as a marker of mitochondrial density) and muscle capillarization. In addition to $\dot{V}O_2$ kinetics, leg blood flow kinetics were measured using Doppler ultrasonography at a work rate requiring ~60% of pre-training $\dot{V}O_{2\,max}$ during single-leg knee-extension exercise. The τ_p was significantly faster post-training in the trained leg (pre-mean: 92 s; post-mean: 48 s) but there was no difference in the 'control' leg (pre-mean: 104 s; post-mean: 109 s). The time constant for mean blood velocity was significantly faster than that of $\dot{V}O_2$ both before and after training in both legs, and was not significantly improved by training. Furthermore, muscle capillarization was not altered by training. However, muscle citrate synthase activity was significantly increased in the trained leg (n = 3). These data indicate that the training-induced speeding of $\dot{V}O_2$ kinetics was related to intra-muscular adaptations and not to an enhancement of O_2 delivery to muscle. Consistent with this interpretation, Bell et al. (1999) reported that hyperoxia did not speed $\dot{V}O_2$ kinetics during exercise at 80% GET in 7 men (aged ~78 years), although the authors cautioned that it is possible that adjustments in blood flow meant that O_2 delivery to muscle was not different between the normoxic and hyperoxic conditions.

In summary to this section, it is unclear whether the faster τ_p with training in older subjects is the result of enhancements in O_2 delivery, O_2 utilization, or both. This will of course depend upon which of these represents the principal limitation in the pre-training condition. While it is more likely that O_2 availability limits $\dot{V}O_2$ kinetics in the elderly than in the young, ageing results in impairments both to the central circulation and muscle metabolism (see Chapter 13). It is therefore difficult to differentiate the key determinants of faster $\dot{V}O_2$ kinetics with training although the available evidence indicates that changes in oxidative enzyme activity may be more important (Bell *et al.*, 2001).

Clinical populations

A variety of disease states (e.g. heart failure, diabetes, obstructive pulmonary disease, peripheral arterial disease, renal disease) result in impairments of oxygen delivery and/or utilization that, in turn, limit the $\dot{V}O_{2\,max}$, LT/GET, $\dot{V}O_2$ kinetics, and functional capacity of patients (Koike *et al.*, 1994; Sietsema *et al.*, 1994; Otsuka *et al.*, 1997; Belardinelli *et al.*, 1998; Regensteiner *et al.*, 1998; Bauer *et al.*, 1999; Koufaki *et al.*, 2002a,b; see Chapter 14). Patient populations are unlikely to perform maximal-intensity exercise in daily life, but are likely to have to cope with abrupt transitions from one metabolic rate to another. Slow $\dot{V}O_2$ kinetics (and the associated greater reliance on substrate-level phosphorylation to meet the energy demand) may be a significant cause of the poor exercise tolerance in such populations. For this reason, there is growing interest in the effect of exercise training on improving $\dot{V}O_2$ kinetics and exercise tolerance in functionally compromised populations. Significantly faster $\dot{V}O_2$ kinetics with training would provide an evidence base for the use of exercise as a therapy in subjects with these conditions.

It is pertinent to point out here that the assessment of $\dot{V}O_2$ kinetics in patient populations presents significant challenges to the investigator (see Chapter 14). Exercise tolerance is often compromised to such an extent that the work rates that can be used are extremely low. With very low amplitude of the $\dot{V}O_2$ response, the signal-to-noise ratio will be very low – as will confidence in the modelled parameters (Lamarra *et al.*, 1987). Also, with a low $\dot{V}O_2$ amplitude above baseline, the Phase I response can represent a large proportion of the total response. A large number of transitions would be required to obtain adequate fitting of the response and sufficient confidence in the modelled parameters; however, this is rarely feasible in patient populations.

Barstow *et al.* (1996b) examined the effect of exercise training (using functional electrical stimulation; 24 sessions of 30-min unloaded cycling for ~8 weeks) in 9 subjects with spinal cord injury. The ability to increase $\dot{V}O_2$ seemed to be associated with the ability to increase heart rate both before and after training. The MRT for $\dot{V}O_2$ was significantly speeded by training both in the on-transient (mean-pre: 154 s; mean-post: 114 s) and the off-transient (mean-pre: 102 s; mean-post: 82 s) to/from unloaded cycling. The $\dot{V}O_{2\,max}$ was also significantly improved as a result of training but there was no correlation between the increase in $\dot{V}O_{2\,max}$ and the speeded $\dot{V}O_2$ kinetics with training, indicating that these responses were influenced by different factors. Spinal cord injured subjects suffer atrophy of the lower limb musculature, a loss of type I muscle fibres, reduced capillary density and lower oxidative enzyme activity (Martin *et al.*, 1992; Round *et al.*, 1993), and it is possible that partial reversal of these changes is responsible for the faster $\dot{V}O_2$ kinetics with functional electrical stimulation.

In end-stage renal disease patients, Koufaki *et al.* (2002a) reported that 12 weeks of moderate-intensity endurance training on 3 days per week resulted in significant improvements in $\dot{V}O_{2\,max}$ and GET, but no significant change in the time constant for the primary $\dot{V}O_2$ kinetics either at the same absolute work rate (33 W; from ~49.6 to ~37.8 s) or at the same relative work rate (90% GET; from ~58.3 to ~51.2 s). Koufaki *et al.* (2002a) reported that the coefficient of variation for the determination of τ_p was ~20% such that the 'speeding' of $\dot{V}O_2$ kinetics that they observed with training was within the variability of the measurement itself. The authors argued that the conclusions drawn in previous studies which reported a quantitatively small but statistically significant speeding of $\dot{V}O_2$ kinetics with training but without reporting the confidence in the determination of the τ_p or MRT of the $\dot{V}O_2$ response should be treated with caution since they may not have physiological or functional significance. In another study, Koufaki *et al.* (2002b) reported that, compared to the pre-training baseline (~68 s), τ_p was significantly shorter at the same relative exercise intensity (90% GET) after three months (~51 s) and six months (~51 s) of the same training regime as described before. However, despite the significant improvement of the group mean response of τ_p to training, the improvement was less than the standard error of the measurement (12.3 s) in 8 of the 18 subjects. While this may also be related to measurement variability, the authors noted that the 'non-responders' were less well nourished than the responders such that differences in the quantity and quality of muscle mass might have been a contributory factor to the difference in response. This demonstrates the importance of variables other than those directly pertaining to the training programme on the physiological response to structured exercise.

Examples of studies that showed significant speeding of $\dot{V}O_2$ kinetics with training in patient populations include those of Brandenburg *et al.* (1999), Otsuka *et al.* (1997) and Puente-Maestu *et al.* (2003). Brandenburg *et al.* (1999) reported that 3 months of supervised exercise training (3 sessions per week of 50 minutes of moderate-intensity exercise) resulted in significant reductions in the MRT at both 20 W and 30 W, though not at 80 W in middle-aged women with type II diabetes. Otsuka *et al.* (1997) reported that τ_p was reduced from ~64 to ~53 s following training (3 days per week for 8 weeks) in patients with chronic obstructive pulmonary disease. Similarly, Puente-Maestu *et al.* (2003) showed that training (45 min/day on 3 days per week for 6 weeks) resulted in a significantly shorter τ_p at 80% GET (from ~84 to ~69 s), which was significantly correlated with the change in muscle citrate synthase activity. To what extent these relatively small improvements reflect meaningful changes in functional capacity (Koufaki *et al.*, 2002b) is debatable. However, in other studies, the positive impact of exercise training on functional capacity is obvious. For example, Casaburi *et al.* (1997) reported that a 6-week training programme involving three 45-min sessions per week resulted in a 77% increase in the time to fatigue during constant work-rate exercise requiring ~80% of pre-training $\dot{V}O_{2\,max}$ in elderly subjects with severe COPD. This was associated with a 17% reduction in the MRT for $\dot{V}O_2$ and a 10% reduction in minute ventilation.

Summary

It is clear both from cross-sectional and longitudinal studies that enhanced 'fitness' is associated with faster $\dot{V}O_2$ kinetics and, for absolute work rates that were at least initially $>LT$, with a reduced amplitude of the $\dot{V}O_2$ slow component. There is a plethora of central and peripheral physiological adaptations to endurance training (Jones and Carter, 2000) that collectively result in improvements in the capacity to deliver O_2 to skeletal muscle and in the capacity of muscle to utilize the O_2 it receives. Which of these factors is decisive in causing the improvement in $\dot{V}O_2$ kinetics observed with training will depend upon whether O_2 availability can be considered limiting in the pre-training situation. This, in turn, will depend upon factors such as the training status, health and age of the subjects studied (Chapters 13 and 14), the exercise modality in which the training is conducted (Chapter 4) and the exercise intensity domains that are considered (Chapter 1), (see Figure 12.3 for further explanation). It should also be considered that the $\dot{V}O_2$ response to exercise represents an integration of factors related to both O_2 delivery and utilization (see Chapter 8). Nevertheless, the available evidence suggests that a speeding of the primary $\dot{V}O_2$ response is essentially limited to exercise which engages the trained musculature (Cerretelli *et al.*, 1979) and is associated with increased oxidative enzyme activity in those muscles (Bell *et al.*, 2001). The reduction of τ_p appears to occur quite soon following the onset of training and may have a similar time course to the rapid increase in oxidative enzyme activity that occurs in the muscle fibres (Gollnick and Saltin, 1982; but see also Phillips *et al.*, 1995). These data therefore suggest that improvements in metabolic potential may play a pivotal role in the reduction of τ_p with training. The mechanism responsible for the reduction in the amplitude of the $\dot{V}O_2$ slow component at the same absolute work rate following training also remains to be determined with certainty but could feasibly involve improvements in muscle O_2 delivery or the homogeneity of its distribution, along with changes in muscle fibre recruitment patterns.

On a practical note, although a large number of studies have demonstrated that endurance training results in improved $\dot{V}O_2$ kinetics, the actual type (i.e. volume, intensity, frequency and duration) of training that optimizes these effects remains to be elucidated. Although individuals with higher 'aerobic fitness' (as judged by $\dot{V}O_{2\,max}$ for example) tend also to have fast $\dot{V}O_2$ kinetics, it appears that the rate and magnitude of improvement in $\dot{V}O_{2\,max}$ and $\dot{V}O_2$ kinetics with training may be dissociated. This suggests that these parameters may be limited by somewhat different physiological factors and therefore be sensitive to different types of training sessions and training programmes. At this point, it is unclear whether $\dot{V}O_2$ kinetics can be improved more by the performance of extensive continuous aerobic training or by more intensive interval-type training. Answers to this, and other fundamental questions, must therefore await further research.

Glossary of terms

ATP   adenosine triphospate
Δ   'delta'; used to express the work rate as a % difference between the work rate at the LT/GET and $\dot{V}O_{2\,max}$
GET   gas exchange threshold
G_p the functional 'gain' of the primary increase in $\dot{V}O_2$ above baseline (i.e. the increase in $\dot{V}O_2$ above baseline at the end of Phase II divided by the increase in work rate)
LT   lactate threshold
MRT   mean response time, time taken for $\dot{V}O_2$ to reach 63% of the 'final' or end-exercise value from the onset of exercise
τ_p time constant of the primary component $\dot{V}O_2$ response
$\dot{V}O_2$ pulmonary oxygen uptake
$\dot{V}O_{2\,max}$ maximal oxygen uptake

References

Aaron, E.A., Johnson, B.D., Seow, C.K. and Dempsey, J.A. (1992). Oxygen cost of exercise hyperpnea: measurement. *Journal of Applied Physiology*, **72**, 1810–917.

Anderson, P. and Henriksson, J. (1977). Capillary supply of the quadriceps femoris muscle of man: adaptive response to exercise. *Journal of Physiology*, **270**, 677–90.

Babcock, M.A., Paterson, D.H. and Cunningham, D.A. (1994a). Effects of aerobic endurance training on gas exchange kinetics of older men. *Medicine and Science in Sports and Exercise*, **26**, 447–52.

Babcock, M.A., Paterson, D.H., Cunningham, D.A. and Dickinson, J.R. (1994b). Exercise on-transient gas exchange kinetics are slowed as a function of age. *Medicine and Science in Sports and Exercise*, **26**, 440–6.

Barstow, T.J. and Molé, P.A. (1991). Linear and nonlinear characteristics of oxygen uptake kinetics during heavy exercise. *Journal of Applied Physiology*, **71**, 2099–106.

Barstow, T.J., Jones, A.M., Nguyen, P.H. and Casaburi, R. (1996a). Influence of muscle fiber type and pedal frequency on oxygen uptake kinetics of heavy exercise. *Journal of Applied Physiology*, **81**, 1642–50.

Barstow, T.J., Scremin, A.M.E., Mutton, D.L., Kunkel, C.F., Cagle, T.G. and Whipp, B.J. (1996b). Changes in gas exchange kinetics with training in patients with spinal cord injury. *Medicine and Science in Sports and Exercise*, **28**, 1221–8.

Barstow, T.J., Jones, A.M., Nguyen, P.H. and Casaburi, R. (2000). Influence of muscle fibre type and fitness on the oxygen uptake/power output slope during incremental exercise in humans. *Experimental Physiology*, **85**, 109–16.

Bauer, T.A., Regensteiner, J.G., Brass, E.P. and Hiatt, W.R. (1999). Oxygen uptake kinetics during exercise are slowed in patients with peripheral arterial disease. *Journal of Applied Physiology*, **87**, 809–16.

Belardinelli, R., Zhang, Y.Y., Wasserman, K., Purcaro, A. and Agostini, P.G. (1998). A four-minute submaximal constant work rate exercise test to assess cardiovascular function class in chronic heart failure. *American Journal of Cardiology*, **81**, 1210–14.

Bell, C., Paterson, D.H., Kowalchuk, J.M. and Cunningham, D.A. (1999). Oxygen uptake kinetics of older humans are slowed with age but are unaffected by hyperoxia. *Experimental Physiology*, **84**, 747–59.

Bell, C., Paterson, D.H., Kowalchuk, J.M., Moy, A.P., Thorp, D.B., Noble, E.G., Taylor, A.W. and Cunningham, D.A. (2001). Determinants of oxygen uptake kinetics in older humans following single-limb endurance exercise training. *Experimental Physiology*, **86**, 659–65.

Billat, V.L., Mille-Hamard, L., Demarle, A. and Koralsztein, J.P. (2002). Effect of training in humans on off- and on-transient oxygen uptake kinetics after severe exhausting intensity runs. *European Journal of Applied Physiology*, **87**, 496–505.

Borrani, F., Candau, R., Millet, G.Y., Perrey, S., Fuchslocher, J. and Rouillon, J.D. (2001). Is the $\dot{V}O_2$ slow component dependent on progressive recruitment of fast-twitch fibers in trained runners? *Journal of Applied Physiology*, **90**, 2212–20.

Brandenburg, S.L., Reusch, J.E.B., Bauer, T.A., Jeffers, B.W., Hiatt, W.R. and Regensteiner, J.G. (1999). Effects of exercise training on oxygen uptake kinetic responses in women with type II diabetes. *Diabetes Care*, **22**, 1640–6.

Carter, H., Jones, A.M., Barstow, T.J., Burnley, M., Williams, C.A. and Doust, J.H. (2000). Effect of endurance training on oxygen uptake kinetics during treadmill running. *Journal of Applied Physiology*, **89**, 1744–52.

Casaburi, R., Storer, T.W., Ben-Dov, I. and Wasserman, K. (1987). Effect of endurance training on possible determinants of $\dot{V}O_2$ during heavy exercise. *Journal of Applied Physiology*, **62**, 199–207.

Casaburi, R., Porszasz, J., Burns, M.R., Carithers, E.R., Chang, R.S. and Cooper, C.B. (1997). Physiologic benefits of exercise training in rehabilitation of patients with severe chronic obstructive pulmonary disease. *American Journal of Respiratory and Critical Care Medicine*, **155**, 1541–51.

Cerretelli, P., Pendergast, D., Paganelli, W.C. and Rennie, D.W. (1979). Effects of specific muscle training on $\dot{V}O_2$ on-response and early blood lactate. *Journal of Applied Physiology*, **47**, 761–9.

Chilibeck, P.D., Paterson, D.H., Petrella, R.J. and Cunningham, D.A. (1996). The influence of age and cardiorespiratory fitness on kinetics of oxygen uptake. *Canadian Journal of Applied Physiology*, **21**, 185–96.

Cleuziou, C., Perrey, S., Borrani, F., Lecoq, A.M., Candau, R., Courteix, D. and Obert, P. (2003). Dynamic responses of O_2 uptake at the onset and end of exercise in trained subjects. *Canadian Journal of Applied Physiology*, **28**, 630–41.

Coggan, A.R., Spina, R.J., King, D.S., Rogers, M.A., Brown, M., Nemeth, P.M. and Holloszy, J.O. (1992). Skeletal muscle adaptations to endurance training in 60- to 70-yr-old men and women. *Journal of Applied Physiology*, **72**, 1780–6.

Convertino, V.A., Goldwater, D.J. and Sandler, H. (1984). $\dot{V}O_2$ kinetics of constant-load exercise following bed-rest-induced deconditioning. *Journal of Applied Physiology*, **57**, 1545–50.

Crow, M.T. and Kushmerick, M.J. (1982). Chemical energetics of slow- and fast-twitch muscles of the mouse. *Journal of General Physiology*, **79**, 147–66.

Davis, J.A., Frank, M., Whipp, B.J. and Wasserman, K. (1979). Anaerobic threshold alterations caused by endurance training in middle-aged men. *Journal of Applied Physiology*, **46**, 1039–46.

Demarle, A.P., Slawinski, J.J., Lafitte, L.P., Bocquet, V.G., Koralsztein, J.P. and Billat, V.L. (2001). Decrease of O_2 deficit is a potential factor in increased time to exhaustion after specific endurance training. *Journal of Applied Physiology*, **90**, 947–53.

Denis, C., Fouquet, R., Poty, P., Geyssant, A. and Lacour, J.R. (1982). Effect of 40 weeks of endurance training on the anaerobic threshold. *International Journal of Sports Medicine*, **3**, 208–14.

Dinenno, F.A., Jones, P.P., Seals, D.R. and Tanaka, H. (1999). Limb blood flow and vascular conductance are reduced with age in healthy humans – relation to elevations in sympathetic nerve activity and declines in oxygen demand. *Circulation*, **100**, 164–70.

Fukuoka, Y., Grassi, B., Conti, M., Guiducci, D., Sutti, M., Marconi, C. and Cerretelli, P. (2002). Early effects of exercise training on on- and off-kinetics in 50-year-old subjects. *Pflugers Archives*, **443**, 690–7.

Gaesser, G.A., Ward, S.A., Baum, V.C. and Whipp, B.J. (1994). Effects of infused epinephrine on slow phase of O_2 uptake kinetics during heavy exercise in humans. *Journal of Applied Physiology*, **77**, 2413–19.

Gollnick, P.D. and Saltin, B. (1982). Significance of skeletal muscle oxidative enzyme enhancement with endurance training. *Clinical Physiology*, **2**, 1–12.

Hagberg, J.M., Hickson, R.C., Ehsani, A.A. and Holloszy, J.O. (1980). Faster adjustment to and recovery from submaximal exercise in the trained state. *Journal of Applied Physiology*, **48**, 218–24.

Harris, S.K., Petrella, R.J., Overend, T.J., Paterson, D.H. and Cunningham, D.A. (2003). Short-term training effects on left ventricular diastolic function and oxygen uptake in older and younger men. *Clinical Journal of Sports Medicine*, **13**, 245–51.

Hepple, R.T. (1997). A new measurement of tissue capillarity: the capillary-to-fibre perimeter exchange index. *Canadian Journal of Applied Physiology*, **22**, 11–22.

Hickson, R.C., Bomze, H.A. and Holloszy, J.O. (1978). Faster adjustment of O_2 uptake to the energy requirement of exercise in the trained state. *Journal of Applied Physiology*, **44**, 877–81.

Hickson, R.C., Hagberg, J.M., Ehsani, A.A. and Holloszy, J.O. (1981). Time course of the adaptive responses of aerobic power and heart rate to training. *Medicine and Science in Sports and Exercise*, **13**, 17–20.

Holloszy, J.O. and Coyle, E.F. (1984). Adaptations of skeletal muscle to endurance exercise and their metabolic consequences. *Journal of Applied Physiology*, **56**, 831–38.

Hultman, E., Bergstrom, J. and Anderson, N.M. (1967). Breakdown and resynthesis of phosphorylcreatine and adenosine triphosphate in connection with muscular work in man. *Scandinavian Journal of Clinical and Laboratory Investigations*, **19**, 56–66.

Jones, A.M. and Carter, H. (2000). The effect of endurance training on parameters of aerobic fitness. *Sports Medicine*, **29**, 373–86.

Karlsson, J., Nordesjo, L.-O., Jorfeldt, L. and Saltin, B. (1972). Muscle lactate, ATP, and CP levels during exercise after physical training in man. *Journal of Applied Physiology*, **33**, 199–203.

Krustrup, P., Hellsten, Y. and Bangsbo, J. (2004). Intense interval training enhances human skeletal muscle oxygen uptake in the initial phase of dynamic exercise at high but not at low intensities. *Journal of Physiology*, **559**, 335–45.

Koike, A., Hiroe, M., Adachi, T., Yajima, T., Yamauchi, Y., Nogami, A., Ito, H., Miyahara, Y., Korenaga, M. and Marumo, F. (1994). Oxygen uptake kinetics are determined by cardiac function at onset of exercise rather than peak exercise in patients with prior myocardial infarction. *Circulation*, **90**, 2324–32.

Koppo, K., Bouckaert, J. and Jones, A.M. (2002). Oxygen uptake kinetics during high-intensity arm and leg exercise. *Respiration Physiology and Neurobiology*, **133**, 241–50.

Koppo, K., Bouckaert, J. and Jones, A.M. (2004). Effects of training status and exercise intensity on phase II $\dot{V}O_2$ kinetics. *Medicine and Science in Sports and Exercise*, **36**(2), 225–32.

Koufaki, P., Mercer, T.H. and Naish, P.F. (2002a). Effects of exercise training on aerobic and functional capacity of end-stage renal disease patients. *Clinical Physiology and Functional Imaging*, **22**, 115–24.

Koufaki, P., Naish, P.F. and Mercer, T.M. (2002b). Assessing the efficacy of exercise training in patients with chronic disease. *Medicine and Science in Sports and Exercise*, **34**, 1234–41.

Lamarra, N., Whipp, B.J., Ward, S.A. and Wasserman, K. (1987). Effect of interbreath fluctuations on characterizing exercise gas exchange kinetics. *Journal of Applied Physiology*, **62**, 2003–12.

Langsetmo, I., Weigle, G.E., Fedde, M.R., Erickson, H.H., Barstow, T.J. and Poole, D.C. (1997). $\dot{V}O_2$ kinetics in the horse during moderate and heavy exercise. *Journal of Applied Physiology*, **83**, 1235–41.

MacDonald, M.J., Shoemaker, J.K., Tschakovsky, M.E. and Hughson, R.L. (1998). Alveolar oxygen uptake and femoral artery blood flow dynamics in upright and supine leg exercise in humans. *Journal of Applied Physiology*, **85**, 1622–8.

Makrides, L., Heigenhauser, G.J.F. and Jones, N.L. (1990). High-intensity endurance training in 20- to 30- and 60- to 70-year old healthy men. *Journal of Applied Physiology*, **69**, 1792–8.

Martin, T.P., Stein, R.B., Hoeppner, P.H. and Reid, D.C. (1992). Influence of electrical stimulation on the morphological and metabolic properties of paralysed muscle. *Journal of Applied Physiology*, **72**, 1401–6.

Meredith, C.N., Frontera, W.R., Fisher, E.C., Hughes, V.A., Herland, J.C., Edwards, J. and Evans, W.J. (1989). Peripheral effects of endurance training in young and old subjects. *Journal of Applied Physiology*, **66**, 2844–9.

Norris, S.R. and Petersen, S.R. (1998). Effects of endurance training on transient oxygen uptake responses in cyclists. *Journal of Sports Sciences*, **16**, 733–8.

Otsuka, T., Kurihara, N., Fujii, T., Fujimoto, S. and Yoshikawa, J. (1997). Effect of exercise training and detraining on gas exchange kinetics in patients with chronic obstructive pulmonary disease. *Clinical Physiology*, **17**, 287–97.

Phillips, S.M., Green, H.J., MacDonald, M.J. and Hughson, R.L. (1995). Progressive effect of endurance training on $\dot{V}O_2$ kinetics at the onset of submaximal exercise. *Journal of Applied Physiology*, **79**, 1914–20.

Poole, D.C., Ward, S.A. and Whipp, B.J. (1990). The effects of training on the metabolic and respiratory profile of high-intensity cycle ergometer exercise. *European Journal of Applied Physiology*, **59**, 421–9.

Powers, S.K., Dodd, S. and Beadle, R.E. (1985). Oxygen uptake kinetics in trained athletes differing in $\dot{V}O_{2\,max}$. *European Journal of Applied Physiology*, **54**, 306–8.

Puente-Maestu, L., Tena, T., Trascasa, C., Perez-Parra, J., Godoy, R., Garcia, M.J. and Stringer, W.W. (2003). Training improves muscle oxidative capacity and oxygenation recovery kinetics in patients with chronic obstructive pulmonary disease. *European Journal of Applied Physiology*, **88**, 580–7.

Regensteiner, J.G., Bauer, T.A., Reusch, J.E., Brandenburg, S.L., Sippel, J.M., Vogelsong, A.M., Smith, S., Wolfel, E.E., Eckel, R.H. and Hiatt, W.R. (1998). Abnormal oxygen uptake kinetic responses in women with type II diabetes mellitus. *Journal of Applied Physiology*, **85**(1), 310–7.

Round, J.M., Barr, F.M.D., Moffat, B. and Jones, D.A. (1993). Fibre areas and histochemical fibre types in the quadriceps muscle of paraplegic subjects. *Journal of Neurological Science*, **116**, 207–11.

Russell, A., Wadley, G., Snow, R., Giacobino, J.-P., Muzzin, P., Garnham, A. and Cameron-Smith, D. (2002). Slow component of $\dot{V}O_2$ kinetics: the effect of training status, fibre type, UCP3 mRNA and citrate synthase activity. *International Journal of Obesity*, **26**, 157–64.

Saunders, M.J., Evans, E.M., Arngrimsson, S.A., Allison, J.D. and Cureton, K.J. (2003). Endurance training reduces end-exercise $\dot{V}O_2$ and muscle use during submaximal cycling. *Medicine and Science in Sports and Exercise*, **35**, 257–62.

Scheuermann, B.W., Bell, C., Paterson, D.H., Barstow, T.J. and Kowalchuk, J.M. (2002). Oxygen uptake kinetics for moderate exercise are speeded in older humans by prior heavy exercise. *Journal of Applied Physiology*, **92**, 609–16.

Shoemaker, J.K., Hodge, L. and Hughson, R.L. (1994). Cardiorespiratory kinetics and femoral artery blood velocity during dynamic knee extension exercise. *Journal of Applied Physiology*, **77**, 2625–32.

Shoemaker, J.K., Phillips, S.M., Green, H.J. and Hughson, R.L. (1996). Faster femoral artery blood velocity kinetics at the onset of exercise following short-term training. *Cardiovascular Research*, **31**, 278–86.

Sietsema, K.E., Ben-Dov, I., Zhang, Y.Y., Sullivan, C. and Wasserman, K. (1994). Dynamics of oxygen uptake for submaximal exercise and recovery in patients with chronic heart failure. *Chest*, **105**, 1693–700.

Stringer, W., Wasserman, K., Casaburi, R., Porszasz, J., Maehara, K. and French, W. (1994). Lactic acidosis as a facilitator of oxyhemoglobin dissociation during exercise. *Journal of Applied Physiology*, **76**, 1462–7.

Wahren, J., Saltin, B., Morfeldt, L. and Pernow, B. (1974). Influence of age on the local circulatory adaptation to leg exercise. *Scandinavian Journal of Clinical and Laboratory Investigations*, **33**, 79–86.

Weltman, A. and Katch, V. (1976). Min-by-min respiratory exchange and oxygen uptake kinetics during steady-state exercise in subjects of high and low max $\dot{V}O_2$. *Research Quarterly*, **47**, 490–8.

Wenger, H.A. and Bell, G.J. (1986). The interactions of intensity, frequency, and duration of exercise training in altering cardiorespiratory fitness. *Sports Medicine*, **3**, 346–56.

Whipp, B.J. (1994). The slow component of O_2 uptake kinetics during heavy exercise. *Medicine and Science in Sports and Exercise*, **26**, 1319–26.

Whipp, B.J., Ward, S.A., Lamarra, N., Davis, J.A. and Wasserman, K. (1982). Parameters of ventilatory and gas exchange dynamics during exercise. *Journal of Applied Physiology*, **52**, 1506–13.

Womack, C.J., Davis, S.E., Blumer, J.L., Barrett, E., Weltman, A.L. and Gaesser, G.A. (1995). Slow component of O_2 uptake during heavy exercise: adaptation to endurance training. *Journal of Applied Physiology*, **79**, 838–45.

Zhang, Y., Johnson, II M.C., Chow, N. and Wasserman, K. (1991). The role of fitness on $\dot{V}O_2$ and $\dot{V}CO_2$ kinetics in response to proportional step increases in work rate. *European Journal of Applied Physiology*, **63**, 94–100.

Index